DAYNA M. MANICCIA

Intervention Mapping

Intervention Mapping

DESIGNING THEORY- AND EVIDENCE-BASED HEALTH PROMOTION PROGRAMS

L. Kay Bartholomew
University of Texas, Houston

Guy S. Parcel
University of Texas, Houston

Gerjo Kok
Maastricht University

Nell H. Gottlieb
University of Texas, Austin

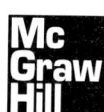

Boston   Burr Ridge, IL   Dubuque, IA   Madison, WI   New York   San Francisco   St. Louis
Bangkok   Bogotá   Caracas   Kuala Lumpur   Lisbon   London   Madrid   Mexico City
Milan   Montreal   New Delhi   Santiago   Seoul   Singapore   Sydney   Taipei   Toronto

This book is dedicated to
Howie and Robert—LKB
Sherry, Jennifer, Steve, Heather, Hannah, and Kate—GSP
Theo—GJK
Paul, Erin, and Marc—NG

McGraw-Hill Higher Education
A Division of The **McGraw-Hill** Companies

INTERVENTION MAPPING, DESIGNING THEORY- AND EVIDENCE-BASED
HEALTH PROMOTION PROGRAMS

Published by McGraw-Hill, a business unit of The McGraw-Hill Companies, Inc., 1221 Avenue of the Americas, New York, NY, 10020. Copyright © 2001, 1994, 1988, by The McGraw-Hill Companies, Inc. All rights reserved. No part of this publication may be reproduced or distributed in any form or by any means, or stored in a database or retrieval system, without the prior written consent of The McGraw-Hill Companies, Inc., including, but not limited to, in any network or other electronic storage or transmission, or broadcast for distance learning.

Some ancillaries, including electronic and print components, may not be available to customers outside the United States.

3 4 5 6 7 8 9 0 DOC/DOC 0 9 8 7 6 5 4 3

ISBN 0-7674-1278-8

Library of Congress Cataloging-in-Publication Data
Intervention mapping : designing theory and evidence-based health promotion programs / L. Kay Bartholomew . . . [et. al.].
    p. cm.
Includes bibliographical references and index.
ISBN 0-7674-1278-8
  1. Evidence-based medicine. 2. Health promotion. 3. Health education.
I. Bartholomew, L. Kay.
RA427.8. I58 2000
613–dc21   00-023290
                                                                        CIP

Sponsoring editor, Michele Sordi; production editor, Windy Johnson; manuscript editor, Karen Dorman; design manager, Jean Mailander; text designer, Joan Greenfield; cover designer, Laurie Anderson; art editor, Rennie Evans; illustrators, Lotus Art; manufacturing manager, Randy Hurst. The text was set in 10.5/13 Minion by TBH Typecast, Inc., and printed on 45# Highland Plus by R.R. Donnelley & Sons Company.

Acknowledgments and copyrights continue at the back of the book on pages 479–480, which constitute an extension of the copyright page.

 This book is printed on acid-free, recycled paper.

BRIEF CONTENTS

PART I: FOUNDATIONS

1 Overview of Intervention Mapping 1

2 Assessment of Community Capacity and Needs 16

3 Core Processes: *Evidence, Theory, and New Research* 47

4 Theories in Health Education and Promotion 74

PART II: INTERVENTION MAPPING

5 Intervention Mapping Step 1:
Preparing Matrices of Proximal Program Objectives 130

6 Intervention Mapping Step 2:
Selecting Theory-Based Intervention Methods and Practical Strategies 171

7 Intervention Mapping Step 3:
Producing Program Components and Materials 228

8 Intervention Mapping Step 4:
Planning Program Adoption, Implementation, and Sustainability 290

9 Intervention Mapping Step 5:
Planning for Evaluation 320

PART III: CASE STUDIES

10 A School AIDS Prevention Program in the Netherlands 353

11 Partners in School Asthma Management Program 387

12 Project Northland: *Alcohol Use Prevention with Older Adolescents* 425

13 Theory and Context in Project PANDA: *A Program to Help Postpartum Women Stay Off Cigarettes* 453

CONTENTS

Preface xvii

About the Authors xxv

PART I: FOUNDATIONS

1 Overview of Intervention Mapping   1

Perspectives   4
   Theory and Evidence   4
   An Ecological Approach to Health Promotion Program Planning   5
   Participation in Planning   7
The Need for Intervention Mapping   8
The Steps of Intervention Mapping   9
   Step 1: Proximal Program Objectives   9
   Step 2: Theory-Based Methods and Practical Strategies   11
   Step 3: Program   11
   Step 4: Adoption and Implementation   12
   Step 5: Evaluation   12
   An Iterative Process   13
Summary   13
References   13

2 Assessment of Community Capacity and Needs   16

Perspectives   16
   Assessment of Both Needs and Strengths   16
   Population at Risk, Environmental Context, and Intervention Groups   17
   Collaborative Planning   19

How to Conduct a Needs Assessment   20
   Combining Qualitative and Quantitative Evidence   20
   Assessing Community Competence, Capacity, and Social Capital   25
   Using PRECEED to Organize and Analyze Needs Data   28
   Understanding Risk Models versus Health-Promoting Models   33
   Deciding Where to Begin the Epidemiological Assessment   36
How to Write Program Goals and Objectives   39
   Health and Quality-of-Life Objectives   40
   Behavioral and Environmental Objectives   41
Summary   41
References   42

3 Core Processes: Evidence, Theory, and New Research   47

Perspectives   48
   Theory: Problem Focus versus Theory Generation   48
   All Theories Are Right   48
Core Processes for Intervention Mapping   50
   Posing Questions   50
   Brainstorming Provisional Answers   53
   Searching the Literature for Empirical Findings   54
   Evaluating the Relevance and Strength of Evidence   55
   Accessing and Using Theory   59
   Identifying and Addressing Needs for New Data   61
   Formulating the Working List of Answers   62
Core Processes Applied: The Case of Child Restraint Devices   62
   Posing the Question   62
   Brainstorming Provisional Answers for Lack of CRD Use   63
   Searching the Literature for Empirical Findings on CRDs   64
   Accessing and Using Theory to Enhance the Provisional List   64
   Identifying and Addressing Needs for New CRD Data   66
   Formulating the Working List of Answers for CRD Use   67
   Posing a New Question   68
Summary   68
References   69

4 Theories in Health Education and Promotion   74

Perspectives   75
   Ecological Interventions   75

Political, Practical, and Habitual Influences on Intervention   77
Overview of Theories   79
   Behavior-Oriented Theories and Environment-Oriented Theories   79
   From Theories of the Problem to Theories of Action   81
Individual Theories   81
   Learning Theories   81
   Theory of Planned Behavior   83
   Transtheoretical Model   86
   Persuasion Communication Model   89
   Goal-Setting Theory   91
   Attribution Theory   92
   Health Belief Model   93
   Self-Regulatory Theories   95
Interpersonal Theories   96
   Social Cognitive Theory   96
   Social Network and Social Support Theories   100
Organizational Change Models and Theories   104
   Stage Theory of Organizational Change   105
   Organizational Development Theory   106
   Interorganizational Relationships Theory   109
Community Organization Models and Theories   111
   Conscientization   111
   Community Organization   112
Societal and Governmental Theories   116
   Public Policy   116
Summary   120
References   120

PART II: INTERVENTION MAPPING

5 Intervention Mapping Step 1: Preparing Matrices of Proximal Program Objectives   130

Perspectives   131
   Importance of Outcomes-Based Planning   131
   Ecology of Cause and Intervention   132
   Tolerance of Complexity   133
Matrix Building Blocks: Behaviors and Environmental Conditions   133
   Identifying Health-Related Behaviors of the At-Risk Group   134
   Stating the Health-Promoting Behaviors   137

Identifying Environmental Conditions   137
Stating the Health-Promoting Environmental Conditions   140
Matrix Building Blocks: Performance Objectives   142
Performance Objectives for Health-Promoting Behaviors   142
Performance Objectives for Environmental Conditions   144
Core Processes for Writing Performance Objectives   145
Validating Performance Objectives   147
Matrix Building Blocks: Personal and External Determinants   148
Matrix Building Blocks: Learning and Change Objectives   150
Selecting Intervention Levels   151
Differentiating the Intervention Population   151
Constructing Matrices and Writing Learning and Change Objectives   158
Clarifying External Determinants and Environmental Conditions   159
Summary   164
References   165

6 Intervention Mapping Step 2: Selecting Theory-Based Intervention Methods and Practical Strategies   171

Perspectives   172
The Case of the Missing Methods   172
Methods at the Different Ecological Levels of Intervention   173
Identifying Methods   174
Work Style   174
Core Processes   174
Translating Theoretical Methods to Practical Strategies   176
An Example of Methods and Strategies   178
Ensuring Effectivness of Methods   180
Basic Methods   180
Successful Communication   180
Relevance, Tailoring, and Individualization   181
Feedback and Reinforcement   183
Facilitation   183
Methods for Personal Determinants   184
Methods to Influence Knowledge   184
Methods to Change Risk Perception, Awareness, and Health Beliefs   187
Methods to Change Attitudes   190

Methods for Changing Social Influence 193
Methods to Influence Skills, Capability, and Self-Efficacy 195
Methods and Strategies to Change External Determinants 199
Looking at Healthful Environments as Outcomes 201
Understanding Power 202
Shifting Social Norms 203
Increasing Social Support and Social Capital 204
Enhancing Access to Resources 207
Summary 220
References 220

7 Intervention Mapping Step 3: Producing Program Components and Materials 228

Perspectives 229
Using Steps 1 and 2 229
Seeking Members of the At-Risk Groups Often and Well 230
Allowing Creativity to Flourish 232
Creating a Program 232
A Summary Program Plan 232
Program Ideas 233
Structure, Themes, and Motifs 233
Channels and Vehicles for Program Methods, Strategies, and Messages 237
Technology 244
Existing Program Materials 250
Designing a Culturally Competent Program 254
Aiming at Cultural Competence 254
Communicating Program Design and Producing Materials 261
Hiring and Working with Creative Resources 261
Writing Design Documents 263
Creating Design Documents for Abstract Vehicles 266
Working with a Print Designer 271
Writing and Organizing to Help the Reader 273
Working with Video Writers and Producers 274
Pretesting and Revising 277
Preproduction Research 277
Pretesting 278
Making Sense of Pretest Data 281

Summary 283
References 283

8 Intervention Mapping Step 4: Planning Program Adoption, Implementation, and Sustainability   290

Perspectives 291
   Planning for Program Use Is Essential 291
   Planned Interventions Can Make a Difference 291
Conceptual Framework 292
   Terms: Adoption, Implementation, and Sustainability 292
   Adoption 292
   Implementation 297
   Sustainability 300
Intervention Mapping Step 4: Planning for Program Use 302
   A Linkage Approach to Program Diffusion 302
   Matrices of Proximal Program Objectives 306
   Selection of Methods and Strategies 314
   Adoption, Implementation, and Sustainability Plan 315
Summary 315
References 316

9 Intervention Mapping Step 5: Planning for Evaluation   320

Perspectives 320
   Evaluation Terms 320
   Reasons for an Evaluation 322
Specifying the Evaluation Model 324
   Evaluating the Program Pathways 328
   Determining an Evaluation Time Frame 328
Focusing the Evaluation and Framing the Questions 331
   Process Evaluation 331
   Effect Evaluation 335
Developing Indicators and Measures 336
   Reliability and Validity 337
   Selecting versus Creating Measures 338
   Effect Measures 338

Designing and Planning the Evaluation 343
    Qualitative Methods for Process Evaluation 343
    The Purpose of Designs for Effect Evaluation 344
    The Evaluation Plan 346
Summary 346
References 349

PART III: CASE STUDIES

10 A School AIDS Prevention Program in the Netherlands 353

Perspectives in This Case 354
Needs Assessment 354
    Behavioral and Environmental Risk Factors 354
    Determinants of Safe Sex 355
Intervention Mapping Step 1: Creating Matrices
  of Proximal Program Objectives 360
    Selection of a Population 360
    Health Behaviors and Environmental Conditions 362
    Performance Objectives, Determinants, and Matrices 362
Intervention Mapping Step 2: Selecting Theory-Based Intervention
  Methods and Practical Strategies 364
    Risk Perception Change 368
    Attitude Change 370
    Change in Perceptions of Social Influences 371
    Self-Efficacy Enhancement 372
Intervention Mapping Step 3: Creating a Coherent Program 373
    Program Plan 373
    Program Scope, Sequence, and Delivery 374
    Pretesting and Production 375
Intervention Mapping Step 4: Specifying Adoption
  and Implementation Plans 376
    Linkage Board 376
    Performance Objectives, Determinants, and Learning Objectives 377
    Implementation Support 378
Intervention Mapping Step 5: Generating an Evaluation Plan 379
    Evaluation Model and Questions 379
    Effect Evaluation Design and Results 379
    Process Evaluation 381

Summary 382
References 382

11 Partners in School Asthma Management Program — 387

Perspectives in This Case 388
   Asthma-Related Health and Quality-of-Life Issues 389
   Environment 390
   Asthma Management 391
   Needs Assessment Summary 393
Intervention Mapping Step 1: Matrices of Proximal Program Objectives 393
   Matrices for the At-Risk Group 394
   Matrices at the Interpersonal and Organizational Levels 397
Intervention Mapping Step 2: Theoretical Methods and Practical Strategies 403
Intervention Mapping Step 3: Program Design 403
   Review of Asthma Management Programs 403
   Program Components and Support Materials 409
   Program Scope and Sequence 414
   Pretesting 414
Intervention Mapping Step 4: Planning Adoption and Implementation 415
   Linkage System 415
   Program Adopters and Implementers 416
Intervention Mapping Step 5: Monitoring and Evaluation Highlights 417
Summary 418
References 418

12 Project Northland: Alcohol Use Prevention with Older Adolescents — 425

Perspectives in This Case 426
Needs Assessment 427
   Health Problems and Quality of Life 427
   Behavioral and Environmental Conditions 428
   Identifying Determinants 428
   Current Programs 430
   Needs Assessment Summary 430

Intervention Mapping Step 1: Matrices
  of Proximal Program Objectives   430
    Health-Related Behaviors and Environmental Conditions   430
    Performance Objectives   431
    Determinants   433
    Population Differentiation   434
    Matrices of Proximal Program Objectives   434
Intervention Mapping Step 2: Theoretical Methods
  and Practical Strategies   440
    Community Organizing Intervention   440
    Youth Development Component   441
Intervention Mapping Step 3: Program Design   442
    Community Program: Direct Action Community Organizing   443
    Community Program: Media Advocacy   445
    Youth Action Teams and Skill Development   445
Intervention Mapping Step 4: Adoption and Implementation   448
    Linkage System   448
    Policy Change Implementation Determinants and Strategies   448
Intervention Mapping Step 5: Evaluation   449
    Effect Evaluation   449
    Process Evaluation   449
Summary   450
References   450

13 Theory and Context in Project PANDA: A Program to Help Postpartum Women Stay Off Cigarettes   453

Perspectives in This Case   454
    Using Theory to Define the Problem   454
    Understanding the Importance of the Context   455
Needs Assessment   456
    Epidemiological Analysis   456
    *Quitting During Pregnancy and the Problem
      of Return to Smoking*   457
    Factors Related to the Return to Smoking   458
    *How to Define the Problem—A Problem of Relapse
      or a Problem of Change?*   459
    Conclusions and Program Objectives   461
Intervention Mapping Step 1: Matrices of Proximal
  Program Objectives   462

Intervention Mapping Step 2: Methods and Strategies   464
Intervention Mapping Step 3: Program Design   470
Intervention Mapping Step 4: Implementation   471
Intervention Mapping Step 5: Evaluation   471
Summary   474
References   474

Credits   479

Name Index   481

Subject Index   499

PREFACE

The practice of health promotion[1] involves three major program planning activities: conducting a needs assessment, developing and implementing a program, and evaluating the program's effectiveness. Over the last 20 years, significant enhancements have been made to the conceptual base and practice of health education and promotion, especially in needs assessment (Green & Kreuter, 1999), program evaluation (Green & Lewis, 1986; Windsor, Baranowski, Clark, & Cutter, 1994), adoption and implementation (Goodman & Steckler, 1989), and the use of theory (Glanz, Lewis, & Rimer, 1997; Glanz, Rimer, & Sutton, 1993; Maibach & Parrott, 1995). However, the health education community has been slow to specify the processes involved in program design and development. Applications of behavioral and social science theories to intervention design are given important consideration, but even in this regard, the processes involved are not typically made explicit in the research or practice literature. Researchers often relegate the discussion of an intervention development and design to a few sentences.

Intervention Mapping is the product of our frustration in teaching health education students the processes involved in planning an intervention. The literature provides helpful models for conducting a needs assessment and program evaluation, and it provides ecological models for conceptualizing the multiple levels of health education intervention (McLeroy, Bibeau, Steckler, & Glanz, 1988; Simons-Morton, Greene, & Gottlieb, 1995; Simons-Morton, Simons-Morton, Parcel, & Bunker, 1988), but it lacks specific frameworks for program development. In our experience, students have been able to understand theories of behavior and social change but have not been able to use them to design a coherent, practical health education intervention. Students frequently ask the following questions: When in the planning process do I use theory to guide my decisions? How do I know what theory to use? How do I make use of the experience of others and the results of other program evaluations? How do I decide what intervention methods to use? How can I get from program goals and objectives to the specific intervention strategies for the program participants? How do I link

---

[1] We use the terms *health education* and *health promotion* interchangeably. We understand that the field has moved to the term *health promotion* to capture both environmental causes of health problems and ecological interventions.

program design with planning for program implementation? How do I address changing the behavior of other people in the environment when they are not at risk for the health problem but are important to changing conditions that affect those at risk?

Motivated by these questions, we began to examine programs we had developed through our work as researchers and practitioners and to identify general principles and procedures in intervention design that were common to most of our work. One of our early case examples was the Cystic Fibrosis Family Education Program, an intervention designed to improve self-management skills, patient–health care provider interaction, health and quality of life of children with cystic fibrosis and their families (Bartholomew et al., 1997; Bartholomew, Czyzewski, et al., 2000; Bartholomew et al., 1991; Bartholomew, Parcel, Swank, & Czyzewski, 1993; Bartholomew, Seilheimer, Parcel, Spinelli, & Pumariega, 1989; Bartholomew, Sockrider, et al., 1993).

To substantiate the steps of Intervention Mapping and to further delineate the tasks required for each, we then conducted a retrospective review of several large demonstration projects in the United States (Mullen & Bartholomew, 1991; Mullen & DiClemente, 1992; Parcel, Eriksen, et al., 1989; Parcel, Taylor, et al., 1989; Perry et al., 1992; Perry et al., 1990) and the Netherlands (De Vries & Dijkstra, 1989; Mesters, Meertens, Crebolder, & Parcel, 1993; Schaalma, Kok, Poelman, & Reinders, 1994; Siero, Boon, Kok, & Siero, 1989). This review led to a working framework for health education program development, the process of Intervention Mapping. Analogous to geographic mapping, Intervention Mapping enables the planner to discover relations, locate desired destinations, plan a route for getting from one place to another, and execute a plan for covering distance. Intervention Mapping also has a visual component, including numerous diagrams and matrices that are used as landmarks to logical program development.

To further evolve the steps of the process, we applied Intervention Mapping prospectively to ongoing projects that involved health education and promotion program development. The following projects are among those that we used to test, revise, and refine our proposed Intervention Mapping steps and tasks: Long Live Love, an HIV prevention program for Dutch adolescents that is described in Chapter 10 (Schaalma & Kok, 1995; Schaalma, Kok, Bosker, et al., 1996; Schaalma, Kok, & Paulussen, 1996); the Asthma Partnership System, a self-management program for children with asthma that is described in Chapter 11 (Bartholomew, Gold, et al., 2000; Bartholomew, Shegog, et al., 2000; Shegog et al., 1999); and Five a Day, a nutrition education program for 9- to 12-year-old girls (Cullen, Bartholomew, & Parcel, 1997; Cullen, Bartholomew, Parcel, & Kok, 1998).

Additional experience with and refinement of the Intervention Mapping process has occurred throughout the course of 5 years of graduate instruction in health promotion planning and implementation at the University of Texas School of Public Health, at the School of Health Sciences, University of Maastricht, The Netherlands, and elsewhere.

Intervention Mapping is presented in this text as an additional tool for the planning and development of health education and promotion programs. It serves as a way to map the path of intervention development from recognition of a need or problem to the identification and testing of potential solutions. The steps and tasks included in Intervention Mapping provide a framework for making and documenting decisions about how to influence change in behavior and conditions to promote health and to prevent or improve a health problem. This documentation provides a means to communicate to everyone involved in the process a logical and conceptual basis for how the intervention is intended to work to make change possible. The level of specificity included in each of the products of Intervention Mapping enhances the possibility that a planned program will be effective in accomplishing its goals and objectives. In addition, by making explicit the pathways and means by which change is expected to occur and by examining the assumptions and decisions made in each step and task of the Intervention Mapping process, program planners, users, and participants can better explain why a program succeeds or fails. It is our hope that this new tool will contribute to more effective health promotion programs and better explication of these programs and will result in an enhanced knowledge base for research and practice.

The first chapter of this text presents the perspective from which Intervention Mapping was conceived as well as its purpose. Before using Intervention Mapping, a planner should have at least an elementary grasp of needs assessment and the use of behavioral science theory in planning. Thus, Chapters 2 through 4 offer an overview of needs assessment, methods for assessing appropriate behavioral science theories and empirical evidence in the planning process, and a brief review of applicable social and behavioral science theories. Chapters 5 through 9 present a step-by-step guide to Intervention Mapping, and Chapters 10 through 13 provide detailed case examples of the application of Intervention Mapping to public health programs.

ACKNOWLEDGMENTS

Many people have been kind enough to offer suggestions and encouragement during the development of this text. Others have contributed through the contributions to health education and promotion from which we have greatly benefited. Still others have allowed us to steer project teams down loosely defined pathways in order to test new ideas. We offer thanks to our friends and colleagues Stuart Abramson, Robin Atwood, Tom Baranowski, Karen Basen-Engquist, Martine Bouman, Lex Bouter, Johannes Brug, Theresa Byrd, Noreen Clark, Jennifer Conroy, Karin Coyle, Karen Cullen, Sharon Cummings, Danita Czyzewski, Evelyne de Leeuw, Hein De Vries, Dirk-Jan den Boer, Elia Diez, Anton Dijker, Aric Dijkstra, Margot Dijkstra, Polly Edmundson-Drane, Michael Eriksen, Alexandra Evans, Maria Fernandez-Esquer, Amy Fetterhoff, Brian Flay, Barbara Giloth, Phyllis Gingiss, Karen Glanz, Gaston Godin, Robert Gold, Bob Goodman, Patricia

Goodson, Larry Green, Merwyn Greenlick, Jan Groff, Jong Long Guo, Karol Kaye Harris, Helen Hill, Jeffrey Hitt, Carole Holahan, Harm Hospers, Dorothy Husky, Aimee James, Ruud Jonkers, Jolanda Keijsers, Doug Kirby, Marshall Kreuter, Cheryl Lackey, Sue Laver, Alexandra Loukas, Barbara Low, Alfred McAlister, Ree Meertens, Ilse Mesters, Barbara Meyer, Anna Meyer-Weitz, Aart Mudde, Nancy Murray, Brian Oldenburg, Theo Paulussen, Bobbie Person, Fred Peterson, Priscilla Reddy, Barbara Rimer, Michael Ross, Rob Ruiter, Ann Saunders, Herman Schaalma, Dale Schunk, Dan Seilheimer, Bruce Simons-Morton, Michele Murphy Smith, Gail Sneden, Marianna Sockrider, Teshia Solomon, Alan Steckler, Mary Steinhardt, Victor Strecher, Paul Swank, Peggy Tate, Wendell Taylor, Mary Tripp, Patricia van Assema, Bart van den Borne, Angelique van der Kar, Pepijn van Empelen, Olga van Rijn, Peter Veen, Marsha Weil, Henk Wilke, and Barry Zimmerman.

We are indebted to our students who allowed us to class-test the text. We attempted to make it better each time we taught it. We also benefited from the review and class-testing by our colleagues Omowale Amuleru-Marshall, Morehouse School of Medicine; Julie Baldwin, Northern Arizona University; Michael Barnes, Brigham Young University; Dan Bibeau, University of North Carolina at Greensboro; Brian Colwell, Texas A&M University; Carolyn Crump, University of North Carolina at Chapel Hill; Debra Krummel, West Virginia University; Michael Pejsach, Central Michigan University; Rick Petosa, Ohio State University; and Ruth Saunders, University of South Carolina.

Janet Reis, University of Illinois, Urbana-Champaign, deserves a special thank you for assigning her students to use the book and to critique each chapter. We read and used those comments and think the book is better for them. Her students who were kind enough to help us were Nicole Berg, Jackie Brunell, Deb Fisher, Heather Lee, Kelley Matlak, Debbie Ng, Kathleen Powell, Trina Ragain, Cressie Suess, and Mickey Trockel.

Our thanks to our colleagues who contributed case studies and other parts of the text: Carlo DiClemente, Maria Fernandez, Randi Bernstein Lachter, Chris Markham, Patricia Dolan Mullen, Cheryl Perry, Karyn Popham, Herman Schaalma, Ross Shegog, Shellie Tyrrell, and Sarah Veblen-Mortenson.

Some of our friends and colleagues provided extraordinary support. Comprehensive reviews by John Allegrante and Kenneth McLeroy enabled us to fine-tune the manuscript. Patricia Dolan Mullen not only contributed her ideas to the book, but unflaggingly believed in the usefulness of Intervention Mapping. Dean Palmer Beasley at the University of Texas School of Public Health maintains an environment in which sustained creative work is possible.

Karen Dorman and Karyn Popham improved the manuscript with intelligent and persistent editing. Thanks to Karen Dorman we rewrote sections that we hadn't previously discerned how to fix. Karyn Popham tracked down seemingly phantom references.

Windy Johnson coordinated a superb production process and caused the authors no headaches. We, on the other hand, caused her many. The entire Mayfield team was exceptional. We appreciate their empathy, encouragement, and responsiveness. Thank you, Michele Sordi.

Finally, the four co-authors thank each other. It seems that every part of Intervention Mapping was discussed, written, argued over, and rewritten. Friendships were developed, tested, and deepened.

Kay Bartholomew
Guy Parcel
Gerjo Kok
Nell Gottlieb

REFERENCES

Bartholomew, L. K., Czyzewski, D. I., Parcel, G. S., Swank, P. R., Sockrider, M. M., Mariotto, M., Schidlow, V., Fink, R., & Seilheimer, D. K. (1997). Self-management of cystic fibrosis: Short-term outcomes of the Cystic Fibrosis Family Education Program. *Health Education and Health Behavior, 24*(5), 652–666.

Bartholomew, L. K., Czyzewski, D. I., Swank, P. R., McCormick, L., & Parcel, G. S. (2000). Maximizing the impact of the Cystic Fibrosis Family Education Program: Factors related to program diffusion. *Family and Community Health, 22*(4), 1–22.

Bartholomew, L. K., Gold, R. S., Parcel, G. S., Czyzewski, D. I., Sockrider, M. M., Fernandez, M., Shegog, R., & Swank, P. (2000). Watch, Discover, Think, and Act: Evaluation of computer-assisted instruction to improve asthma self-management in inner-city children. *Patient Education and Counseling, 39*(2–3), 269–280.

Bartholomew, L. K., Parcel, G. S., Seilheimer, D. K., Czyzewski, D., Spinelli, S. H., & Congdon, B. (1991). Development of a health education program to promote the self-management of cystic fibrosis: Application of a diagnostic framework. *Health Education Quarterly, 18*(4), 429–443.

Bartholomew, L. K., Parcel, G. S., Swank, P. R., & Czyzewski, D. I. (1993). Measuring self-efficacy expectations for the self-management of cystic fibrosis. *Chest, 103*(5), 1524–1530.

Bartholomew, L. K., Seilheimer, D. K., Parcel, G. S., Spinelli, S. H., & Pumariega, A. J. (1989). Planning patient education for cystic fibrosis: Application of a diagnostic framework. *Patient Education and Counseling, 13*(1), 57–68.

Bartholomew, L. K., Shegog, R., Parcel, G. S., Gold, R. S., Fernandez, M., Czyzewski, D. I., Sockrider, M. M., & Berlin, N. (2000). Watch, Discover, Think, and Act: A model for patient education program development. *Patient Education and Counseling, 39*(2–3), 253–268.

Bartholomew, L. K., Sockrider, M. M., Seilheimer, D. K., Czyzewski, D. I., Parcel, G. S., & Spinelli, S. H. (1993). Performance objectives for the self-management of cystic fibrosis. *Patient Education and Counseling, 22*(1), 15–25.

Cullen, K., Bartholomew, L. K., Parcel, G. S., & Kok, G. (1998). Intervention Mapping: Use of theory and data in the development of a fruit and vegetable nutrition program for Girl Scouts. *Journal of Nutrition Education, 30*(4), 188–195.

Cullen, K. W., Bartholomew, L. K., & Parcel, G. (1997). Girl Scouting: An effective channel for nutrition education. *Journal of Nutrition Education, 29*(2), 86–91.

De Vries, H., & Dijkstra, M. (1989). Non-smoking, your choice, a Dutch smoking prevention programme. In C. James, J. Balding, & D. Harris (Eds.), *World yearbook of education* (pp. 20–31). London: Kogan Page.

Glanz, K., Lewis, F. M., & Rimer, B. K. (Eds.). (1997). *Health behavior and health education: Theory, research, and practice* (2nd ed.). San Francisco: Jossey-Bass.

Glanz, K., Rimer, B. K., & Sutton, S. M. (1993). *Theory at a glance: A guide for health promotion practice.* Bethesda, MD: National Cancer Institute of the National Institutes of Health.

Goodman, R. M., & Steckler, A. (1989). A model for the institutionalization of health promotion programs. *Family and Community Health, 11*(4), 63–78.

Green, L. W., & Kreuter, M. W. (1999). *Health promotion planning: An educational and ecological approach* (3rd ed.). Mountain View, CA: Mayfield.

Green, L. W., & Lewis, F. M. (1986). *Measurement and evaluation in health education and health promotion.* Palo Alto, CA: Mayfield.

Maibach, E., & Parrott, R. L. (Eds.). (1995). *Designing health messages: Approaches from communication theory and public health practice.* Thousand Oaks, CA: Sage.

McLeroy, K. R., Bibeau, D., Steckler, A., & Glanz, K. (1988). An ecological perspective on health promotion programs. *Health Education Quarterly, 15*(4), 351–377.

Mesters, I., Meertens, R., Crebolder, H., & Parcel, G. (1993). Development of a health education program for parents of preschool children with asthma. *Health Education Quarterly, 8*(1), 53–68.

Mullen, P. D., & Bartholomew, L. K. (1991). Project PANDA: development of a program to reduce return to smoking by new mothers. Paper presented to the Society for Health Education, Atlanta, GA.

Mullen, P. D., & DiClemente, C. (1992). Sustaining women's non-smoking postpartum. Paper presented to the 8th World Conference on Tobacco and Health, Buenos Aires, Argentina.

Parcel, G. S., Eriksen, M. P., Lovato, C. Y., Gottlieb, N. H., Brink, S. G., & Green, L. W. (1989). The diffusion of a school-based tobacco-use prevention program: Project description and baseline data. *Journal of Health Education Research, 4*(1), 111–124.

Parcel, G. S., Taylor, W. C., Brink, S. G., Gottlieb, N. H., Engquist, K. E., O'Hara, N. M., & Eriksen, M. P. (1989). Translating theory into practice: Intervention strategies for the diffusion of a health promotion innovation. *Family and Community Health, 12*(3), 1–13.

Perry, C. L., Parcel, G. S., Stone, E., Nader, P., McKinlay, S. M., Luepker, R. V., & Webber, L. S. (1992). The Child and Adolescent Trial for Cardiovascular Health (CATCH): Overview of the intervention program and evaluation methods. *Cardiovascular Risk Factors, 2*(1), 36–44.

Perry, C. L., Stone, E. J., Parcel, G. S., Ellison, R. C., Nader, P., Webber, L. S., & Luepker, R. V. (1990). School-based cardiovascular health promotion: The Child and Adolescent Trial for Cardiovascular Health (CATCH). *Journal of School Health, 60*(8), 406–413.

Schaalma, H., & Kok, G. (1995). Promoting health through education: The surplus value of a systematic approach. *Odyssey, 1,* 44–51.

Schaalma, H. P., Kok, G., Bosker, R. J., Parcel, G. S., Peters, L., Poelman, J., & Reinders, J. (1996). Planned development and evaluation of AIDS/STD education for secondary school students in the Netherlands: Short-term effects. *Health Education Quarterly, 23*(4), 469–487.

Schaalma, H., Kok, G., & Paulussen, T. (1996). HIV behavioural interventions in young people in The Netherlands. [Review]. *International Journal of STD and AIDS, 7*(Suppl. 2), 43–46.

Schaalma, H., Kok, G., Poelman, J., & Reinders, J. (1994). The development of AIDS education for Dutch secondary schools: A systematic approach based on research, theories, and co-operation. In D. R. Rutter (Ed.), *The social psychology of health and safety: European perspectives* (pp. 175–194). Aldershot, UK: Avebury Publishers.

Shegog, R., Bartholomew, L. K., Gold, R. S., Pierrel, E., Parcel, G. S., Sockrider, M. M., Czyzewski, D. I., Fernandez, M., Berlin, N., Combes, R., & Abramson, S. (1999). Self-management education for pediatric chronic disease: A description of the Watch, Discover, Think, and Act asthma computer program. Manuscript submitted for publication.

Siero, S., Boon, M. E., Kok, G., & Siero, F. (1989). Modification of driving behavior in a large transport organization: A field experiment. *Journal of Applied Psychology, 74*(3), 417–423.

Simons-Morton, B. G., Greene, W. H., & Gottlieb, N. H. (1995). *Introduction to health education and health promotion* (2nd ed.). Prospect Heights, IL: Waveland Press.

Simons-Morton, D. G., Simons-Morton, B. G., Parcel, G. S., & Bunker, J. F. (1988). Influencing personal and environmental conditions for community health: A multilevel intervention model. *Family and Community Health, 11*(2), 25–35.

Windsor, R., Baranowski, T., Clark, N., & Cutter, G. (1994). *Evaluation of health promotion, health education, and disease prevention programs* (2nd ed.). Mountain View, CA: Mayfield.

ABOUT THE AUTHORS

L. KAY BARTHOLOMEW is associate director of the Center for Health Promotion and Prevention Research at the University of Texas Health Science Center in Houston. She serves as associate professor of behavioral sciences in the School of Public Health. Dr. Bartholomew has worked in the field of health education and health promotion since her graduation from Austin College more than 25 years ago, first at a city-county health department and later at Texas Children's Hospital. In her current research center and faculty roles she teaches courses in health-promotion intervention development and conducts research in chronic disease self-management. Dr. Bartholomew received her M.P.H. from the University of Texas–Houston School of Public Health and her Ed.D. from the University of Houston. Dr. Bartholomew has won the Society for Public Health Education (SOPHE) Program Excellence Award for the Cystic Fibrosis Family Education Program as well as numerous other professional association and media awards.

GUY S. PARCEL, the John P. McGovern Professor of Health Promotion, is director of the Center for Health Promotion and Prevention Research at the University of Texas Health Science Center in Houston. He serves as professor of behavioral sciences and associate dean for research in the School of Public Health. Dr. Parcel has directed research projects to develop and evaluate programs to address sexual risk behavior for adolescents, diet and physical activity in children, self-management of childhood chronic diseases, smoking prevention, sun protection for preschool children, and the diffusion of health promotion programs. Dr. Parcel received his B.S. and M.S. degrees in health education at Indiana University and his Ph.D. at Pennsylvania State University with a major in health education and a minor in child development and family relations. Dr. Parcel has authored or co-authored more than 180 scientific papers and received the American School Health Association (ASHA) 1990 William A. Howe Award for outstanding contributions and distinguished service in school health.

GERJO KOK is dean of the Faculty of Psychology at Maastricht University, the Netherlands. He also holds the Dutch AIDS Fund endowed chair for AIDS prevention and health promotion. Currently a professor of applied psychology, from 1984 to 1998 he was professor in health education at Maastricht University. A social psychologist, he received his doctorate in social sciences from the University of Groningen, the Netherlands. His main interest is in the social psychology of health education.

NELL H. GOTTLIEB is professor and coordinator of health education programs in the Department of Kinesiology and Health Education at the University of Texas at Austin and professor of behavioral science at the University of Texas–Houston School of Public Health. Dr. Gottlieb is author of numerous articles and two textbooks. She received her Ph.D. in sociology from Boston University. Her interests are in multi-level health-promotion intervention development and evaluation, particularly in the area of tobacco prevention and control. Dr. Gottlieb has served as chair of the Health Education and Promotion Section of the American Public Health Association (APHA) and as the president of the Society for Public Health Education (SOPHE).

CHAPTER 1

Overview of Intervention Mapping

READER OBJECTIVE

- Gain an overview of the Intervention Mapping process

In this chapter we present the perspective from which Intervention Mapping was conceived as well as its purpose. We also present a preview of the program-planning framework, which is detailed in the remaining chapters.

The purpose of Intervention Mapping is to provide health education program planners with a framework for effective decision making at each step in intervention planning, implementation, and evaluation. A health education or promotion intervention is a planned combination of theoretical methods delivered through a series of strategies organized into a program. An intervention can be designed to change environmental or behavioral factors related to health, but the most immediate impact of an intervention is on a set of well-defined antecedents or determinants of behavior and environmental conditions.

Imagine a health educator in a city health department. The city's mayor, who has recently received strong criticism for inattention to a number of critical health issues, has just announced that $500,000 of the annual budget will be used to address these issues. Youth violence, adolescent smoking and other substance abuse, and the high incidence of HIV/AIDS are among the issues competing for the mayor's attention. Not only does the allocated sum of money represent a gross underestimation of what is needed to address these issues, but also the city council is strongly divided on which health issue should receive priority. Council members do agree, however, that to excessively dilute effort among the different issues would be a questionable decision likely resulting in little or no impact on any single issue. As a response to increasing political pressures, the mayor makes a bold political move and presents a challenge to the interest groups lobbying for public assistance. The mayor signs a contract with the city agreeing to continue allocation of funds, on a yearly basis, contingent on demonstration by the designated planning group of significant, measurable improvements in the issues at hand by the end of each fiscal year.

(continued)

Chapter 1
Overview of Intervention Mapping

The head of the health promotion division of the city health department is a social psychologist. She intends to use the mayor's challenge as a testing ground for her favorite behavioral science theory, but she has appointed the health educator to lead the planning group. Although apprehensive about the professional challenge as well as the complications inherent in facilitating a powerful group, the health educator is encouraged by the prospect of working with community and public health leaders.

The composition of the city's planning group is professionally diverse, and spurred by the mayor's challenge, group members are enthusiastic to contribute their expertise. With this early momentum, the group devotes several weeks to a needs assessment, guided by the PRECEDE/PROCEED model (Green & Kreuter, 1999). The members consider the various quality-of-life issues relevant to each of the health problems, the segments of the population affected by each issue, associated environmental and behavioral risk factors for each health problem, and determinants of the risk factors.

The members recognize the relative importance of all three issues, but select youth violence because they are challenged by the lack of effective or evaluated violence prevention programs in the field (Tolan & Guerra, 1994, 1996) and also because of the interests and expertise of the individual group members. The results of the needs assessment indicate that violence is the leading cause of death among young people aged 15 to 24 in the United States, and the primary cause of death among Hispanics and African Americans in this age group ("Advance Report," 1994; Singh & Yu, 1996). Moreover, for every violent death, conservative estimates suggest that 100 nonfatal injuries result from violence (U.S. Department of Justice, 1994). The group reviews the literature to identify the behavioral and environmental causes of violence and finds that the factors related to violence are diverse. For example, socioeconomic status, education, and job mobility are all factors that may predispose a person to violence. The lack of conflict resolution and communication skills are enabling factors related to personal violence. At the same time, the sudden occurrence of situational antagonism, such as verbal or physical assault, is a contextual factor that is also likely to incite violent behavior (Reiss, Miczek, & Roth, 1993). The planning group reviews a long list of determinants. They recognize that certain skills can be addressed in their one-year program. However, they also recognize that broad social problems such as poverty and unemployment must be taken into account as determinants of behavior even though they are not easily addressed in a single-year intervention. Further investigation reveals that little empirical evidence is available on the effectiveness of existing programs that address a broad array of determinants of violent behavior (Tolan & Guerra, 1994).

The planning committee appoints a community liaison subgroup to begin meeting with members of various communities within the city that have been disproportionately affected by violence. This subgroup wants to understand community members' perceptions of their needs, but it is equally concerned with understanding the strengths of the communities and their unique potential contributions to a violence prevention partnership. The subgroup invites members of each interested neighborhood to join the planning group. Jointly, the planning group, the communities, and the funders agree to select this problem as the focus of a health education and promotion intervention.

Working on the needs assessment facilitated group cohesion and cultivated even greater enthusiasm about generating a solution for the health problem. Several members of the group even begin to imagine the victory that would be had were the group to produce a change in half the allotted time because so much of the needed background information had already been gathered. The health educator remains apprehensive about the time frame, yet comfortable with the pace and productivity of the group. Now that the group has decided which issue will be addressed, it faces the challenge of moving to the program-planning phase. In previous work, the health educator had implemented and evaluated programs designed by others, but had not created new programs. However, bolstered by its good work, the group schedules the first program-planning meeting.

What the health educator hadn't anticipated was that in the course of conducting the needs assessment, each group member had independently begun to conceive of the next step in the planning process as well as to visualize the kind of intervention that would be most suitable to address the problem.

The day of the meeting arrives, and the agenda is a discussion of how the group should begin program planning. What follows is a snapshot of dialogue from the planning group that illustrates several differing perspectives.

"As we see from the needs assessment, violence is a community problem. According to community development techniques, we have to start where the people are—I think we should begin by conducting a series of focus groups and have the kids tell us what to do."

"But why do you use the kids to develop a program for the community? I say we address violence at the family level, using a series of conflict resolution training workshops for kids and their parents."

"Community and family are only two dimensions of the problem. The literature says you have to address multiple levels in a comprehensive approach. Plus, one-time workshops have no long-term impact. I say we find a nonprofit group to serve as a community coordinating center from which various interventions and services can be implemented. That way programs are sustainable and a variety of activities can be offered."

"One of the national violence prevention centers has great brochures and videos—in three languages. We have numerous testimonials from kids, teachers, and parents about how motivated they were by these interventions. This approach is quick and easy, it's low cost, and I've already made sure we can get the materials. Plus, if the materials come from a national specialty center, they must be effective."

"But is that idea really feasible? How would you get people to participate? And how would you address the different levels of the community? Moreover, violence is a human problem. The root of the problem is that kids don't have

Overview of Intervention Mapping

(continued)

anyone or anything they can relate to. In nursing school we always started with learning objectives that reflect the needs of the specific patient population."

"Yes, but we know it takes more than learning information to change behavior. We have to address factors such as attitudes and self-efficacy. But how do we measure a change in attitudes? I think we should measure behavior directly."

"Well, clearly we have to begin by designing a curriculum. What are our learning objectives?"

The health educator in our example must first consider what steps to follow to construct the intervention, and then must consider how each step might be designed to incorporate the needs, ideas, training, and experience of the various members of the planning group. The planning group began well by completing a comprehensive needs assessment using an effective model that has been applied to many health issues (Green & Kreuter, 1999). The members began the program-planning phase armed with an ecological perspective, that is, the need to intervene at individual, organizational, community, and societal levels in a problem (McLeroy, Bibeau, Steckler, & Glanz, 1988; Simons-Morton, Greene, & Gottlieb, 1995). But, as can be seen in the group dialogue and as planners often experience in group activities, each group member brought a different set of experiences and professional training to the meeting. Although group members may become critical of other perspectives, each member makes an important and relevant contribution worthy of consideration in the creation of the intervention. The difficulty planners encounter is in delineating tasks for the development of health education programs that are based on theory, empirical findings from the literature, and data collected from the at-risk population.

Existing literature, appropriate theories, and additional research data are basic tools for any health educator, but often it is unclear how and where these tools are to be used in program planning. In Intervention Mapping, these tools are systematically applied in the steps of program development.

PERSPECTIVES

Theory and Evidence

We agree with Kurt Lewin's adage that nothing is as useful as a good theory (Hochbaum, Sorenson, & Lorig, 1992), especially in health promotion planning. Still, given this assertion, more guidance is needed regarding the application of theory in health education practice. Few teachers of health education would debate the importance of teaching behavioral and social science theories, but many would question whether they use effective methods to teach students to use theory. Hochbaum and colleagues argue that many practitioners find theory practically irrelevant to their practices. Furthermore, health educators approach intervention and the use of theory in a way that is fundamentally different from either the theory generation or the single theory testing often done by scientists. Practitioners are likely to confront a problem and bring to it multiple theoretical and experiential perspectives rather than to define a practice or research agenda around a theoretical approach. Teachers of health education suggest that health educators could be served better through guidance in how to use theory to understand health and social problems (Burdine & McLeroy, 1992; Earp & Ennett, 1991; Glanz, Lewis, & Rimer, 1997; Hochbaum et al.; Kok, Schaalma, de Vries, Parcel, & Paulussen, 1996).

To understand the problem, the health educator begins with a question about a specific health or social issue (Veen, 1985). The health educator then accesses social and behavioral science theories of causation at multiple levels. These or other theories may suggest intervention points and methods, and the health educator proceeds to accumulate evidence for the effectiveness of these methods. By evidence we mean not only data from research studies as represented in the scientific literature, but also opinion and experience of community members and planners. In this way theoretical and empirical evidence are brought to bear on meeting a health or social need. Intervention Mapping provides a detailed framework for this process.

An Ecological Approach to Health Promotion Program Planning

Intervention Mapping uses a social ecological approach in which health is viewed as a function of individuals and of the environments in which individuals are embedded, including family, social networks, organizations, communities, and societies (Stokols, 1996). Individual behavior is influenced by determinants at these various environmental levels. The social ecological paradigm focuses on the interrelationships among individuals with their biological, psychological, and behavioral characteristics and their environments. These environments include physical, social, and cultural aspects that exist across the individual's life domains and social settings. A nested structure of environments allows for multiple influences both vertically across levels and horizontally within levels. The picture that emerges is a complex web of causation as well as a rich context for intervention. Looking for the most effective leverage points within this web, across levels, reduces the complexity and is necessary for the development of effective multilevel interventions.

Health educators can look at the relationship between individuals and their environments in two ways. First, mechanistically, the individual and the environment can be viewed as cogs in a general system in which small changes in the social environment, for example, can lead to large changes in individual behavior (Green, personal communication, February 26, 1997). This view tends toward an emphasis on higher order intervention leverage points as external determinants of the individual's behavior, health, and quality of life. Second, the various levels are viewed as embedded systems. In Figure 1.1, higher order systems set constraints and provide inputs to lower order systems, and the lower order systems provide inputs to systems at a higher level. New properties emerge at each system level, but each level incorporates the lower levels of embedded systems. For example, social norms exist independently of the individual even though the individual perceives them. An intervention may influence both levels (i.e., the actual norms and the individual perception), and these may in turn influence both health behavior and health. Figure 1.1 denotes embedded reciprocal systems with individual, group, organization, community, society, and supranational levels. This figure indicates that the individual exists within groups, which in turn are embedded within organizations and higher order systems; the individual is influenced by, and can influence directly or through groups and organizations, the higher order systems. We acknowledge the hazards of trying to plan from such a complex formulation, but we judge the hazards of oversimplicity to be greater. Nevertheless, we agree with

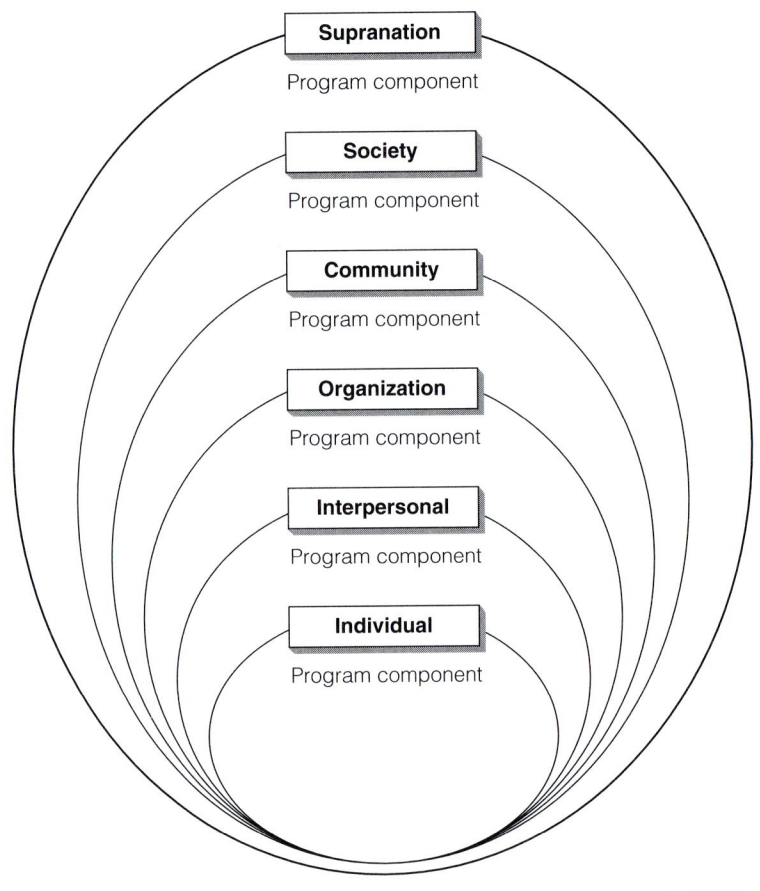

FIGURE 1.1 Schematic of the Ecological Approach in Health Promotion Programs (*Note.* Adapted from "Assessment of the Integration of the Ecological Approach in Health Programs," by L. Richard, L. Potvin, N. Kishchuk, H. Prlic, and L. W. Green, 1996, *American Journal of Health Promotion, 10*[4], pp. 318–328.)

Green that complexity can breed despair, and we encourage the reader to bear with the process (Green, Richard, & Potvin, 1996).

The World Health Organization (WHO) defines health as an instrumental value in service of a full, gratifying life (World Health Organization, 1978, 1986). We recognize the interaction of health and quality of life, and as Robertson and Minkler (1994) point out, "there is both a micro level or individual dimension to health and a macro level structural dimension."

Our primary focus, consonant with health education and health promotion, is that of health as it is mediated by both behavior and environment (Parcel et al., 1987). In addition to having an impact on multiple levels of causation and leverage points, health promotion programs must integrate plans for adoption and implementation. The potential impact of any health education program depends on both the efficacy of the intervention to influence change and the proportion of the intended population exposed to the program. A program with modest effectiveness could have a great impact if it reached the entire population. Health education programs may be difficult to implement and sustain because they are innovations that cause change in organizational systems. Program planning must include strategies to ensure that those people who will use it with the intended populations adopt the program (Orlandi, 1987; Smith, Steckler, & McCormick, 1995). In addition, there is a difference between the potential program efficacy and actual program effectiveness when interventions are transported from their developers to extended use in practice. Program implementation may tend to decline in amount and quality over time. Practitioners must know what is an acceptable level of implementation (Ottoson & Green, 1987) and must plan strategies for program maintenance. As a result of increasing awareness of problems with program diffusion, implementation, and maintenance, health educators have recently been giving more attention to the factors affecting program use (Basen-Engquist et al., 1994; Gingiss, Gottlieb, & Brink, 1994; Goodman & Steckler, 1989; Mullen & Mullen, 1983; Oldenburg, Hardcastle, & Kok, 1997; Orlandi, Landers, Weston, & Haley, 1990; Ottoson & Green; Paulussen, Kok, & Schaalma, 1994; Paulussen, Kok, Schaalma, & Parcel, 1995; Scheirer, 1990; Scheirer & Rezmovic, 1983).

Participation in Planning

Our last perspective is an emphasis on participation in planning. Our commitment is to bringing both a community and a multidisciplinary professional perspective to the process of planning health promotion. Despite the hazards faced by the health educator in our scenario, work groups are a fact of life for health educators. Programs cannot be developed in a vacuum, nor can they be developed from a position of expertise or authority that does not allow full participation of all stakeholders (Wallerstein, 1992). Health educators develop programs as group participants and group leaders, and as such should have a goal of encouraging full participation to bring multiple perspectives to bear on a problem and to create the most intelligent, productive consensus possible.

No matter how many "experts" are involved in program development, the individuals for whom the intervention is intended can best convey the subjective meaning of the health problem and its antecedents. The people who will deliver the program can best convey the realities of the program setting. Ongoing interaction between program planners and potential program users and participants is necessary for the planner to fully understand and convey the "real world" program context.

THE NEED FOR INTERVENTION MAPPING

When the authors of the often-used PRECEDE/PROCEED model began development more than 25 years ago, they were concerned with the focus of the field of health education on intervention. Health education programs often did not have firm epidemiological foundations, and outcomes sometimes were not documented in terms of change in behavior, environment, health, or quality of life. Green, Kreuter, and colleagues intentionally steered away from a focus on intervention (Green, personal communication, February 26, 1997). After 25 years of developments in the field, we believe that we can cautiously steer back toward an intervention focus.

In the last two decades, health education and related fields have adopted more sophisticated planning processes, including a refined needs assessment process, the creation of multilevel interventions, the acknowledgment of the importance of theory in understanding the determinants of behavior and behavior change, and the assurance of adequate program implementation. The innovations that have enhanced health education practice have made for complex program development that demands a sophisticated systematic approach. Simplistic or poorly designed processes cannot effectively lead to the creation of multilevel interventions that use needs assessment data, that involve the intended recipients and program users, that are based on theory, and that use multiple methods and strategies. As health education continues to develop as a field with a wealth of methods and with expectations for sophisticated program development, there is a need for a system or model for the creation of interventions. We believe that every health educator must have the knowledge and skills to develop effective interventions. Anyone with the responsibility to help individuals or communities change health risk behavior, initiate health-promoting behavior, change environmental factors, or manage illnesses must design or adapt existing effective health education interventions and develop plans to implement them. Yet there remains some confusion about how planners can integrate the wealth of information, theories, ideas, and models to develop interventions that are logical and appropriate in their foundations and are practical and acceptable in their administration. The complexity of intervention development is, for the most part, overlooked in health education training. Seldom do health educators write in depth about the process of intervention development, and complicated interventions are often reduced to several sentences in evaluation articles.

Intervention Mapping also enables health educators to create programs that are feasible and that have a high likelihood of being effective. Good program planning not only provides the basis for creative health education practice but also provides the vehicles for communicating program specifications to production specialists such as writers and artists. Thorough planning at the beginning of a project can lead to creative developmental and production processes, can enhance the intervention's deliverability, and can result in the desired outcomes. Intervention Mapping provides a guide for everyone involved in program planning and development to travel a common path from start to finish.

THE STEPS OF INTERVENTION MAPPING

Each step of Intervention Mapping comprises several specific tasks (Figure 1.2). The completion of the tasks in a step creates a product that is the guide for the subsequent step. The Intervention Map is the result of the completion of all the tasks for each of the steps. The Intervention Map is a blueprint for the design, implementation, and evaluation of an intervention based on a foundation of theoretical, empirical, and practical information. The five fundamental steps of the Intervention Mapping process are

- the creation of matrices of proximal program objectives based on the determinants of behavior and environmental conditions
- the selection of theory-based intervention methods and practical strategies
- the translation of methods into organized programs
- the integration of adoption and implementation plans
- the generation of an evaluation plan

Figure 1.2 shows how Intervention Mapping fits in the health education and promotion planning and intervention process. Before starting the process of Intervention Mapping, planners summarize their knowledge with respect to the health problem, to related behavior and environmental conditions, and to associated determinants for different populations. Three processes underlie each step: review and application of relevant theory, inclusion of empirical evidence, and revision with new qualitative and quantitative data obtained in interaction with the intended program recipients.

Step 1: Proximal Program Objectives

Step 1 (Chapter 5) provides the foundation for the intervention by specifying who and what will change as a result of the intervention. The product of Step 1 is a series of matrices of selected ecological levels (i.e., individual through societal) that merges performance objectives for each level with selected personal and environmental determinants to produce a set of proximal program objectives. In

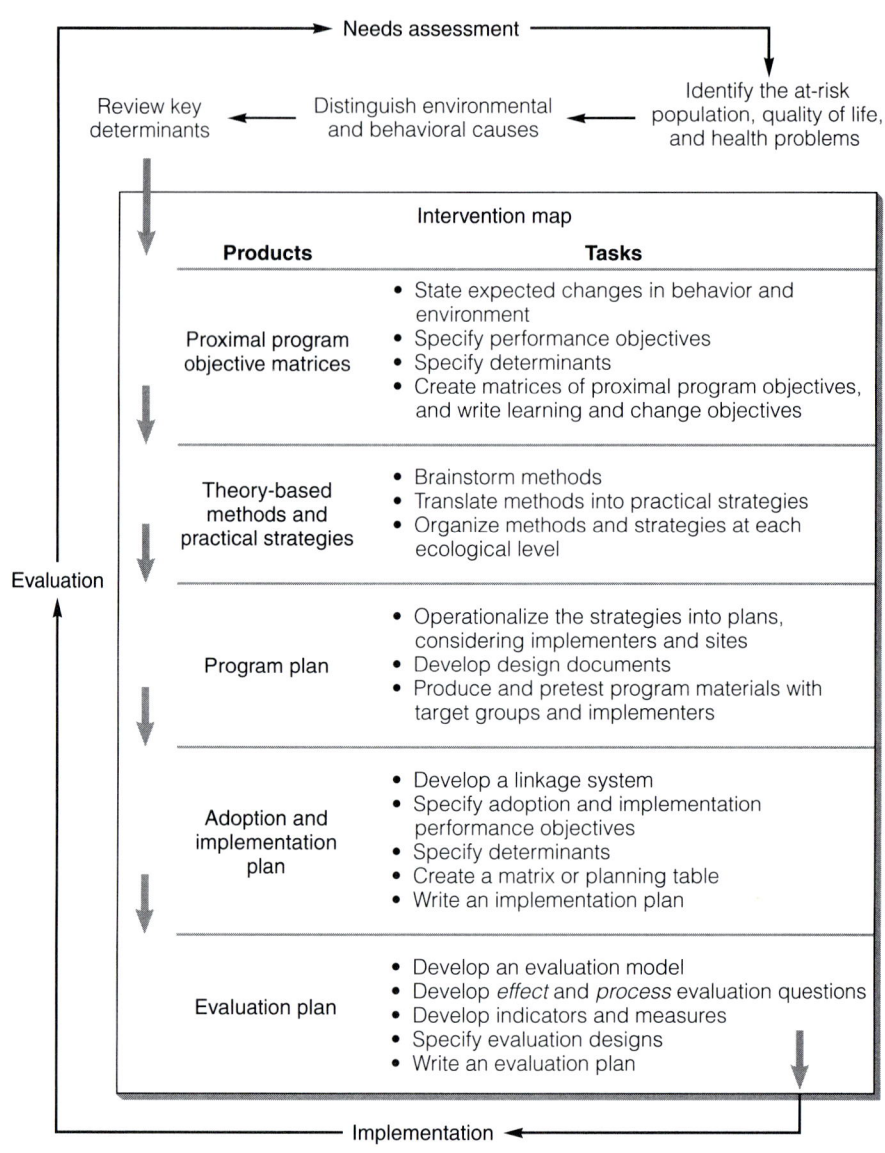

FIGURE 1.2 Intervention Mapping

order to develop performance objectives beyond the individual, roles are identified at each selected ecological level. For example, superintendents, principals, and teachers may have roles for school environmental change. Proximal program objectives, that is, statements of what must be changed at each ecological level and who must do the changing, are more specific intervention foci than are traditional program goals and objectives. For example, the mayor's planning committee constructed matrices that focused on the school environments in the city, on neighborhood environments including supervised youth activities and community cohesion, and on the behavior of the youth themselves. For another example, in a program to increase fruit and vegetable consumption by elementary school children, matrices would be created for both the child and the food services. The food service matrix might contain more than one role: for example, the manager's purchasing practices and the cooks' recipe choices. These matrices do not include objectives concerning the dissemination, adoption, implementation, and maintenance of the program because these objectives require additional planning (Chapter 8).

Step 2: Theory-Based Methods and Practical Strategies

Health education and health promotion seek to effect changes in the health behavior of individuals and related small groups and to change organizational and societal factors to affect the environment. An intervention method is a defined process by which theory postulates how change may occur in the behavior of an individual, a small group, or other social structure. One example of a theory-based method is modeling, which is frequently used to facilitate behavior change. In Step 2, intervention methods that correspond to the proximal program objectives developed in Step 1 are listed. These are then used to begin to formulate program activities that will result in change in the proximal program objectives (Chapter 6). Step 2 produces the intervention methods and strategies that match Step 1's proximal program objectives.

Whereas a method is a theory-based technique to influence behavior or environmental conditions, a strategy is a way of organizing and operationalizing the intervention methods. The translation of selected methods into action is completed through the development of strategies. Examples of strategies include a meeting with community members to form community development task forces, a diary for self-monitoring, role-model stories for modeling, a pledge for commitment, and self-talk for cognitive-behavioral rehearsal. A planner working from the food service matrix mentioned in Step 1 might use the methods of persuasion and modeling to influence purchasing practices of the food services manager. Strategies might include testimonials by food service personnel who had incorporated healthier buying practices. If the planner discovered that school district policy was a barrier to changing purchasing practices, he or she would return to Step 1, identify roles at the district level that could influence the policy, write performance objectives for these roles, specify determinants, and construct matrices. These district-level policy changes would then functionally be methods for change at the next lower ecological level, the food service managers and cooks.

Step 3: Program

The product in Step 3 includes a description of the scope and sequence of the components of the intervention, the completion of program materials, and protocols for implementation. This step demands the careful reconsideration of the intended program participants and the program context as well as pilot testing of program strategies and materials with intended implementers and recipients (Chapter 7). This step also gives specific guidance for communicating program intent to producers (e.g., graphic designers, videographers, and writers). The planners of the food service change might organize all their change methods and strategies into a "Creative Cooks for Healthy Kids Cooking School." The "school," however, might include on-the-job training, policy change, newsletters featuring role models, and social reinforcement—or whatever was planned in Step 2 to produce the changes specified in Step 1.

Step 4: Adoption and Implementation

The focus of this step is program adoption and implementation (including consideration of program sustainability). Matrices similar to those in Step 1 are developed with adoption and implementation objectives juxtaposed to personal and external determinants. The synthesis of each objective with a determinant produces a proximal objective. These proximal objectives are then operationalized using methods and strategies to form concrete and comprehensive theory-based plans for adoption and implementation. For example, the promoters of the food service change would ask the following questions: Who is in charge of food service at the school district and at individual schools? Who would perceive a need, develop awareness of a program, and choose to adopt changes in the food service? Who would be in charge of implementation? What, specifically, would these people have to do? For example, a principal might have to order the program for review, ask the food service manager for his or her opinion of the program, and form a task force for food service change. The planner then uses theory and evidence to hypothesize determinants of the principal's adoption and implementation performance objectives. The product for Step 4 is a detailed plan for accomplishing program adoption and implementation by influencing behavior of individuals or groups who will make decisions about adopting and using the program (Chapter 8).

Step 5: Evaluation

In the process of Intervention Mapping, planners make decisions about learning and change objectives, methods, strategies, and implementation. The decisions, although based on theory and evidence from research, still may not be optimal or may even be completely wrong. Through effect and process evaluation, planners can determine whether decisions were correct at each mapping step (Green & Lewis, 1986; Rossi, Freeman, & Lipsey, 1999; Windsor, Baranowski, Clark, & Cutter, 1994). To evaluate the effect of an intervention, researchers analyze the reduction of the health and social problems, changes in behavior and environment, and changes in determinants of performance objectives. All these variables have been defined in a measurable way during the preceding steps. Effect evaluation may show positive, negative, or mixed effects or show no effect at all. Planners want to understand the reasons behind the effects that were achieved, regardless of what those effects were. They need to know more about the process and the changes in intermediate variables; they ask such questions as, Were determinants well specified? Were strategies well matched to methods? How many people did the program reach? Was the implementation complete and appropriate? The product of Step 5 is a plan for answering these questions (Chapter 9).

An Iterative Process

Even though we present Intervention Mapping as a series of steps, the process is iterative rather than completely linear. Program developers move back and forth between tasks and steps as they gain information and perspective from various activities, tasks, or steps. However, the process is also cumulative. Developers base each step on the previous steps, and inattention to a step can jeopardize the potential effectiveness of the intervention by narrowing the scope and compromising the validity with which later steps are conducted. Sometimes planners can get carried away by momentum in the process of the planning group and forget a step or they may perform a step with less rigor than may be optimal. Fortunately, most of the time, planners can backtrack and include, repeat, or elaborate on a neglected step.

SUMMARY

Intervention Mapping is a systematic process that explicates a series of steps and procedures for the development of health education programs based on theory, empirical findings from the literature, and data collected from the population. Intervention Mapping provides health promotion program planners with a guide for effective decisions in each step of program development. The steps and procedures included in Intervention Mapping are not new to the experienced health educator, but the specification of the tasks in each step and the organization of these tasks into a systematic, interrelated approach to intervention development represent an innovation for the practice of health education.

REFERENCES

Advance report of final mortality statistics. (1994). *Mortality Vital Statistics Reports, 45*(3).

Basen-Engquist, K., O'Hara-Tompkins, N. M., Lovato, C. Y., Lewis, M. J., Parcel, G. S., & Gingiss, P. L. (1994). The effect of two types of teacher training on implementation of Smart Choices: A tobacco prevention curriculum. *Journal of School Health, 64*(8), 334–339.

Burdine, J. N., & McLeroy, K. R. (1992). Practitioners' use of theory: Examples from a workgroup. *Health Education Quarterly, 19*(2), 331–340.

Earp, J. A., & Ennett, S. T. (1991). Conceptual models for health education research and practice. *Health Education Research: Theory and Practice, 6*(2), 163–171.

Gingiss, P. L., Gottlieb, N. H., & Brink, S. G. (1994). Increasing teacher receptivity toward use of tobacco prevention education programs. *Journal of Drug Education, 24*(2), 163–176.

Glanz, K., Lewis, F. M., & Rimer, B. K. (Eds.). (1997). *Health behavior and health education: Theory, research, and practice* (2nd ed.). San Francisco: Jossey-Bass.

Goodman, R. M., & Steckler, A. (1989). A model for the institutionalization of health promotion programs. *Family and Community Health, 11*(4), 63–78.

Green, L. W., & Kreuter, M. W. (1999). *Health promotion planning: An educational and ecological approach* (3rd ed.). Mountain View, CA: Mayfield.

Green, L. W., & Lewis, F. M. (1986). *Measurement and evaluation in health education and health promotion.* Palo Alto, CA: Mayfield.

Green, L. W., Richard, L., & Potvin, L. (1996). Ecological foundation of health promotion. *American Journal of Health Promotion, 10*(4), 270–281.

Hochbaum, G. M., Sorenson, J. R., & Lorig, K. (1992). Theory in health education practice. *Health Education Quarterly, 19*(3), 295–314.

Kok, G., Schaalma, H., De Vries, H., Parcel, G., & Paulussen, T. (1996). Social psychology and health education. In W. Stroebe & M. Hewstone (Eds.), *European review of social psychology* (pp. 241–282). New York: Wiley.

McLeroy, K. R., Bibeau, D., Steckler, A., & Glanz, K. (1988). An ecological perspective on health promotion programs. *Health Education Quarterly, 15*(4), 351–377.

Mullen, P. D., & Mullen, L. R. (1983). Implementing asthma self-management education in medical care settings: Issues and strategies. *Journal of Allergy and Clinical Immunology, 72*(5, Pt. 2), 611–622.

Oldenburg, B., Hardcastle, D., & Kok, G. (1997). Diffusion of health promotion and education programs. In K. Glanz, F. M. Lewis, & B. K. Rimer (Eds.), *Health behavior and health education: Theory, research, and practice* (2nd ed., pp. 270–286). San Francisco: Jossey-Bass.

Orlandi, M. A. (1987). Promoting health and preventing disease in health care settings: An analysis of barriers. *Preventive Medicine, 16*(1), 119–130.

Orlandi, M. A., Landers, C., Weston, R., & Haley, N. (1990). Diffusion of health promotion innovations. In K. Glanz, F. M. Lewis, & B. K. Rimer (Eds.), *Health behavior and health education: Theory, research and practice* (pp. 288–313). San Francisco: Jossey-Bass.

Ottoson, J. M., & Green, L. W. (1987). Reconciling concept and context: Theory of implementation. In W. B. Ward, S. Simonds, P. D. Mullen, & M. H. Becker (Eds.), *Advances in health education and promotion* (pp. 353–382). Greenwich, CT: JAI Press.

Parcel, G. S., Simons-Morton, B. G., O'Hara, N. M., Baranowski, T., Kolbe, L. J., & Bee, D. E. (1987). School promotion of healthful diet and exercise behavior: An integration of organizational change and Social Learning Theory interventions. *Journal of School Health, 57*(4), 150–156.

Paulussen, T., Kok, G., & Schaalma, H. (1994). Antecedents to adoption of classroom-based AIDS education in secondary schools. *Health Education Research: Theory and Practice, 9*(4), 485–496.

Paulussen, T., Kok, G., Schaalma, H., & Parcel, G. S. (1995). Diffusion of AIDS curricula among Dutch secondary school teachers. *Health Education Quarterly, 22*(2), 227–243.

Reiss, A., Miczek, K., & Roth, J. (1993). *Understanding and preventing violence.* Washington, DC: National Academy Press.

Richard, L., Potvin, L., Kishchuk, N., Prlic, H., & Green, L. W. (1996). Assessment of the integration of the ecological approach in health promotion programs. *American Journal of Health Promotion, 10*(4), 318–328.

Robertson, A., & Minkler, M. (1994). New health promotion movement: A critical examination. *Health Education Quarterly, 21*(3), 295–312.

Rossi, P. H., Freeman, H. E., & Lipsey, M. W. (1999). *Evaluation: A systematic approach* (6th ed.). Newbury Park, CA: Sage.

Scheirer, M. A. (1990). The life cycle of an innovation: Adoption versus discontinuation of the fluoride mouth rinse program in schools. *Journal of Health and Social Behavior, 31*(2), 203–215.

Scheirer, M. A., & Rezmovic, E. L. (1983). Measuring the degree of program implementation: A methodological review. *Evaluation Review, 7*(5), 599–633.

Simons-Morton, B. G., Greene, W. H., & Gottlieb, N. H. (1995). *Introduction to health education and health promotion* (2nd ed.). Prospect Heights, IL: Waveland Press.

Singh, G. K., & Yu, S. M. (1996). Trends and differentials in adolescent and young adult mortality in the United States, 1950 through 1993. *American Journal of Public Health, 86*(4), 560–564.

Smith, D. W., Steckler, A. B., McCormick, L. K., & McLeroy, K. R. (1995). Lessons learned about disseminating health curricula to schools. *Journal of Health Education, 26*(1), 37–43.

Stokols, D. (1996). Translating social ecological theory into guidelines for community health promotion. *American Journal of Health Promotion, 10*(4), 282–298.

Tolan, P. H., & Guerra, N. G. (1994). *What works in reducing adolescent violence: An empirical review of the field.* Boulder, CO: Center for the Study and Prevention of Violence.

Tolan, P. H., & Guerra, N. G. (1996). Progress and prospects in youth violence-prevention evaluation. *American Journal of Preventive Medicine, 12*(5 Suppl.), 129–131.

U.S. Department of Justice. (1994). *Criminal victimization in the United States, 1994: A National Crime Victimization Survey Report.* Washington, DC: Bureau of Justice Statistics.

Veen, P. (1985). *Sociale psychologie toegepast: Van probleem naar oplossing* [Applying social psychology: From problem to solution]. Alphen aan den Rijn, The Netherlands: Samson.

Wallerstein, N. (1992). Powerlessness, empowerment, and health: Implications for health promotion programs. *American Journal of Health Promotion, 6*(3), 197–205.

Windsor, R., Baranowski, T., Clark, N., & Cutter, G. (1994). *Evaluation of health promotion, health education, and disease prevention programs* (2nd ed.). Mountain View, CA: Mayfield.

World Health Organization. (1978). *Primary health care: Report of the International Conference on Primary Health Care, Alma-Ata, USSR, Sept. 6–12, 1978* (Health for All Series, No. 1). Geneva, Switzerland: Author.

World Health Organization. (1986). Ottawa charter for health promotion. *Health Promotion International, 1,* iii–iv.

CHAPTER 2

Assessment of Community Capacity and Needs

READER OBJECTIVES

- Decide where to enter a needs assessment model
- Describe at-risk populations and potential program participants
- Include quality of life, health, behavioral, environmental, and determinant data in a needs assessment
- Balance a needs assessment with an assessment of community capacity
- Use the assessment to begin thinking about intervention points
- Use both qualitative and quantitative data to understand the needs and capacity of the community
- Work from the assessment to write program objectives

Intervention Mapping or any other health education program planning must be based on a thorough assessment of community capacity and needs. This assessment encompasses two components: a scientific, epidemiologic, behavioral, and social perspective of a community and its problems; and an effort to "get to know," or begin to understand, the character of the community, its members, and its strengths. The purpose of this chapter is to enable the reader to understand the necessity for and the requirements of performing both capacity and needs assessments.

PERSPECTIVES

Assessment of Both Needs and Strengths

A needs assessment is a systematic study of quality of life and health status and those factors that influence them, such as health behavior and environment. A need indicates a difference between what currently exists and a more desirable state. Gilmore and colleagues suggest that planners not worry too much about the difference between need and "perceived need," because needs are always changing in character and quantity and because needs are always interpreted by someone (Gilmore, Campbell, & Becker, 1989). Inevitably in the assessment process, needs will be interpreted by both the intended population and program planners.

Needs assessments of health problems include an analysis of the physiological risk factors and behavioral and environmental risks to health, even when the actual health problems have not yet manifested. For example, cardiovascular disease is a health problem, high-cholesterol levels are a physiological risk factor, eating high-fat foods is a behavioral risk factor, and poor access to healthy diet is an environmental risk factor. Finally, needs assessments include study of the determinants of behavior and environmental contributors to health problems or health risks. By determinants, we mean those factors that have been found to be associated with the at-risk behavior or the environmental condition. The implication for intervention is that determinants are causally related to the conditions. However, even though the logic is causal, the empirical evidence most often is not.

The study of a community from a capacity, or resources and strengths, perspective rounds out the assessment (Fawcett, 1991; Goeppinger & Baglioni, 1985; Goodman, Steckler, Hoover, & Schwartz, 1993; Kretzmann & McKnight, 1993). Studying the strengths of a community can help the health educator keep in mind a community's unique character and ability to plan its own interventions. An attitude of partnership between health professionals and community members will more likely prevent a top-down or outsider planning approach (Minkler & Wallerstein, 1997). For example, a school of public health class began an assessment of the Acres Homes Community in Houston, Texas, an area that had originated as a community that was not served by many city services. Community residents made it clear to planners that needs had to be understood in a context of both current and historical community pride, entrepreneurship, and leadership. Despite a host of urban problems, inconsistent support from the city, and deficits in health services, the community maintained a strong African American culture that had begun attracting new resources. From a needs perspective the community had a certain profile, and from a capacity perspective it had another look entirely.

Furthermore, a focus on community competencies and resources from the outset of program planning directs attention to the need for enhancement of capacity in the program development and implementation. All too often health education and other social programs, especially research and demonstration efforts, have entered communities only to leave them unchanged when funding ended (Goodman & Steckler, 1989). Program goals that include enhanced capacity as a program aim at the start of planning can make this scenario less likely to develop.

Population at Risk, Environmental Context, and Intervention Groups

The designation "population at risk" means a group with a definable boundary and shared characteristics that have, or are at risk for, certain health and quality-of-life problems. To lay the foundation for intervention, planners should also be concerned with the environmental context of the at-risk group. The environment may contribute directly to the health problem, in the case, for example, of contaminated water and diarrhea. Or it can be a more indirect influence, such as the contribution of social networks to the continuation of smoking. We suggest four levels of analysis of the environmental context: interpersonal, organizational, community, and societal. These levels are similar to the ones proposed by Richard, Potvin, Kishchuk, Prlic, and Green (1996). We have added interpersonal in order to facilitate thinking about intervention, and we have incorporated the supranational level into our societal level for the same reason.

Organizations are "systems with a formal multi-echelon decision process operating in pursuit of specific objectives. Schools, stores, companies, and professional associations are a few examples" (Richard et al., 1996, p. 320). Communities are restricted in Richard's description to a geographical area comprising persons and organizations. Neighborhoods, cities, villages, or groups of towns are examples of communities (p. 320). However, we include in communities other groups that exhibit relationships among the members of a certain population in addition to shared characteristics and boundaries (Fellin, 1995). In addition to geopolitical boundaries, there are demographic boundaries (e.g., socioeconomic status, gender, age, and family structure) and demographic-ethnic boundaries (e.g., Latino, European American, African American). There are also groups with shared characteristics, such as persons with a certain disease, or those served by the same agency. A community may also be a group coming together for a cause or political agenda (Eng & Parker, 1994). Societies are larger systems possessing means to control several aspects of the lives and development of their constituent systems. They also are more self-contained than are communities. Examples of societies are provinces, states, and countries (Richard et al., 1996). We also include in this environmental level multinational organizations such as the European Union.

Often, in an assessment of a health problem, the relatedness in a population at risk is that all the members have a risk factor or health problem in common, for example, cystic fibrosis, cardiovascular disease, AIDS. Sometimes these individuals come together in organizations for mutual support—the Tourette Syndrome Association, the Multiple Sclerosis Society, Mothers Against Drunk Driving. Of course, the population may be defined by a combination of variables, such as adults with cystic fibrosis who are English speaking and living in North America, or adolescents age 11 to 16 who live in the inner city and are at risk for HIV and other STDs. The important issue is that the population or populations are well defined during the process of the assessment (Gilmore et al., 1989; Soriano, 1995; Witkin & Altschuld, 1995).

The broad scope of environmental context suggests not only complex causation of health problems, but also the need for health education and promotion intervention on a variety of levels and at a variety of venues (e.g., work sites, schools, communities, and health care organizations). However, we do not believe that these different types of communities need a substantively different type of planning process. They do need a systematic planning process that allows for the incorporation of their unique qualities.

The first task in performing a needs assessment is to describe the individuals who are the potential recipients of the health promotion intervention. There may be several groups in a comprehensive multilevel program, and the recipients are not necessarily the population at risk. They could be environmental agents, such as the health care provider in a case of chronic disease management, or organizations and government in a case of primary prevention policy. There are often multiple groups, some who are populations at risk and others who influence the environment. The at-risk population always is the intended recipient of program benefits such as risk reduction or improvements in health status or quality of life.

Designating people as a "target" group might be criticized on the basis of health promotion's concern for participation, inclusion, and power distribution. However, the term does not imply that the people we work with are not full partners from social, philosophical, and political perspectives. The need to define an intervention group means a programmatic need for an epidemiologically and demographically defined population in order to plan effective programs and to measure their effects on health and quality of life. Precisely defining the various groups who will benefit from the program enables the planner to know both the numerator, the people who get the program, and the denominator, the population for whom the program is intended (Glasgow, Vogt, & Boles, 1999).

Collaborative Planning

A final perspective is our emphasis on collaborative planning. The philosophy of health education is built on the principle of self-determination, an individual's governance of his or her own behavior. Health education has a history of community participation in program development. The frequently cited passage from the 1974 Alma-Ata Declaration proclaims "people have the right and the duty to participate individually and collectively in the planning and implementing of their health care" (World Health Organization [WHO], 1978). Green has asserted that participation increases the probability that health improvement goals will be achieved; that listening to people and freely sharing information will improve their participation and consensus; and that feedback on the progress of programs they have planned increases trust in the process (Green, 1986; Kreuter, Lezin, Kreuter, & Green, 1997). Currently, there is considerable work taking place on the impact of participatory planning, implementation, and evaluation on individual and community empowerment. For example, community health worker activities have affected community competence (Eng & Young, 1992; Ovrebo, Ryan, Jackson, & Hutchinson, 1994). Others have described the empowering effects of involving community members in the documentation of needs (Wang & Burris, 1994) and in the development of their own program materials (Rudd & Comings, 1994).

The second task in performing a needs assessment is to form a planning group with broad participation. We conceptualize the participation as a linkage system similar to that discussed by Orlandi and colleagues (Orlandi, 1986, 1987; Orlandi, Landers, Weston, & Haley, 1990). In the development of every project there is a resource system (developers), an intermediate user system (implementers), and an end user system (participants or intervention groups). For successful implementation, a planner must develop a linkage between these three systems. The development of this linkage system should begin as early in the project development as possible, optimally in project funding development and needs assessment. The linkage process is further discussed in Chapter 8. The linkages can be defined on a continuum from minimum involvement with the health educator accessing the community and the implementers for information or consultation through a full partnership model in which the community members are the planners and the planning becomes a part of the intervention, as in a community empowerment model (Fisher, Auslander, Sussman, Owens, & Jackson-Thompson, 1992; Fisher et al., 1994; Hugentobler, Israel, & Schurman, 1992).

Whatever the level of participation, the health promoter cannot be sure that the resource system fully represents the end users. Efforts to represent the community should be ongoing. Even when health promoters work in a collaborative community participation mode that is as pure as possible, they should never assume that they "understand" the community; understanding is a process. Therefore, they must keep asking whether they know whom the intervention is meant to affect, and they must continue to build relationships based on listening in order to move to ever-higher levels of understanding. They must also be sure that they access various members of communities, not simply those members who have been recruited to be part of the resource team; they must be sure that they are not working only with information that is filtered by members of the planning group.

In addition to at-risk population partnerships, health educators must build linkages with the intermediate users, or program implementers. Even though the intermediate users are not usually the focus of the needs assessment, they may be one important source of data. That the program implementers are not the focus may seem self-evident. However, the person who works with a health problem, rather than the individuals who have the health problem, may be the first contact for the health educator—the physician or nurse for a chronic disease, the emergency medical service for injuries, the HIV counselor for AIDS. This care provider perspective can overwhelm the assessment picture if care is not taken to maintain balance between the views of the provider and the clients. The concept of implementers, or intermediate users, is discussed more in Chapter 8, which covers adoption and implementation. In this chapter we concentrate on the at-risk population and related environmental participants.

HOW TO CONDUCT A NEEDS ASSESSMENT

Combining Qualitative and Quantitative Evidence

The third task in performing a needs assessment is to use both qualitative and quantitative data. A full community assessment considers both objective assessment of the difference between the current status and an optimal one and

How to Conduct a Needs Assessment

The health educator from Chapter 1 is in a meeting with the department head. The two are struggling with how to get the planning group started. The health educator is worried that, although the planning group was handpicked by the mayor, it is not representative enough of the neighborhoods in which the group wants to focus their violence project. The health educator wants permission to add to the group as they encounter interested community residents during the needs assessment.

"Adding more community people will be good for the group, good for planning, and (politically) good for the mayor," the health educator points out.

"Yes, but too large a committee is too hard to handle," argues the department head.

"These will be the people who understand the problem firsthand," counters the health educator, "and they are also the people who will ensure the implementation of whatever program we come up with. Besides, people who don't feel included can sabotage our efforts." At this point the health educator turns to the cartoon hanging on the wall (Illustration 2.1). "Haven't you ever encountered this?"

"Okay, I'll get the mayor's approval, but I trust you to really manage this group. Better review your group skills books" (Bradford, 1976; Daniels, 1986; Toseland & Rivas, 1984). "Make sure your group leadership is not rusty. I don't have to tell you how anxious the mayor is to see something happening. I know, I know! You say we have to do a needs

(continued)

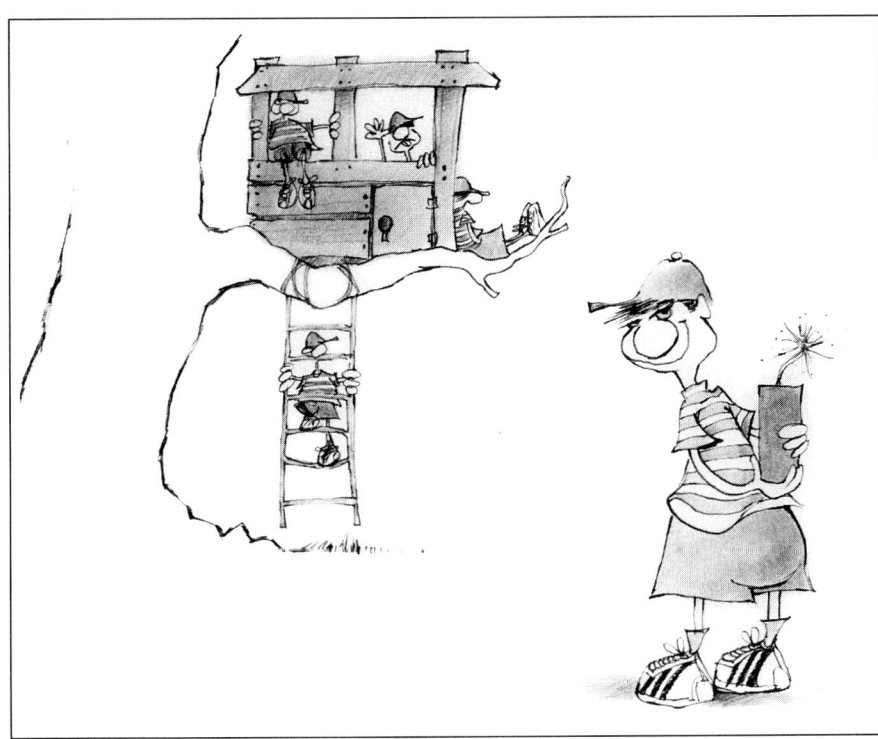

ILLUSTRATION 2.1 Task Group Sabotage

assessment. I am convinced, but is that going to give us the visibility we need? Can we just think of how to do this in such a way that it is clear to everyone that we are doing something?"

"Yes," the health educator responded. "I've been thinking about that. We need both qualitative and quantitative evidence about this problem. We also need information from our own community as well as from studies conducted elsewhere. We need information about violence and its context, but we also need a real feel for the strengths of these communities. What if we could make the complexity work for us in two ways? Let's break the group into teams. Some people will go after the scientific literature. We have some real library moles in the bunch. Another group will get out into the community and talk to people. That will keep us visible. It also will help with the needs versus strengths issue. We'll structure short reports based on our PRECEDE model and present them to the mayor as we go along."

"That sounds good. Now that we have that settled, let's get started."

subjective assessment, or the actual felt needs or meaning of certain needs to members of a community. As Hancock and Minkler (1997) suggest, "a balance of studies and stories make up the information needed to assess communities and community health." Furthermore, using both qualitative and quantitative data allows planners to increase confidence in the validity of their results. Quantitative methods such as surveys and disease registries enable the planner to estimate the incidence and prevalence of health problems and related behaviors in the at-risk population. Quantitative methods also enable estimates of the strength of the correlation of determinants with risk behaviors. On the other hand, qualitative methods such as ethnographic interviews (Bauman & Adair, 1992; Braithwaite, Bianchi, & Taylor, 1994), focus groups (Basch, 1987; Kreuger, 1988; Morgan, 1988), the problem-posing methods from Freire's education for critical consciousness (1973), critical incident technique (McNabb, Wilson-Pessano, & Jacobs, 1986), and nominal group process (Delbecq, Van de Ven, & Gustafson, 1975) help health educators to understand communities, health problems, behavioral and environmental causes, and determinants from the perspectives of the people involved.

Qualitative and quantitative approaches to problem analysis are not simply two different techniques to arrive at the same answer. They are essentially different, even in their philosophical origins and approaches to knowledge—so different that some researchers would argue that they cannot be used together. The health education field, although dominated by quantitative work, is adopting a paradigm integrating the two approaches. We think the two methods used together produce a more usable, comprehensive, and accurate assessment product (as well as better information about and from members of the intended community throughout Intervention Mapping). However, each approach must be used with its own assumptions, and the reader is referred to other texts for instruction in quantitative (Cook & Campbell, 1979; Green & Lewis, 1986) and qualitative (Berg, 1989; Miles & Huberman, 1994; Patton, 1990; Strauss, 1988; Wolcott, 1994) methods.

The methods in each tradition differ in the research object and in design, data collection, and analysis (De Vries, Weijts, Dijkstra, & Kok, 1992). In general, qualitative approaches are (Patton, 1990)

- inductive
- discovery oriented, iterative
- question and theory generating
- subjective and valid with the self as the instrument
- not usually amenable to counting
- case oriented
- not generalizable

Quantitative methods are

- deductive
- theory verification oriented
- question answering
- objective and reliable, subject to reliable counting
- population oriented
- generalizable

Steckler, McLeroy, Goodman, Bird, and McCormick (1992) present a useful diagram of four ways that qualitative and quantitative methods can be used in program evaluation (Figure 2.1). Those research models are equally appropriate in needs assessment. In Model 1, the planner uses qualitative data gathering methods such as focus groups, nominal group technique, observation, ethnographic interviews, or semi-structured interviews in order to begin to hear perceptions of health problems, related behavioral and environmental causes, determinants, and quality of life in the community. Then surveys are developed to document the prevalence of the issues discussed in the group or individual interviews (Desvousges & Frey, 1989; O'Brien, 1993). Beginning with qualitative methods in this case gives the planner a better chance of asking pertinent and intelligible questions during a survey phase. This sequence of using qualitative methods to inform survey design may also enable the researcher to develop new hypotheses or to refine hypotheses before the quantitative phase of the research. For example, O'Brien used focus groups in a study of the social relationships of gay and bisexual men to inform questionnaire development. He learned the language that the men in the groups used to discuss relationships and sexual experiences. His discussions led to a survey that contained careful definitions of the terms *primary relationship* and *safer sex,* two very important and potentially

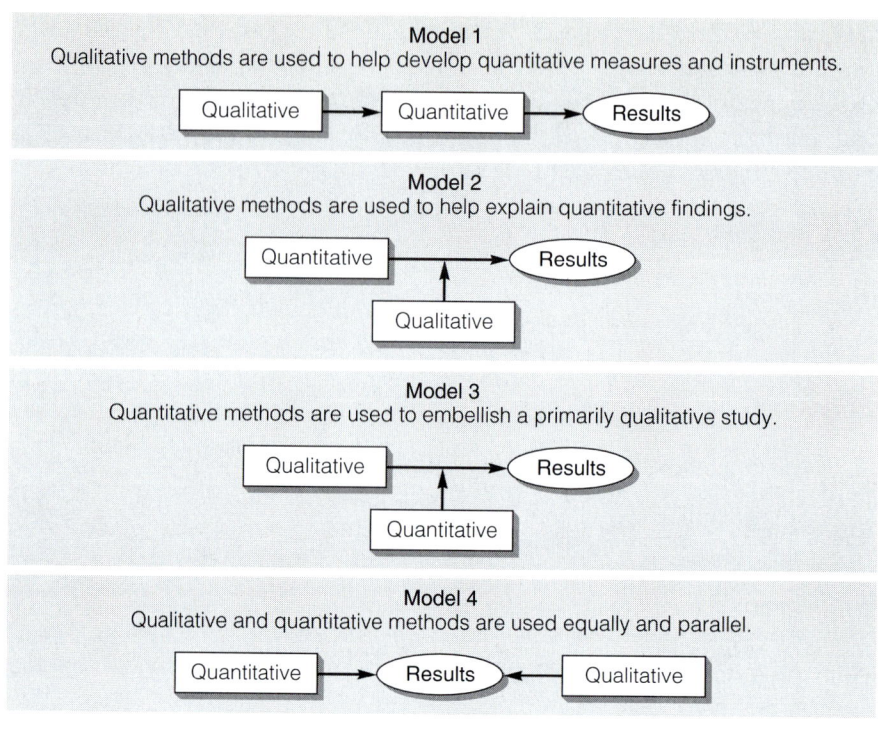

FIGURE 2.1 Integrating Qualitative and Quantitative Methods (*Note.* From "Toward Integrating Qualitative and Quantitative Methods: An Introduction," by A. Steckler, K. R. McLeroy, R. M. Goodman, S. T. Bird, and L. M. McCormick, 1992, *Health Education Quarterly,19*(1), 1–8.)

ambiguous concepts. The focus groups also led to the addition of several questions to be addressed by the larger study.

In Model 2, planners use qualitative techniques to better understand the meaning of their quantitative findings. In a needs assessment, health educators might use census or epidemiologic data to describe the health problem, behavioral or environmental risk, or determinants. They might then conduct qualitative research to better understand the perceptions of the at-risk group (Wingood, Hunter-Gamble, & DiClemente, 1993). For example, in 1992 in the United States more than 100,000 women of childbearing age had been infected with HIV. The prevalence of HIV was much higher in women of color than in White women; African American women accounted for 52.8% and Latinas 23% of the cases in the United States (Centers for Disease Control and Prevention [CDC], 1999). The cumulative incidence of AIDS in African American women was more than 10 times higher than in same-age European American women (Bakeman, McCray, Lumb, Jackson, & Whitley, 1987). Part of the transmission was due to IV drug use, but a larger proportion seems to have been accounted for by sexual intercourse with infected partners. Wingood and colleagues used the focus group technique to better understand the determinants of HIV-associated risk behaviors in African American women. They found that the women they spoke with could bring up with their partners the conversational topic of safer sex, but they could not effectively negotiate condom use. Demanding that a partner use condoms could imply lack of trust in a relationship, violate a woman's conflict-avoiding stance, and prove difficult or even dangerous to a woman. In another study of Latinas and African American women, Ehrhardt, Yingling, Zawadzki, and Martinez-Ramirez (1992) found that women understood HIV transmission but did not perceive themselves to be at risk, had idiosyncratic ways of attributing risk to partners, thought asking long-term partners to use condoms implied lack of trust, and found condoms to be at odds with both sexual pleasure and desire for pregnancy. These studies provide examples of defining a problem with epidemiologic data and then trying to better understand the risk behavior (unsafe sex) using qualitative methods.

In Model 3, the health educator conducts a qualitative study in order to document the problems or needs in a community and then uses quantitative data to verify and establish the magnitude of the primarily qualitative needs assessment. In the final model, both qualitative and quantitative methods are used in parallel to shed light on an issue or a problem (Saint-Germain, Bassford, & Montano, 1993).

De Vries and colleagues (1992) suggest an iterative or spiral approach for use in intervention development. In their description, a planner alternates qualitative and quantitative approaches both in the development of interventions and in their evaluation. Figure 2.2 presents the approach to alternating qualitative and quantitative methods used in the various stages of the Cystic Fibrosis Family Education Program. Though not entirely categorized as assessment at each stage of the project, qualitative and quantitative processes were alternated and used to stimulate each phase of the program development, evaluation, and diffusion process (Bartholomew et al., 1997; Bartholomew, Czyzewski, Swank, McCormick, & Parcel, 2000; Bartholomew, Seilheimer, Parcel, Spinelli, & Pumariega, 1989; Bartholomew et al., 1993).

Assessing Community Competence, Capacity, and Social Capital

The fourth task in performing a needs assessment is to survey the community for resources and capacities. There is increasing interest in the definition and measurement of aspects of community that are important in three ways: as inputs and context for health promotion planning and programs; as throughputs, or factors related to successful program implementation; and as outputs, or impact of health promotion programs. As a matter of fact, one World Health Organization (WHO) document describes a healthy community as one that is continually creating and improving resources in its physical and social environments that enable people to mutually support each other in performing all the functions of life (Hancock & Duhl, 1986). Community competence is focused on how a community is currently functioning. Iscoe (1974) emphasized the ability to obtain and use resources. Cottrell (1977) defined eight dimensions based on the ability of a community to collaborate effectively to identify problems and needs; to achieve a

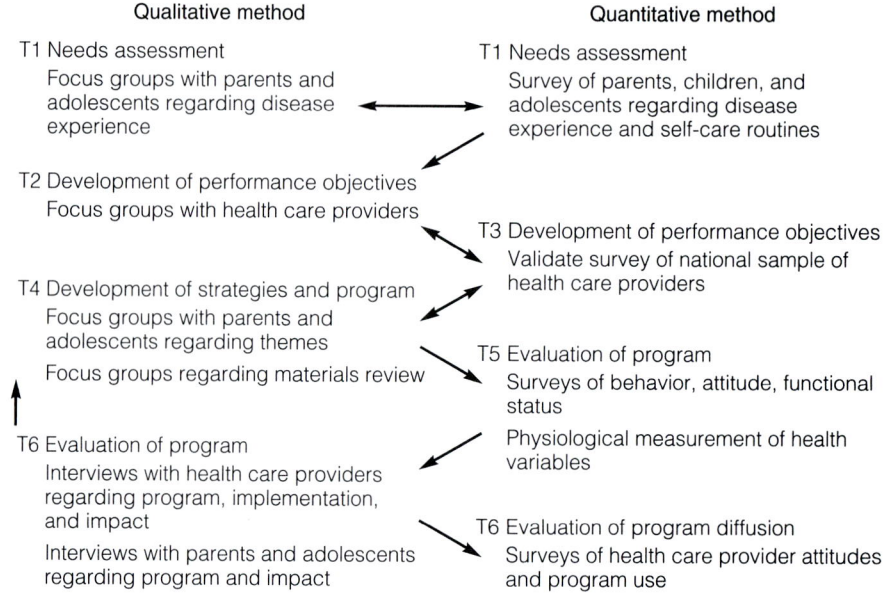

FIGURE 2.2 Iterative Use of Qualitative and Quantitative Methods in the Development of the Cystic Fibrosis Family Education Program

working consensus on priorities, ways, and means; and to implement actions. Eng and Parker (1994) developed a measure of dimensions of community competence: social support; management of relations with the wider society; conflict containment and accommodation; articulation of collective views; awareness of stance on issues and comparison to other community parts; participation; commitment; and ability to establish formal means of ensuring representative input in decision making.

A closely related construct is community capacity—current competence as well as existing resources and aptitude for future performance (Centers for Disease Control and Prevention [CDC], 1997). Community capacity refers to "the characteristics of communities that affect their ability to identify, mobilize and address social and public health problems" (McLeroy, 1996). Goodman and colleagues (1998) have identified several aspects of community capacity. One is community participation, the depth and breadth of citizen involvement in defining and resolving needs. Participation is highly interrelated with inclusivity and encouragement by community leaders. Both participation and leadership are predicated on the third dimension of capacity—a skill base that includes group process, conflict resolution, collection and analysis of data, problem solving, program planning and evaluation, resource development, policy formulation, and media advocacy. Another dimension of capacity is a social network characterized by multiple and overlapping ties between organizations and individuals as well as the capability to form new ties. The link between the neighborhood residents and individuals and institutions outside the neighborhood also is important. A number of dimensions of the community's sense of itself also seem to be important. Central to these are the community's ability to analyze its own thinking processes and change efforts; its sense of connection among people and to community rituals; an awareness of previous change efforts and current conditions; and community power—the ability to create change, values, and critical reflection. Goodman and colleagues describe resources as both physical and social capital resources from inside and outside the community. Social capital is the ability of community members to cooperate and to form new ties based on trust (Kreuter et al., 1997; Putnam, 1993).

Kretzmann and McKnight (1993), in their guide to mapping community capacity, identify three types of resources. The first type are resources located in the community and largely under community control:

- Personal capacity
- Personal income
- Gifts of labeled people (such as the physically challenged)
- Individual local businesses
- Home-based enterprises
- Citizen associations
- Associations of businesses
- Financial institutions (e.g., the Gameen bank in Bangladesh and the South Shore Bank in Chicago)
- Cultural organizations
- Communications organizations
- Religious organizations

They also include a protocol for assessing personal capacity in areas such as construction, office equipment operation and repair, food preparation, transportation, and child care. Many other domains of individual competence can be imagined, including leadership, group process, problem-solving and participation skills.

The second type of resources are assets located within the community but largely controlled by outsiders:

- Institutions of higher learning
- Hospitals
- Social service agencies
- Public schools
- Police
- Fire departments

- Libraries
- Parks
- Land—unused land and buildings
- Energy and waste resources

Finally, there are resources originating outside the neighborhood and controlled by outsiders:

- Welfare expenditures
- Capital improvement expenditures
- Public information

Using PRECEDE to Organize and Analyze Needs Data

The fifth task in performing a needs assessment is to conduct an epidemiological assessment. As planners move from a view of the resources of communities to a view of their needs, they need guidance to incorporate important predictors of health problems as well as their consequences. The model health planners use most often is PRECEDE/PROCEED, a population-based epidemiological model that is also ecological in its perspective. The model directs planners to determine health problem characteristics such as morbidity, mortality, disease risk, and burden of disease in groups of people, and to describe causation of these problems at multiple levels. The model also takes into account multiple determinants of health-related behavior and environment. Health problems such as coronary artery disease have both behavioral risk factors, such as eating high-cholesterol foods, and environmental causes, such as the unavailability of exercise facilities. The subsequent updates of PRECEDE (Green & Kreuter, 1991, 1999) clarified and amplified the important role of both social and physical environment in the causation of health problems.

PRECEDE has been used as the basis for health education planning in hundreds of programs (Bartholomew, Koenning, Dahlquist, & Barron, 1994; Bartholomew et al., 1989; Green et al., 1994). When developed in the 1970s, PRECEDE was not intended to guide the health education field through all of the steps of intervention, but to lead the field to a more outcome-based approach to planning (Green, personal communication, February 26, 1997).

The model (Figure 2.3) begins on the right with descriptions of quality of life and health problems. Changes in these dimensions should be the intention of a health education or promotion intervention. It then guides the planner to explore the scientific evidence to build logical, empirical, and theoretical links between the levels of causation. For example, if premature mortality and morbidity from cardiovascular disease is the health problem, loss of productive years and burden of heart disease begin to define the quality-of-life issues for society and the individual. Next, the planner must support these relationships with data and then begin to find evidence of behavioral and environmental causes. Chapter 3 de-

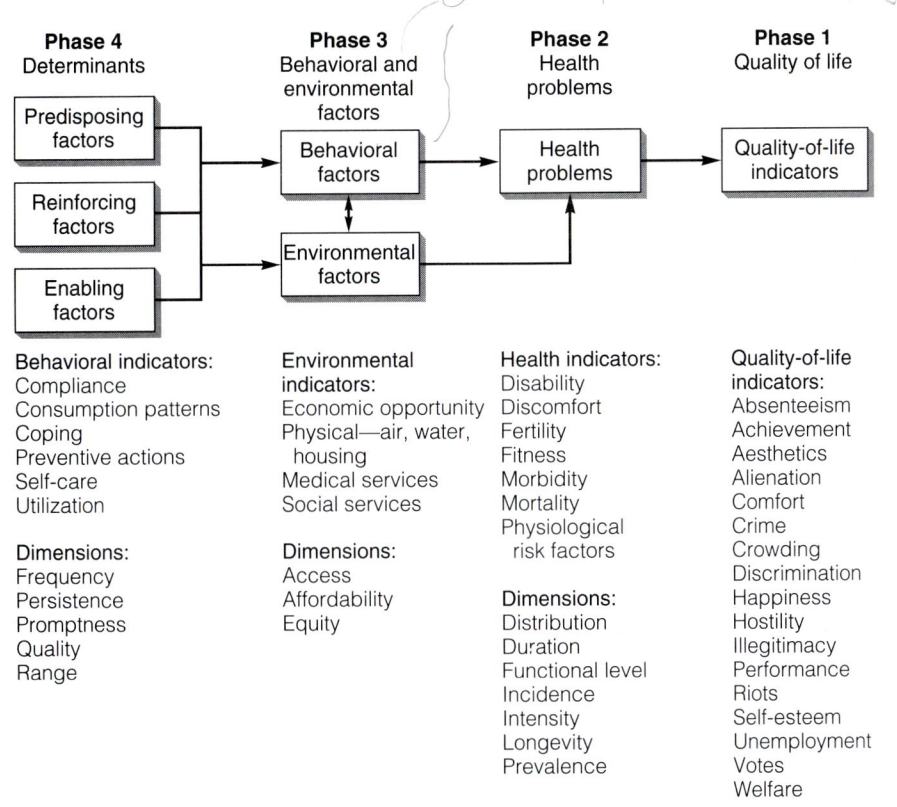

FIGURE 2.3 PRECEDE (*Note.* Modified from *Health Promotion Planning: An Educational and Ecological Approach* [3rd ed.], by L. W. Green and M. W. Kreuter, 1999, Mountain View, CA: Mayfield Publishing.)

scribes in greater detail the core processes for using information from the literature, theory, and new research to develop the needs assessment model (and for Intervention Mapping).

The PRECEDE model begins with health and quality-of-life indicators. In a community, for a specific health problem, the planner can describe morbidity and mortality rates, risk factor prevalence and incidence, and the social costs of these disease dimensions. For example, in a program development effort for reducing morbidity from stroke, we were interested in the incidence and prevalence of stroke in the United States and specifically in east Texas (Table 2.1). Then we wanted to understand the implications of stroke for quality of life of the individual and society as well as the meaning of these burdens for the stroke victims and their social networks, for example, loss of cognitive functioning, loss of financial and physical independence, and medical care costs.

The behavioral analysis typically includes what the at-risk individuals are doing that increases their risk of the health problem. In the case of secondary and tertiary prevention, the analysis investigates what individuals are doing that increases the risk of disability or death from the health problem. In our stroke

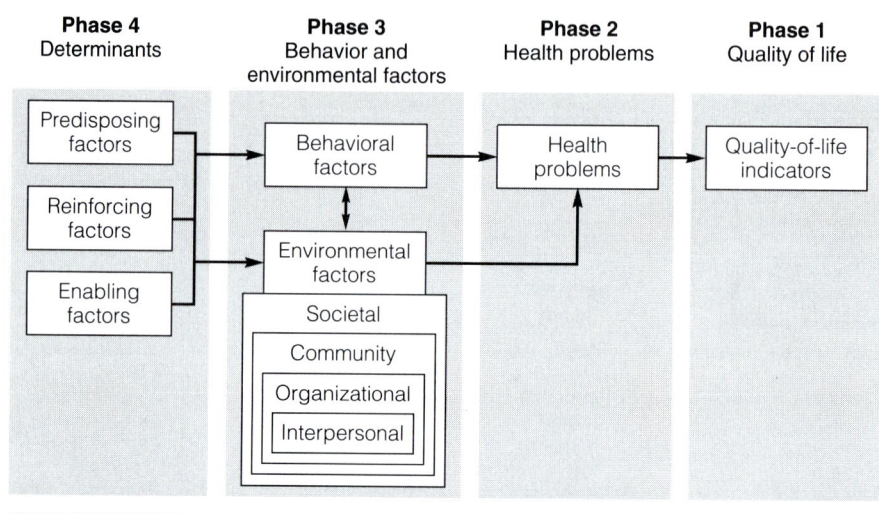

FIGURE 2.4 Levels of Environment in PRECEDE

example, it was apparent from the literature that, with the advent of acute stroke therapy with a 3-hour administration window, an important behavior of the stroke victim and witnesses was waiting before transporting the stroke victim to an emergency department. Factors related to the delay included being assessed by a primary care doctor and arriving by personal car rather than by ambulance (Alberts, Bertels, & Dawson, 1990; Bratina, Greenberg, Pasteur, & Grotta, 1994; Feldmann et al., 1993; National Institute of Neurological Disorders and Stroke [NINDS], 1997).

The environmental analysis includes conditions in the social and physical environment that are related to the health problem directly or to its behavioral causes. In the stroke example, the stroke patient can only receive treatment if the community emergency department is prepared to give acute stroke therapy and if they conduct a neurological examination and specific radiologic and laboratory tests within a certain time frame. Likewise, the emergency department can only perform its function in the chain of events if the emergency medical service transports the individual quickly and contributes to a speedy evaluation (NINDS, 1997).

In many analyses of health problems the environment plays a significant and modifiable role in the causation of the problem either directly, such as air pollution in lung disease, or indirectly, such as availability of condoms and the social norms to use them in safer sex. A diagram by Richard and colleagues (1996) has been modified in Chapter 1 (Figure 1.1) to depict individuals embedded in multiple, interacting levels of environment. When this concept is transferred to PRE-CEDE (Figure 2.4), it is apparent that each of the four levels of environment (interpersonal, organizational, community, and societal) can influence both individual behavior and any lower level of environment.

Table 2.1
PRECEDE Model: Increasing Opportunity for Acute Stroke Therapy

PREDISPOSING, ENABLING, AND REINFORCING FACTORS	BEHAVIOR AND ENVIRONMENT	HEALTH AND QUALITY-OF-LIFE OUTCOMES
Persons in proximity or person with stroke	**Persons in proximity or person with stroke**	**Persons with stroke**
Lack of perceived susceptibility and seriousness of stroke	Do not note symptoms and compare to those for possible stroke	Discharge functional status
		Hospital case fatality
Not knowing signs of stroke, that time is critical, how to call 911	Wait to see if symptoms resolve	Receipt of TPA
	Do not call 911 immediately	Time from ED contact to acute stroke therapy (time in hospital to CT scan, time to physician neuro exam, time to ready for acute therapy)
Outcome expectations—nothing can be done for stroke so that disability is less	Call primary care provider	
	Wait in ER without treatment	
Barriers: cost of calling 911, being female, being male without a partner		
Social norms: friends would not call 911		
Do not live with someone or is retired		
EMS	**EMS**	
Do not believe that they can make a difference in stroke as they can in trauma and heart attack	Dispatcher:	
	Does not triage to highest priority	
Do not see stroke as urgent	Does not convey stroke possibility and urgency	
No knowledge or skills to treat in transit	Responder:	
Lack stroke protocol for dispatcher and responders	Does not "load and go"	
	Gives blood pressure lowering meds	
	Does not call ahead to the hospital	
Payers	**Payers**	
Cost	Do not approve ER treatment with TPA	
Cost/benefit		
Hospital ED	**Hospital ED**	
Believe TPA is dangerous despite trial results	Does not complete the evaluation in 60 minutes	
Lack knowledge, skills, and self-efficacy for administering TPA	Does not make a differential diagnosis of stroke (perform a neurological exam using modified NIH scale/protocol)	
Lack skills and self-efficacy to determine onset time	Does not order CT scan, lab work immediately	
Lack skills to perform diagnosis and neurologic exam	Cannot document onset time	
Perceive inadequate acute treatment as normative	Lacks stroke protocol, designated stroke team, brain box, access to TPA in emergency room	
Self-efficacy for stroke treatment		

(continued)

Table 2.1 PRECEDE Model: Increasing Opportunity for Acute Stroke Therapy (continued)

PREDISPOSING, ENABLING, AND REINFORCING FACTORS	BEHAVIOR AND ENVIRONMENT	HEALTH AND QUALITY-OF-LIFE OUTCOMES
Hospital ED		
Outcome expectations for treatment—does not equate study results to real-life quality of life for stroke patients		
No protocol in ER		
Perception that cost is greater than benefit		
Primary care providers	**Primary care providers**	
Perceive inadequate acute stroke treatment as normative, in other words, as standard of care	Demand to consult on ER patients before treatment of stroke	
Outcome expectations for treatment—do not equate study results to real-life quality of life for stroke patients	Do not come immediately to ER when called for stroke	
No protocol in office	Do not warn high-risk patients to call 911 for stroke symptoms	
	Do not train office staff on protocol for phone call with stroke symptoms	
	Tell patients with symptoms of stroke to wait or to come to the office	

Note. ED = emergency department; EMS = emergency medical service; ER = emergency room; TPA = tissue plasminogen activator.

Beginning in the needs assessment and continuing in Intervention Mapping, the planner is faced with choosing what should be changed from an array of behavioral and environmental factors. The planner must decide whether the environmental factors are important to the problem and whether they are changeable in the scope of the program mandate. Once the environmental factors are chosen, the planner must discover the agents at each level for each environmental change objective. These agents are the people (and the social or organizational roles assigned to them) who are in positions to change the environment. For the stroke example, the hospital emergency departments and the emergency medical services (EMS) are the organizations, and the agents able to make change are a variety of health care providers and administrators such as the medical director of the emergency department, the director of the EMS, and the chair of the critical care committee. In another example, this one concerning adolescent sexual risk taking, parents might be in a position to change something about the immediate environment of adolescents, such as the amount of unsupervised time at home (related to the opportunity to have sexual intercourse).

The MATCH model presents the environment in this way, where environmental levels are chosen for intervention whether or not they have been directly implicated in health problem causation (Simons-Morton, Greene, & Gottlieb, 1995; Simons-Morton, Simons-Morton, Parcel, & Bunker, 1988). Environmental agents often are not responsible for the original environmental condition, but can create change. For example, legislators or city counsel representatives may not be responsible for violence that occurs in unsafe streets or parks, but they might be in roles where they can change the environment of their cities. Therefore they are leverage points for citizen efforts to change the parks and streets, thereby reducing the probability of violent acts in these environments.

The next phase of the PRECEDE model is an analysis of the determinants of behavioral and environmental factors. Because the evidence for these "determinants" is usually associational rather than causal, these determinants are somewhat hypothetical. Health educators think in terms of what factors or variables are related to the behaviors and environment. Green and Kreuter (1999) describe factors affecting behavior as reinforcing, enabling, and predisposing. Predisposing factors "include a person or population's knowledge, attitudes, beliefs, values, and perceptions that facilitate or hinder motivation for change" (p. 40). Existing skills can, through the self-efficacy factor, predispose an individual to take action, but such skills are usually classified as an enabling factor. Enabling factors facilitate action by individuals or organizations. These factors often are conditions of the environment and may not appear in an analysis if the environmental factors have been thoroughly analyzed. Enabling factors are "those skills, resources, or barriers that can help or hinder the desired behavioral changes as well as environmental changes" (p. 40). Reinforcing factors are events that occur after a behavior that make the behavior more likely to reoccur. This category may include punishment, an event that occurs after an action that makes the reoccurence less probable.

Theory can be immensely helpful in exploring factors that are useful in explaining behavior and environment. For example, the concepts of reinforcement just described came originally from the learning theory of operant conditioning (Kazdin, 1989; Skinner, 1963) and then were further articulated in social cognitive theories (Bandura, 1986). Knowing the exact definitions of these constructs from theory is important in order to garner their full explanatory power. In Chapter 3 we explain in detail about the processes for applying theoretical thinking to determinants of behavior and environment as well as to other questions of intervention development.

In the discussion of needs assessment, the need for quantities of data—both qualitative and quantitative—is evident. Table 2.2 is intended to give some sense of what kind of information is needed and where these data may be found. However, we refer the reader to comprehensive sources on health data, such as the Behavioral Risk Factor Surveillance System (Centers for Disease Control and Prevention) or the National Health Interview Survey (National Center for Health Statistics).

Understanding Risk Models Versus Health-Promoting Models

So far the discussion of PRECEDE has been presented as a risk model—a model of health and quality-of-life problems and their antecedents. However, we have also used PRECEDE in our work to formulate disease management models that are couched in terms of health-promoting behavior and environment (Bartholomew et al., 1994; Bartholomew, Parcel, & Czyzewski, 1996; Bartholomew et al., 1989). In other words we analyzed what patients and families as well as their environments would have to "do" in order to manage disease and minimize the health and quality-of-life consequences of a chronic illness. In an example of asthma in children (Figure 2.5), the quality of life for children with asthma often includes considerations of ability to attend school regularly and to participate in physical activities. Health includes indicators of morbidity such as symptom days and medical care utilization (emergency room visits and hospitalizations). These indicators are quite different than those for acute stroke, where hospital services are seen as critical rather than as an indicator of excess symptoms and lack of control as they are in asthma.

To use PRECEDE for planning self-management programs such as asthma, we ask what at-risk or ill individuals could do to decrease their risk of the health and quality-of-life problems related to the illness. In the case of asthma, the child takes both relief and control medicines, avoids triggers, and maintains primary health care. Asthma has particularly compelling environmental components because elements of both the physical environment (indoor and outdoor allergens and irritants) and the health care environment (behavior of health care providers) affect the behavior required of patients and families and affect health directly (see Chapter 11).

Table 2.2
Sources of Data for Needs Assessment

	EXAMPLES OF INDICATORS	EXAMPLES OF QUALITATIVE DATA SOURCES	EXAMPLES OF QUANTITATIVE DATA SOURCES
Quality of life	Absenteeism, psychological adaptation and coping, income, housing, employment, crime, discrimination, alienation, cost	Ethnographic interviews and observation, focus groups, nominal group techniques, Freirian question posing, critical incident technique	Census data, agency studies, school records, data from other governmental units
Health	Morbidity, mortality, functional status, fertility, physiological risk factors, health care utilization	Ethnographic interviews and observation, focus groups, nominal group techniques, Freirian question posing, critical incident technique	Surveillance statistics from governmental health units (e.g., ministries, U.S. DHHS, CDC), surveys, medical records
Behavior and environment	Risk behaviors, adherence, self-management, coping, prevention, pollution, policy setting, provision of supplies and services	Ethnographic interviews and observation, focus groups, nominal group techniques, Freirian question posing, critical incident technique	Risk factor surveys (e.g., BRFSS), environmental measurement
Determinants	Behavioral capability, reinforcement, self-efficacy, outcome expectations, cues, barriers, awareness, incentives, availability	Ethnographic interviews and observation, focus groups, nominal group techniques, Freirian question posing, critical incident technique	Surveys

Note. BRFSS = Behavioral Risk Factor Surveillance System

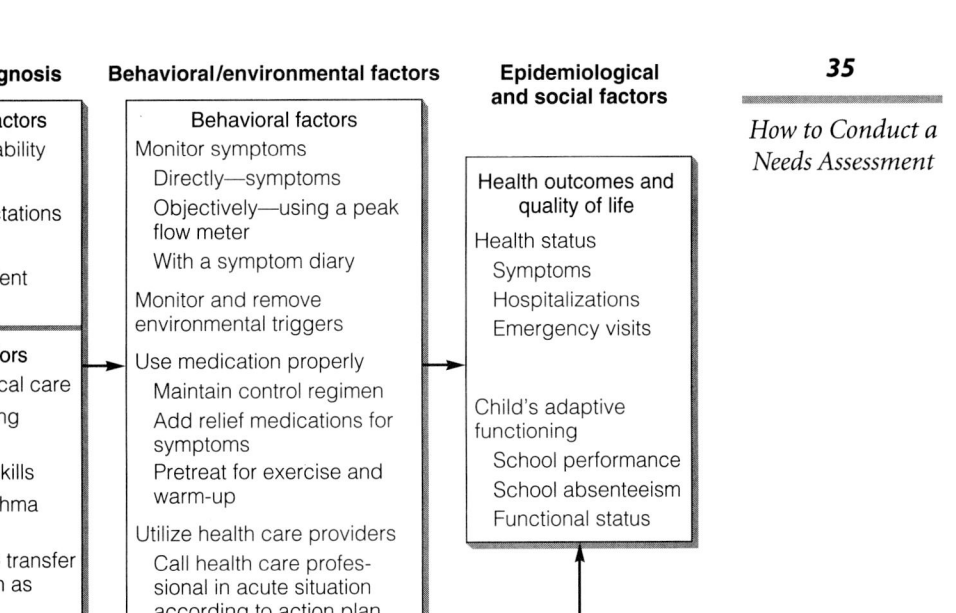

FIGURE 2.5 Asthma Management PRECEDE

Any problem can be analyzed in this positive direction, but for most issues of health risk, we suggest understanding the risk model first and then making the transition to a health promotion model. Much can be learned from fully understanding a causal model of a health problem before translating the problem behavior and environment (and their determinants) into health-promoting factors. In cardiovascular disease, for example, one of the risk factors is sedentary lifestyle and one health-promoting behavior is to increase exercise. Of course, the determinants of increasing exercise are different from the determinants of sedentary lifestyle, and understanding the determinants of sedentary lifestyle will help us understand some of the barriers to exercise. This analysis might not occur if we began directly by looking only at the health-promoting behavior. This process of translating the negative behavior and environment into positive must be completed as we enter Intervention Mapping.

Deciding Where to Begin the Epidemiological Assessment

A major consideration in completing the PRECEDE model—the problem-focused part of the assessment—is at what level to begin. With the quality of life in the community? With health problems or risks? With behavioral or environmental risks? Because so many agencies that employ health educators are funded, at least in part, with categorical funds designated for one disease or risk (e.g., cardiovascular disease, lung disease), health educators often are directed to look at needs and problems in terms of whatever is the focus of the funding or of the employer. The health educator who works for a cancer agency looks at cancer. The health educator who works for an AIDS agency looks at HIV. These are health problems, and the health educators have entered the assessment model at the level of health. Perhaps, though, the health educator works for a substance abuse agency; then the needs assessment would begin at the behavior of substance abuse. The health educator has entered the model at behavior.

It can be confusing to think that planners must begin the PRECEDE model with a quality-of-life diagnosis, as if it were always possible to begin in a community and determine the most salient quality-of-life issues for that community and work back to health, further back to behavioral and environmental causes, and even further back to the determinants of that behavior or those environmental conditions. Some planners will be entering the needs assessment with wide parameters for the issues they are empowered to work on, even as wide as license to work with the community as a whole to designate needs and choose issues. These planners will begin by assessing quality-of-life indicators. Many other planners will have an assigned task that is related to a specific health problem, health risk behavior, or environmental problem. No matter where a health educator begins the needs assessment, he or she will need to cover all the phases of the model, including the relation of health to quality of life. The emphasis on covering all levels of the model regardless of where health educators begin is based on the assumption that health and behavior are instrumental values, that is, that they are valuable because of their relation to other values. Health is related to quality of life; behavior is related to health.

BEGINNING WITH QUALITY OF LIFE   Some planners conduct a broad assessment of a community beginning with quality of life and moving through health, behavior, environment, and determinants (Figure 2.6). The study would include

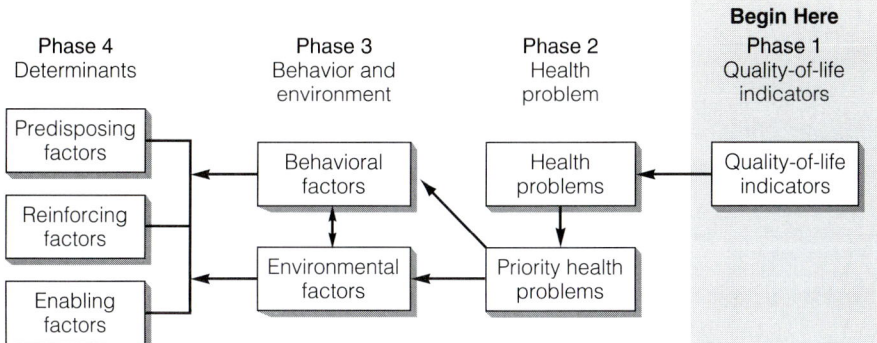

Note. The arrows in this model are the direction of the analysis, *not* the direction of the implied causation.

FIGURE 2.6 Entering the Model with Quality of Life

not only community problems but also resources in the community. Once quality-of-life issues are described for a community, health educators move to health and describe health problems related to the quality-of-life issues they have documented. Because they will have uncovered a wide range of quality-of-life issues, they then will have a long list of health problems that they need to prioritize. Once they choose the health problem or problems that will be the focus of their work, they can move to the right in the model and analyze quality-of-life factors that are specifically tied to the health problem or problems that are priorities. Then they can move to the left and analyze behavior, environment, and determinants that are all related to the same health problem.

For example, a health educator is working with a group of homeless youth, street teens. She conducts a survey with youth who congregate at certain hangouts in a neighborhood of about ten square blocks in a large inner city. The health educator conducts individual interviews and observations, and she relies on agency, city, and state data for her quantitative data set. She finds that the quality-of-life issues for these youth include lack of family and other social support, alienation, lack of role models and life goals, fear of HIV/AIDS, depression and hopelessness, fear of violence and aggression, and victimization. In terms of health, they have a high prevalence of unwanted pregnancy, STDs, and HIV. She also finds drug addiction, malnutrition, and disordered sleep. Based on the prevalence estimates in the literature and the priorities of the youth, she narrows the health problem that she will work on to violence and victimization. Then she works backward through quality of life, this time as it relates only to violence, and forward to behavior and determinants, again as they predict violent acts and the probability of becoming a victim.

BEGINNING WITH A HEALTH PROBLEM If health educators begin with a specific health problem, they then move to the right in the needs assessment to

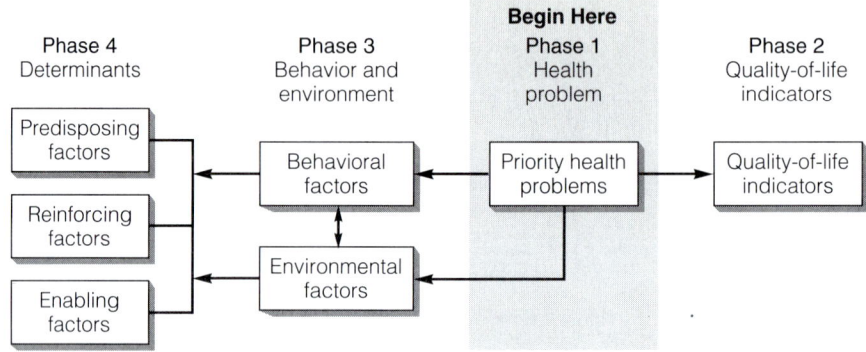

Note. The arrows in this model are the direction of the analysis, *not* the direction of the implied causation.

FIGURE 2.7 Entering the Model with the Health Problem

include an analysis of the impact of the health problem on the quality of life in the at-risk population before moving on to study the behavioral, environmental, and determinant factors that contribute to the health problem (Figure 2.7). The health educator from our previous example is working with the same population. This time, however, she is working for an AIDS agency. Her supervisor convenes a meeting during the first week to clarify her job description. The supervisor says not only that the health educator should work on HIV prevention among homeless youth, but that she should focus on the risk factor of multiple sexual partners. As the health educator begins her needs assessment she is confused; she thinks that the HIV prevention focus suggests that she is beginning on the health level, but she heard from her supervisor a mandated emphasis on a certain risk behavior, sexual intercourse with multiple partners. She wonders if she is beginning with behavior. After thinking for a while, she enters the model with data on the health problem. She reasons that if she starts with health, then she frees herself to consider risk factors other than multiple sexual partners.

The health educator begins her assessment with HIV transmission and AIDS in the population of youth between the ages of 11 and 21 years who are living on inner-city streets. She uses data from the CDC to find the U.S. prevalence rates of HIV in this age group. She then looks at local figures for HIV incidence and prevalence obtained from the city health department and at figures from other cities with comparable groups of street youth. Once she has a picture of HIV transmission as a problem in this group, she works forward to the implications of HIV for quality of life and backward to behavior, environment, and determinants. When she analyzes behavior, she finds that multiple sexual partners is one factor, but more important factors are condom use and needle sharing. When the health educator reports her needs assessment data to her supervisor, she is able to present all the risk behaviors and gain support to work on them. She is not limited by her supervisor's original bias.

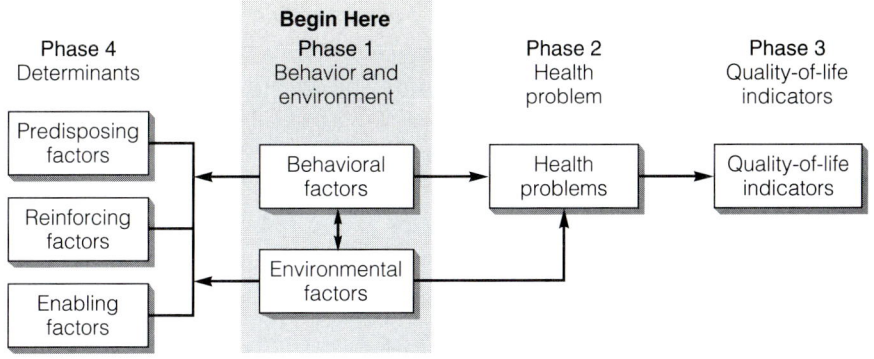

Note. The arrows in this model are the direction of the analysis, *not* the direction of the implied causation.

FIGURE 2.8 Entering the Model with Behavior and the Environment

BEGINNING WITH A BEHAVIOR OR AN ENVIRONMENTAL CONDITION In this option, health educators begin with specific behavioral risk factors, such as unsafe sexual behavior, or an environmental condition, such as polluted drinking water, and move to the right in the model to include the impact of these factors on health and quality-of-life indicators for the population (Figure 2.8). Then health educators will look at determinants of the risk behavior or environmental condition. In our example of the person working with the street youth, where might she begin the needs assessment if she were working for an agency concerned with the risky behaviors of early sexual intercourse, intercourse with multiple partners, and intercourse without the protection of a condom? The educator would probably go to the literature to establish estimates of these behaviors in similar populations. She might also use survey techniques to establish estimates of these behaviors in her population and qualitative methods such as ethnographic interviews and focus groups to understand the context and meaning of the behaviors to the youth. She then would move to establishing the relation of these behaviors to health problems and quality of life and, finally, to determinants of the behaviors.

HOW TO WRITE PROGRAM GOALS AND OBJECTIVES

The last task in performing a needs assessment is to write program goals and objectives. Statements of objectives based on the needs and capacity assessments can be important planning tools, and writing clear and measurable ones can be a very useful skill. Green and Kreuter (1991) state that "objectives are crucial: they form a fulcrum, converting diagnostic data into program direction" (p. 118). We approach this topic with a caveat: The alternative title for this section is "If it walks like a duck and quacks like a duck, it probably is a duck, but it might be called a goose." Both in funding agency requests for proposals and in the literature, references to the terms *goals, objectives,* and *program aims* do not share common definitions. The words have different meanings to different users. Therefore we have carefully defined several types of goals and objectives to use in Intervention Mapping. They work for this purpose and may be generalizable to other planning. However, we strongly advise the reader always to find out what others mean when they use the terms and to respond with objectives as required by the requester—especially when the "other" is an employer, a funding agency, or a reviewer. The important issue is not what these planning tools are called but what information they contain.

For use in the Intervention Mapping framework, we define program goals as general or broad statements of the desire to reduce the gap between the current status and the optimal status of a situation, whereas an objective is stated in terms that are operationally defined, in other words, that can be measured (Rossi, Freeman, & Lipsey, 1999, p.121). Program objectives are quantified statements from different levels of the needs assessment (i.e., quality of life, community capacity, health, behavior, or environment). In Chapter 5 we present performance objectives for intervention groups including members of the at-risk population and individuals in the environment. We also present proximal program objectives (statements of learning and change objectives) that concern both determinants and performance objectives. In Chapter 8 we deal again with performance objectives, this time for program adopters and implementers.

Health and Quality-of-Life Objectives

Health and quality-of-life objectives may be thought of as the desired outcomes from a program. Health objectives are stated as indicators of health status, such as morbidity, mortality, incidence, prevalence, disability, and physiological risk factors (Green & Kreuter, 1999). An objective includes a statement (with a strong verb) of what will change in a specified population, by how much, and by what period of time. The amount of expected change and the time frame must be empirically justifiable. For example, the health educator working with street youth established objectives related to the incidence of HIV infection in her population. She set an objective of a 10% decrease in the incident rate of these infections in the first two years of the program based on other intensive work with this population reported in the literature. She stated her health objective as follows: The program will reduce the incidence rate of HIV infection 10% in the population during the first two years of the program. Some programs also seek to improve quality of life, and Green and Kreuter list many examples of quality-of-life indicators, including employment, crowding, absenteeism, achievement, alienation, discrimination, happiness, and self-esteem. Some of these factors are defined at the societal level and may change only over long periods of time, whereas others are more individual and can be measured in the time periods more typical for program evaluation. Another point about indicators of quality of life is that they often are constructs that require operational definition and sometimes psychological or sociological measurement instruments. For example: What is happiness? How does one define and measure it? What is crowding? How does one define and measure it?

Behavioral and Environmental Objectives

Behavioral and environmental program objectives address the changes that need to be made in behaviors or environment in order to effect the health and quality-of-life objectives. As a matter of fact, sometimes because of time required for change to occur, this level of objective is written as the main outcome instead of health or quality-of-life objectives (see Chapter 9). This only can be done, however, when there is an empirically documented link between the behavior or environment and the health outcome. For example, someone working in tobacco control among youth might have objectives regarding smoking rates and access to tobacco that can be measured in the short run rather than health objectives regarding incidence of cardiovascular disease and cancer that could only be observed after many years. This level of program objective also is stated as what must change, how much, and by when. The program objectives for the street youth included reduction of the rate of unprotected sexual intercourse by 45% in the first year of the program.

SUMMARY

The crucial components of a community assessment are the epidemiology of needs and an inventory of the capacities of the community. Both assessments should include qualitative evidence as well as quantitative data that allow the health educator to get an idea of the magnitude of both the problems and their causes. Of course, all community assessment depends on the definition of the community and potential intervention groups.

Knowing where to begin in an assessment is also important because health educators are sometimes given assignments that could lead to incorrect assumptions. Being clear about where to begin and then completing all parts of the PRECEDE model will allow the planner to correct assignments when they are wrong, expand horizons when they are too narrow, and narrow tasks when they are too wide.

> *Tasks in Performing a Needs Assessment:*
> - Describe a tentative intervention population
> - Put together a planning group with broad participation
> - Use both qualitative and quantitative data
> - Survey the community for resources and capacities
> - Conduct an epidemiological assessment. Be clear about where the PRECEDE model is being entered
> - Write program goals and objectives

REFERENCES

Alberts, M. J., Bertels, C., & Dawson, D. V. (1990). An analysis of time of presentation after stroke. *Journal of the American Medical Association, 263*(1), 65–68.

Bakeman, R., McCray, E., Lumb, J. R., Jackson, R. E., & Whitley, P. N. (1987). The incidence of AIDS among blacks and Hispanics. *Journal of the National Medical Association, 79*(9), 921–928.

Bandura, A. (1986). *Social foundations of thought and action: A social cognitive theory.* Englewood Cliffs, NJ: Prentice Hall.

Bartholomew, L. K., Czyzewski, D. I., Parcel, G. S., Swank, P. R., Sockrider, M. M., Mariotto, M., Schidlow, V., Fink, R., & Seilheimer, D. K. (1997). Self-management of cystic fibrosis: Short-term outcomes of the Cystic Fibrosis Family Education Program. *Health Education and Behavior, 24*(5), 652–666.

Bartholomew, L. K., Czyzewski, D. I., Swank, P., McCormick, L., & Parcel, G. S. (2000). Maximizing the impact of the Cystic Fibrosis Family Education Program: Factors related to program diffusion. *Family and Community Health, 22*(4), 1–22.

Bartholomew, L. K., Koenning, G., Dahlquist, L., & Barron, K. (1994). An educational needs assessment of children with juvenile rheumatoid arthritis. *Arthritis Care and Research, 7*(3), 136–143.

Bartholomew, L. K., Parcel, G. S., & Czyzewski, D. I. (1997). Planning health education programs for self-management of pediatric chronic disease and disability. In H. M. Wallace, R. Biehl, J. MacQueen, & J. Blackman (Eds.), *Mosby's resource guide to children with disabilities and chronic illness: A comprehensive community and clinical approach.* St. Louis: Mosby–Year Book.

Bartholomew, L. K., Seilheimer, D. K., Parcel, G. S., Spinelli, S. H., & Pumariega, A. J. (1989). Planning patient education for cystic fibrosis: Application of a diagnostic framework. *Patient Education and Counseling, 13*(1), 57–68.

Bartholomew, L. K., Sockrider, M. M., Seilheimer, D. K., Czyzewski, D. I., Parcel, G. S., & Spinelli, S. H. (1993). Performance objectives for the self-management of cystic fibrosis. *Patient Education and Counseling, 22*(1), 15–25.

Basch, C. E. (1987). Focus group interview: An underutilized research technique for improving theory and practice in health education. *Health Education Quarterly, 14*(4), 411–448.

Bauman, L. J., & Adair, E. G. (1992). The use of ethnographic interviewing to inform questionnaire construction. *Health Education Quarterly, 19*(1), 9–23.

Berg, B. L. (1989). *Qualitative research methods for the social sciences.* Boston: Allyn & Bacon.

Bradford, L. P. (1976). *Making meetings work: A guide for leaders and group members.* San Diego, CA: University Associates.

Braithwaite, R. L., Bianchi, C., & Taylor, S. E. (1994). Ethnographic approach to community organization and health. *Health Education Quarterly, 21*(3), 407–417.

Bratina, P., Greenberg, L., Pasteur, W., & Grotta, J. (1994). Current emergency department management of stroke in Houston, Texas. *Stroke, 26*(3), 409–414.

Centers for Disease Control and Prevention. (1999). *HIV/AIDS Surveillance Report, 11*(1), 1–24.

Centers for Disease Control and Prevention and Agency for Toxic Substances and Disease Registry, Committee on Community Engagement. (1997). *Principles of community engagement.* Atlanta, GA: Public Health Practice Program Office. Available: http://www.cdc.gov/phppo/pce/index.htm

References

Cook, T. D., & Campbell, D. T. (1979). *Design and analysis issues for field settings.* Boston: Houghton Mifflin.

Cottrell, L. (1977). The competent community. In R. Warren (Ed.), *New perspectives on the American community: A book of readings* (3rd ed.). Chicago: Rand McNally College Publications.

Daniels, W. R. (1986). *Group power I: A manager's guide to using task-force meetings.* Erlanger, KY: Pfeiffer.

Delbecq, A., Van de Ven, A. H., & Gustafson, D. H. (1975). *Group techniques for program planning: A guide to nominal and delphi processes.* Glenview, IL: Scott, Foresman.

Desvousges, W. H., & Frey, J. H. (1989). Integrating focus groups and surveys: Examples from environmental risk studies. *Journal of Official Statistics, 5,* 349–363.

De Vries, H., Weijts, W., Dijkstra, M., & Kok, G. (1992). The utilization of qualitative and quantitative data for health education program planning, implementation, and evaluation: A spiral approach. *Health Education Quarterly, 19*(1), 101–115.

Ehrhardt, A. A., Yingling, S., Zawadzki, R., & Martinez-Ramirez, M. (1992). Prevention of heterosexual transmission of HIV: Barriers for women. *Journal of Psychology and Human Sexuality, 5*(1–2), 37–67.

Eng, E., & Parker, E. (1994). Measuring community competence in the Mississippi Delta: The interface between program evaluation and empowerment. *Health Education Quarterly, 21*(2), 199–220.

Eng, E., & Young, R. (1992). Lay health advisors as community change agents. *Family and Community Health, 15*(1), 24–40.

Fawcett, S. B. (1991). Some values guiding community research and action. *Journal of Applied Behavior Analysis, 24*(4), 621–636.

Feldmann, E., Gordon, N., Brooks, J. M., Brass, L. M., Fayad, P. B., Sawaya, K., Nazareno, F., & Levine, S. R. (1993). Factors associated with early presentation of acute stroke. *Stroke, 24*(12), 1805–1810.

Fellin, P. (1995). Understanding American communities. In E. J. Rothman, J. Erlich, & J. Tropman (Eds.), *Strategies of community intervention* (5th ed.). Itasca, IL: Peacock.

Fisher, E. B., Jr., Auslander, W., Sussman, L., Owens, N., & Jackson-Thompson, J. (1992). Community organization and health promotion in minority neighborhoods. *Ethnicity and Disease, 2*(3), 252–272.

Fisher, E. B., Jr., Sussman, L. K., Arfken, C., Harrison, D., Munro, J., Sykes, R. K., Sylvia, S., & Strunk, R. C. (1994). Targeting high risk groups: Neighborhood organization for pediatric asthma management in the Neighborhood Asthma Coalition. *Chest, 106*(4 Suppl.), 248s–259s.

Freire, P. (1973). *Education for critical consciousness.* New York: Seabury Press.

Gilmore, G. D., Campbell, M. D., & Becker, B. L. (1989). *Needs assessment strategies for health education and health promotion.* Madison, WI: Brown and Benchmark.

Glasgow, R. E., Vogt, T. M., & Boles, S. M. (1999). Evaluating the public health impact of health promotion interventions: The RE-AIM Framework. *American Journal of Public Health, 89*(9), 1322–1327.

Goeppinger, J., & Baglioni, A. J. (1985). Community competence: A positive approach to needs assessment. *American Journal of Community Psychology, 13*(5), 507–523.

Goodman, R. M., Speers, M. A., McLeroy, K., Fawcett, S., Kegler, M., Parker, E., Smith, S., & Sterling, T. (1998). Identifying and defining the dimensions of community capacity to provide a basis for measurement. *Health Education and Behavior, 25*(3), 258–278.

Goodman, R. M., & Steckler, A. (1989). A model for the institutionalization of health promotion programs. *Family and Community Health, 11*(4), 63–78.

Goodman, R. M., Steckler, A., Hoover, S., & Schwartz, R. (1993). A critique of contemporary community health promotion approaches: Maine—A multiple case study. *American Journal of Health Promotion, 7*(3), 208–220.

Green, L. W. (1986). Theory of participation: A qualitative analysis of its expression in national and international health policies. In W. B. Ward (Ed.), *Advances in health education and promotion* (Vol. 1, Pt. A, pp. 211–236). Greenwich, CT: JAI Press.

Green, L. W., Glanz, K., Hochbaum, G. M., Kok, G., Kreuter, M. W., Lewis, F. M., Lorig, K., Morisky, D., Rimer, B. K., & Rosenstock, I. M. (1994). Can we build on, or must we replace, the theories and models in health education? *Health Education Research: Theory and Practice, 9*(3), 397–404.

Green, L. W., & Kreuter, M. W. (1991). *Health promotion planning: An educational and environmental approach* (2nd ed.). Mountain View, CA: Mayfield.

Green, L. W., & Kreuter, M. W. (1999). *Health promotion planning: An educational and ecological approach* (3rd ed.). Mountain View, CA: Mayfield.

Green, L. W., & Lewis, F. M. (1986). *Measurement and evaluation in health education and health promotion.* Palo Alto, CA: Mayfield.

Hancock, T., & Duhl, L. (1986). *Healthy cities: Promoting health in the urban context.* Copenhagen, Denmark: WHO Europe.

Hancock, T., & Minkler, M. (1997). Community health assessment or healthy community assessment: Whose community? Whose health? Whose assessment? In M. Minkler (Ed.), *Community organizing and community building for health* (pp. 139–156). New Brunswick, NJ: Rutgers University Press.

Hugentobler, M. K., Israel, B. A., & Schurman, S. J. (1992). An action research approach to workplace health: Integrating methods. *Health Education Quarterly, 19*(1), 55–76.

Iscoe, I. (1974). Community psychology and the competent community. *American Psychologist, 29*(8), 607–613.

Kazdin, A. E. (1989). *Behavior modification in applied settings* (4th ed.). Pacific Grove, CA: Brooks/Cole.

Kretzmann, J. P., & McKnight, J. L. (1993). *Building communities from the inside out: A path toward finding and mobilizing a community's assets.* Chicago, IL: ACTA Publications.

Kreuger, R. A. (1988). *Focus groups: A practical guide for applied research.* Newbury Park, CA: Sage.

Kreuter, M. W., Lezin, N. A., Kreuter, M. W., & Green, L. W. (1997). *Community health promotion ideas that work: A field-book for practitioners.* Sudbury, MA: Jones and Bartlett.

McLeroy, K. (1996). *Community capacity: What is it? How do we measure it? What is the role of the Prevention Centers and CDC?* Paper presented at the Sixth Annual Prevention Centers Conference, Centers for Disease Control and Prevention, National Center for Chronic Disease Prevention and Health Promotion, Atlanta, GA.

McNabb, W. L., Wilson-Pessano, S. R., & Jacobs, A. M. (1986). Critical self-management competencies for children with asthma. *Journal of Pediatric Psychology, 11*(1), 103–117.

Miles, M. B., & Huberman, A. M. (1994). *Qualitative data analysis: An expanded source book* (2nd ed.) Thousand Oaks, CA: Sage.

Minkler, M., & Wallerstein, N. (1997). Improving health through community organization and community building: A health education perspective. In M. Minkler (Ed.), *Community organizing and community building for health* (pp. 30–52). New Brunswick, NJ: Rutgers University Press.

Morgan, D. L. (1988). *Focus groups as qualitative research.* Newbury Park, CA: Sage.

National Institute of Neurological Disorders and Stroke. (1997). *Proceedings of a national symposium of rapid identification and treatment of acute stroke, December 12–13, 1996* (NIH Pub. No. 97-4239). Bethesda, MD: Author.

O'Brien, K. (1993). Using focus groups to develop health surveys: An example from research on social relationships and AIDS-preventive behavior. *Health Education Quarterly, 20*(3), 361–372.

Orlandi, M. A. (1986). The diffusion and adoption of worksite health promotion innovations: An analysis of barriers. *Preventive Medicine, 15*(5), 522–536.

Orlandi, M. A. (1987). Promoting health and preventing disease in health care settings: An analysis of barriers. *Preventive Medicine, 16*(1), 119–130.

Orlandi, M. A., Landers, C., Weston, R., & Haley, N. (1990). Diffusion of health promotion innovations. In K. Glanz, F. M. Lewis, & B. K. Rimer (Eds.), *Health behavior and health education: Theory, research, and practice* (pp. 288–313). San Francisco: Jossey-Bass.

Ovrebo, B., Ryan, M., Jackson, K., & Hutchinson, K. (1994). The Homeless Prenatal Program: A model for empowering homeless pregnant women. *Health Education Quarterly, 21*(2), 187–198.

Patton, M. Q. (1990). *Qualitative evaluation and research methods* (2nd ed.). Beverly Hills, CA: Sage.

Putnam, R. D. (1993). The prosperous community: Social capital and public life. *American Prospect, 143,* 35–42.

Richard, L., Potvin, L., Kishchuk, N., Prlic, H., & Green, L. W. (1996). Assessment of the integration of the ecological approach in health promotion programs. *American Journal of Health Promotion, 10*(4), 318–328.

Rossi, P. H., Freeman, H. E., & Lipsey, M. W. (1999). *Evaluation: A systematic approach* (6th ed.). Newbury Park, CA: Sage.

Rudd, R. E., & Comings, J. P. (1994). Learner developed materials: An empowering product. *Health Education Quarterly, 21*(3), 313–327.

Saint-Germain, M. A., Bassford, T. L., & Montano, G. (1993). Surveys and focus groups in health research with older Hispanic women. *Qualitative Health Research, 3*(3), 341–367.

Simons-Morton, B. G., Greene, W. H., & Gottlieb, N. H. (1995). *Introduction to health education and health promotion* (2nd ed.). Prospect Heights, IL: Waveland Press.

Simons-Morton, D. G., Simons-Morton, B. G., Parcel, G. S., & Bunker, J. F. (1988). Influencing personal and environmental conditions for community health: A multilevel intervention model. *Family and Community Health, 11*(2), 25–35.

Skinner, B. F. (1963). Operant behavior. *American Psychologist, 18,* 503–515.

Soriano, F. I. (1995). *Conducting needs assessments: A multidisciplinary approach.* Thousand Oaks, CA: Sage.

Steckler, A., McLeroy, K. R., Goodman, R. M., Bird, S. T., & McCormick, L. (1992). Toward integrating qualitative and quantitative methods: An introduction. *Health Education Quarterly, 19*(1), 1–8.

Strauss, A. L. (1988). *Qualitative analysis for social scientists.* Cambridge, UK: Cambridge University Press.

Toseland, R. W., & Rivas, R. F. (1984). *An introduction to group work practice.* New York: Macmillan.

Wang, C., & Burris, M. A. (1994). Empowerment through photo novella: Portraits of participation. *Health Education Quarterly, 21*(2), 171–186.

Wingood, G. M., Hunter-Gamble, D., & DiClemente, R. J. (1993). A pilot study of sexual communication and negotiation among young African American women: Implications for HIV prevention. *Journal of Black Psychology, 19*(2), 190–203.

Witkin, B. R., & Altschuld, J. W. (1995). *Planning and conducting needs assessments: A practical guide.* Thousand Oaks, CA: Sage.

Wolcott, H. F. (1994). *Transforming qualitative data: Description, analysis, and interpretation.* Thousand Oaks, CA: Sage.

World Health Organization. (1978). *Primary health care: Report of the International Conference on Primary Health Care, Alma-Ata, USSR, September 6–12, 1978* (Health for All Series No. 1). Geneva, Switzerland: Author.

CHAPTER 3

Core Processes: Evidence, Theory, and New Research

READER OBJECTIVES

- Pose planning problems as questions that facilitate finding answers from theory, the existing literature, and new research
- Brainstorm answers to planning questions
- Use the issue, construct, and general theories approaches to accessing theory and empirical evidence to answer the questions and generate potential solutions to health education problems
- Critically reflect on information from the literature

Health educators deal with problems of defining behavior, finding determinants of behavior, differentiating the intended recipients, selecting methods, creating strategies, and developing implementation plans. They answer these questions with the wealth of information available in the existing empirical and theoretical literature related to health and health behavior and with new research. In this chapter we focus on finding and using appropriate theories in the planning of health education programs. Though the review of existing literature and collection of new data have been described extensively elsewhere, we also touch briefly on both, because all three processes are interdependent. We encourage the reader to consult other sources for guidance on literature synthesis and on qualitative and quantitative research and evaluation (Cooper & Hedges, 1994; De Vries, Weijts, Dijkstra, & Kok, 1992; Green & Lewis, 1986; Greenbaum, 1988; Huberman & Miles, 1994; Krueger, 1988; Lorig & Holman, 1993; Merriam, 1988; Morgan, 1988; Mullen & Ramirez, 1987; Patton, 1990; Rossi, Freeman, & Lipsey, 1999; Stake, 1995; Windsor, Baranowski, Clark, & Cutter, 1994; Yin, 1994).

The health educator from Chapter 1 knows that as the violence prevention planning group moves toward intervention development it will need effective processes for defining problems. Group members must ask questions about what causes violence, using an ecological perspective that includes environmental, social, and psychological determinants. They must ask questions about who is at risk for perpetrating violence and about who is likely to be a victim. They must formulate ideas of how to intervene with the determinants of violence in their community.

They know that a simple answer that suggests the need to intervene on a single behavioral or environmental risk factor (e.g., more parental supervision) probably would be inadequate. They also wonder if theory might help them understand determinants, and they think about planning new research. The health educator knows that once the planning group understands determinants of the behavior and environmental conditions and decides on program objectives, it must ask equally important questions about effective intervention methods. The group members who searched the literature in the needs assessment uncovered some articles that used theory, but they were left with more questions than answers. They wonder whether theory or new research would be useful, but they don't know which theory or theories to explore. The way they structure the questions related to these issues and the processes they use to formulate the answers will underlie the success of their program-planning efforts.

PERSPECTIVES

Theory: Problem Focus Versus Theory Generation

A behavioral or social scientist who wants to find a solution to a problem has a different task than one who wants to test a theory in practice. More forcefully stated: A scientist testing a theory in practice will contribute to theory development but should not assume to contribute directly to practical problem solving. Problem-driven applied behavioral or social science uses problem definition, application of theory and empirical evidence, and new research to solve a problem. It often uses a multiple theory approach, that is, applying many theories to solve one problem. In this approach, the main focus is on problem solving, and the criteria for success are formulated in terms of the problem rather than the theory. Resulting contributions to theory development are probably useful, but remain peripheral to the problem-solving process. In Intervention Mapping we are always working from a problem-driven perspective. Choices have to be made in the process of developing an intervention, and theories are one tool to enable us to make better choices.

All Theories Are Right

In a problem-driven context, then, all theories are "right," within the parameters that the theory describes, and the challenge is to find the best theory or combina-

> When the mayor's planning group met to discuss the causes of violence and to decide how to intervene in their community, one member wanted to focus on the impact on children of violence in the media (Centerwall, 1993; Eron, Huesman, Lefkowitz, & Walder, 1996). The group discussed the importance of this idea and the social cognitive theory construct of modeling as it helps explain the effects of media violence, but they did not stop their discussion of determinants of violence with this one construct or theory.
>
> The group did not find in their literature search a unified theoretical model describing the relationship between the risk factors for perpetrating violence or describing the determinants of those factors in children and adolescents (American Psychological Association Commission on Youth Violence, 1993). However, they did come up with mounds of theoretical and empirical evidence that helps explain or describe the causes of violence. They wanted to understand what all the information meant and to try to develop a comprehensive perspective on the predictors of violence. They analyzed many possible determinants of aggressive behavior in children and adolescents and sorted them into personal, behavioral, and social-environmental factors (Perry & Jessor, 1985).
>
> Some of the theory-related personal factors were beliefs that support aggression and aggressive attributional bias (Dodge & Coie, 1987; Slaby & Guerra, 1988). Theory-related behavioral risk factors discussed were inadequate problem-solving skills and watching media with violent role models (Centerwall, 1993; Eron et al., 1996; Slaby & Guerra). Social-environmental factors related to theories of parenting included coercive family interactions, hostile or rejecting parenting, inconsistency, permissiveness, disintegrated family unit, and little parental monitoring (Patterson, 1986; Patterson & Stouthamer-Loeber, 1984; Perry, Perry, & Boldizar, 1990; Yoshikawa, 1994).
>
> Because the focus in this chapter is on theory, we are interested in the group's list of theoretical concepts. However, it should be noted that the group's understanding of violence included other determinants that were not clearly related to theory, for example, the effects of brain injury, lead exposure, low academic achievement, poverty, easy access to weapons, family violence, and parental criminality (Baker, O'Neill, Ginsburg, & Li, 1992; Farrington, 1995; Loeber & Dishion, 1983; Loeber, Stouthamer-Loeber, Nan Kammen, & Farrington, 1991; Needleman, Reiss, Tobin, Biesecker, & Greenhouse, 1996; Webster, Wilson, Duggan, & Pakula, 1992; Yoshikawa).

tion of theoretical constructs to understand or solve the problem at hand. A limited focus on one or only a few theories may lead to an inadequate solution of a practical problem, or worse, to conclusions that are counterproductive.

With the beginnings of a comprehensive picture of what causes violence in youth, the planning group in our example could begin to figure out important and changeable determinants and proceed with planning an intervention. They have quite a bit more work to do, and we would have suggested undertaking the work via a slightly different approach, as we describe in the remainder of this chapter. However, the example serves to show how different this problem-focused approach is from the approach they would have taken had they been theory-centered—applying one set of theoretical constructs to violence and measuring predictive validity, for example—or had they failed to search for causation of violence and launched directly into an intervention, as often seems to happen in the field.

CORE PROCESSES FOR INTERVENTION MAPPING

Sometimes the processes involved in understanding a problem or answering a question with empirical data and theory are complex and time consuming. Many health educators do not persevere through the difficulties. Consequently understanding often is incomplete or inadequate, and intervention is faulty. Therefore we provide considerable detail about how to undertake these core processes (Figure 3.1).

Posing Questions

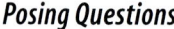

The first task for the core processes is to pose a question. The best way to clarify the problem is to go to the literature to find what others know about the problem (which is what the mayor's planning group did in our violence prevention example). This basic tool of going to the literature will remain a first step through all the stages of bringing theory and research to bear on a problem. To facilitate the problem analysis, Veen (1985) and Kok (1991) suggest a number of questions to clarify the problem. Even though these questions overlap considerably, they provide good insight into all aspects of the problem. They include the following: What is the problem? Why is it a problem? To whom is it a problem? What are the aspects of the problem? What may be the causes of the problem? Is the problem likely to be resolved? Is it desirable to solve the problem? Careful consideration of multiple dimensions of the problem may prevent time spent on irrelevant problems or on problems that require approaches from other disciplines, such as economics, law, or engineering.

Although these questions are concerned with, among other things, explanations and solutions, they are not meant to offer adequate answers at this stage, but simply to clarify the problem. For example, if a solution to a problem appears to be quite obvious, it may give cause for an examination of why this solution has not been tried in the past. It is possible that the organization responsible for solving the problem was resistant to the most obvious solution. This resistance puts the problem in another light and calls for redefining the problem in terms of both questions about the causes of the problem and questions about proposed solutions.

A common mistake that health educators make in defining a problem is allowing the problem to be defined by another person or organization and accepting that definition just the way it has been presented. In 1980, one of us was involved in a campaign about road safety in a small Dutch town. The town

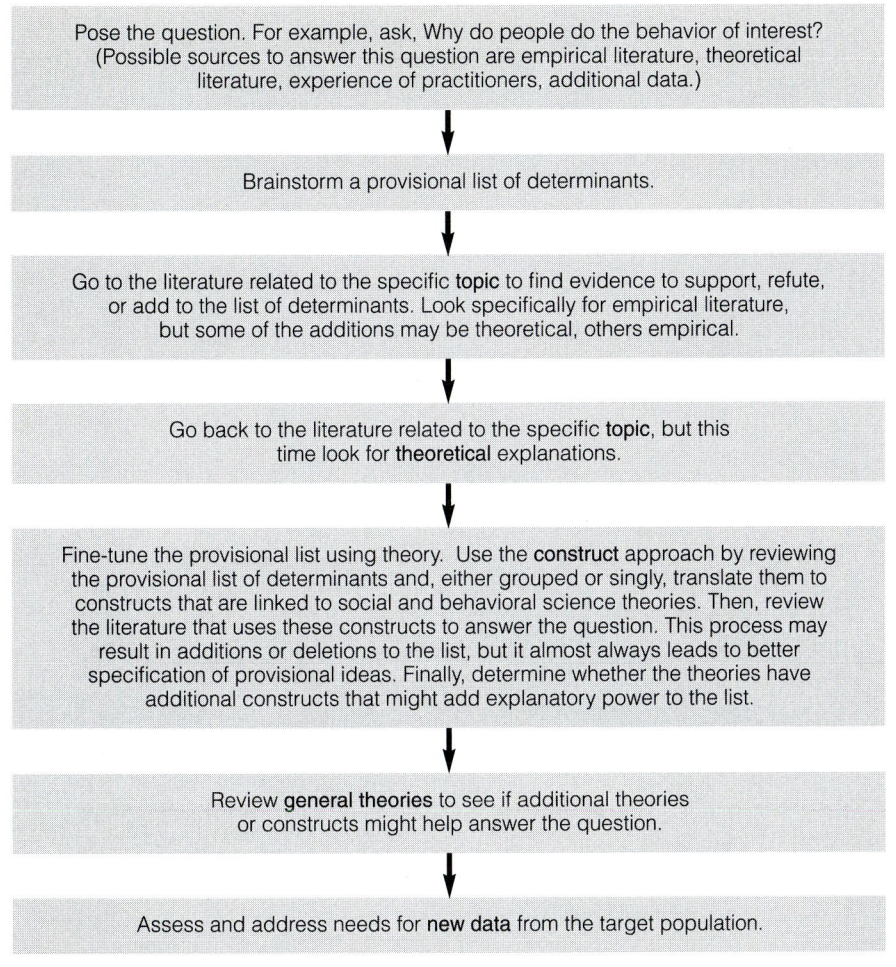

FIGURE 3.1 How to Use Theory, Literature, and New Data

undertook this campaign when it noticed that its rate of accidents at intersections was higher than in similar towns. The health educators working on the problem allowed it to remain defined in health terms—there is an excess of mortality and morbidity resulting from traffic accidents—and accepted the question as, What can be done regarding public education to solve the health problem? They began a local campaign about right-of-way rules. They failed, however, to ask additional questions about the accidents, specifically, questions about the environmental causes. In the middle of the education campaign, the health educators discovered that the majority of all right-of-way accidents happened at only one point: the exit of the parking lot near the supermarket. The problem could have been solved with an environmental intervention such as pruning the shrubs that obscured the view or introducing a traffic light at a single intersection. In this case, the planning group would have had to ask questions to determine the environmental cause of the problem and the agents who could effect these changes. A careful and thorough analysis of the given problem that began with more information about the problem (where, for whom, how much) and a definition of the problem in terms of causes (Why do drivers have accidents in this town?) might have saved wasted money and effort.

In Intervention Mapping, we first define the problem, then question the causes of the problem, and later examine methods and strategies used to influence the determinants of behavioral and environmental causes. It is important to state the problem as a question using *what, why,* or *how* and to state a new question or questions for each step of the program-planning process: health problems, behavior and environmental conditions, determinants, methods, strategies, adoption, and implementation.

For example, a work group in one of our health education methods classes began work on a project to promote adolescent condom use, and the first thing they did was to define the health problem as the increasing incidence of HIV, other STDs, and pregnancy in adolescents. They found that of the 441,528 reported AIDS cases in 1994, there were 1,965 cases among the 13 to 19 age group and 16,575 cases among the 20 to 24 age group (CDC, 1994). The incidence of AIDS in young adults indicated that adolescents had been infected with HIV. Other STDs were also a significant problem, as was adolescent pregnancy (Metzler, Noell, Biglan, Ary, & Smolkowski, 1994). The work group then asked, What is an important risk behavior for the transmission of HIV and STDs and for pregnancy among adolescents? The answer, failure to use condoms, is in interaction with other behaviors such as initiating sexual intercourse at an early age and having multiple sexual partners.

After defining the health problem and the behavioral risks, the group asked a question concerning determinants of the risk behavior of failing to use condoms. They posed a question to elicit the explanation (i.e., determinants): Why do adolescents fail to use condoms during sexual intercourse? As they worked through the processes for addressing questions about the causes of the problem, they began to formulate and address questions about potential solutions (i.e., methods and strategies): How can we ensure that adolescents use condoms? Over the course of Intervention Mapping, as the work group began to understand more about the problem (i.e., determinants), attention shifted to more specific questions about solutions (intervention methods and strategies for influencing determinants): What methods can be used to influence the determinants of condom use?

The questions may also be different for subgroups of the intervention population. For example, the work group might have found that some adolescents have higher rates of condom use than others do, or that some adolescents begin condom use at higher rates than others in response to behavior change interventions. The group also might have found that the age at first intercourse varies by ethnicity (Nodora, 1995). So, in regard to causes of the problem or determinants, the group asked, Why do some adolescents use condoms and others do not? and Why do some adolescents begin to use condoms as a result of health education interventions and others do not? Then the focus of the questions could shift to potential solutions or methods: How can we help specific subgroups of adolescents to use condoms?

Finally, the problem shifted to the implementation process. The problem was defined in this way: Some health professionals do not adopt programs to help adolescents begin condom use. The work group asked about determinants: What influences health professionals to adopt and implement programs that help adolescents learn to use condoms? Shifting to the intervention, the group asked: How can we motivate and train health professionals to implement programs that help adolescents use condoms? These questions are answerable with theory, empirical evidence from the literature, and new data from the at-risk population.

Brainstorming Provisional Answers

The second task for the core processes is to brainstorm a provisional list of answers. Before searching the literature for empirical evidence and theory, health educators should formulate possible explanations for a problem. Making a provisional list of answers to a question is a creative process that primarily involves free association (Veen, 1985). It is important to start with as many explanations as possible in response to a question. At the end, poor explanations are dropped, but it is definitely not good to get stuck on a single explanation too soon. In formulating these provisional explanations, health educators as applied behavioral scientists always use specific theoretical knowledge, whether consciously or not. It is unavoidable to do so in this stage, but the list should not be limited to either explicitly data- or theory-based items. The brainstorming should be as open as possible.

The group of students working on condom use generated the provisional list in Table 3.1. The work group brainstormed determinants based on what they knew from many sources about condom use. They stimulated creativity by taking the perspective of the sexually active adolescent and by narrowing the question to certain populations and situations. When they became stuck, they reversed perspectives and asked themselves the radical question, How can the problem be increased—how would we *reduce* the use of condoms? Reversing perspective helped them get in touch with the barriers to condom use.

At this stage of the brainstorming there is no reason to favor one explanation over another. However, in the subsequent steps, health educators should begin to take into account two criteria for good answers: an explanation should describe a process, and it should be plausible. A process explanation provides an answer to the question, Why? and provides insight into the variations among variables as well as between the variables and the problem, environment, or behavior. In this respect, a useful aid is to represent the explanation in a schematic model consisting of boxes with arrows between them (Earp & Ennett, 1991). A plausible explanation is one that can survive when it is depicted graphically and examined with common sense.

Table 3.1
Provisional List: Determinants of Lack of Condom Use Among Sexually Active Adolescents

ORIGINAL PROVISIONAL LIST	ADDITIONS FROM EMPIRICAL LITERATURE	ADDITIONS FROM THEORY
Personal determinants		
Lack of knowledge of HIV transmission	Alcohol and drug use	Intention to use condoms (theory of planned behavior)
Lack of knowledge of STDs	Girls' lack of anticipation of a sexual encounter	Subjective norms (perception of significant other and motivation to comply)
Perceived group norms		
Perceived benefits of condoms		Perceived barriers to condom use (health belief model)
Attitudes toward condom use		
Experience with condom use		Self-efficacy and skills for putting on condoms
Gender		
Salience—knowing someone with AIDS		Self-efficacy and skills regarding negotiation of condom use
Lack of confidence to use condoms		
External determinants		
Partner's insistence on not using condoms	Living in a poor neighborhood	
Mass media portrayal of sexual activity	Coercive relationship with parents	
Availability of condoms	Association with deviant peers	

The next steps are to reinforce provisional explanations with empirical evidence, theoretical foundations, and new research. This focused literature review will yield new explanations, cause deletion of some explanations from the provisional list, and raise new questions to be answered by means of additional research (Kok, Schaalma, De Vries, Parcel, & Paulussen, 1996).

Searching the Literature for Empirical Findings

The third task for the core processes is to search the literature for empirical evidence and evaluate the strength of the evidence. Once a question is posed and a provisional list of answers is generated, health educators should focus on the topic at hand and search the literature for empirical findings. The student group in our example looked for what others had found regarding condom use in adolescents. In this topical approach to the literature, broadening the topic to include related issues and different populations is important. Mindful of this, the group also looked for information on other risk-taking behaviors in adolescents (Bishop-Townsend, 1996; Donovan, Jessor, & Costa, 1991) and for other behaviors related to sexual activity, such as contraception use (Costa, Jessor, Fortenberry, & Donovan, 1996; Levinson, 1995). From the topical review, the provisional list of answers to the posed question is refined. From their search, the student work group added to Table 3.1 the relation of lack of condom use with other risky behaviors, such as alcohol and drug use, and the difficulty for young women in the United States of premeditating sexual intercourse, that is, of anticipating a sexual encounter.

Evaluating the Relevance and Strength of Evidence[1]

The approach to selecting the primary sources for a literature review that many planners learned is the equivalent of saying, "Look up everything you can find on the subject." And yet, setting study selection criteria in a literature review or synthesis is as important as setting criteria for a primary study. For example, the selection criteria for studies of interest to an intervention development project with the overall goal of increasing use of condoms by high-risk adolescents might include the age range encompassing "adolescence" as well as any combination of socio-demographic, institutional, or behavioral markers of "risk," such as social class, ethnicity, residence in a public housing project, or sexual contact with multiple partners. Planners must also decide whether to seek information from studies of volunteers who may already be motivated to change risky behavior and who are likely to comply with all study requirements or to seek information from an intact population that includes individuals who may be quite resistant to change.

As planners search for and find evidence to guide intervention development, they weigh many aspects of "the literature." They should address two overarching questions: Which evidence is relevant to my questions? and What conclusions can safely be drawn regarding the nature of the relationships between variables of interest?

Setting selection criteria for a literature search is a conceptual and somewhat intuitive activity, based on the aims of the search and the expected availability and characteristics of the literature. Criteria should be specific, appropriate, and efficient. A search should be specific and replicable. The boundaries can be narrow or broad, so long as they are clear. An example of a broad criterion for a search for interventions of interest is "any educational intervention conducted in a group format that includes a social inoculation approach and has the objective of increasing use of protection during sex." Because of the diverse interventions that could meet this criterion, it would be essential to code or categorize the various intervention characteristics that could affect the outcome, such as contact time, type of contact, content, and whether the objective was protection against pregnancy or STDs/HIV. These variables could even be used in a meta-analysis multivariate procedure (Cooper & Hedges, 1994) to help sort out the relative effectiveness of intervention features. Figure 3.2 presents a checklist for judging the quality of literature reviews.

---

[1] Contributed by Patricia Dolan Mullen, DrPH, University of Texas–Houston.

Another approach might emphasize population characteristics, modifying the broad criterion just mentioned to be "any educational intervention conducted in a group format [regardless of techniques, number of sessions, or aim] with low-income Mexican American boys in middle school/junior high." Alternatively, the health educator could set narrow boundaries based on other considerations, such as any educational intervention conducted with a subpopulation identified by their stage of change, for example, "precontemplators," that is, individuals who are not thinking about beginning to use condoms.

Specific criteria are not sufficient, however. They must also be *appropriate* for the questions that are guiding a particular search. A group of planners, for example, are researching for a sun protection intervention. For the sake of this example, let's say that it is already well known that sales of sunscreens with sun protection factor (SPF) of 15 are a significant part of total product sales. Through brainstorming other areas in which one of the desired behaviors was product substitution (in this case, to a sunscreen with an SPF greater than 15), the group's search would include reports of interventions to discourage use of full-fat dairy products in favor of low-fat or nonfat products. After reading about such interventions, the group would likely come up with the strategy of point-of-purchase labeling (e.g., shelf labels) of both desirable and undesirable products, with the insight that such strategies and the implied method, mild fear-arousal with simultaneous presentation of a means of reducing risk, might be usefully applied to one segment of the intended group, individuals who already purchase sunscreen. Further, once the group considered the point-of-purchase labeling strategy for use in pharmacies, this same strategy might also be applied to another change objective—increase perceived susceptibility to the negative consequences of sun exposure when using over-the-counter photosynthesizing products commonly sold in pharmacies, for example, shaving creams or painkillers. Thus, shelf labels might also be considered for such products and were actually tested in a randomized trial (Palmer, Mayer, Eckhardt, & Sallis, 1998).

Finally, criteria should be set with conservation of resources in mind: they should be efficient. For example, health educators who are researching "what's been tried" to reduce HIV/STD risk among adolescents who attend school unfortunately could encounter studies of motivational speeches at school assemblies or of pamphlets mailed to every student's home. Scanning abstracts from a computer search sounds easy, but such searches frequently turn up even more unrelated studies, and there may be hundreds of abstracts. If these studies are simply scanned and not retrieved, the cost of research may be low, and they might provide a basis for a conclusion not to use these common methods. More likely, however, including these studies will waste time and other resources, resources that might be better spent comparing the relative effectiveness of a limited set of interventions with highest promise of success, lowest cost, or widespread use.

To develop the study selection criteria, we recommend two tools: the questions that the intervention development team has identified, and the framework suggested in the synthesis literature by Bryant and Wortman (1984), advocated by Mullen and Ramirez (1987), and used by others (Mullen et al., 1997; Tabak et al.,

- ❏ What was the **purpose** of the review? Ask, What were the questions to be answered? What was the hypothesis? Is the question, hypothesis, or objective clearly stated?

    Ideally, the reviewers did not attempt to address too broad a question, for example, What methods have been effective in patient education programs? This question covers a vast territory, and the reviewers are likely to take a highly selective view of that territory with little description of the biases that shaped the selection. More useful reviews have more specific objectives, for example, to test alternative explanations for "mixed results."

- ❏ Are the **criteria** for including or excluding studies clearly stated? Ask, What is the rationale for these criteria? Is this an appropriate rationale in my context?

    Looking at the criteria plus search strategies (see next item) should ensure that the review produced a fair representation of the available evidence.

- ❏ How was the **search** done that located the studies? Ask, Was the search systematic? Is it fully described so that it can be replicated? Did it go beyond computerized databases (e.g., experts, bibliographies of articles already retrieved, bibliographies of other relevant written materials such as government reports, books, monographs)?

    The search should usually go beyond published sources to avoid publication bias, or the tendency (on the parts of both investigators and editors) to avoid publishing negative findings (Cooper & Hedges, 1994). Note: Some reviewers restrict the studies they will include to those that have been peer reviewed. This restriction appears to be a higher standard, and it is, in some journals; in others, however, no independent statistical review is required, and published articles can vary markedly in quality on statistical and many other aspects of study design.

- ❏ Are **study characteristics** clearly noted? Study characteristics include study design, sample, variables, and measures.

    Are tables and charts or a structured narrative used to display important study characteristics for all the included studies? To interpret the review's conclusions, the same information must be obtained about every study.

- ❏ Is the **intervention** well specified? Interventions include intended methods and strategies; vehicles and communication channels; and participant group contact points, frequency, and duration.

- ❏ Is a common **metric** used (e.g., standard deviation units)? Does the reviewer avoid relying on tests of significance (e.g., the percent achieving some behavior in the control or comparison group and in the experimental group; or the mean difference and confidence interval)?

    Most important, does the reviewer avoid relying on tests of significance to tell the outcome of the studies and allow an opportunity to see a measure of effect size so that meaningful, consistent differences can be separated from problems of low study power and that small, unimportant differences can be separated from large numbers (excessive power)?

- ❏ Are **dependent variables** examined separately?

    Some reviews, particularly quantitative reviews or meta-analyses, have combined knowledge and belief measures with measures of behavior and physiologic effects as if these were all measuring the same construct.

- ❏ Are **findings** interpreted in depth? Are nonaverage findings, positive and negative, examined closely? Are the lessons that can be derived from such outliers clearly articulated? Does the reviewer pursue the "whys"?

FIGURE 3.2 Considerations in Evaluating Reviews: A Checklist (*Note.* Adapted from "Using the Research Base to Improve Program Design," by P. D. Mullen, 1993, in B. E. Giloth, Ed., *Managing Hospital-Based Patient Education* [pp. 313–326], Chicago: American Hospital Association.)

1991). This framework is based on the four major types of validity described by Cook and Campbell (1979, pp. 37–91):

- Construct validity
- External validity
- Statistical conclusion validity
- Internal validity

These validity types form two pairs: Construct and external validity refer to the validity of generalizations about a study's intervention and measurement operations to target interventions and outcomes and from a study's sample, setting(s), and times to target populations, settings, and times. Statistical conclusion and internal validity refer to the validity of conclusions about the strength and direction of relationships. For health educators who are perusing the threats to each of these types of validity, Cook and Campbell (1979) are helpful in identifying areas in which criteria should be developed; for a characteristic in which the criterion is broad, the threats will suggest a hierarchy of evidence.

Decisions about generalizations are captured by the question, Is this study relevant to our questions? For example, the threat of experimenter expectancies under construct validity reminds planners to prefer studies in which those researchers who are collecting and analyzing data are blinded to study group assignment. A more fundamental threat is inadequate preoperational explication of constructs. This seemingly impenetrable term refers to the match between the intended construct—the outcome or the determinant or method or strategy being investigated—and the specific operations used in a particular study. To use a common, problematic example, a search of the intervention literature for studies evaluating the use of peer educators will net a wide range of definitions of the term *peer educator*, from individuals selected by students from their own group to honors students selected by school personnel as exemplary in their eyes. If the results of this broad range of operations are to be interpreted in designing an intervention, it is essential to be clear about what constitutes the construct of "peer." Inevitably, some of the studies should be discarded from the group, lest their negative results be misunderstood as indicating that peer educators are ineffective.

Another example of relevance, one in which a conceptual bridge had to be built to a different population, comes from the PANDA case study in Chapter 13. The problem was to develop an intervention to reduce the number of women who stop smoking successfully during pregnancy but who return to smoking after the birth. One issue was that no such programs had been reported in the published literature. So, the task of identifying populations that would be relevant meant that those populations would have to be conceptually relevant, not relevant in a concrete sense, that is, not a sample of pregnant women who had stopped smoking during pregnancy. The development team asked for suggestions from colleagues who knew the smoking literature, which led to a search of the literature on preventing return to smoking by victims of heart attacks who, largely because of hospital policy, were not able to smoke while they were hospitalized. The idea of stopping smoking because of a temporary, acute event and external constraints had some parallels; on the other hand, the population was older and primarily male. Nevertheless, some of these studies revealed the importance of attributions for stopping smoking and other hypotheses regarding moderating variables that would be important in developing the PANDA intervention (Mullen et al., 1999). Thus, fortunately, relevance may be achieved without a perfect match to the topic or the question at hand.

The second pair of validity types, statistical conclusion and internal validity, pertain to study rigor, or, as described by Bryant and Wortman (1984), study "acceptability." The issue in this validity pair is, Does the design of this study provide valid evidence for a causal relation?

Many studies from which "determinants" are identified are actually cross-sectional rather than prospective. For example, the observation that adolescents whose friends smoke were also likely to smoke gave rise to "social influence" explanations and "social inoculation" interventions. The evidence, however, was primarily an association with plausible, bidirectional interpretations. Although it may be true that joining a social group preceded smoking, switching directions also yielded a plausible explanation that could be described using the construct "social affiliation." Thus, it may be the case that adolescents who smoke are more likely to choose friends who smoke, and "social inoculation" may not be an appropriate intervention.

We are not suggesting that the only possibility is to follow the Cochrane Collaboration's policy of excluding all but randomized trials (1999). We are, however, cautioning health educators to be wary of overenthusiastic authors who may describe their findings in terms that exaggerate their strength. Also, several literature synthesis projects have set different criteria for rigor of design, depending on the level at which the intervention took place, so that the searchers recognize that community-wide interventions will be evaluated with different designs than individual-level interventions are. A review of the threats to the second pair of validity types will temper over-reliance on randomized designs.

Accessing and Using Theory

The next task for the core processes is to reinforce provisional explanations with theoretical concepts. We suggest three approaches—issue, concept, and general theories—to search the literature for applicable theories (Veen, 1985).

With the topic or issue approach, planners again look at the literature through the subject or issue. But this time they specifically look for theories and constructs in answer to their question. For example, the student group working on HIV as a health problem had posed a question about the predictors of condom use and had searched for provisional explanations in the literature specifically related to HIV and condom use. They then used the topic of condom use to approach the literature and found studies that used the health belief model (Lux & Petosa, 1994) and Ajzen's theory of planned behavior (Basen-Engquist & Parcel, 1992). From these theories, they considered adding to their list any of the constructs that were not already present, such as barriers from the health belief model and intention to perform the behavior from the theory of planned behavior. Also from Ajzen's (1988) theory the group redefined perceived norms as subjective norms to include both perception of whether significant others support performance of a behavior and the motivation to comply with the wishes of those others. If the work group had had a low yield through this narrow search, they would also have looked for theories in the literature on contraception (Levinson, 1995) as a related behavior and in the literature on risk-taking behavior by adolescents (Bishop-Townsend, 1996) as a more general subject.

As a matter of fact, the group did expand its search to the issues of adolescent pregnancy and STD prevention in general because they wanted to think about the problem slightly more broadly before they were satisfied with focusing on condom use. They chose to expand because they noticed, as they worked with their provisional list, that a focus on condom use narrowed their list of determinants to those determinants within the individual or quite close to the individual. The group was also interested in the wider social context of why adolescents might be underconcerned about pregnancy and STDs. They found that researchers had demonstrated that, controlling for ethnicity and family background, living in a poor neighborhood increases the likelihood of early pregnancy (Jencks & Mayer, 1990). Under conditions of poverty and lack of adult role models, babies provide young girls with proof that they are successful adults (Anderson, 1990; Musick, 1991). The group also found evidence that lack of parental supervision, association with deviant (i.e., participating in other risk behavior) peers, and coercive parenting were associated with engaging in sexual risk taking (Metzler et al., 1994). (See Table 3.1, column 2.)

The concept approach enables planners to track the concepts on the provisional list to theoretical constructs and then to their parent theories. Going to the construct enables full understanding of the meaning of a concept on the list and orientation to other constructs from the theory. For example, "confidence" on the student work group's provisional list (Table 3.1) is similar to the construct of self-efficacy in the social cognitive theory (Bandura, 1986; Mulvihill, 1996). When the group explored the construct of self-efficacy in lieu of confidence, they found considerable useful information. This new information guided them to split self-efficacy: self-efficacy for negotiating condom use as separate from self-efficacy for applying a condom. The work group also found that self-efficacy is closely related to skills, so they added skills to the list. Further, they encountered methods for influencing self-efficacy and began to think ahead about the intervention. None of this useful information would have been available if the group had not gone beyond the concept of confidence.

Working with the construct-related approach also means that planners may apply the theory fully. In other words, most of the time, a theory will have constructs in addition to the constructs on the provisional list that led to the theory. For instance, the work group found the construct of self-efficacy by exploring the concept of confidence. They also found that social cognitive theory contained other constructs, such as outcome expectation, expectancies, skills, reciprocal determinism, and modeling. Some of these constructs were then added to their provisional list.

In the general theories approach, planners look at their question through the lens of a determinants theory or a change theory, depending on the question. They also think about how the specific constructs in that theory apply to their question. If the question concerns determinants of behavior, as in the case of condom use, they may go to the theory of planned behavior, for example, and consider subjective norms, attitudes, self-efficacy expectations, and behavioral intentions, in the unlikely event that they haven't encountered this theory through the earlier processes (Ajzen & Madden, 1986). Clearly, the construct and general theories approach is limited by the number of theories with which a planner is familiar, and we devote the next chapter to a brief review of multiple theories commonly used in health education. We suggest also that the reader review theories from more complete sources (Glanz, Lewis, & Rimer, 1990). However, applying the construct approach—for instance, by using the index of a textbook—may lead planners to theories with which they are not yet familiar. That is the reason we strongly advise planners to first apply the construct approach before going to the general theories with which they are familiar.

Identifying and Addressing Needs for New Data

At this point the planner will have found a number of theoretical approaches that fit with, or add to, the provisional explanations. In some cases, these theories provide insight into the exact processes of the provisional answers, and at the same time, they give cause for further examination of some variables and raise questions that the planning team had not thought of before. For example, they would want to know whether theoretical constructs that look promising were actually explanatory in their population. They would also want to know the particular way a factor is expressed in their group.

In general, a combination of qualitative and quantitative techniques is used to explore the question of interest in the population (De Vries et al., 1992; Steckler, McLeroy, Goodman, Bird, & McCormick, 1992). During this process, the theories that have been applied to this point can serve as a guide for the qualitative and quantitative study questions. For a question regarding determinants, for example, planners first search the available theoretical and empirical literature on the cause of the behavior or environmental condition of interest to find theories and data. They might then use a qualitative method to find out the population's own ideas about determinants of their behavior and follow with a structured questionnaire with questions that are based on the results of the qualitative phase. Some factors cannot be measured by just asking the population because perceptions may be different from realities, so planners need information from key persons and through observations. Of course in some situations qualitative and quantitative methods are used independently rather than sequentially to shed light on a question, or qualitative methods are used later in the research process to better understand the findings from a quantitative approach (Steckler et al.).

Formulating the Working List of Answers

At this point the planning team is ready to summarize their provisional list of determinants and finalize this list of answers into a list of indicators for solutions. They already have considered the criteria of plausibility and process. Now, two further general criteria are used: What is the strength of the association between the determinant and the behavior or environmental condition in question or between the method and change? Also, how easy is it to influence the determinant, or to use the method, in a health education intervention? The latter criterion requires health educators to consider that some determinants may be changed by interventions directed at the individual and others by interventions directed at the environment. For determinant questions, answers that remain on the list will be factors that are both important and changeable. For a solutions or methods question, answers that remain on the list will be processes that have been shown to produce significant change in similar situations and determinants and that are within the realm of possibility for a particular project.

CORE PROCESSES APPLIED: THE CASE OF CHILD RESTRAINT DEVICES

Posing the Question

The Dutch Foundation for Traffic and Safety has a long history of educating parents on the consistent use of child restraint devices (CRDs) in cars to protect young children against the consequences of an accident. However, there remained a high number of car accidents in which children were injured (problem). The Foundation board decided to find out why their educational programs did not work and how they could be improved. The board engaged a consulting team. However, when the team began thinking about the problem as conceptualized by the Foundation board, the members realized that no question regarding determinants had ever been asked. The team's perspective shifted somewhat from a question of program failure to a determinant analysis. This perspective helped the team reformulate the questions: What are the reasons parents do not always use CRDs? (question to the explanation or determinants) and, How can we promote the use of CRDs? (question to the solution or methods and strategies). With this redirection, the team focused itself away from simply looking at the failure of the Foundation's education campaigns. The remainder of this example presents the process the team used for finding answers to the first question, the question to the explanation.

Brainstorming Provisional Answers for Lack of CRD Use

The consulting team brainstormed a provisional list of answers to the question regarding why parents don't use CRDs (Table 3.2). They discussed the possibility that parents may not have been exposed to information and have never heard of CRDs. It is also possible that parents do not know that CRDs are especially meant to prevent serious injury from accidents. Parents may think that they can prevent serious injury in other ways, such as by tightly holding the child, and they may underestimate their risks. Perhaps they think they do not run any risks themselves, for example, because they do not expect to be involved in an accident or because they expect to be able to hold the child in case of an accident (risk perception). There may be practical problems involved. For example, parents may find approved CRDs too expensive or that they take too much space. It is also possible that parents have actually bought a CRD, but do not use it consistently, for example, because they have two cars or because various children have to be transported at the same time. This discussion highlighted the difference between acquisition of a CRD and its use. Finally, the group discussed the possible effect of

Table 3.2
Provisional List: Determinants of Lack of CRD Use

ORIGINAL PROVISIONAL LIST	ADDITIONS FROM EMPIRICAL LITERATURE AND THEORY	ADDITIONS FROM NEW DATA
Parents' educational level	Outcome expectations	Delete lack of exposure to information
Practical problems, such as having two cars or having the child ride in cars of relatives or other caretakers	Risk perception—unrealistic optimism based on perception of control, stereotypical perception of the "type" of parents who run risks, overestimation of comparative efforts to take precautions	Self-efficacy specifically for handling the child's behavior
CRDs are too expensive to acquire		Outcome expectations regarding handling the child's behavior
Lack of exposure to information that CRDs prevent serious injury to children		Skills to handle the child's behavior
Lack of knowledge of CRDs (lack of understanding that CRDs are especially meant to avoid serious injury from accidents)	Response efficacy	
	Perception of control	
	Delete parent education—not a process, no evidence	
Underestimation of child's risk in an accident	Self-efficacy and behavioral effectiveness	
Underestimation of risk of being in an accident (risk perception)	Subjective norms	
Overestimation of the benefits of other ways of protecting the child, such as holding or using seat belts	Parents have tried and stopped using CRDs	

the parents' level of education. The next steps were to enhance the provisional list with theoretical explanations and new data when necessary.

Searching the Literature for Empirical Findings on CRDs

Once the group clarified its question and generated a provisional list of answers about why parents do not use CRDs, they searched the literature for empirical findings regarding CRD use. Because they found very little research, they also looked for information on seat belt use. Concerning CRDs and seat belts, they found information on prevalence of use- and nonuse-related injury (Johnston, Hendricks, & Fike, 1994; Kaplan & Cowley, 1991; Russell, Kresnow, & Brackbill, 1994), risk factors (Thompson & Russell, 1994), and the effects of regulation (Escobedo et al., 1991; Walter & Kuo, 1993). However, they learned little about their actual question and almost nothing that brought theory to bear on the problem.

Accessing and Using Theory to Enhance the Provisional List

The consultants had already entered the literature through their topic or issue and had found little that was theory related. This situation is a good example of the usefulness of the brainstorming and provisional list. With their provisional list in hand, the group moved on to the next approach to finding theories.

From the list, the team pursued the concepts of risk and found that theories such as the protection-motivation model (Rogers, 1983), health belief model (Janz & Becker, 1984), social learning theory (Mullen, Gottlieb, Biddle, McCuan, & McAlister, 1988; see also Allen & Bergman, 1976; Goebel, Copps, & Sulayman, 1984), and risk perception theories (Weinstein, 1988) have explained other risk-taking phenomena. Weinstein's precaution adoption theory explains why some people wrongfully think they do not run any risk. According to this theory, people tend to underestimate risks when they think they control the situation. A parent driving the car may believe he or she controls the child's risk, as may the parent who plans to hold the child in case of an accident. In addition, people believe they run less risk than others (unrealistic optimism). This belief is partly because they have a stereotypical perception of parents who actually run risks. It also is because they overestimate their efforts to take precautions compared to what other parents undertake (Van der Pligt, Otten, Richard, & Van der Velde, 1993). From this review, the consultants were able to clarify and further delineate the concept of risk on their list (see Table 3.2).

The process of clarifying concepts on the provisional list with the theoretical explanations can stimulate creative thinking. For example, when the team discussed the process of unrealistic optimism, they began to think about answers to questions to the solutions. In other words, they began to think of what they might do to intervene. They posed learning objectives to help parents become more aware of the real risks and consequently to use the CRD more consistently. One learning objective suggested by the team was that parents should see other parents take measures to protect their children and thus be persuaded that car accidents are partly uncontrollable and unpredictable. In a way, the group members "got ahead of themselves" here and addressed a question that should only have been asked once a working list (rather than a partial provisional list) of answers to their question was available. On the other hand, creative thinking is very important to the process and should be encouraged as long as the task group records its ideas for future reference and soon returns to its provisional list and completes the core processes.

Other risk perception models, such as the health belief model (Becker, 1974; Janz & Becker, 1984; Rosenstock, Strecher, & Becker, 1988) and the protection motivation theory (Rogers, 1983), cover more than just risk perception. They indicate under what circumstance risk perception leads to adequate action. They add the constructs of behavioral effectiveness and self-efficacy expectations. The threat of risk motivates parents to acquire and use a CRD provided that they are convinced that such a seat constitutes an effective means of protection (behavioral effectiveness) and that they believe they are able to acquire such a seat and use it consistently (self-efficacy).

Other constructs in the list of provisional explanations have to do with the costs and inconvenience of CRDs. The cost-benefit balance often occurs in the description of attitude (Ajzen, 1988). This attitude theory in turn is part of a model of behavioral determinants that suggests three types of determinants: attitude (risk perception, behavioral effectiveness, costs, and inconvenience), social influence, and self-efficacy. The consultants noticed that the provisional explanations at first considered neither social influence nor self-efficacy. Working from Ajzen's theory, the consultants explored social influence effects and found possible importance of subjective norms (the partner's expectation that a CRD should be used and the motivation to comply) as well as the overt behavior of other parents (modeling). In addition, the team assumed that a number of people would be motivated (favorable attitude) but probably would not be able to adopt the behavior (low self-efficacy). The group returned to social influence and self-efficacy in the course of additional research, when they were trying to find out what reference persons were important and what the difficulties were of performing the behavior.

Even though this team encountered Ajzen's model via a concept on their list, the application of the model is an example of the third possible strategy for accessing theories, namely, the approach through general theories. Because they had encountered quite a productive set of theories and theoretical constructs via the concept approach, the consultants completed their analysis with review of only one general theory. They applied McGuire's persuasion communication model (McGuire, 1985) as it is used in public health education (Kok et al., 1996) to address their question of why parents don't use CRDs, even though the model usually is used for questions related to mass media campaign failure. McGuire has distinguished a sequence of steps from a first exposure to a health education message to the maintenance of the advocated behavior, in this case, always using CRDs. By means of McGuire's model, the team listed several possible reasons why parents do not use CRDs: (a) attention: they have never heard of CRDs; (b) comprehension: they do not understand the purpose of the CRD; (c) attitude: they are not convinced of the advantages of the CRD; (d) social support: the partner does not consider it necessary; (e) self-efficacy: it is too much trouble when they have two cars; (f) behavioral change: they do not think of it at the moment; (g) behavior maintenance: they tried, but do not sustain the behavior.

This list suggests various reasons why health education had not produced the desired effect so far. Some of these reasons were already included in the provisional explanations and also came up via the other two approaches, but some are new. From this list, the team added behavior maintenance to their provisional list.

Identifying and Addressing Needs for New CRD Data

We can offer three reasons why the consultants needed to collect new data after reviewing the literature. It may be obvious that the group might not know enough about the possible reasons for not using CRDs. Even if they have listed all the reasons, they do not know which are the most important or how determinants are expressed in their particular population. Finally, they had uncovered little empirical evidence supporting the theoretical constructs they had discussed as possible predictors (determinants) of CRD or seat belt use. The reader will recall that the theoretical constructs did not come from research articles on CRD or seat belt use (the issue or subject approach), but from the construct and general theory approaches. Therefore, the planning group could not be certain that those theoretical constructs applied to CRDs or seat belts. The consultants were fortunate to have the time and resources to conduct a study (Pieterse, Kok, & Verbeek, 1992). They questioned parents at the exit to a parking lot about their reasons for acquiring and using CRDs (or not). The consultants were guided by the constructs on their provisional list, particularly the components of attitudes derived from Ajzen (1988). They paid particular attention to practical barriers. In short, the researchers discovered that the safety of the children (risk perception, attitude) is the main reason that parents acquired CRDs and that more than 90% of parents were positively disposed to use CRDs.

However, the most important reason for not using the CRD for these parents was the child's response. If a child becomes restless and disruptive while riding in a seat, parents often do not know how to cope with the behavior and consequently remove the child from the seat. In theoretical terms, the child's behavior is punishing feedback to the parents for using the CRDs. These negative consequences may result in low perceived self-efficacy to continue the behavior. The consultants realized that the impact of emphasizing the risks of not using CRDs without raising the parents' skills and self-efficacy for dealing with unruly children might have a contrary effect. Research has demonstrated that increasing negative outcome expectations, or risk perception, under conditions of low self-efficacy results in a condition, similar to learned helplessness, in which individuals are unlikely to acquire and perform the behavior (Hale & Dillard, 1995). In this case high self-efficacy for using CRDs and managing children would be an important requisite for effectively coping with risk information. Again the consultants began to think about solutions. With this additional information, they realized that the intervention emphasis should be on increasing self-efficacy rather than only on risk perception. From new research the group's provisional explanations were substantially improved.

Formulating the Working List of Answers for CRD Use

In general, it seems that the determinants of CRD use center around motivational issues related to risk perception and around self-efficacy issues related most importantly to dealing with the behavior of a child restrained in a car seat. The group first deleted some items based on the criteria of process and plausibility. For example, the explanation that more highly educated parents use CRDs more often than do less educated parents does not reflect a process. A process explanation might be that higher educated parents are relatively more convinced of the use of CRDs. Another might be that they are relatively less concerned about the high price of these seats. But the group had no data to bear this explanation out. In terms of plausibility, the group knew that in health centers parents consistently receive health education about CRDs. Therefore, that most parents are unaware of the existence of CRDs would not be a very plausible explanation. However, it might be a plausible explanation for a group of parents with special characteristics, for example, immigrant parents having difficulties with the language and consequently with health care facilities.

The group of consultants completed their working list of answers (Table 3.2) and discussed which were the most important predictors of CRD use and which were the most changeable. The resultant causal diagram (Figure 3.3) depicts their decisions. As the reader can see in the figure, it seemed to the consultants at the

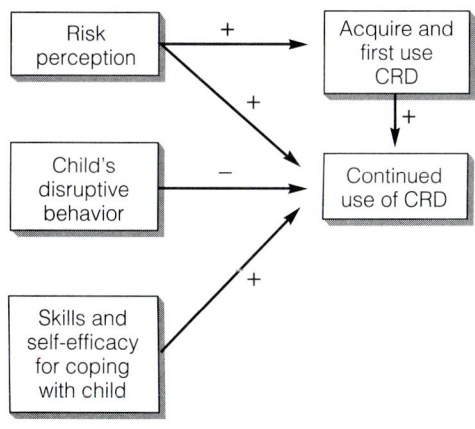

FIGURE 3.3 Hypothetical Causal Model for CRD Use

end of their analysis that parents obtain and try to use car seats because they perceive their children to be at risk from car accidents. However, they discontinue use because they are unable to manage their children's behavior. Therefore, intervention solutions might increase the intensity of the risk perception while providing skills and self-efficacy for managing children who are riding in car seats.

Posing a New Question

The team immediately thought of two kinds of solutions: a change in the environment, that is, improving the quality of seats to make children feel more comfortable; and a behavioral change, that is, training and guiding parents in coping with obstinate children. However, at this point they paused and asked a question to the solution: How can parents develop the knowledge and skills to cope with unruly children? And they worked back through the core processes, this time with a focus on methods. Through the issue-related approach, they could not find any study on training parents for this particular situation. Through the construct-related approach, they found theories on training, on coping, and on the combination of those two, with Bandura's social cognitive theory (1986) as the most applicable one. Methods that may be used would be modeling with guided enactment, for instance, in group meetings with parents. Through the general theories approach, the team found theories on relapse prevention (Marlatt & Gordon, 1985) that suggest ways to help parents continue to use CRDs over time by preparing them to deal with difficult situations that would tempt them to return to nonuse of the CRD. For instance, parents may be taught that if they wait five minutes the child will often stop crying.

The consultants also looked at learning theory (operant conditioning and contingency management) and found that learning theory would suggest that a child who is rewarded for unruly behavior by being transported without a car seat would have unruly behavior more frequently. They reasoned that parents would have to be trained to prevent children from ever being transported without the CRD. The other possible solution, improvement of the quality of the CRDs, is a different type of solution in the sense that the intervention would not be directed at the behavior of the parents or the child but at the environment. A change in the environment has to be organized systematically through (the behavior of) various agents, such as parents, consumer organizations, industry, and retailers. Theories that may help in the development of such an intervention include, for instance, theories on community development, media advocacy, coalition formation, and empowerment, but in this case the consultants had no clear evidence to support deficits in the comfort of car seats.

SUMMARY

In this chapter we presented some techniques for thinking with theory and evidence. These techniques included defining the problem and related questions, brainstorming provisional explanations, and then using empirical evidence from the literature, theory, and new data to add to and tighten the logic in the provisional list. These techniques are core intellectual and academic processes for use in program planning, and the Intervention Mapping framework provides the structure for when and how to use them. The continual solicitation and integration of information from a broad range of sources, using a broad range of techniques, is an essential exercise in maintaining a dynamic discourse between problem and solution. The more vigorously and comprehensively the problem can be expressed at initial stages of research and throughout the research process, the more robust and far-reaching will be the solution.

The major contributions of the constant application of these processes is that they divert health educators from always relying on only a favorite theory and they expand the number and type of potential solutions for a question. In the examples given in this chapter, the planning teams and consultants used the core processes to greatly expand their thinking on determinants questions and to lay a solid foundation for intervention.

Tasks for the Core Processes:

- Pose a question
- Brainstorm a provisional list of answers
- Search the literature for empirical evidence
- Evaluate the strength of the evidence
- Use the issue, concept, and general theories approaches for finding empirical and theoretical literature related to the question
- Address needs for new data
- Formulate a working list of answers and ask a new question

REFERENCES

Ajzen, I. (1988). *Attitudes, personality, and behavior.* Chicago: Dorsey Press.

Ajzen, I., & Madden, T. J. (1986). Prediction of goal-directed behavior: Attitudes, intentions, and perceived behavioral control. *Journal of Experimental Social Psychology, 22*(5), 453–474.

Allen, D. B., & Bergman, A. B. (1976). Social learning approaches to health education: Utilization of infant auto restraint devices. *Pediatrics, 58*(3), 323–328.

American Psychological Association Commission on Youth Violence. (1993). *Violence and youth: Psychology's response.* Washington, DC: Author.

Anderson, E. (1990). Neighborhood effects on teenage pregnancy. In C. Jencks & P. E. Peterson (Eds.), *The urban underclass.* Washington, DC: The Brookings Institution.

Baker, S. P., O'Neill, M., Ginsburg, M. J., & Li, G. (1992). *The injury fact book.* New York: Oxford University Press.

Bandura, A. (1986). *Social foundations of thought and action: A social cognitive theory.* Englewood Cliffs, NJ: Prentice Hall.

Basen-Engquist, K., & Parcel, G. S. (1992). Attitudes, norms, and self-efficacy: A model of adolescents' HIV-related sexual risk behavior. *Health Education Quarterly, 19*(2), 263–277.

Becker, M. H. (1974). The health belief model and sick role behavior. *Health Education Monographs, 2*, 409–419.

Bishop-Townsend, V. (1996). STDs: Screening, therapy, and long-term implications for the adolescent patient. *International Journal of Fertility and Menopausal Studies, 41*(2), 109–114.

Bryant, F. B., & Wortman, P. M. (1984). Methodological issues in the meta-analysis of quasi-experiments. In W. H. Yeaton & P. M. Wortman (Eds.), *New directions for program evaluation: No. 24. Issues in data synthesis.* San Francisco: Jossey-Bass.

Centers for Disease Control and Prevention. (1994). *HIV/AIDS surveillance report.* Atlanta, GA: Author.

Centerwall, B. S. (1993). Television and violent crime. *Public Interest, 111*, 56–71.

Cochrane Collaboration Web Site. (4 January 1999). Available: http://www.update-software.com/ccweb/default.html

Cook, T., & Campbell, D. (1979). *Quasi-experimentation: Design and analysis issues for field settings.* Boston: Houghton Mifflin.

Cooper, H., & Hedges, L. V. (1994). *The handbook of research synthesis.* New York: Russell Sage Foundation.

Costa, F. M., Jessor, R., Fortenberry, J. D., & Donovan, J. E. (1996). Psychosocial conventionality, health orientation, and contraceptive use in adolescence. *Journal of Adolescent Health, 18*(6), 404–416.

De Vries, H., Weijts, W., Dijkstra, M., & Kok, G. (1992). The utilization of qualitative and quantitative data for health education program planning, implementation, and evaluation: A spiral approach. *Health Education Quarterly, 19*(1), 101–115.

Dodge, K. A., & Coie, J. D. (1987). Social information processing factors in reactive and proactive aggression in children's peer groups. *Journal of Personality and Social Psychology, 53*(6), 1146–1158.

Donovan, J. E., Jessor, R., & Costa, F. M. (1991). Adolescent health behavior and conventionality-unconventionality: An extension of problem-behavior theory. *Health Psychology, 10*(1), 52–61.

Earp, J. A., & Ennett, S. T. (1991). Conceptual models for health education research and practice. *Health Education Research: Theory and Practice, 6*(2), 163–171.

Eron, L. D., Huesman, L. R., Lefkowitz, M. M., & Walder, L. O. (1996). Does television violence cause aggression? In D. F. Greenberg (Ed.), *The international library of criminology, criminal justice, and penology: Vol. 2. Criminal careers* (pp. 311–321). Aldershot, UK: Dartmouth.

Escobedo, L. G., Chorba, T. L., Remington, P. L., Anda, R. F., Sanderson, L., & Saidi, A. A. (1991). State laws and the use of car seat belts [letter]. *New England Journal of Medicine, 325*(22), 1586–1587.

Farrington, D. P. (1995). The Twelfth Jack Tizard Memorial Lecture: The development of offending and antisocial behavior from childhood. Key findings from the Cambridge study in delinquent development. *Journal of Child Psychology and Psychiatry and Allied Disciplines, 36*(6), 929–964.

Glanz, K., Lewis, F. M., & Rimer, B. K. (1990). Theory, research, and practice in health education: Building bridges and forging links. In K. Glanz, F. M. Lewis, & B. K. Rimer (Eds.), *Health behavior and health education: Theory, research, and practice* (pp. 17–32). San Francisco: Jossey-Bass.

Goebel, J. B., Copps, T. J., & Sulayman, R. F. (1984). Infant car seat usage: Effectiveness of a postpartum educational program. *JOGN Nursing, 13*(1), 33–36.

Green, L. W., & Lewis, F. M. (1986). *Measurement and evaluation in health education and health promotion.* Palo Alto, CA: Mayfield.

Greenbaum, T. L. (1988). *The practical handbook and guide to focus group research.* Lexington, MA: Lexington Books.

Hale, J. L., & Dillard, J. P. (1995). Fear appeals in health promotion campaigns: Too much, too little, just right? In E. Maibach & R. L. Parrott (Eds.), *Designing health messages: Approaches from communication theory and public health practice* (pp. 65–81). Thousand Oaks, CA: Sage.

Huberman, A. M., & Miles, M. B. (1994). Data management and analysis methods. In N. K. Denzin & Y. S. Lincoln (Eds.), *Handbook of qualitative research* (pp. 428–444). Thousand Oaks, CA: Sage.

Janz, N. K., & Becker, M. H. (1984). The health belief model: A decade later. *Health Education Quarterly, 11*(1), 1–47.

Jencks, C., & Mayer, S. E. (1990). Residential segregation, job proximity, and black job opportunities. In L. E. Lynn and M. McGeary (Eds.), *Inner-city poverty in the United States.* Washington, DC: National Academy Press.

Johnston, J. J., Hendricks, S. A., & Fike, J. M. (1994). Effectiveness of behavioral safety belt interventions. *Accident Analysis and Prevention, 26*(3), 315–323.

Kaplan, B. H., & Cowley, R. A. (1991). Seatbelt effectiveness and cost of noncompliance among drivers admitted to a trauma center. *American Journal of Emergency Medicine, 9*(1), 4–10.

Kok, G. (1991). Health education theories and research for AIDS prevention. *Hygie, 10*(2), 32–39.

Kok, G., Schaalma, H., De Vries, H., Parcel, G., & Paulussen, T. (1996). Social psychology and health education. *European Review of Social Psychology, 7,* pp. 241–282. Chichester, UK: Wiley.

Krueger, R. A. (1988). *Focus groups: A practical guide for applied research.* Newbury Park, CA: Sage.

Levinson, R. A. (1995). Reproductive and contraceptive knowledge, contraceptive self-efficacy, and contraceptive behavior among teenage women. *Adolescence, 30*(117), 65–85.

Loeber, R., & Dishion, T. (1983). Early predictors of male delinquency: A review. *Psychological Bulletin, 94,* 68–99.

Loeber, R., Stouthamer-Loeber, M., Nan Kammen, W., & Farrington, D. P. (1991). Initiation, escalation, and desistance in juvenile offending and their correlates. *Journal of Criminal Law and Criminology, 94,* 68–99.

Lorig, K., & Holman, H. (1993). Arthritis self-management studies: A twelve-year review. *Health Education Quarterly, 20*(1), 17–28.

Lux, K. M., & Petosa, R. (1994). Using the health belief model to predict safer sex intentions of incarcerated youth. *Health Education Quarterly, 21*(4), 487–497.

Marlatt, G. A., & Gordon, J. R. (1985). *Relapse prevention: Maintenance strategies in the treatment of addictive behaviors.* New York: Guilford.

McGuire, L. W. (1985). Attitudes and attitude change. In G. Lindzey & E. Aronson (Eds.), *The handbook of social psychology* (3rd ed., pp. 233–346). New York: Random House.

Merriam, S. B. (1988). *Case study research in education: A qualitative approach.* San Francisco: Jossey-Bass.

Metzler, C. W., Noell, J., Biglan, A., Ary D., & Smolkowski, K. (1994). The social context for risky sexual behavior among adolescents. *Journal of Behavioral Medicine, 17*(4), 419–438.

Morgan, D. L. (1988). *Focus groups as qualitative research.* Newbury Park, CA: Sage.

Mullen, P. D. (1993). Using the research base to improve program design. In B. E. Giloth (Ed.), *Managing hospital-based patient education* (pp. 313–326). Chicago: American Hospital Association.

Mullen, P. D., DiClemente, C. C., Carbonari, J. P., Nicol, L., Richardson, M. A., Sockrider, M. M., & Taylor, W. C. (1999). Project PANDA: Maintenance of prenatal smoking abstinence 12 months postpartum. Manuscript submitted for publication.

Mullen, P. D., Gottlieb, N. H., Biddle, A. K., McCuan, R. A., & McAlister, A. L. (1988). Predictors of safety belt initiative by primary care physicians: A social learning theory perspective. *Medical Care, 26*(4), 373–382.

Mullen, P. D., & Ramirez, G. (1987). Information synthesis and meta-analysis. In W. Ward, M. H. Becker, P. D. Mullen, & S. Simonds (Eds.), *Advances in health education and promotion* (Vol. 2, pp. 201–239). Greenwich, CT: JAI Press.

Mullen, P. D., Simons-Morton, D. G., Ramirez, G., Frankowski, R. F., Green, L. W., & Mains, D. A. (1997). A meta-analysis of trials evaluating patient education and counseling for three groups of preventive behaviors. *Patient Education and Counseling, 32*(3), 157–173.

Mulvihill, C. K. (1996). AIDS education for college students: Review and proposal for a research-based curriculum. *AIDS Education and Prevention, 8*(1), 11–25.

Musick, J. S. (1991). The high-stakes challenge of programs for adolescent mothers. In P. B. Edelman & J. Ladner (Eds.), *Adolescence and poverty: Challenge for the 1990s.* Washington, DC: Center for National Policy Press.

Needleman, H. L., Reiss, J. A., Tobin, M. J., Biesecker, G. E., & Greenhouse, J. B. (1996). Bone lead levels and delinquent behavior. *Journal of the American Medical Association, 275*(5), 363–369.

Nodora, J. (1995). *Ethnic comparisons of adolescent sexual risk-taking and preventive behavior.* Unpublished doctoral dissertation, University of Texas-Houston School of Public Health.

Palmer, R. C., Mayer, J. A., Eckhardt, L., & Sallis, J. F. (1998). Promoting sunscreen in a community drugstore [Research letter]. *American Journal of Public Health, 88*(4), 681.

Patterson, G. R. (1986). Performance models for antisocial boys. *American Psychologist, 41*(4), 432–444.

Patterson, G. R., & Stouthamer-Loeber, M. (1984). The correlation of family management practices and delinquency. *Child Development, 55*(4), 1299–1307.

Patton, M. Q. (1990). *Qualitative evaluation and research methods* (2nd ed.). Thousand Oaks, CA: Sage.

Perry, C. L., & Jessor, R. (1985). The concept of health promotion and the prevention of adolescent drug abuse. *Health Education Quarterly, 12*(2), 169–184.

Perry, D. G., Perry, C. L., & Boldizar, J. P. (1990). Learning of aggression. In M. Lewis & S. M. Miller (Eds.), *Handbook of developmental psychopathology: Perspectives in developmental psychology* (pp. 135–146). New York: Plenum.

Pieterse, M. E., Kok, G., & Verbeek, J. (1992). Determinants of the acquisition and utilization of automobile child restraint devices: A survey among Dutch parents. *Health Education Research: Theory and Practice, 7*(3), 349–358.

Rogers, R. (1983). Cognitive and physiological processes in fear-based attitude change: A revised theory of protection motivation. In J. T. Cacioppo & R. E. Petty (Eds.), *Social psychophysiology: A sourcebook*. New York: Guilford Press.

Rosenstock, I. M., Strecher, V. J., & Becker, M. H. (1988). Social learning theory and the health belief model. *Health Education Quarterly, 15*(2), 175–183.

Rossi, P. H., Freeman, H. E., & Lipsey, M. W. (1999). *Evaluation: A systematic approach* (6th ed.). Newbury Park, CA: Sage.

Russell, J., Kresnow, M. J., & Brackbill, R. (1994). The effect of adult belt laws and other factors on restraint use for children under age 11. *Accident Analysis and Prevention, 26*(3), 287–295.

Slaby, R. G., & Guerra, N. G. (1988). Cognitive mediators of aggression in adolescent offenders: 1. Assessment. *Developmental Psychology, 24*(4), 580–588.

Stake, R. E. (1995). *The art of case study research*. Thousand Oaks, CA: Sage.

Steckler, A., McLeroy, K. R., Goodman, R. M., Bird, S. T., & McCormick, L. (1992). Toward integrating qualitative and quantitative methods: An introduction. *Health Education Quarterly, 19*(1), 1–8.

Tabak, E. R., Mullen, P. D., Simons-Morton, D. G., Green, L. W., Mains, D. A., Eilat-Greenberg, S., Frankowski, R. F., & Glenday, M. C. (1991). The definition and yield of inclusion criteria for a meta-analysis of patient education studies in clinical services. *Evaluation and the Health Professions, 14*(4), 388–411.

Thompson, E. J., & Russell, M. L. (1994). Risk factors for non-use of seatbelts in rural and urban Alberta. *Canadian Journal of Public Health. Revue Canadienne de Sante Publique, 85*(5), 304–306.

Van der Pligt, J., Otten, W., Richard R., & Van der Velde, F. (1993). Perceived risk of AIDS: Unrealistic optimism and self-protective action. In B. J. Pryor & G. D. Reeder (Eds.), *The social psychology of HIV infection* (pp. 39–58). Hillsdale, NJ: Erlbaum.

Veen, P. (1985). *Sociale Psychologie Toegepast: van Probleem Naar Oplossing* [Applying social psychology: From problem to solution]. Alphen aan den Rijn, The Netherlands: Samson.

Walter, R. S., & Kuo, A. R. (1993). Taxicabs and child restraint. *American Journal of Diseases of Children, 147*(5), 561–564.

Webster, D. W., Wilson, M. E., Duggan, A. K., & Pakula, L. C. (1992). Parents' beliefs about preventing gun injuries to children. *Pediatrics, 89*(5, Pt 1), 908–914.

Weinstein, N. D. (1988). The precaution-adoption process. *Health Psychology, 7*(4), 355–386.

Windsor, R., Baranowski, T., Clark, N., & Cutter, G. (1994). *Evaluation of health promotion, health education, and disease prevention programs* (2nd ed.). Mountain View, CA: Mayfield.

Yin, R. (1994). *Case study research: Design and methods* (2nd ed.). Newbury Park, CA: Sage.

Yoshikawa, H. (1994). Prevention as cumulative protection: Effects of early family support and education on chronic delinquency and its risks. *Psychological Bulletin 115*(1), 28–54.

CHAPTER 4

Theories in Health Education and Promotion

READER OBJECTIVES

- Describe a social ecological approach to health-related behavior and environments
- Identify theories that describe determinants and change at each ecological level
- Select theoretical constructs that explain influences on individual behavior and on interpersonal, organizational, community, and societal conditions
- Select theoretical methods to change determinants of these behaviors and conditions

The purpose of this chapter is to identify theories that are applicable to health education and promotion problems. The primary focus is health-related behavior, the supporting social and physical environments for this behavior, and the environments related directly to health. We review theories that help to explain or to change health-related behavior or environments.

Chapter 2 showed how to define health and quality-of-life problems, describe who has the problem and who is at risk for it, and explore behavioral, social, and physical contributors to the problem. Planners of health education and promotion programs then must search for determinants or causes of the behaviors or conditions and choose methods to influence those determinants. In this process, the health educator can look to theory for help with

- describing the at-risk and intervention groups
- understanding the health-promoting behavior and environmental conditions
- defining determinants of healthful behavior and environments
- finding methods to promote change in the determinants, behavior, and environmental conditions

Table 4.1
When to Use Theory in Intervention Planning

TASK	EXAMPLES
To describe and select intervention groups	Transtheoretical model Diffusion of innovations theory[a] Agenda-building theory
To define behaviors	Self-regulatory theories Organizational change theory Diffusion of innovations theory[a]
To define environmental conditions	Social cognitive theory Social support theory Organizational development theory
To understand and select determinants of behaviors and environmental conditions	Theory of planned behavior Social cognitive theory Health belief model
To choose methods to promote change and to translate the theoretical methods into practical strategies	Persuasion communication model Organizational development theory Conscientization

[a]See Chapter 8.

Table 4.1 presents uses of theory and examples of each use. An understanding of theoretical constructs applicable to health education can broaden the planner's ability to do all these tasks. In a general sense, theory in health promotion and health education planning falls into two broad categories of use: first to understand the problem, both its behavioral and external or environmental causes (theory of the problem); next to understand the possible mechanisms for change (theory of action).

PERSPECTIVES

Ecological Interventions

Once a health educator understands a health problem—including the behavior, the environmental conditions, and their determinants—the next use of theory is to identify intervention levels and methods. The choice of environmental levels can depend on the level of the problem and its determinants (Steuart, 1993). Richard, Potvin, Kishchuk, Prlic, and Green (1996) identified five potential levels: individuals, groups or the interpersonal environment, organizations to which individuals belong, communities, and political players that may be at community or societal levels (see Chapter 1, Figure 1.1). All levels other than the individual are called environmental levels, and interventions that include levels beyond the individual are called environmental interventions. Health promotion interventions can involve the direct transformation of an entity (e.g., the individual or the organization) or may involve the creation of a network among two or more entities (e.g., development of a coalition of organizations or a self-help group of individuals). Consonant with this approach, the model by Richard and colleagues also assumes that the ultimate focus of health promotion interventions is the health of at-risk individuals, even though the intervention may not directly address these persons.

Multiple levels may be influenced by an intervention at one level. For example, a program aimed at convincing organizations to conduct health-related lobbying may influence a legislature to pass laws that may influence individual health behavior. In one case, one of our colleagues worked with a coalition in a large metropolitan area to use media and social advocacy to influence the police department and the U.S. Department of Labor to crack down on the use of young Hispanic children as dancers in bars and nightclubs (an activity that can lead to health risk behaviors of substance abuse and prostitution). In this example, intervention at the individual or interpersonal levels would have been difficult. Families felt helpless to control the girls' activities, and the monetary incentives to dance were strong in impoverished neighborhoods. However, once social change began to occur, parents expressed more empowerment to manage their children. A program may be aimed at any ecological level and have effects on that level and all the levels nested within it.

Green (personal communication, February 26, 1997) suggests that higher order change may sometimes be more powerful from a systems perspective. He gives a simple but nevertheless clear conceptualization of various levels of change fitting together like wheels with cogs. When change can be made on the big, societal wheel, then faster change is stimulated by the meshing of the cogs of the smaller wheels with the bigger. Direct intervention to influence higher level systems, such as policy or social norms, is often assumed to have effects downstream on population health, either through behavior or, less frequently, through the environment independent of behavior. However, more research is needed to demonstrate such causal linkages.

We draw the approach to change at the various ecological levels from three traditions. The first is that of Kurt Lewin, who focused on the gatekeepers within channels (McGrath, 1995). The second is social exchange theory, which focuses on the positions or roles of persons within the social system (Coleman, 1990), and the third is the MATCH model that has been used to plan multilevel interventions for health education (B. G. Simons-Morton, Greene, & Gottlieb, 1995; D. G. Simons-Morton, Simons-Morton, Parcel, & Bunker, 1988).

In each of these views, the key to understanding social reality at each of the ecological levels and how to change conditions at each level is tied to understanding the positions that comprise the level and exert influence on its conditions. For example, Lewin described two channels by which food gets to a family's table: the grocery channel and the garden channel (McGrath, 1995). In the grocery channel, various gatekeepers act to influence what foods are selected to move along the channel, from the food manufacturer product line managers to the buyers at the wholesale grocers, to the grocery chain buyers, to the individual store managers, to the shopper for the family. At each point an array of forces help or hinder passage through the gates along the channel. The product line manager, for example, acts on findings from consumer marketing surveys, cost and availability of ingredients, and fit to the company's manufacturing facilities. Consumer demand for low-fat products could influence the food manufacturer to produce these foods. Moving down the channel to the end of the line, the family shopper may be influenced by forces that include motivations to provide healthful food for the family, to please the family, to save money, and to purchase food that is easily prepared. By understanding the determinants of these gatekeeper behaviors at several levels, the health educator is better able to plan where to intervene to create the most effective and efficient interventions for change.

We have adopted the approach of D. G. Simons-Morton and colleagues (1988) of looking at agents (decision makers or role actors) at each systems level: interpersonal (e.g., parents), organizational (e.g., managers of school food services), community (e.g., newspaper editors), or societal (e.g., legislators). The focus of interventions at the various levels are agents (individuals or groups, such as boards or committees) in positions that exercise control over the behaviors of others, for example, school boards who control the managers of school food services.

This focus on agents allows planners to start with a social psychological view of the decision-making agent. The planner asks, What influences the decision-making agent to make the healthful decision? Why, for example, does the decision-making agent buy fruits and vegetables for the home? purchase or modify healthful foods for the school cafeteria? develop feature articles on how families are changing the way they eat for health and well-being? pass legislation subsidizing healthful school meals for low-income children? As with individual health behavior, agent decision making is influenced by personal and external determinants.

At the higher order system levels, however, the complexity increases and different variables come into play. For example, a legislator will be concerned with the cost and effectiveness of the policy; with how constituents, key interest groups, and other legislators view it; with how it relates to the party platform; and with how it will influence the health of the population. These concerns are all personal determinants. External determinants would include reinforcement, punishment, and social pressure through campaign contributions, feedback from legislative colleagues, and telephone calls and letters from constituents. From an intervention perspective, lobbying and advocacy activities from concerned organizational and individual constituents change these internal and external determinants.

Political, Practical, and Habitual Influences on Intervention

Health educators often work within settings—such as public health departments, schools, work sites, hospitals, or community agencies—with particular missions and funded projects. Also, health educators may have specialization of training or special skills and talents that influence them to focus on a particular level, or even type, of intervention, for example, community organization, media advocacy, small group facilitation, or counseling. In addition, health educators often have their own favorite theories or ways of understanding health problems, risk factors, and determinants. Health educators and those who direct their work may intervene habitually with methods and strategies based on the one or two theories with which they are most comfortable. However, using a favorite explanation for every problem and intervening in every situation with the same method may be like knowing only grandmother's recipe for soup. It is familiar, and sometimes it

---

The mayor's planning committee found itself in a predicament. Everyone in the planning group had his or her favorite recipe for intervention. They had brainstormed some determinants of violent behavior and used the core processes (Chapter 3), but the health educator seemed hard-pressed to get the group members to see beyond their own pet theories. Some group members thought that theoretical eclecticism was forbidden to academically well-trained individuals. (And don't forget the health educator's boss was among this crowd.) What to do? The health educator was determined to help the group construct a useful multitheoretical model of the problem, an approach which had been effective at the health educator's previous job—and then to decide, based on this hypothetical causal model, about intervention levels and methods. But how to get the group to come along?

The health educator approached the group management problem like any other planning process question. What are the determinants of *the group members'* behavior? What was holding them back from really working with theory? The health educator brainstormed a list: Some group members knew only one theory; some of them wanted a venue for theory testing; some of them just wanted to get the intervention done—they weren't sure theory was helpful at all. Looking at this short list, the health educator decided that if the group had better knowledge of multiple theories and how to apply them to the problem of violence, they might be more willing to continue with the planning process. The health educator took all the literature that the group had gathered and divided the articles by the underlying theories; then by whether the articles discussed causes of violence or interventions. With each set of violence-related articles, the health educator put a review article of the relevant theory. Small groups from the task force then were assigned to summarize a set of articles and present them to the larger group. The small groups answered the following questions: What do these articles say about the causes of violent behavior? Which of these causes are psychosocial determinants of individual behavior and which are environmental conditions? If the causes are environmental, does the article contain data or theories that suggest the determinants of the environmental cause? With crossed fingers and held breath, the health educator awaited the results.

works, depending on what ingredients the cooks have at hand and on their skill in the kitchen. But sometimes it doesn't work, and the cook needs both new ingredients and new recipes.

This chapter is a review of theories and perhaps a diagnostic tool for the need for further reading in a particular theory. Our list of theories is only a selection of possible theories; we refer the reader to textbooks on theories (Conner & Norman, 1996; Gilbert, Fiske, & Lindzey, 1998; Glanz, Lewis, & Rimer, 1997; Sabini, 1992). A brief description of each theory is followed by a summary of the contribution of the theory to understanding intended programs recipients, behaviors, the environment, determinants, and methods.

OVERVIEW OF THEORIES

We have organized this chapter by mapping theories onto ecological levels, as presented in Table 4.2 (Glanz et al., 1997; McLeroy, Bibeau, Steckler, & Glanz, 1988). This presentation is a simplification because theories often link systems levels. For example, social cognitive theory includes determinants from the social and physical environments, and the theory of planned behavior has as a key predictor of behavior the normative expectations of others as perceived by the individual. The health educator can look outside the more obvious boundaries of a particular theory and work with the causal determinants from higher order levels. For example, a planner working with concepts from the theory of planned behavior could think about the sources of the normative beliefs and, moving to a more sociological frame of reference or to communications theory, look at how social norms are created and transmitted. Thus, even though individual theory may not explicitly link levels of analysis, an eclectic approach to the use of theory can be used to develop hypothetical causal maps of how systems work to determine specific behavior or environmental changes.

Behavior-Oriented Theories and Environment-Oriented Theories

In this chapter, we present social science theories that may be applied in health education. We describe two types: behavior-oriented theories, mostly from behavioral sciences, and environment-oriented theories, mostly from the sociopolitical sciences.

Theories may be used primarily for one type of application, but many theories are potentially applicable to all ecological levels and also to adoption and implementation. When available, we give examples of applications outside the theory's standard application. The theory of planned behavior, for example, is often applied to individual health behavior (Godin & Kok, 1996) but can be applied to explain the behavior of politicians (B. S. Flynn et al., 1998; N. H Gottlieb et al., 1999) and program implementers (Paulussen, Kok, Schaalma, & Parcel, 1995).

Table 4.2
Theories Arrayed by Level

PROBLEM AND INTERVENTION LEVELS	THEORIES
Individual	Theory of planned behavior
	Transtheoretical model
	Persuasion communication model
	Goal-setting theory
	Attribution theory
	Health belief model
	Self-regulatory theories
Interpersonal environment	Social cognitive theory
	Diffusion of innovations theory[a]
	Social network and social support theories
Organization	Stage theory of organizational change
	Organizational development theory
	Interorganizational relationship theory
Community	Conscientization
	Community organization
Society and government	Agenda-building theory
	Policy windows theory

[a]See Chapter 8.

The behavioral science theories that try to explain behavior and behavior change have two roots: health and health education in particular, or behavior and behavior change in general (the last being mainly social psychological theories). Health and health education–oriented theories, for example, the health belief model, are often related to perceptions of health risks. Some other theories, such as the transtheoretical model of stages of change, were developed in a health setting but evolved into a general theory. Most general social psychological models such as social cognitive theory were developed for a broad range of behaviors but are easily applicable to health behavior and change.

We also present organization, community, and society level theories that have been used in the field of health education. These theories are primarily change-oriented theories rather than theories of determinants. At the organizational level, the stage theory of organizational change, organizational development theory, and interorganizational theory provide a toolbox for the health educator to plan and conduct interventions for organizational change.

At the community and society levels we first present the classic models of community organization and community development and describe the current perspectives being used for health promotion. Issues of power, participation, and goals have received much discussion among health educators in recent years (Minkler, 1997b). In selecting the constructs to use for community change, planners must clarify their assumptions and values about the nature of the change process and select and implement strategies congruent with these assumptions. Finally, we examine theories of policy making that have been used primarily at the national, state, and governmental level.

From Theories of the Problem to Theories of Action

The link between theories of the problem and theories of action is often not very clear. Some theories provide both explanations of behavior and how to change it; most theories give only one or the other. Theories of the problem suggest what to change; theories of action ideally tell how to change it. In practice, the jump from objectives to methods may be neither clear nor easy.

Witte (1995) suggests an interesting approach to this challenge. She organizes the results of the determinants analysis in a list of relevant categories (e.g., beliefs, social influences, self-efficacy, values) and then decides which determinants need to be changed, which need to be reinforced, and which need to be introduced. For example, in a program for HIV prevention for Hispanic men, their belief that condoms were unclean needed to be changed, the importance of family values needed to be reinforced, and the belief that condoms could prevent HIV infection needed to be introduced. Witte also suggests that the health educator address cues such as cultural values, source preferences, and audience characteristics based on the persuasion communication model described later in this chapter (McGuire, 1985).

Intervention Mapping suggests a link between theories of the problem and theories of action through the link between the first two steps: objectives and methods. Theories of the problem help planners formulate appropriate objectives ordered by determinant; theories of action point to methods that fit with the determinants. For example, using the theory of planned behavior, the educator may have formulated a program objective in terms of perceived social expectations; using social cognitive theory, the educator may select modeling and guided practice to improve resistance to social pressure.

INDIVIDUAL THEORIES

Learning Theories

Learning refers to any enduring change in the way an organism responds based on its experience (Westen, 1996). Learning theories assume that experiences shape behavior and that learning is adaptive. Learning theory is the foundation of most behavioral science theories. Two major learning theory perspectives are classical conditioning and operant conditioning.

Classical conditioning refers to the association of an unconditioned stimulus (UCS) with a conditioned stimulus (CS). A UCS produces a response that does not have to be learned (e.g., nausea as a result of chemotherapy). A conditioned response is a response that people learn as a result of the association of the CS with the UCS (e.g., certain food aversions in cancer patients who have experienced nausea during chemotherapy). The association is most effective when the time interval is short and the CS precedes the UCS. People generalize from one CS to another, similar CS (e.g., fear of one dog to fear of another dog), but they also discriminate between CS (e.g., fear of dogs but not of cats). Extinction (unpairing of the stimuli, forgetting, or unlearning) will occur when the CS is repeatedly presented without the UCS.

Operant conditioning refers to the reinforcement of a behavior, resulting in its recurrence. Presentation of a positive reinforcer makes a behavior more likely to occur, whereas the removal of a negative reinforcer (e.g., a loud noise) has the same effect. Punishment decreases the probability that a behavior will recur. Positive feelings may serve as positive reinforcements. The more continuous the reinforcement schedule is, the faster the learning process; however, the less continuous the reinforcement schedule is, the stronger the resistance to extinction. A shorter time interval between the behavior and the reinforcer leads to a faster learning process. People learn to discriminate between situations that lead to the reinforcement and situations that do not. What is actually reinforcing may be different for individuals and for cultures.

The reinforcing effects of positive feelings form the basis for social cognitive theories. The basic assumption of social cognitive theories is that what is crucial to learning is not the environmental stimulus per se, but the perception of the environmental stimulus. Perceptions of environmental stimuli include, for instance, outcome expectations and self-efficacy expectations (see "Social Cognitive Theory" later in this chapter).

Zajonc (1980) showed that people become more positive about stimuli the more times they are exposed to them, even when people are not consciously aware of that process. One way to change people's attitudes in a more positive direction would be to expose them repeatedly to the new behavior or object. For instance, adolescents may be shown condoms repeatedly in classroom HIV preventive education. Probably, this effect is limited to stimuli that are associated with a relatively neutral attitude at the start.

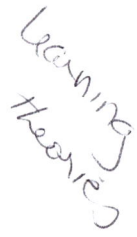

Uses in Problem Analysis and Intervention Methods

Appropriate focus: Groups of people with the same learning history

Behaviors: All (human) behavior

Environment: Many stimuli originate from the physical and social environment

Determinants: Association of conditioned stimuli with unconditioned stimuli; responses to short-term positive reinforcement, negative reinforcement, punishment; attitude

Methods: Short-term dissociation or association of CS with UCS; short-term positive reinforcement for healthful behaviors; removal of negative reinforcement for healthful behaviors; punishment of unhealthful behaviors; and repeated exposure

Theory of Planned Behavior

CONSTRUCTS Ajzen's (1988) theory of planned behavior (TPB) is an extension of the theory of reasoned action (Conner & Sparks, 1996; Fishbein & Ajzen, 1975; Godin & Kok, 1996; Montaño, Kasprzyk, & Taplin, 1997). Both theories focus primarily on determinants of behavior. Although they do not give specific methods for behavior change, they do help health educators understand the specific variables that need to be changed (Witte, 1995). The theory should be applied in situations in which people are aware of the negative consequences of their behavior, for instance, when they realize they are eating a high-fat diet (Brug, Hospers, & Kok, 1997; Brug, Lechner, & De Vries, 1995). When people are not aware, they first have to become aware of the problem before determinants can be analyzed. TPB postulates that intention, the most proximal determinant of behavior, is determined by three conceptually independent constructs: attitude, subjective norms, and perceived behavioral control. Ajzen's names for these constructs can be somewhat confusing in relation to other theories. We prefer using other terms: perceived social expectations for Ajzen's subjective norms, and self-efficacy for Ajzen's perceived behavioral control. Ajzen (1991) indicates that his perceived behavioral control is not really different from Bandura's (1986) self-efficacy (Salovey, Rothman, & Rodin, 1998).

TPB describes an attitude as a disposition to respond favorably or unfavorably to an object, behavior, person, institution, or event. In health promotion, it is mostly the attitude toward a behavior, "the individual's positive or negative evaluation of performing the particular behavior of interest" (Ajzen, 1988, p. 117), that health educators are concerned about. To understand attitudes toward a behavior, there must be correspondence, meaning that attitudes may predict behavior when both concepts are assessed at identical levels of action, context, and time.

The attitude toward the behavior is determined by salient beliefs about that behavior. Each behavioral belief links the behavior to a certain outcome or to an attribute (going on a low-fat diet reduces my blood pressure). Beliefs are weighted by the evaluations of those outcomes (a reduced blood pressure is very good for me). Fishbein and Ajzen (1975) distinguish between direct and indirect measures of the attitude. The direct attitude is measured by asking evaluative judgments about the behavior, for instance, always using a condom is [good versus bad, harmful versus beneficial, pleasant versus unpleasant]. The indirect attitude is the sum of the multiplication of each belief by its evaluation, for example, "always using a condom protects me from getting infected with an STD, [likely versus unlikely]" times "protecting me against infection with an STD is [good versus bad]." Direct and indirect attitudes are similar to Bandura's social cognitive constructs of outcome expectations and expectancies (Bandura, 1986).

The construct of perceived social expectations (subjective norms) is a function of beliefs that specific, important individuals or groups approve or disapprove of performing the behavior. The direct measure would be, for example, "most people around me think that I definitely should (or definitely should not) eat a low-fat diet." When given the specific social referents ("my partner thinks..." or "my mother thinks..."), the beliefs are termed normative beliefs. They are weighted by the motivation to comply with the referent person or group ("how much do you care what your partner thinks you should do?"). The indirect perceived social expectations are the sum of the multiplication of each normative belief by the motivation to comply. Some authors distinguish between social expectations and social pressure, the latter being described as a much stronger influence (De Vries, Backbier, Kok, & Dijkstra, 1995; Evans et al., 1978).

Self-efficacy (Bandura, 1986), or perceived behavioral control (Ajzen, 1988), refers to the subjective probability that a person is capable of executing a certain course of action. In TPB, this variable is directly measured by a number of questions in terms of "complete versus little control" or "easy versus difficult" ("for me to go on a low-fat diet would be [easy versus difficult]"). The indirect measure of perceived behavioral control would be the summed multiplication of control beliefs (e.g., "when eating out, there is a limited choice of fruit available [likely versus unlikely]") and power statements (e.g., "the limited choice of fruit makes my eating fruit... [likely versus unlikely]"; see Conner and Sparks, 1996). Ajzen sees perceived behavioral control as influencing behavior through intention and as influencing behavior directly (Montaño et al., 1997).

Other authors have suggested determinants in addition to the three that are currently in the theory. One suggestion is the addition of personal moral norms and anticipated regret. Personal moral norms are measured, for instance, as "I personally think I should always use a condom" (Godin, Fortin, Michaud, Bradet, & Kok, 1997; Godin, Savard, Kok, Fortin, & Boyer, 1996; Manstead & Parker, 1995). Anticipated regret is measured, for instance, as "how would you feel afterward if you had unprotected sex?" (Richard et al., 1996). Another current development is attention to the relation between intention and behavior. Studies on implementation intention show that helping people make plans to behave in a certain way (e.g., "exactly when and how do you think you will...") can improve the intention-behavior link (Orbell, Hodgkins, & Sheeran, 1997).

MEASUREMENT OF DETERMINANTS TPB gives very clear guidelines for measuring the determinants of behavior—starting with open, qualitative methods such as interviews and focus groups—to find all the salient factors, the prevalence and strength of which are then summarized through quantitative methods (De Vries et al., 1994). One well-researched topic, for example, is the onset of smoking in youth (various studies by De Vries and colleagues; see Kok, Schaalma, De Vries, Parcel, & Paulussen, 1996, for a summary). First, young people age 10 to 15 were asked about smoking, nonsmoking, and regular smoking in interviews or open response questionnaires to elicit salient outcome beliefs, normative beliefs, self-efficacy expectations, and intentions. Based on this eliciting procedure, structured questionnaires were developed, which consisted of

- beliefs and evaluations of the consequences of smoking (e.g., "if I smoke or should start to smoke, this is very [sociable versus unsociable]")

- normative beliefs and corresponding motivations to comply with respect to various social referents (e.g., mother, father, brothers, sisters, friends, classmates)
- self-efficacy expectations (e.g., students' perceived ability to refuse offers of cigarettes, to provide arguments against smoking, to resist social pressures to smoke)
- intentions regarding both initial and regular smoking (e.g., smoking with friends, smoking at parties)

The answers to these questions differentiated smoking from nonsmoking youth. For example, nonsmokers are more likely than smokers to endorse that smoking causes bad health consequences (e.g., cancer, coughing, nausea); that smoking has other bad effects (e.g., bad smell, high cost, tendency to offend others); and that there are negative social expectations regarding smoking (e.g., from parents, other relatives, friends, and classmates). Smoking students are more likely than nonsmokers to endorse the personal advantages of smoking (e.g., increased sociability; a good way to be nice, to show off, to relax, or to relieve boredom) and conformity, or the importance of belonging to a group and doing what others do.

Regular smoking was more closely connected with long-term effects such as health, whereas initial smoking was associated with short-term effects such as taste. Nonsmokers had higher self-efficacy for not smoking when friends smoke, refusing cigarettes, staying a nonsmoker, and explaining that they do not want to smoke. As a matter of fact, smokers reported negative self-efficacy about stating reasons to refuse a cigarette, not smoking when friends smoke, and becoming a nonsmoker.

USE AT HIGHER ECOLOGICAL LEVELS TPB is most often applied at the individual level. However, it can be applied to other ecological levels as well. For example, TPB has been used to examine the voting intentions of state legislators in North Carolina, Vermont, and Texas (B. S. Flynn et al., 1998; N. H. Gottlieb et al., 1999). General attitudes and norms concerning cigarette tax increases were predictive of legislators' intentions to vote for a cigarette tax increase (B. S. Flynn et al.). Normative influences that were significant were tobacco industry interests, constituent interests, legislative interests, and health interests (B. S. Flynn et al.). Legislators who intended to vote for enforcement of the minors' access legislation held strong outcome beliefs and evaluations about public health impact. The strongest normative beliefs were for health and medical lobbyists (e.g., "medical lobbyists expect me to . . ."), and motivation to comply was strongest for voters and medical lobbyists (e.g., "I care about what voters and lobbyists expect me to do").

The perceived impact of the cigarette tax legislation on retail sales, public health, and loss of political support for the next election—along with perceived behavioral control for getting the bill out of committee, voting for it, and passing it—were each associated with voting intention. These types of TPB findings can provide guidance to health educators in planning messages for advocacy efforts.

TPB has also been used to plan the implementation of health education program innovations (Paulussen, Kok, & Schaalma, 1994; Paulussen et al., 1995). Differences in beliefs, perceived social expectations, and self-efficacy were associated with different rates of diffusion, adoption, and implementation of an HIV prevention program by teachers. Diffusion was associated with social influence of colleagues through professional networks; adoption, with outcome expectations such as expected student satisfaction; implementation, with self-efficacy expectations about the proposed teaching strategies and with teacher's moral opinions on sexuality. Surprisingly, the effectiveness of the program had no influence on teachers' implementation decisions.

Uses in Problem Analysis and Intervention Methods

Intervention groups: Groups that can be differentiated according to their beliefs and intentions

Behaviors: Useful for understanding health risk behaviors when people are aware of the (negative) outcomes associated with continuing the behavior

Environment: Helps explain environmental barriers in relation to perceived self-efficacy; all its constructs can be used to explain behavior of agents at every ecological level

Determinants: Beliefs, attitudes, perceived social expectations, perceived self-efficacy

Methods: Does not suggest methods; other theories can be accessed for methods to change TPB-explained beliefs and intentions

Transtheoretical Model

The transtheoretical model (TTM) has two major sets of constructs: stages of change and processes of change (Prochaska & DiClemente, 1984; Prochaska, DiClemente, & Norcross, 1997). This model has been used to describe cessation of addictive behaviors and, more recently, to predict uptake of health-promoting behaviors. Further, both the stages of change and the processes of change are suggestive of intervention methods to stimulate change.

In the stages of change, people are thought to move from no motivation to change to internalization of the new behavior. The early stages are defined by the intention to change a problem behavior, whereas the later stages are defined by engaging in the new behavior. The first stage is precontemplation, in which people have no intention to change their behavior. In a successful change process, people make the transition to contemplation, in which they are thinking about changing the problem behavior in the next six months. Ideally, people then move to preparation, in which they are planning to change this behavior in the short term (one month). People who have recently changed the behavior are in the action stage, whereas people who have performed the new behavior for more than six months are in the maintenance stage. People in the action or maintenance stages may lapse and then recycle to action or relapse to contemplation or even precontemplation. A similar conceptualization, presented in Weinstein's (1988) precaution adoption model, includes (a) unaware; (b) aware, but not thinking about changing; (c) thinking; (d) intention; (e) action; and (f) maintenance.

TTM can be used to describe, explain, and predict behavior. As such, it is a model of behavioral determinants as well as a model of behavior change. An important contribution of the model is the specific tailoring of educational efforts to include different methods for individuals in different stages of change. Prochaska et al. (1997) describe processes of change that may be stimulated by different methods (see Chapter 6). Other authors have suggested processes for the various stages as well. Processes sometimes are clearly determinants of moving to the next stage; at other times they are very close to methods for promoting change. Holtgrave, Tinsley, and Kay (1995) suggest methods based on risk perception theories for the first two steps. Maibach and Cotton (1995) suggest methods based on social cognitive theory. De Vries and Backbier (1994) and Marlatt and Gordon (1985) provide additional methods. Table 4.3 defines the processes suggested by the authors of TTM and by others.

Table 4.3
Change Processes in the Transtheoretical Model

PROCESSES	DEFINITION
From precontemplation to contemplation	
Consciousness raising[a]	Finding and learning new facts, ideas, and tips to support a behavior change
Dramatic relief[a]	Experiencing the negative emotions (fear, anxiety, worry) that go along with the unhealthy behavioral risks
Environmental re-evaluation[a]	Realizing the negative impact of the unhealthful behavior and the positive impact of the healthful behavior
Risk comparison[b]	Comparing risks with similar dimensional profiles: dread, control, catastrophic potential, and novelty
Cumulative risk[b]	Processing cumulative probabilities instead of single incident probabilities
Qualitative and quantitative risks[b]	Processing both qualitative and quantitative expressions of risks
Positive framing[b]	Focusing on success framing instead of failure framing
Self-examination related to risk[c]	Risk perception: likelihood information, personalization, impact on others
Re-evaluation of outcomes[c]	Emphasizing positive outcomes of alternative behaviors and re-evaluating outcome expectancies
Perception of benefits[d]	Perceiving advantages of the healthy behavior and disadvantages of the risk behavior
From contemplation to preparation for action	
Self–re-evaluation[a]	Realizing that the behavioral change is an important part of a person's identity
Self-efficacy and social support[d]	Mobilizing social support; skills training on coping with emotional disadvantages of change

(continued)

Table 4.3 Change Processes in the Transtheoretical Model (continued)

PROCESSES	DEFINITION
Decision-making perspective[b]	Focusing on a decision-making perspective
Tailoring on time horizon[b]	Incorporating personal time horizons
Focus on important factors[b]	Incorporating factors with the highest importance
Trying out new behavior[c]	Changing something about oneself and gaining experience with that behavior
Persuasion of positive outcomes[c]	Promoting new positive outcome expectations and reinforcing existing ones
Modeling[c]	Showing models to effectively overcome barriers
From preparation to action	
Self-liberation[a]	Making a firm commitment to change
Skill improvement[c]	Restructuring environments to contain important, obvious, socially supported cues for the new behavior
Coping with barriers[c]	Identifying barriers and planning solutions to the behavior-change obstacles
Goal setting[c]	Setting specific and incremental goals
Modeling[c]	Perceiving models who receive social reinforcement of healthy behaviors
From action to maintenance	
Helping relationships[a]	Seeking and using social support for the healthy behavior change
Counterconditioning[a]	Substituting healthier alternative behaviors and cognitions for the unhealthy ones
Contingency management[a]	Increasing the rewards for the positive behavioral change and decreasing the rewards for the unhealthy behavior
Stimulus control[a]	Removing reminders or cues to engage in the unhealthy behavior and adding cues or reminders to engage in the healthy behavior
Social liberation[a]	Realizing that the social norms are changing in the direction of supporting the healthy behavior change
Skill enhancement[c]	Restructuring cues and social support; anticipating and circumventing obstacles; modifying goals
Dealing with barriers[c]	Understanding that setbacks are common and can be overcome
Self-rewards for success[c]	Feeling good about progress; reiterating positive consequences
Maintenance	
Coping skills[e]	Identifying high-risk situations; selecting solutions; practicing solutions; coping with lapses

[a]Prochaska, DiClemente, & Norcross, 1997; [b]Holtgrave, Tinsley, & Kay, 1995; [c]Maibach & Cotton, 1995; [d]De Vries & Backbier, 1994; [e]Marlatt & Gordon, 1985.

Uses in Problem Analysis and Intervention Methods

Individual Theories

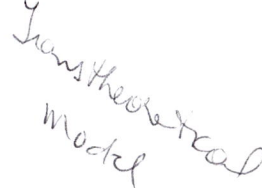
Transtheoretical Model

Intervention groups: People in precontemplation, contemplation, preparation, action, and maintenance should be differentiated

Behaviors: Originally helpful for addictive behaviors; currently work is being done for a variety of behaviors

Environment: Suggests environmental barriers for change; is also relevant for considering behavior change of agents at the various environmental levels

Determinants: Stages help define the determinants of various behaviors, which are different for each stage

Methods: Suggests that intervention might be necessary for people not to remain stuck in early stages, and methods should be tailored to stages; processes of change provide guidance for the selection of methods

Persuasion Communication Model

One general theory for behavior change is McGuire's (1985) Persuasion Communication Model (PCM). It is used in public health education somewhat differently from the way McGuire originally intended (Kok et al., 1996). In the original model, McGuire distinguishes the following stages: exposure to the message, attention to the message, comprehension of the arguments and conclusions, acceptance of the arguments, retention of the content resulting from information integration, and attitude change (Hamilton & Hunter, 1998). Health educators use this model to describe an individual's progression from an initial response to an educational message, through intermediate processes, to change of behavior in the desired direction.

Table 4.4 presents McGuire's (1985) persuasion communication matrix. The first steps posit that successful communication should result in attention and comprehension by the receiver. The subsequent steps refer to the receiver's changes in attitudes, social influences, self-efficacy, and behavior, and the last step refers to the maintenance of that behavior change. McGuire argues that educational interventions should match each step. Choices of the content of the message, the program audience, the communication context, and the message source depend on the step that is addressed. For instance, certain mass media

---

The mayor's health educator has an enlarged persuasion communication matrix on the office wall. When creating a health education intervention, the health educator refers to the matrix so as to consider all important elements of successful communication. No subgroup of the committee is reviewing the contribution of the persuasion communication model to the understanding of violence, but the health educator plans to make sure the committee reviews its program plans from McGuire's perspective.

messages, such as statements by famous sports heroes, may attract a lot of attention but may have negative effects on self-efficacy. An important contribution of PCM is that every method that uses communication will have to go through the steps for successful communication in order to have any effect at all. Protocols for pilot testing or pretesting of educational materials should apply these steps, and in practice, most of them do (National Cancer Institute, 1989).

PCM can accommodate a host of social psychological variables that have been found to influence attitude and behavior (McGuire, 1985). However, for many of these variables, the relationship to attitude and behavior change is ambiguous. McGuire explains this ambiguity by distinguishing differential effects on reception of the message (i.e., successful communication) and yielding to the message (i.e., attitude and behavior change). One variable—for instance, the use of celebrities in persuasive messages—can have a positive effect on reception but a negative effect on yielding. Almost no variables have a universal, unidirectional effect on attitude and behavior change.

Petty and Cacioppo (1986) have caused a dramatic new perspective on persuasion effects with their elaboration likelihood model (ELM). The basic idea of ELM is that people differ in the ability and motivation for thoughtful information processing of educational messages. These authors explain two ways of information processing: central or peripheral (also called systematic versus heuristic; Chaiken, 1987). Central processing occurs when a message is carefully considered and compared against other messages and beliefs. Peripheral processing occurs when a message is processed without thoughtful consideration or comparison. For example, a student learning about self-efficacy for the first time can process the information centrally by comparing his or her own self-efficacy

Table 4.4
Persuasion Communication Matrix

	MESSAGE CONTENT	GROUP	COMMUNICATION CONTEXT	MESSAGE SOURCE
ATTENTION				
COMPREHENSION				
ATTITUDES				
SOCIAL INFLUENCES				
SELF-EFFICACY				
BEHAVIOR				
MAINTENANCE				

for several different behaviors. He or she can continue the central processing by trying to find situations wherein self-efficacy seems to be important in choosing to attempt a behavior or in choosing to maintain effort. Pollay and colleagues (1996) suggest that peripheral cues are systematically used in tobacco advertisements for youth because these cues tend to bypass logical analysis. A variable—for instance, source credibility of a sports hero as a role model—may have a positive effect when receivers process the message through the peripheral route but a negative effect when they follow the central route, because people realize that their behavioral capabilities are different from those of the sports hero. The same variable, source credibility, may also influence the motivation and ability to think, thus shifting people from the peripheral route to the central route or vice versa (Petty & Wegener, 1997). ELM has been very successful in explaining persuasion effects retrospectively, but is as yet less successful in predicting persuasion effects prospectively.

Research findings suggest that thoughtful information processing is related to a higher persistence of attitude change, a higher resistance to counterpersuasion, and a stronger attitude-behavior consistency (Petty & Cacioppo, 1986). Health educators would thus like to promote thoughtful information processing as much as possible. ELM suggests two ways to stimulate motivation to think about the message: make the message more personally relevant and unexpected, and repeat it.

Uses in Problem Analysis and Intervention Methods

Intervention groups: Points out that intended program recipients may be at different stages at which they have (or have not) reached awareness, comprehension, attitude change, social support, sufficient self-efficacy, behavior change, or maintenance, and that they may tend to process the messages with either high or low elaboration likelihood; therefore, health educators should either differentiate by stage or include all stages in intervention

Behaviors: Applicable to any behavior that can be influenced by communication

Environment: Complexity of the available information hinders information processing; information processing can also be disturbed by external factors

Determinants: Different by stage

Methods: Principles of increasing thoughtful information processing, of tailoring intervention methods to stage, and of successful communication; effects by stage; use of the matrix to plan all communication decisions

Goal-Setting Theory

Goal setting leads to better performance because people with goals exert themselves more, persevere in their tasks, concentrate more, and if necessary, develop strategies for carrying out the behavior. Goal-setting theory is clearly a theory of action and describes a particular method for behavior change. In AIDS prevention, for example, the health educator may attempt to associate safe sex with important goals of students, such as careers that might be threatened by consequences of unsafe sex. In this way, safe sex becomes part of the strategy to attain long-term goals.

Goal setting in health education also may be directly related to the health behavior. In the Cystic Fibrosis Family Education Program, for example, parents and children work with health care providers to set goals regarding self-care, such as increasing calories a certain amount or keeping a record of symptom change (Bartholomew et al., 1991). To provide the context for the self-care goals, health care providers also work with the families to clarify life goals seemingly unrelated to health. For example, a child may set a goal to try out for the school tennis team. She may need to improve weight and fitness to do so; therefore, she sets specific eating and exercise goals.

A goal should be behaviorally specific and measurable or observable. Strecher and colleagues (1995) advise that goals should be stated in terms of behavior (e.g., exercise behavior and food intake) instead of health outcomes (e.g., weight loss). Locke and Latham (1991) have demonstrated that setting a challenging goal, in other words, a goal that is difficult though feasible, leads to a better performance than does setting an easy goal or no goal at all. This positive effect of difficult goals occurs only if a person accepts the challenge and has sufficient experience, self-efficacy, and feedback to be able to perform adequately. The rewards for reaching the goal are not only the expected outcomes but also a sense of self-satisfaction. Goal setting may not be effective when the task is too complex. In that case the educator can provide subgoals and suggest strategies (e.g., not to quit smoking permanently, but first to abstain for one week and then set a new goal).

Uses in Problem Analysis and Intervention Methods

Intervention groups: People who are high or low in self-efficacy and skills need different goals

Behaviors: All behaviors in which feedback is feasible

Environment: Complexity or difficulty of goals should match the individual's skills

Determinants: Self-efficacy and skills

Methods: Goal setting through difficult goals, acceptance of goal, and feedback

Attribution Theory

An important variable in many models that try to explain determinants of behavior is self-efficacy. But what are the determinants of self-efficacy? Weiner (1986) suggests that self-efficacy (Weiner calls this *expectancy of success,* but we prefer *self-efficacy*) is determined by the perceived stability of the attributions for success and failure. Attribution theory describes the impact of the way people attribute the outcomes of behavior on their future cognition and behavior. Weiner distinguishes attributional dimensions. For the understanding of self-efficacy expectations for health behavior change, stability is the relevant dimension. A person attributing a failure to a stable cause (e.g., ability) will have a lower self-efficacy for performing the same task again compared to somebody who attributes a failure on the same task to an unstable cause (e.g., bad luck). For success, this effect is reversed. Furthermore, attribution theory suggests that lower self-efficacy leads to a less adaptive task behavior; people will invest less energy in the task at hand. Hospers, Kok, and Strecher (1990) report an attribution explanation of health behavior. They found in their study that success of participants in a weight reduction program was positively related to the participants' self-efficacy at the start of the program. Self-efficacy was inversely related to stability of attributions for earlier failures, and both relationships were independent of the number of failures.

A method for changing attributions to improve self-efficacy is called attributional retraining, or reattribution (Kok et al., 1992). The health educator or counselor tries to help people reinterpret previous failures in terms of unstable attributions ("you were in a very difficult situation there") and previous successes in terms of stable attributions ("you have been able to stay off cigarettes during your whole pregnancy!"). Attributional retraining is an often-used method in attempts to prevent relapse (Marlatt & Gordon, 1985). Relapses are caused by a lack of coping response when a person lapses in a high-risk situation. Relapse prevention theory suggests that people can learn adequate coping responses by identifying high-risk situations and practicing personal coping responses.

Uses in Problem Analysis and Intervention Methods

Intervention groups: People who make stable versus unstable attributions for failure

Behaviors: All behaviors with success or failure characteristics

Environment: Real barriers that may be too difficult even with high self-efficacy

Determinants: Stable versus unstable attributions for failure

Methods: Attributional retraining; relapse prevention training

Health Belief Model

Historically, a number of theories have focused directly on health and risk-related behavior (Weinstein, 1988). A model that has been used in a wide range of health-related contexts is the health belief model (HBM; Becker, 1974; Janz & Becker, 1984; Rosenstock, Strecher, & Becker, 1988; Strecher & Rosenstock, 1997). The basic components of the HBM are based on psychological expectancy-value models. These models hypothesize that human behavior depends mainly on the value placed by an individual on a particular goal, and on an estimate of the likelihood that a given action will achieve that goal. With respect to health, the components are the desire to avoid illness or to get well and the belief that specific behavior will prevent or reduce illness.

HBM consists of four psychological variables (Janz & Becker, 1984). Perceived susceptibility refers to a person's subjective perception of the risk of contracting a particular condition or illness (perceived personal risk). Perceived severity is a person's feelings concerning the seriousness of contracting an illness. Perceived benefits is a person's belief regarding the effectiveness of various actions available to reduce the threat of a disease. Perceived barriers refers to potential negative aspects of a particular health action. In other words, an individual's decision to engage in a health action is determined by perceptions of personal susceptibility to, and the severity of, a particular condition or illness. The specific action taken is based on an informal cost-benefit analysis of perceived benefits and barriers. According to HBM, this decision-making process is triggered by a cue to action, which may be internal (e.g., symptoms of a disease) or external (e.g., a health education message). However, the influence of the cue to action has not been studied empirically.

Although an impressive body of research findings has linked HBM dimensions to health actions (Harrison, Mullen, & Green, 1992; Janz & Becker, 1984), recent research has demonstrated the importance of factors that were not originally examined in the context of the model. For example, many health-related behaviors are undertaken for ostensibly nonhealth reasons, suggesting that people's cost-benefit analysis should include benefits other than health beliefs. Current general social psychological models suggest that an individual's behavior, including health-related behavior, is also determined by perceptions of social influences and self-efficacy (Ajzen, 1988; Bandura, 1986). In later descriptions of HBM, these variables were incorporated, self-efficacy specifically and the role of social influences more generally (Rosenstock et al., 1988; Strecher, DeVellis, Becker, & Rosenstock, 1986). HBM may be most helpful in understanding relatively simple health behaviors, such as mammography screening or immunization. However, HBM has been shown to have some predictive validity for other problems, such as diabetes self-care.

HBM is a descriptive model of determinants of behavior and does not suggest specific methods for behavioral change, except for the cue to action, which is the weakest concept in the theory so far. HBM does give clear guidelines for the factors that should be changed, but not on how they may be changed.

An alternative model that has the same basic ingredients is the protection motivation theory (PMT; Boer & Seydel, 1996; Rogers, 1975, 1983, 1985; Salovey et al., 1998). PMT suggests that people will try to control the danger, but they will also try to control the associated fear. Low response efficacy and low self-efficacy may lead to maladaptive behavior. The person at risk may avoid the health education message but not the behavior. Empirical studies show that a high threat may result in health-promoting behavior, but only in combination with high self-efficacy (Ruiter, Kok, & Abraham, 1999).

Uses in Problem Analysis and Intervention Methods

Intervention groups: Groups can be differentiated according to their beliefs

Behaviors: Originally for health protective behaviors; currently for all health-promoting behaviors

Environment: Perceived environmental barriers in relation to perceived benefits

Determinants: Perceived susceptibility, perceived severity, perceived benefits (e.g., outcome expectations), and perceived barriers (e.g., self-efficacy)

Methods: Principle of tailoring to determinants; cues to action

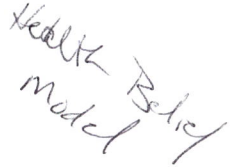

Health Belief Model (handwritten)

Self-Regulatory Theories

Self-regulatory conceptualizations have to do with how individuals function to behaviorally self-correct. Various authors' descriptions of this process are presented in Table 4.5. The general procedure is (a) the monitoring of some aspect of behavior or health; (b) comparing one's observations with baseline or normal, describing a problem or divergence from normal, and analyzing the causes of the problem; and (c) trying a behavioral correction. The entire process recycles with a return to monitoring (Clark & Zimmerman, 1990). This theory, like coping theory (Lazarus, 1993; Lazarus & Folkman, 1991), is useful for the designation of health-promoting behaviors for the self-management of chronic disease. For example, in a pediatric asthma self-management program, Bartholomew and

Table 4.5
Self-Regulatory Theory

AUTHORS	CONSTRUCT NAMES		
	Monitoring	Evaluation	Action
Clark & Zimmerman, 1990	Self-observation	Self-judgment	Self-reaction
Kotses, Lewis, & Creer, 1990	Monitoring	Comparing to personal best	Normal activity Control of the disease
Creer, Kotses, & Wigal, 1992	Information collection	Information processing and evaluation	Self-management skills Self-instruction Treatment steps
Lazarus & Folkman, 1991	Appraisal	Problem description	Generation of flexible solutions
Thoresen & Kirmil-Gray, 1983	Self-monitoring	Self-evaluation	Action Self-reinforcement

colleagues conceptualized both asthma-specific skills (e.g., taking control medications) and self-regulatory skills (e.g., monitoring for symptoms of asthma) (see Chapter 11; Bartholomew, Gold, et al., 2000; Bartholomew, Shegog, et al., 2000; Shegog et al., 1999). The teaching of self-regulatory skills has been demonstrated in the school setting (Schunk, 1998; Schunk & Zimmerman, 1994). In the asthma program the skills were called Watch, Discover, Think, and Act. Children were taught to watch or monitor their asthma symptoms, discover whether there was a problem and what might be causing it, decide on a plan of action to solve the problem or to prevent a future problem, and take action.

In another example of the application of self-regulatory theory to the delineation of self-management behavior, Cox, Gonder-Frederick, Julian, and Clarke (1994) taught diabetics to prevent both hypoglycemia and hyperglycemia by providing self-regulatory skill training and practice. They increased sensitivity to symptoms, promoted identification of external events such as insulin administration or food intake that can change the likelihood of blood sugar peaks and dips, and helped participants create effective responses to internal and external cues.

In the Cystic Fibrosis Family Education Project, Bartholomew and colleagues (1993) used coping theory to delineate performance objectives for the self-management of cystic fibrosis. Applying work by Lazarus (1993) that suggests coping is situation specific, should be judged by its effectiveness, and depends on accurate appraisal of situations and flexibility in problem-solving alternatives, the cystic fibrosis project team specified the coping objectives in Table 4.6.

Uses in Problem Analysis and Intervention Methods

Intervention groups: People who are trying to incorporate complex behaviors into their lifestyle

Behaviors: Performance objectives for self-regulatory behaviors, that is, monitoring, evaluation, action

Environment: Helps the learner explicitly consider the role of the environment in the performance of certain behaviors, for example, to appraise the environment in the monitoring phase

Determinants: Particularly useful in the definition of behavior and performance objectives (Chapter 5); therefore, can be seen as a determinant of behavioral capability

Methods: Does not suggest methods; however, skill training is important to teach self-regulation, and motivation is a prerequisite

INTERPERSONAL THEORIES

Social Cognitive Theory

Bandura's (1986) social cognitive theory (SCT) covers both determinants of behavior and the process of behavior change (Bandura, 1997; Baranowski, Perry, & Parcel, 1997). SCT explains human behavior "in terms of a model of reciprocal

Table 4.6
What Family Members Will Do to Cope with Cystic Fibrosis

Recognize need to cope with CF
    Accept CF as the medical diagnosis (e.g., genetics, prognosis, variable course)
    Acknowlege potential extent of the physical effects of CF
    Acknowledge that disease-related problems may occur at any time
    Recognize need for adjustment by child and family to the demands of self-care
    Accept the occurrence of emotional distress to the child and family as a periodic consequence of CF

Appraise situations for potential problems related to CF
    Identify sources of stress
    Identify personal and family signs of stress
    Estimate likelihood of undesirable outcomes from stressful situations

Generate multiple coping alternatives, including categories of action, stopping action, information seeking, and thinking or feeling about things differently
    Acknowledge the value of using a variety of coping strategies (flexibility)
    Generate alternatives to solve problems, including strategies of seeking information and of social support
    Generate alternatives to ameliorate emotional distress, such as seeking distraction and social support and practicing anxiety management

Use selected alternatives from the coping strategies that were generated
    Use a variety of strategies to solve problems
    Use a variety of strategies to ameliorate emotional distress

Evaluate effectiveness of coping strategies used
    Judge whether problem has been solved
    Judge whether new problems have been created through application of coping strategies
    Judge whether emotional distress has been reduced
    Recycle to appraisal if coping strategy not judged effective

Note. CF = cystic fibrosis.

determinism in which behavior, cognitive and other personal factors, and environmental events all operate as interacting determinants of each other" (Bandura, 1986, p.18). Major determinants of behavior described by SCT are outcome expectations, self-efficacy, behavioral capability, perceived behavior of others, and environment.

CONSTRUCTS   An outcome expectation is a judgment of the likely consequence that a certain behavior will produce ("when I use a condom consistently, I will prevent STDs"). Outcome expectancies are the values that individuals place on a certain outcome. Outcome expectations are comparable to behavioral beliefs in TPB, and outcome expectancies are comparable to evaluations.

Self-efficacy is a judgment of a person's capability to accomplish a certain level of performance ("I am confident that I can use a condom consistently"). Bandura (1986) is very explicit about the interrelation between outcome expectations and self-efficacy: "The types of outcomes people anticipate depend largely on their judgments of how well they will be able to perform in given situations" (p. 392). So, when people are not confident that they can use a condom consistently, they may also not expect to prevent STDs. Some studies have found an interaction effect between self-efficacy and outcome expectations. When a person is in a situation in which outcome expectations are positive and strong but self-efficacy for that behavior is low, a situation of avoidance or denial may occur and the person is unlikely to attempt the behavior.

The concept of behavioral capability is that if people are to perform a particular type of behavior, they must know what the behavior is (knowledge of the behavior) and how to perform the behavior (skill). Self-efficacy is a person's perception; capability is the real thing. Health education programs should go beyond knowledge to provide behavioral capability, which is closer to actual performance. The development of behavioral capability is the result of the individual's training, intellectual capacity, and learning style. The behavioral training technique called mastery learning provides cognitive knowledge of what is to be performed, practice in performing those activities, and feedback about successful performance.

Most human behavior is learned by observation through modeling, or vicarious learning. By observing others, a person forms rules of behavior, and on future occasions this coded information serves as guides for action. Four constituent processes govern modeling:

- Attention to and perception of the relevant aspects of modeled activities (including characteristics of the observer and the model)
- Retention and representation of learned knowledge and remembering
- Production of appropriate action
- Motivation as a result of observed positive incentives and reinforcement

When providing models to encourage the learning of certain behaviors, the health educator should find a role model from the community or at-risk group that will encourage identification. The model should present a coping model (e.g., "I tried to quit smoking several times and was not successful, then I . . . Now I have been off cigarettes for . . .") rather than a mastery model (e.g., "I just threw my pack away and that was it"). Models also should be observed being reinforced for their behavior (e.g., being congratulated by friends for staying off cigarettes, having a partner say how fresh the ex-smoker smells).

Perceived behavior of others has to be distinguished from perceived social expectations (TPB): smoking parents may be contributing to their child taking up smoking (a model) while they may expect their child not to smoke (perceived social expectation). The term *environment* refers to an objective notion of all the factors that can affect a person's behavior but that are physically external to that person. The social environment includes, for instance, family members, peers, and neighbors. The physical environment includes, for instance, availability of certain foods, indoor and outdoor air quality, and restrictions for smoking. Individuals may or may not be aware of the strong influence that the environment has on their behavior. Likewise, health educators may underutilize the role of environment in their program planning; keeping the concept of reciprocal determinism in mind will help planners avoid this pitfall.

COLLECTIVE EFFICACY   In addition to personal self-efficacy, Bandura (1997) describes perceived collective efficacy, belief in the performance capability of a social system as a whole. Defined as "a group's shared belief in its conjoint capabilities to organize and execute the courses of action required to produce given levels of attainments" (p. 477), collective efficacy may be applied to the levels of family, community, organizations, social institutions, and nation. Although related to personal self-efficacy, it is an emergent group-level attribute that is more than the sum of members' perceived personal efficacies. It emerges from the social interdependence of individuals performing tasks and carrying out roles. Specific types of collective efficacy include perceived organizational efficacy (employees' beliefs that their work team or organization can accomplish its goals) and perceived political efficacy (people's beliefs that they can influence the political system). As with personal efficacy, specificity with collective efficacy is important, and collective efficacy should be measured for particular behaviors rather than globally. For example, collective efficacy in organizations might be specific to scanning the environment for trends, to product development, or to marketing. Political efficacy has subcomponents such as efficacy for voting, fund-raising, voter registration, and lobbying.

Collective efficacy has been less well researched than has personal efficacy. However, teachers' collective efficacy has been linked to the academic performance of students in elementary schools; workers' collective efficacy has been linked to the performance of self-managing work teams; and players' collective efficacy has been linked to athletic teams' performance. Perceived protest efficacy (a specific form of political efficacy) along with strong outcome expectations of harm were found to be predictive of people's willingness to protest the placement of a chemical plant in their community (Bandura, 1997).

Change in collective efficacy comes through the same mechanisms that change does in personal efficacy. The most effective way to enhance a community's collective efficacy is through success at accomplishing a particular goal, for example, lobbying the city council to pass a clean indoor air act for the city. Models of how other communities accomplished similar goals could also enhance efficacy, as might community leaders challenging the community members to take action.

SCT AND BEHAVIOR CHANGE   SCT integrates determinants of behavior with methods for behavior change. All SCT interventions are based on active learning that promotes performance during the learning process. Perceived behavior of others is not only a determinant of behavior, it is also a very effective method for behavior change: modeling. A general method of SCT is reinforcement, of which modeling is a specific case: A person may experience vicarious reinforcement by observing a model receiving reinforcement. Reinforcements (or incentives) may be external (receiving money) or internal (doing something that is perceived as right). Self-efficacy and behavioral capability may be improved through

- enactive mastery experiences with feedback to serve as indicators of capability
- vicarious experiences (modeling) that alter efficacy expectations through perception of competencies and comparison with the attainment of others
- verbal persuasion and allied types of social influences that suggest the person, agent, or group possesses certain capabilities
- enhancement or reduction of physiological and affective states (e.g., anxiety) from which people partly judge their own capability, strength, and vulnerability to dysfunction (Bandura, 1997)

Uses in Problem Analysis and Intervention Methods

Intervention groups: No specification

Behaviors: Any behavior; but is usually applied to behaviors that are complex and require extensive behavioral capability

Environment: Real barriers may be too difficult even with high self-efficacy; there is a strong impact of the social and the physical environment

Determinants: Outcome expectations, self-efficacy expectations, behavioral capability, perceived behavior of others; social and physical environment

Methods: Active learning, reinforcement, modeling and guided practice, persuasion

Social Network and Social Support Theories

SOCIAL NETWORKS Social relationships are the foundation for human existence. The concept of social network is an analytic framework for understanding relationships among members of social systems. Networks are classified as personal, based on the ties an individual has with other persons, or whole network, based on the relationships among a defined group of people. Personal, or egocentric, networks are particularly useful for the study of social support, whereas the whole network approach allows the identification of cliques of individuals and the identification of roles, such as occupational positions, that extend across networks (boundary spanners). Networks can be horizontal or vertical and provide a way to understand power relationships in organizations. Community can be understood metaphorically as networks of networks in which the nodes of the larger network comprise smaller-scale networks (B. H. Gottlieb, 1985; N. H. Gottlieb & McLeroy, 1994; Hall & Wellman, 1985).

Sociologists have referred to the actual and potential resources available to an individual through a network as social capital. Individuals are able to secure benefits through membership in networks—such as those defined by kinship, ethnicity, or friendship—or through other social structures. Portes (1998) points out that such social capital may result not only in positive consequences, such as observance of norms, family support, and network-mediated benefits, but also in potentially negative consequences of restricted access to opportunities, constraints on individual freedom, and excessive claims on group members. The focus on social capital, like social support, has been on the positive outcomes of these social networks. Putnam (1993, 1995) has extended the concept of social capital to communities and described it as "civicness"—involvement and participatory behavior. Within health education, Green and Kreuter (1999) have defined social capital as structures and processes among people and organizations that lead to accomplishing goals with outcomes of mutual social benefit. High social capital is manifest in high levels of four interrelated constructs: trust, cooperation, civic engagement, and reciprocity. Social capital and the aggregate effect of social connections seem to be related to increased community problem solving and have been discussed as aspects of community capacity by Goodman and colleagues (1988). (See Chapter 2.)

Social networks consist of nodes (individuals, groups, or organizations) that are joined by ties (the relationships among nodes). Networks can be defined by their content—whether they are primarily friendship, kinship, communication, or task-oriented organizational networks. The network also has a structure, including the number of members, how similar they are to each other, how they are connected, and their links to other networks. Definitions of key structural properties of social networks are seen in Table 4.7. An individual can play several roles in a network: a group member, a linking agent, or an isolate with few ties to other network members (Fulk & Boyd, 1991). Linking agents are especially important because, as members of other networks, they bring information across network boundaries.

SOCIAL SUPPORT The egocentric social network, defined as a person-centered web of social relationships, is the structure through which social support may be provided. Social support is defined as "aid and assistance exchanged through social relationships and interpersonal transactions" (Heaney & Israel, 1997, p. 181). In contrast to other types of interpersonal interactions, such as criticism and domination, social support is always intended by the sender to be helpful. Four main types of social support have been identified: emotional (affective), instrumental (tangible), informational (cognitive), and appraisal (Heaney & Israel). Emotional support includes love, caring, and empathy. Instrumental support includes aid or service, such as babysitting or lending a person money. Informational support is the giving of information, advice, or suggestions. Appraisal support, a special form of cognitive support, merits its own category; it is self-evaluative information that is important for maintenance of a person's identity. This information includes constructive feedback, affirmation of beliefs

Table 4.7
Structural and Relationship Properties of Social Networks

STRUCTURAL PROPERTIES

Range	The number of network members
Density	The extent to which a network is connected; measured by the proportion of direct ties that exist among network members out of all possible ties that could exist among them
Degree	The extent to which a network member has direct ties with other network members
Boundedness	The proportion of all ties of network members that stay within the network's boundaries
Reachability	The average number of ties required to link any two network members
Homogeneity	The extent to which network members have similar characteristics (age, race, gender, economic status, etc.)
Cliques	Portions of networks in which all members are tied directly
Clusters	Portions of networks in which not all members are tied directly
Components	Portions of networks in which all members are tied directly or indirectly

RELATIONSHIP PROPERTIES

Strength	The quantity of resources between two network members
Frequency	The quantity of contact between two network members
Multiplexity	The number of different types of social support exchanged between two network members
Duration	The length of time a relationship has existed
Symmetry	The extent to which social support is both given and received between two network members
Intimacy	The perceived emotional closeness between two network members

Note. From "Social Health," by N. H. Gottlieb and K. R. McLeroy, 1994, in M. P. O'Donnell and J. S. Harris, Eds., *Health Promotion in the Workplace* (2nd ed., pp. 459–493), Albany, NY: Delmar; from "Social Networks and Social Support," by A. Hall and B. Wellman, 1985, in S. Cohen and L. Syme, Eds., *Social Support and Health,* New York: Academic Press; and from "Social Networks and Health Status: Linking Theory, Research, and Practice," by B. A. Israel, 1982, *Patient Counseling and Health Education,* 4(2), pp. 65–79.

and values, and social comparison (N. H. Gottlieb & McLeroy, 1994; Heaney & Israel).

Different types of social networks are associated with specific types of social support. Small, dense, geographically close, intense networks provide affective and appraisal support. These networks typically do not have access to the larger society or to information outside the network's domain. On the other hand, large, diffuse, and less intense networks provide more informational support and social outreach. Different types of social support are important at different times in the experience of stressors. For example, with loss of a job, affective support that the individual is still loved and his or her self is intact is most important at first. Later, informational support regarding other job opportunities or possible career changes is needed. Tangible support, such as loans, transportation, or child care, may also help people when they are job hunting.

The extent and nature of social relationships has been linked to health status in a number of studies, and we refer the reader to comprehensive reviews (Heaney & Israel, 1997; House, Umberson, & Landis, 1988; Israel & Rounds, 1987). The mechanisms underlying this epidemiological finding have been hypothesized to include modeling and reinforcement of positive health-related behaviors, buffering of the effects of stress on health, and providing access to resources to cope with stress (Heaney & Israel; House et al.).

The health benefits of social support have been studied extensively in the area of breast cancer, where social network interventions have been specifically designed to increase health. Spiegel, Bloom, Kraemer, and Gottheil (1989) conducted a study in which the researchers assessed the effects of support groups on the emotional state of women with advanced breast cancer. In addition to finding that the support groups helped the women emotionally, they discovered that the women lived an average of 18 months longer than did women with comparable severity of breast cancer and medical care who did not attend support groups. Other studies investigating the effects of social support on cancer have found similar positive relationships (Ell, 1984; Funch & Mettlin, 1982; Northouse, 1988; Peter-Golden, 1982). Although support from intervention groups is beneficial, the emotional support provided by the woman's partner and family has been shown to be the most significant predictor of physical and psychological well-being of women with breast cancer (Lichtman, Taylor, & Wood, 1987).

SOCIAL SUPPORT INTERVENTIONS   Heaney and Israel (1997) identify four types of intervention to increase social support. First is the enhancement of existing social network linkages, which can be accomplished by training network members in skills for providing support and by training members of the target group to mobilize and maintain their networks. For example, family members may be trained to provide support to individuals who are in smoking cessation programs (Cohen & Lichtenstein, 1990; Mermelstein, Cohen, Lichtenstein, Baer, & Kamarck, 1986). In another example of enhancing existing linkages, the STOP AIDS Project in San Francisco worked through existing formal and informal social groups to enhance social support for safe sex as part of its community-organizing strategy. Many groups that the organizers approached were reluctant to provide an organized discussion about AIDS and the role friends play in encouraging safe sex and discouraging unsafe sex, because their goals were unrelated. However, organizations as diverse as a gay marching band, a gay Catholic group, and informal social networks participated in the STOP AIDS workshops and discussions (Wohlfeiler, 1997). A media campaign, "Good Friends Make Good Medicine," focused on informing people about the influence of social support on health and encouraging them to connect with their friends and family by phone or in person and to trade favors and share feelings with them (Hersey, Kibanoff, Lam, & Taylor, 1984).

The second type of intervention develops new social network linkages through mentor programs, buddy systems, and self-help groups. Groups such as Alcoholics Anonymous, Overeaters Anonymous, and Weight Watchers provide access to new social networks designed to provide cognitive, instrumental, and affective support for behavioral and life change. Third, indigenous or natural helpers have been employed to enhance networks, particularly around health issues. They are identified from the community and provided with training to increase their knowledge and skills on health topics, resources, and social support. Such helpers have focused on prenatal care (Meister, Warrick, de Zapien, & Wood, 1992), health promotion (Eng & Hatch, 1991), breast cancer screening (Eng & Smith, 1995; Skinner et al., 1998), stress of urban women with children (Parker, Schulz, Israel, & Hollis, 1998), and hunger (Eng & Parker, 1994). Finally, networks can be enhanced at the community level through participatory problem-solving processes. In the Tenderloin Senior Organizing Project, networks of elderly residing in single-room occupancy hotels received leadership training and consultation for problem solving and advocacy around such topics as housing policies and security (Minkler, 1997a).

> *Uses in Problem Analysis and Intervention Methods*
>
> Intervention groups: Networks of individuals are the focus for social support interventions; networks of organizations and individuals are the focus for interventions to increase social capital
>
> Behaviors: Provision of emotional, instrumental, informational, and appraisal support by the network and, for individuals, the mobilization of support from their networks; for community social capital, relevant behaviors include citizen participation, information sharing, and volunteering
>
> Environment: Social networks are an environmental characteristic themselves
>
> Determinants: Network characteristics of reciprocity, intensity, complexity, density, and homogeneity
>
> Methods: Methods to enhance existing networks include training members in skills to provide support and training individuals to mobilize and maintain their networks; includes training of indigenous natural helpers and using participatory problem-solving processes; methods to develop new social networks include mentor programs, buddy systems, and self-help groups

ORGANIZATIONAL CHANGE MODELS AND THEORIES

In this section, we introduce several theories and models underlying organizational change, which may include changes in organizational norms and structures. We begin with a model of the stages through which changes are made and then move to a general discussion of organizational development and the processes that can facilitate changes.

Stage Theory of Organizational Change

In their work on the establishment of employee assistance programs in U.S. government agencies, Beyer and Trice (1978) developed a stage theory of organization change that has been used in health education practice (Goodman, Steckler, & Kegler, 1997; see Chapter 8). An organization moves sequentially through seven stages as a health promotion innovation is adopted and institutionalized. The stages are as follows:

- Sensing unsatisfied demands on the system, in which a problem is noted and brought to the surface
- Searching for possible responses, in which solutions to the demand are sought
- Evaluating alternatives, in which the potential solutions are judged
- Deciding to adopt a course of action, in which one of a number of alternative responses is selected
- Initiating action within the system, which requires policy changes and resources necessary for implementation
- Implementing the change, which includes actually putting the innovation into practice and usually requires some organization members to change their work behaviors and relationships
- Institutionalizing the change, in which the change is included in strategic plans, job descriptions, and budgets so that it is a routine part of organizational operations

The key actors involved in change have been found to differ from stage to stage (Miles & Huberman, 1999). Senior-level administrators with political skills are important in the early stages—in which a problem is surfaced, alternative solutions discussed, and a choice made and initiated within the organization—and at the stage of institutionalization. Mid-level administrators are active during adoption and the early implementation stages, in which administrative skills to introduce procedures and provide training on the innovation are critical. The people who need to make changes in their practice are the focus of the implementation process. Examples are teachers for curriculum innovation or food service workers for an innovation in cafeteria food preparation. The focus here is on people's professional and technical skills. Of course, because the agents and behaviors are different at different stages, the determinants change as well. For example, at the decision stage organizational leaders might be persuaded by the characteristics of the intervention, whereas implementation might be determined to a great extent by skills, feedback, and reinforcement.

Organizational development approaches have taken into account stages in the diffusion of a tobacco prevention curriculum to school districts by Goodman and colleagues (Goodman, Smith, Dawson, & Steckler, 1991; Goodman et al., 1997; Smith, Steckler, McCormick, & McLeroy, 1995). Different organizational development interventions were used at different stages of diffusion. One intervention consisted of meetings with senior district administrators to raise their awareness of tobacco use prevention and to encourage them to adopt the project. Another was to help districts address concerns associated with potential adoption of the project combined with intensive training of teachers for curriculum implementation. The project also provided pretraining and post-training consultation with teachers and process consultation with program champions and administrators to address program institutionalization.

Uses in Problem Analysis and Intervention Methods

Intervention groups: Organizations and specific agents (role incumbents) who have responsibility for the organizational process at each stage of organizational change

Behaviors: Sensing of unsatisfied demands on the system, search for possible responses, evaluation of alternatives, decision to adopt a new course of action, initiation of action with the system, implementation of the change, and institutionalization of the change; the agents initiate and coordinate the change

Environment: Availability of organizational processes to enable the behavior and organizational resources

Determinants: Motivation and behavioral capability of the role agents vary by stage

Methods: Must be matched to stage; informational and motivational in the earlier stages, and skills training and reinforcement in the later stages

Organizational Development Theory

ACTION PLANNING Organizational development generally seeks to improve the quality of work life through organizational diagnosis, structure modification, or human process change. Its origins in applied social psychology can be traced to the action research model developed by Lewin and his colleagues in the 1940s (Bowditch & Buono, 1994). Organizational development is primarily a theory of action, organized around four basic steps: diagnosis, action planning, intervention, and evaluation.

Diagnosis includes the identification of organizational issues or problems related to the "environment factors; the organization's mission, goals, policies, procedures, structures, technologies, and physical setting; social and interpersonal factors; desired outcomes; and readiness to take action" (Goodman et al., 1997, p. 293). Action planning includes identification of possible interventions to address the issues or problems identified and then selecting the interventions based on organizational readiness, the availability of leverage points within the organization, and the skill of the planner. Organizational development interventions of three general types are then employed: laboratory training, survey research and feedback, and sociotechnical systems (Bowditch & Buono, 1994). Laboratory training, often referred to as T-groups, uses purposefully unstructured small group activities designed for participants to learn about their own interactions and about the group dynamic. In survey research and feedback, findings from management and employee attitude surveys are fed back to the client group, often assembled in work teams, for discussion, emergence of new perspectives, and development of action plans. Sociotechnical interventions use a systems approach to change an organization's context, climate, and methods for performing work. These interventions can include changes in job designs; organizational authority and reporting relationships; personnel recruitment, training, and compensation; strategic planning and forecasting; strategy implementation; and leadership development. Evaluation assesses the outcome of the change effort and of the current organizational state.

CHANGING ORGANIZATIONAL CULTURE Some organizational development theorists have focused on organizational culture. Schein (1992) defines culture as a pattern of basic assumptions invented, discovered, or developed by a given group as it learns to cope with its problems of external adaptation and internal integration. For the pattern to be "culture," it must have worked well enough to be considered valid and is therefore taught to new members as the way to perceive, think, and feel. Organizational interventions are most effective when they are compatible with the culture, so it is important to understand the culture of the organization in which a health promotion program is being developed and implemented (see also Chapter 6 and Chapter 7 on culture and culturally competent practice).

It is also possible to facilitate changes in organizational culture, although this process is slow and evolutionary. Culture changes with the group's learning and experience over time, as organizational members react to environmental shifts and crises within the organization. Schein (1992) describes the importance of leaders' behavior in shaping organizational culture—what leaders pay attention to, how they react to critical incidents, their modeling and coaching, and the criteria set for allocating rewards, personnel recruitment, and promotion. As seen in Table 4.8, Schein refers to leader behaviors as primary culture-embedding mechanisms. The culture is reinforced by organizational design, structure, and formal statements. In a young organization, leaders create the culture, and the organizational systems reinforce the culture. In mature organizations, the organizational systems become primary, constraining future leaders' behavior.

Worksite programs have applied culture change interventions specifically to health (J. Allen & Bellingham, 1994; R. Allen & Kraft, 1984). These programs intend for individuals to achieve their personal goals facilitated by the culture, with the condition that the culture allow for individual differences and freedom of choice. The intervention includes assessment of what the work-site norms are and what employees would like these norms to be for health-related behaviors such as physical fitness, smoking cessation, stress reduction, nutrition, substance

Table 4.8
Culture-Embedding Mechanisms

PRIMARY EMBEDDING MECHANISMS	SECONDARY ARTICULATION AND REINFORCEMENT MECHANISMS
What leaders pay attention to, measure, and control on a regular basis	Organization design and structure
	Organizational systems and procedures
How leaders react to critical incidents and organizational crises	Design of physical space, facades, and buildings
Observed criteria by which leaders allocate scarce resources	Stories, legends, and myths about people and events
Deliberate role modeling, teaching, and coaching	Formal statements of organizational philosophy, values, and creed
Observed criteria by which leaders allocate rewards and status	
Observed criteria by which leaders recruit, select, promote, retire, and excommunicate organizational members	

Note. From *Organizational Culture and Leadership* (2nd ed., p. 231), by E. H. Schein, 1992, San Francisco: Jossey-Bass.

abuse, safety, mental health, and human relations. Employees report perceptions of the health behaviors of organizational members (e.g., a work-site norm for people to be a few pounds overweight) and opinions about work-site support for health-promoting endeavors (e.g., whether the organization has facilities for physical activity; R. Allen & Kraft).

Organizational support factors are then examined: modeling, training, rewards and recognition, communication, orientation, relationships and interaction, resource allocation and commitment, confrontation, and rituals, myths, and symbols. These data are obtained using document review, participant observation, focus group interviews, and surveys. Strengths and opportunities for improvement are identified. Examples of findings for a company might include the following observations: that the leader often works out at the company's fitness facility during lunch; that the executive dining room serves alcohol; that new employees are invited to join company-sponsored exercise programs; and that new employee orientation does not include the company health promotion program as a primary benefit, but instead focuses on medical coverage and sick leave (J. Allen & Bellingham, 1994).

The facilitators then convene small groups for employees and managers to develop a shared vision of the desired norms and to develop both individual and organizational plans for change. Self-help educational materials, support group programs, periodic work group discussions, and health promotion task forces are put into place. A group leader or buddy keeps in touch with the participants. Positive behavioral modeling by participants, especially the organizational leaders, and incentives compatible with the culture are also key components of this intervention. Evaluation, feedback, and goal setting continues to sustain the change (J. Allen & Bellingham, 1994).

Uses in Problem Analysis and Intervention Methods

Intervention groups: Organizations and the agents who influence them

Behaviors: Structure, norms, and behaviors of the organization related to the health of its constituents

Environment: Seeing the organization as the environment that is healthy (or not) in itself and that promotes (or does not promote) healthy living; helps elucidate not only ways for change, but the why of the organization's current status

Determinants: Not well developed

Methods: Laboratory training, survey research and feedback, sociotechnical systems change, and modeling and coaching; assessment of norms; small group work on visioning new norms

Interorganizational Relationships Theory

Organizations form partnerships to manage their environments. These interactions may be informal and transient or highly structured with shared decision making and leadership. The interactions have been viewed as forming a hierarchy from cooperation, through coordination, to collaboration in which the interorganizational relationships become more refined and complex with an increasing degree of organizational participation and decreasing organizational independence (Daka-Mulwanda, Thornburg, Filbert, & Klein, 1995; Kagan, 1991). For cooperation, two or more organizations maintain autonomous programs but agree to work together to make all programs more successful (Hoyt, 1978). Coordination is information sharing and joint planning (Lugg & Boyd, 1993). In collaboration, resources, power, and authority are shared to reach joint goals (Kagan). The most effective form of partnership depends on the task to be accomplished and the context of the situation. However, organizations must collaborate to address the complex health and education issues currently faced by communities.

COALITIONS Coalitions have been defined as "an organization of individuals representing diverse organizations, factions or constituencies who agree to work together in order to achieve common goals" (Feighery & Rogers, 1989, p. 1). The form of interaction may be cooperation, coordination, or collaboration. Coalitions' compositions may vary. Grassroots coalitions are volunteers banding together, often in times of crisis, to achieve a goal; professional coalitions are composed of professional organizations seeking to coordinate their activities to maximize their power and influence; community-based coalitions of professionals and grassroots leaders are formed to influence the health and welfare of their community (Butterfoss, Goodman, & Wandersman, 1993).

Coalitions develop through specific stages, each of which requires a different set of skills and resources and thus different strategies for training and technical assistance by staff and consultants. Butterfoss and colleagues (1993) term these stages formation, implementation, maintenance, and the accomplishment of goals or outcomes. Their review identifies factors contributing to the success of each stage. Factors effective for formation include recognition of the need to collaborate and the advantages of collaboration, scarcity of resources, mandate to collaborate, history of collaboration, a motivated catalyst organization, and compatibility among organizations. For implementation and maintenance, the factors of formalized rules, roles and procedures, competent leadership, diverse and committed membership with skills to participate fully, and linkage to external resources in the environment are key to effective functioning over time. Thorough evaluation and feedback of the short-term and long-term effects of its activities are necessary to keep the program on track and to indicate whether the coalition has achieved its goals. Habana-Hafner and Reed (1989) point out that, for a coalition to function optimally, compatibility should exist in comprehensiveness and complexity of purpose, nature of leadership, decision making, communication, formality of agreements, and amount of centralization of authority. For example, coalitions that survive over time are more structured and task oriented and have more offices, committees, and regular meetings than do coalitions that are not sustained (Chavis, Florin, Rich, & Wandersman, 1987). Butterfoss, Goodman, and Wandersman (1996) examined the relationship of coalition characteristics to effectiveness in a community coalition to reduce alcohol, tobacco, and other drug abuse in a three-county area. They found that effective leadership, shared decision making, linkages with other organizations, and a positive organizational climate were key to member participation and satisfaction. However, these variables were not related to the quality of the plans produced by the coalition subcommittees.

FACILITATING EMPOWERMENT Coalitions and partnerships are an important method for facilitating empowerment, which is broadly defined as influencing conditions that are relevant to people who share neighborhoods, workplaces, or concerns (Fawcett et al., 1995).

Fawcett and colleagues (1995) describe four primary methods for enabling the empowerment process in partnerships: (a) enhancing experience and competence, (b) improving group structure and capacity, (c) removing social and environmental barriers, and (d) increasing environmental support and resources. Strategies to enhance experience and competence include listening sessions and surveys to identify local issues, an inventory of community assets, guidelines for selecting leadership and membership, training on leadership skills, and technical assistance on action planning and early projects. Strategies to improve group structure and capacity include technical assistance with strategic planning, development of an organizational structure, inclusion of key members and volunteers, and financial development. For removing social and environmental barriers, suggested strategies include focus groups, social marketing to promote adoption of new programs, and training in conflict resolution. Strategies to increase environmental support and resources include information and feedback about community change; development of ties to existing community sectors, organizations, and groups; opportunities for networking; and the promotion of policies and resource allocations.

Uses in Problem Analysis and Intervention Methods

Intervention groups: Organizations are the focus for formation of coalitions; coalitions themselves are the focus for implementation, maintenance, and action

Behaviors: Coalition formation, implementation, maintenance, and action

Determinants: Motivation to collaborate, organizational capacity, models of coalitions, barriers to collaboration, community capacity, and community resources

Methods: Enhancing experience and competence, enhancing group structure and capacity, removing social and environmental barriers, and enhancing environmental support and resources

COMMUNITY ORGANIZATION MODELS AND THEORIES

Communities may be based on geography; on gender, ethnic, or cultural identity; or on an issue such as the environment, animal rights, or public health. A shared reality or identity is key to the construct (Labonte, 1997). In this section we discuss conscientization and several models of community organization, all aimed at empowering people in their lives and the lives of their communities (Minkler & Wallerstein, 1997b). We then turn to models of community organization from the United States, beginning with a description of Rothman's (1979) classic models of community organization and next discussing the approach of Minkler and Wallerstein, who extend earlier models to include an explicit focus on community strengths and capacity.

Conscientization

The work of the Brazilian Paulo Freire (1973) in liberation education has formed the basis for empowerment models (Wallerstein, Sanchez-Merki, & Dow, 1997). Individuals in small groups are led through a consideration of their own realities and the constraints they experience to an understanding of the social forces underlying the problem and their responsibility to act. In this model, the facilitator participates in a dialogue with the learners to uncover the root social causes of the problems in their own life experiences. Through a cyclical process of listening, dialogue, and action, participants develop an understanding of their social and political reality and how to transform these conditions. To facilitate the dialogue, learning materials such as drawings, photographs, or songs are used to focus on common themes that are discussed collectively. These discussions lead the participants to understand their own reality, including the constraints placed on their lives, and to take action for social change. In a particular application of this process, photo novellas produced by program participants have been used to assist New England farm workers, a New York neighborhood, building trades workers, and rural Chinese women to influence programs and policies affecting their lives (Rudd & Comings, 1994; Wang & Burris, 1994).

From their work with the Adolescent Social Action Program that focused on alcohol and substance abuse prevention, Wallerstein and Sanchez-Merki (1994) have identified three stages through which an individual passes from apathy to a social responsibility to act (see Figure 4.1). The first stage involves individuals beginning to care about the problem, each other, and their ability to act in the world. This stage is accomplished through dialogue and self-disclosure in small groups and through the use of questioning. At the next stage, individual responsibility to act, individuals' self-efficacy to talk and help others increases as a result of engaging in participatory and caring dialogue with community members who have experienced problems with alcohol or drugs. The final stage, social responsibility to act, involves critical thinking about the social forces that underlie the problem, and a commitment to engage in self and community change. This three-stage transformation results in individual and community empowerment.

> *Uses in Problem Analysis and Intervention Methods*
>
> Intervention groups: Community groups, especially marginalized populations
>
> Behaviors: To become politically and socially active
>
> Environment: Community groups can become empowered to confront the larger social and political environments
>
> Determinants: Collective self-efficacy and an understanding of the root causes of problems
>
> Methods: Freirian methods are reflection-action-reflection, nonjudgmental small group discussion of learning materials, question posing, and self-disclosure

Community Organization

Building on the three types of social change identified by Bennis, Benne, and Chin (1969), Rothman (1979) developed three models of community organization: locality development, social planning, and social action. Locality development utilizes normative–re-educative change, which involves raising consciousness about underlying causes of problems and identifying strategies of action. It is heavily process oriented with an emphasis on consensus, cooperation, and building a sense of community. This model is most akin to the community development tradition in health education. Social planning, based on rational-empirical change, uses information derived from empirical research. It is heavily task oriented with

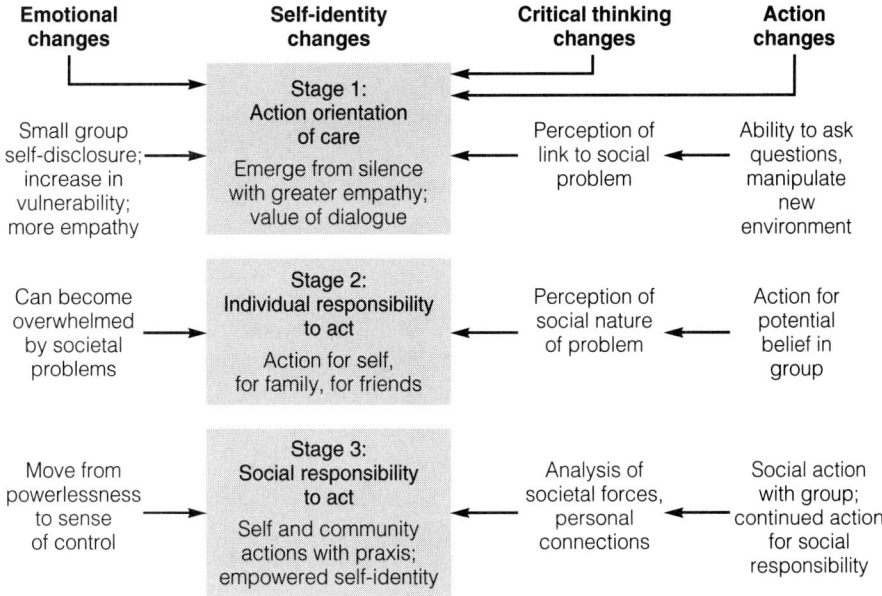

FIGURE 4.1 Stages to Responsibility to Act (*Note.* From *Community Organizing and Community Building for Health,* by M. Minkler, Ed., 1997, New Brunswick, NJ: Rutgers University Press.)

an emphasis on expert consultation as a means to solve problems. Social action is based on coercive change and seeks to redress imbalances of power. It relies on conflict methods of change, such as demonstrations and boycotts, and the change agent is an activist and partisan. The skillful organizer assesses the context of the community and of the problem at hand and mixes and matches the change models (Rothman).

Minkler and Wallerstein (1997a, 1997b) extend Rothman's (1979) work, presenting a typology of community organization based on change method (consensus vs. conflict) and view of the community (needs-based vs. strengths-based). In their typology, diagrammed in Figure 4.2, earlier models of community organization—both community development and social action—are viewed as needs-based, centering around the organizer "helping" the community. Current community organization practice is seen as centered on the community, building on community strengths and assets. The form of practice differs with whether consensus or conflict is the change strategy. Community-building approaches use consensus and inclusiveness, a concept of power as "power with," whereas empowerment-oriented social action uses conflict and challenges "power over." Both types of community change are directed toward increased community competence, leadership development, and critical awareness within the community. Methods and strategies in their typology include grassroots organizing, professionally driven organizing, coalitions, lay health workers, building community identity, political and legislative actions, and culturally relevant practice.

Chapter 4
Theories in Health Education and Promotion

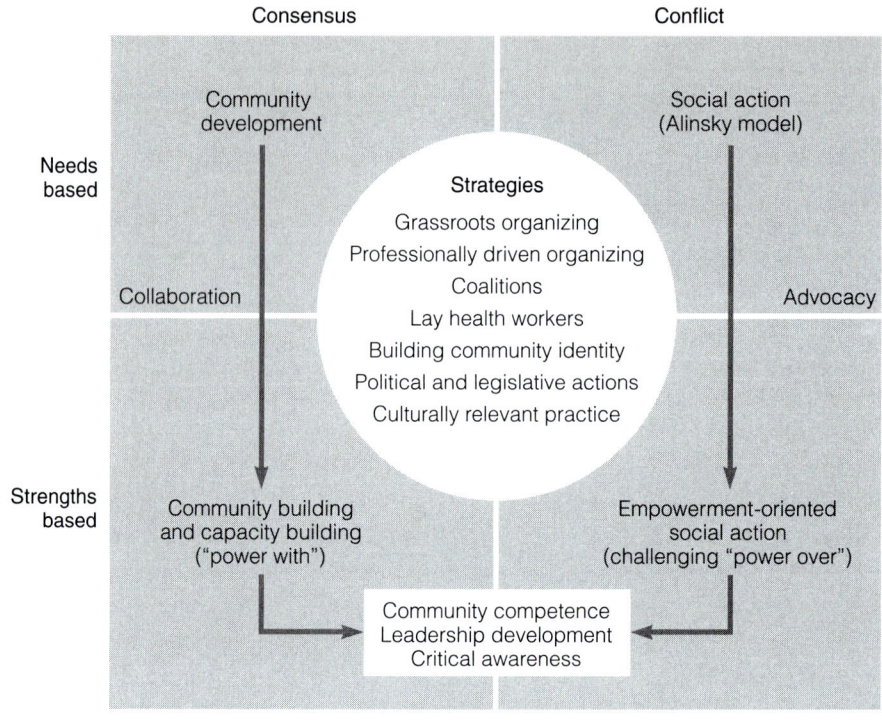

FIGURE 4.2 Community-Organizing and Community-Building Typology (*Note.* From "Improving Health Through Community Organization and Community Building," by M. Minkler and N. Wallerstein, 1997, in K. Glanz, F. M. Lewis, and B. K. Rimer, Eds., *Health Behavior and Health Education: Theory, Research, and Practice* (2nd ed.), San Francisco: Jossey-Bass.)

Empowerment is a process through which individuals, communities, and organizations change their social and political environments. In so doing, they gain a sense of mastery, improved equity, and enhanced quality of life (Minkler & Wallerstein, 1997b). At the individual level, the results of empowerment are psychological, including increased perception of control over one's destiny, political efficacy, and motivation to act (Syme, 1988; Zimmerman, 1990). This type of empowerment occurs when people take action to gain power and control through organizational and community involvement and to critically understand their environment (see discussions of conscientization and of social networks earlier in this chapter) (Zimmerman, 1995).

At the organizational and community levels, empowerment involves collective problem solving, shared leadership and decision making, and accessible government, media, and resources. Zimmerman (1990) describes individual level outcomes as perceived control and behavioral capability to gain power and control and higher ecological level outcomes as organizational networks, resource acquisition, policy development, evidence of pluralism, and accessible community resources (see the discussion of collective efficacy earlier in this chapter) (Bandura, 1997).

The Contra Costa County (California) Health Services Department, through its Healthy Neighborhoods Project, worked with the El Pueblo neighborhood, a public housing development, to identify and train neighborhood health advocates. The advocates received training in health, tobacco, and nutrition using Freirian popular education methods and in aspects of community organization, including door-to-door interviewing, community asset mapping, cross-cultural communication, and media and policy advocacy. Then, using the health department coordinator as a facilitator and broker for resources, the neighborhood health advocates assessed the capacities of residents and residents' perceptions of their community, and organized a community mapping day on which trained adult and youth volunteers mapped the neighborhood's positive and negative physical and institutional features. The findings were presented at a community forum, and an action plan was developed by the residents who attended. They organized the painting of a mural by local children that showed the residents' vision for the community (El-Askari et al., 1998).

To achieve the top priority of installation of speed humps to slow traffic and reduce drug dealing, a residential council talked with the police chief, lobbied the city council, spoke at public meetings, organized demonstrations, and involved the media. These actions resulted in a consensus decision by the housing advisory commission to approve the speed humps. Better street lighting and increased police patrol, two other priorities, were also accomplished. Residents organized to have a neighborhood tobacco billboard removed and to have a community-based organization offer healthful cooking classes.

The residents council became larger, better organized, and more representative of the residents. Members began to visit other San Francisco Bay Area public housing residents councils to share experiences. The council then wrote and received funding for three grants: a tenant opportunities grant to establish computer classes, job training classes, and job search workshops; a drug elimination grant; and a youth sports grant. Over the course of the project, initial successes motivated residents to take leadership roles in addressing other issues and led to a strong sense of control. Residents reported increased energy and life satisfaction, and strong social ties developed. Residents also began involvement in broader policy-making initiatives, such as the county's public and environmental health advisory board (El-Askari et al., 1998).

Uses in Problem Analysis and Intervention Methods

Intervention groups: Communities

Behaviors: Taking action to change community conditions related to health

Environment: Community capacity and enabling structures

Determinants: Motivation to act, political efficacy, and enabling community structures

Methods: Grassroots organizing, professionally driven organizing, coalitions, lay health workers, building community identity, political and legislative actions, and culturally relevant practice

SOCIETAL AND GOVERNMENTAL THEORIES

Public Policy

Health policy is directly related to public health and health services. Other public policies directed to issues such as economics, housing, or public safety also have much potential to influence health. Milio (1981) views economic policy as acting directly on people's biophysical and socioeconomic environments and indirectly through various areas for public policy, such as environmental safety policy, energy policy, income maintenance policy, and health and human services delivery policy (see Figure 4.3). This framework shows policy as a determinant of health behavior and of health.

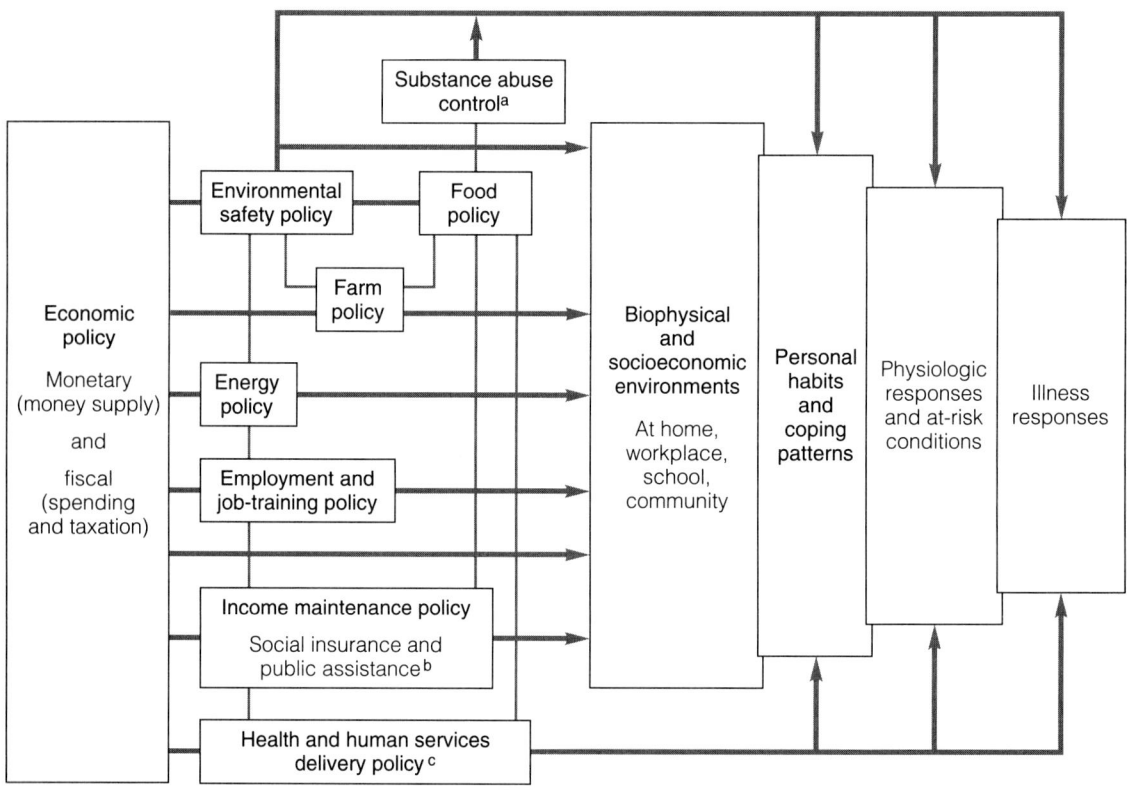

[a]cigarettes, alcohol, other drugs; [b]includes food stamps and Medicaid; [c]includes education, legal assistance, day care, counseling

FIGURE 4.3 Public Socio-Environmental Policy That Shapes American Environments, Personal Behavior, and Prospects for Health (*Note.* From *Promoting Health Through Public Policy,* by N. Milo, 1981, Philadelphia: F. A. Davis.)

Public policy sets options for organizations and for individuals, both directly and indirectly through organizations. According to Milio (1981), policy components should make "the creation and maintenance of healthful environments and personal habits the easiest—the 'cheapest' and most numerous—choices for selections by governmental units and corporations, producers and consumers, among all the options available to them" (p. 83). Policy instruments include direct spending, such as grants and contracts and the production of goods and services; regulation and monitoring; and fiscal incentives such as subsidies, taxation, and tax deductions.

HEALTHY CITIES The Healthy Cities program is an intersectoral political program that is focused on change in the power relations between community sectors regarding health and illness (Davies & Kelley, 1993). It grew within the context of health promotion as viewed by the World Health Organization (WHO) in the Ottawa Charter—"the process of enabling people to increase control over, and to improve, their health" (World Health Organization, 1986)—and through a positive or health-promoting approach to health (Hancock, 1993). The process includes both the development of mechanisms through which local government departments could work collaboratively to improve health and an emphasis on community mobilization and participation. The Healthy Cities projects in Europe, Canada, the United States, and Australia differ according to their contexts but share the philosophic view of health as social and ecological rather than biomedical. Some projects are more bureaucratic in orientation; others are more community oriented. Some are closely linked to national and supranational health objectives, for example, the U.S. Objectives for the Nation and the WHO 38 European targets, whereas others are more locally determined (Cutrice, 1993; B. C. Flynn, 1993).

Much has been written about how policy is made and how to influence the process. Decision-making models include assessment of the likelihood of various policy outcomes and their values. In a rational or economic decision-making model, the policy maker selects the most efficient alternative to maximize the most valuable output. However, in most cases, there is not sufficient information to make these decisions, and there is not only one set of goals or values among policy stakeholders. In the bounded rationality model, rationality is limited by the task environment and personal motivation; this leads the policy maker to accept a feasible or "good enough" solution (Gustafson, Cats-Baril, & Alemi, 1992, pp. 32–33.) In the political model, goals are inconsistent because of pluralistic interest groups, and incrementalism through compromise is the approach to a solution. Decision analysis examines the outcomes of various actions, their values, and the probability that the outcomes will occur, and this information is used to evaluate policy options (Gustafson et al., 1992; Patrick & Erickson, 1993).

SETTING THE POLICY AGENDA Other theorists have examined how an issue is placed on the policy agenda. Cobb and Elder (1983) have presented three models of how policy is set. The process for influencing policy depends on whether the policy is initiated (a) outside the government, (b) from within the government as an inside initiative not requiring public support, and (c) from within the government but requiring support from the outside for passage. Kingdon's (1995) model is less rational: political events, social problems, and policy solutions float in independent streams, with "windows" opening between the stream so that policy can be made.

Leeuw (2000) raises the important question of who determines which policy is to be formulated. She suggests that the social planning model underlies traditional hierarchical policy formulation in which government sets policy. In comparision, locality development and social action community processes are most relevant to current policy agenda-setting models. Who sets the policy is that entity—individuals or organizations—who best uses these processes. Social entrepreneurs such as academicians, nongovernmental organizations, and community activists who value social justice and seek innovative solutions for social problems can have a significant impact on policy (Catford, 1998; Duhl, 1990; Leeuw).

According to Laumann and Knoke (1987), influential organizations with specific national policy interests and fluid resources and who are embedded within communication and resource-exchange networks are the main actors in the national policy process. These organizations include corporate entities, such as trade associations, professional societies, labor unions, corporations, public interest groups, government bureaus, and congressional committees. The policy process begins when one or more of these organizations recognizes a condition as a problem or an issue and alerts other organizations to it. Options are then generated by the interested organizations, often as solutions in search of issues. The alternative options are then narrowed to get the policy option onto the governmental agenda for consideration. Each step is a product of negotiation and advocacy.

AGENDA-BUILDING THEORY According to Cobb and Elder (1983), there are two policy agendas. The systemic agenda contains issues that politicians see as meriting public attention and as within the legitimate jurisdiction of existing governmental authority. The institutional agenda contains issues that are available for the active and serious consideration of political decision makers. These theorists propose three models for agenda building. In the outside-initiative model, public support for an issue and the idea that the issue requires action that falls within governmental authority brings the issue first to the systemic agenda and then, with continued public pressure, to the institutional agenda. In the inside-initiative model, the initiative comes from within the government system and does not involve the larger public; it often moves quickly from the systemic agenda to the institutional agenda. In the mobilization model, policy proposals are developed within government and then support is sought among the public for formal policy passage and successful implementation.

Methods to influence the policy process depend on which model best describes a process and where in the process an issue is. A group who wishes to get its issue on the policy agenda must gain media attention as well as the support of opinion leaders and political leaders. Media advocacy (Wallach, Dorfman, Jernigan, & Themba, 1993) provides a framework and set of tools for a community group to use to influence policy. The three steps of media advocacy are setting the agenda, or framing it for access to the media and thus to specific opinion leaders; shaping the debate, or framing the content to highlight social definitions and solutions to problems; and advancing the policy by articulating the solutions and placing pressure on policy makers.

When an issue is on the systemic agenda, Cobb and Elder (1983) suggest that it is more likely to be placed by politicians on the institutional agenda if it has high and long-term social relevance, is not technical or technocratic, and is unique. These criteria suggest how advocates should frame the policy and messages concerning it.

An issue being initiated from the inside does not need to gain widespread public support. In this case, a smaller group of inside stakeholders is reviewing the proposal. The health educator can work with legislative staff to frame the issue so that it will both support the health policy being sought and reach the institutional agenda. In the mobilization model, the problem is for the government to generate support from the public on issues of importance to the government. Here the role of the health educator would be to influence public support for a policy.

POLICY WINDOW THEORY Kingdon (1995) has also investigated how issues reach systemic or governmental agenda status. He views this process in terms of three streams: politics, problems, and policies. The political stream includes changes in administration, party platforms, elections, and national mood regarding government. The problem stream includes issues within the various policy sectors, such as global warming, the national debt, health care costs, teenage pregnancy, specific diseases, and poor housing infrastructure. Policy solutions, such as pollution controls, universal health insurance, school-based clinics, or cooperative housing, "float around in or near government, searching for problems to which to become attached or political events that increase their likelihood of adoption" (Kingdon, p. 118). Events and ideas in these streams move along independently until there is a change in one stream, such as a change in government, emergence of a large problem, or advocacy of new policies. At this point a "window" between the streams opens up so that a problem may enter the political stream or a policy may become linked to a problem. The role of the policy advocate is to create, monitor, and capitalize on these opportunities.

Policy advocates or entrepreneurs promote their proposals and the associated problems and facilitate coupling between the streams, linking problems, policies, and political opportunities together when the windows are open. Characteristics of effective policy advocates are recognized authority; visibility; strong political, communication, and negotiation skills; ability to engage in strategic planning; creativity; persistence; relative independence in resources and structure; and persistence (Duhl, 1990; Kingdon, 1995; Milio, 1988).

Intervention groups: Policy makers

Behaviors: Enactment of health-promoting legislation, regulation, and policy

Environment: Political, problem, and policy streams

Determinants: Motivation and behavioral capability

Methods: Include advocacy, persuasion, communication, and negotiation; are tailored to whether the issue is initiated from within or outside the government or requires community mobilization for enactment and implementation; are used by policy advocates to create support for issues when policy windows are open for solutions to meet problems.

SUMMARY

In this chapter we provided an overview of some of the most relevant theories for health educators. These theories are from behavioral, social, and policy sciences. We distinguish between theories at the individual level and theories at multiple environmental levels: groups, organizations, communities, and societies. We also distinguish between theories for understanding the problem and theories for understanding the intervention action.

Use of Theories in Intervention Mapping:

- Define the health, behavioral, and environmental problems
- Describe and select groups of potential program participants
- Describe determinants of behaviors and environmental conditions that are related to health problems
- Choose methods to promote change
- Translate the theoretical methods into practical strategies and programs

REFERENCES

Ajzen, I. (1988). *Attitudes, personality, and behavior.* Chicago: Dorsey Press.

Ajzen, I. (1991). The theory of planned behavior. *Organizational Behavior and Human Decision Process, 50,* 179–211.

Allen, J., & Bellingham, R. (1994). Building supportive cultural environments. In M. P. O'Donnell & J. S. Harris (Eds.), *Health promotion in the workplace* (2nd ed., pp. 204–216). Albany, NY: Delmar Publishers.

Allen, R., & Kraft, C. (1984). The importance of cultural variables in program design. In M. P. O'Donnell & T. H. Ainsworth (Eds.), *Health promotion in the workplace* (pp. 69–95). New York: Wiley.

Bandura, A. (1986). *Social foundations of thought and action: A social cognitive theory.* New York: Prentice Hall.

Bandura, A. (1997). *Self-efficacy: The exercise of control.* New York: Freeman.

Baranowski, T., Perry, C. L., & Parcel, G. S. (1997). How individuals, environments, and health behavior interact: Social cognitive theory. In K. Glanz, F. M. Lewis, & B. K. Rimer (Eds.), *Health behavior and health education: Theory, research, and practice* (2nd ed., pp. 153–178). San Francisco: Jossey-Bass.

Bartholomew, L. K., Gold, R. S., Parcel, G. S., Czyzewski, D. I., Sockrider, M. M., Fernandez, M., Shegog, R., & Swank, P. R. (2000). Watch, Discover, Think, and Act: Evaluation of computer-assisted instruction to improve asthma self-management in inner-city children. *Patient Education and Counseling, 39*(2–3), 269–280.

Bartholomew, L. K., Parcel, G. S., Seilheimer, D. K., Czyzewski, D. I., Spinelli, S. H., & Congdon, B. (1991). Development of a health education program to promote the self-management of cystic fibrosis. *Health Education Quarterly, 18*(4), 429–443.

Bartholomew, L. K., Shegog, R., Parcel, G. S., Gold, R. S., Fernandez, M., Czyzewski, D. I., Sockrider, M. M., & Berlin, N. (2000). Watch, Discover, Think, and Act: A model for patient education program development. *Patient Education and Counseling, 39*(2–3), 253–268.

Bartholomew, L. K., Sockrider, M. M., Seilheimer, D. K., Czyzewski, D. I., Parcel, G. S., & Spinelli, S. H. (1993). Performance objectives for the self-management of cystic fibrosis. *Patient Education and Counseling, 22*(1), 15–25.

Becker, M. H. (1974). The health belief model and sick role behavior. *Health Education Monographs, 2,* 409–419.

Bennis, W. G., Benne, K. D., & Chin, R. (Eds.). (1969). *The planning of change* (2nd ed.). New York: Holt, Rinehart, & Winston.

Beyer, J. M., & Trice, H. M. (1978). *Implementing change: Alcoholism programs in work organizations.* New York: Free Press.

Boer, H., & Seydel, E. R. (1996). Protection motivation theory. In M. Conner & P. Norman (Eds.), *Predicting health behaviour: Research and practice with social cognition models* (pp. 95–120). Buckingham, UK: Open University Press.

Bowditch, J. L., & Buono, A. F. (1994). *A primer on organizational behavior* (3rd ed.). New York: Wiley.

Brug, J., Hospers, H. J., & Kok, G. (1997). Differences in psychosocial factors and fat consumption between stages of change for fat reduction. *Psychology and Health, 12*(5), 719–727.

Brug, J., Lechner, L., & De Vries, H. (1995). Psychosocial determinants of fruit and vegetable consumption. *Appetite, 25*(3), 285–296.

Butterfoss, F. D., Goodman, R. M., & Wandersman, A. (1993). Community coalitions for prevention and health promotion. *Health Education Research, 8*(3), 315–330.

Butterfoss, F. D., Goodman, R. M., & Wandersman, A. (1996). Community coalitions for prevention and health promotion: Factors predicting satisfaction, participation, and planning. *Health Education Quarterly, 23*(1), 65–79.

Catford, J. (1998). Social entrepreneurs are vital for health promotion—but they need supportive environments too [Editorial]. *Health Promotion International, 13*(2), 95–98.

Chaiken, S. (1987). The heuristic model of persuasion. In M. P. Zanna, J. M. Olson, & C. P. Herman (Eds.), *The Ontario Symposium: Social influence* (Vol. 5, pp. 3–39). Hillsdale, NJ: Erlbaum.

Chavis, D., Florin, P., Rich, R., & Wandersman, A. (1987). *The role of block associations in crime control and community development: The Block Booster project.* Final report to the Ford Foundation, New York.

Clark, N. M., & Zimmerman, B. J. (1990). A social cognitive view of self-regulated learning about health. *Health Education Research: Theory and Practice, 5*(3), 371–379.

Cobb, R. W., & Elder, C. D. (1983). *Participation in American politics: The dynamics of agenda building.* Baltimore: Johns Hopkins University Press.

Cohen, S., & Lichtenstein, E. (1990). Partner behaviors that support quitting smoking. *Journal of Consulting and Clinical Psychology, 58*(3), 304–309.

Coleman, J. S. (1990). *Foundations of social theory.* Cambridge, MA: Harvard University Press.

Conner, M., & Norman, P. (1996). *Predicting health behaviour: Research and practice with social cognition models.* Buckingham, UK: Open University Press.

Conner, M., & Sparks, P. (1996). The theory of planned behaviour and health behaviours. In M. Conner & P. Norman (Eds.), *Predicting health behaviour: Research and practice with social cognition models* (pp. 121–162). Buckingham, UK: Open University Press.

Cox, D. J., Gonder-Frederick, L., Julian, D. M., & Clarke, W. (1994). Long term follow-up evaluation of blood glucose awareness training. *Diabetes Care, 17*(1), 1–5.

Creer, T. L., Kotses, H., & Wigal, J. K. (1992). A second-generation model of asthma self-management. *Pediatric Asthma, Allergy, and Immunology, 6*(6), 143–165.

Cutrice, L. (1993). Strategies and values: Research and the WHO Healthy Cities project in Europe. In J. K. Davies & M. P. Kelley (Eds.), *Healthy Cities: Research and practice* (pp. 34–54). London and New York: Routledge.

Daka-Mulwanda, V., Thornburg, K. R., Filbert, L., & Klein, T. (1995). Collaboration of services for children and families: A synthesis of recent research and recommendations. *Family Relations, 44*(2), 219–223.

Davies, J. K., & Kelley, M. P. (1993). Healthy Cities: Research and practice. In J. K. Davies & M. P. Kelley (Eds.), *Healthy Cities: Research and practice* (pp. 1–13). London and New York: Routledge.

De Vries, H., & Backbier, E. (1994). Self-efficacy as an important determinant of quitting among pregnant women who smoke: The Phi-pattern. *Preventive Medicine, 23*(2), 167–174.

De Vries, H., Backbier, E., Dijkstra, M., Van Breukelen, G., Parcel, G., & Kok, G. (1994). A Dutch social influence smoking prevention approach for vocational school students. *Health Education Research: Theory and Practice, 9*(3), 365–374.

De Vries, H., Backbier, E. Kok, G., & Dijkstra, M. (1995). The impact of social influences in the context of attitude, self-efficacy, intention, and previous behaviour as predictors of smoking onset. *Journal of Applied Social Psychology, 25*(3), 237–257.

Duhl, L. (1990). *The social entrepreneurship of change.* New York: Pace University Press.

El-Askari, G., Freestone, J., Irizarry, C., Kraut, K. L., Mashiyama, S. T., Morgan, M. A., & Walton, S. (1998). The Healthy Neighborhoods Project: A local health department's role in catalyzing community development. *Health Education and Behavior, 25*(2), 146–159.

Ell, K. (1984). Social networks, social support, and health status: A review. *Social Service Review, 58*(1), 133–145.

Eng, E., & Hatch, J. W. (1991). Networking between agencies and black churches: The lay health education model. *Prevention in Human Services 10*(1), 123–146.

Eng, E., & Parker, E. (1994). Measuring community competence in the Mississippi Delta: The interface between program evaluation and empowerment. *Health Education Quarterly, 21*(2), 199–220.

Eng, E., & Smith, J. (1995). Natural helping functions of lay health advisors in breast cancer education. *Breast Cancer Research and Treatment, 35*(1), 23–29.

Evans, R. I., Rozelle, E. M., Mittelmark, M. B., Hansen, W. B., Bane, A. L., & Havis, J. (1978). Deterring the onset of smoking in children: Knowledge of immediate physiological effects and coping with peer pressure, media pressure, and parental modeling. *Journal of Applied Social Psychology, 8*(2), 126–135.

Fawcett, S. B., Paine-Andrews, A., Francisco, V. T., Schultz, J. A., Richter, K. P., Lewis, R. K., Williams, E. L., Harris, K. J., Berkley, J. Y., & Fisher, J. L. (1995). Using empowerment theory in collaborative partnerships for community health and development. *American Journal of Community Psychology, 23*(5), 677–697.

Feighery, E., & Rogers, T. (1989). *Building and maintaining effective coalitions.* Palo Alto, CA: Stanford Center for Research in Disease Prevention, Health Promotion Resource Center.

Fishbein, M., & Ajzen, I. (1975). *Belief, attitude, intention, and behavior: An introduction to theory and research.* Reading, MA: Addison Wesley.

Flynn, B. C. (1993). Healthy Cities within the American context. In J. K. Davies & M. P. Kelley (Eds.), *Healthy Cities: Research and practice* (pp. 112–126). London and New York: Routledge.

Flynn, B. S., Goldstein, A. O., Solomon, L. J., Bauman, K. E., Gottlieb, N. H., Cohen, J. E., Munger, M. C., & Dana, G. S. (1998). Predictors of state legislators' intentions to vote for cigarette tax increases. *Prevention Medicine, 2*(2), 157–165.

Freire, P. (1973). *Pedagogy of the oppressed.* New York: Seabury Press.

Fulk, J., & Boyd, B. (1991). Emerging theories of communication in organizations. *Journal of Management, 17,* 407–446.

Funch, D. P., & Mettlin, C. (1982). The role of support in relation to recovery from breast surgery. *Social Science and Medicine, 16*(1), 91–98.

Gilbert, D. T., Fiske, S. T., & Lindzey, G. (1998). *The handbook of social psychology* (4th ed.). Boston: McGraw-Hill.

Glanz, K., Lewis, F. M., & Rimer, B. K. (Eds.). (1997). *Health behavior and health education: Theory, research, and practice* (2nd ed.). San Francisco: Jossey-Bass.

Godin, G., Fortin, C., Michaud, F., Bradet, R., & Kok, G. (1997). Use of condoms: Intention and behavior of adolescents living in juvenile rehabilitation centres. *Health Education Research: Theory and Practice, 12*(2), 289–300.

Godin, G., & Kok, G. (1996). The theory of planned behavior: A review of its applications to health-related problems. *American Journal of Health Promotion, 11*(2), 87–98.

Godin, G., Savard, J., Kok, G., Fortin, C., & Boyer, R. (1996). HIV seropositive gay men: Understanding adoption of safe sex practices. *AIDS Education and Prevention, 8*(6), 529–545.

Goodman, R. M., Smith, D. W., Dawson, L., & Steckler, A. (1991). Recruiting school districts into a dissemination study. *Health Education Research: Theory and Practice, 6*(3), 373–385.

Goodman, R. M., Speers, M. A., McLeroy, K., Fawcett, S., Kegler, M., Parker, E., Smith, S. R., Sterling, T. D., & Wallerstein, N. (1988). Identifying and defining the dimensions of community capacity to provide a basis for measurement. *Health Education and Behavior, 25*(3), 258–278.

Goodman, R. M., Steckler, A., & Kegler, M. C. (1997). Mobilizing organizations for health enhancement: Theories of organizational change. In K. Glanz, F. M. Lewis, & B. K. Rimer (Eds.), *Health behavior and health education: Theory, research, and practice* (2nd ed., pp. 287–312). San Francisco: Jossey-Bass.

Gottlieb, B. H. (1985). Social networks and social support: An overview of research, practice, and policy implications. *Health Education Quarterly, 12*(1), 5–22.

Gottlieb, N. H., Goldstein, A. O., Flynn, B. S., Cohen, J. E., Bauman, K. E., Solomon, L. J., Munger, M. C., & Dana, G. S. (1999). *Legislators' intentions, attitudes, and normative beliefs relative to voting on youth tobacco prevention legislation: Implications for health education practice at the policy level.* Manuscript submitted for publication.

Gottlieb, N. H., & McLeroy, K. R. (1994). Social health. In M. P. O'Donnell & J. S. Harris (Eds.), *Health promotion in the workplace* (2nd ed., pp. 459–493). Albany, NY: Delmar Publishers.

Green, L. W., & Kreuter, M. W. (1999). *Health promotion planning: An educational and ecological approach* (3rd ed.). Mountain View, CA: Mayfield.

Gustafson, D. H., Cats-Baril, W. L., & Alemi, F. (1992). *Systems to support health policy analysis: Theory, models, and uses.* Ann Arbor, MI: Health Administration Press.

Habana-Hafner, S., & Reed, H. B. (1989). *Partnerships for community development: Resources for practitioners and trainers.* Amherst, MA: University of Massachusetts at Amherst, Center for Organizational and Community Development.

Hall, A., & Wellman, B. (1985). Social networks and social support. In S. Cohen & L. Syme (Eds.), *Social support and health.* New York: Academic Press.

Hamilton, M. A., & Hunter, J. E. (1998). A framework for understanding meta-analyses of the persuasion literature. In M. Allen & R. W. Preiss (Eds.), *Persuasion: Advances through meta-analysis* (pp. 1–28). Cresskill, NJ: Hampton.

Hancock, T. (1993). The Healthy City from concept to application: Implications for research. In J. K. Davies & M. P. Kelley (Eds.), *Healthy Cities: Research and practice* (pp. 14–24). London and New York: Routledge.

Harrison, J. A., Mullen, P. D., & Green, L. W. (1992). A meta-analysis of studies of the health belief model with adults. *Health Education Research: Theory and Practice, 7*(1), 107–116.

Heaney, C. A., & Israel, A. (1997). Social networks and social support. In K. Glanz, F. M. Lewis, & B. K. Rimer (Eds.), *Health behavior and health education: Theory, research, and practice* (2nd ed., pp. 179–205). San Francisco: Jossey-Bass.

Hersey, J. C., Kibanoff, L. S., Lam, D. J., & Taylor, R. L. (1984). Promoting social support: The impact of California's "Friends Can Be Good Medicine" campaign. *Health Education Quarterly, 11*(3), 293–311.

Holtgrave, D. R., Tinsley, B. J., & Kay, L. S. (1995). Encouraging risk reduction: A decision-making approach to message design. In E. Meibach & R. L. Parrot (Eds.), *Designing health messages: Approaches from communication theory and public health practice* (pp. 24–40). Thousand Oaks, CA: Sage.

Hospers, H. J., Kok, G., & Strecher, V. (1990). Attributions for previous failures and subsequent outcomes in a weight reduction program. *Health Education Quarterly, 17*(4), 1–47.

House, J. S., Umberson, D., & Landis, K. R. (1988). Structures and processes of social support. *Annual Review of Sociology, 14*, 293–318.

Hoyt, K. B. (1978). *The concept of collaboration in career education.* Washington, DC: U.S. Office of Education.

Israel, B. A. (1982). Social networks and health status: Linking theory, research, and practice. *Patient Counseling and Health Education, 4*(2), 65–79.

Israel, B. A., & Rounds, K. A. (1987). Social networks and social support: A synthesis of health educators. *Advances in Health Education and Promotion, 2,* 311–351.

Janz, N. K., & Becker, M. H. (1984). The health belief model: A decade later. *Health Education Quarterly, 11*(1), 1–47.

Kagan, S. L. (1991). *United We Stand: Collaboration for child care and early education services.* New York: Teachers College Press.

Kingdon, J. W. (1995). *Agendas, alternatives, and public policies* (2nd ed.). New York: HarperCollins College Publishers.

Kok, G., Den Boer, D-J., De Vries, H., Gerards, F., Hospers, H. J., & Mudde, A. N. (1992). Self-efficacy and attribution theory in health education. In R. Schwartzer (Ed.), *Self-efficacy: Thought control of action* (pp. 245–262). Washington, DC: Hemisphere.

Kok, G., Schaalma, H., De Vries, H., Parcel, G., & Paulussen, T. H. (1996). Social psychology and health education. *European Review of Social Psychology, 7* (pp. 241–282).

Kotses, H., Lewis, P., & Creer, T. L. (1990). Environmental control of asthma self-management. *Journal of Asthma, 27*(6), 375–384.

Labonte, R. (1997). Community, community development, and the forming of authentic partnerships: Some critical reflections. In M. Minkler (Ed.), *Community organizing and community building for health* (pp. 88–102). New Brunswick, NJ: Rutgers University Press.

Laumann, E. O., & Knoke, D. (1987). *The organizational state: Social choice in national policy domains.* Madison, WI: University of Wisconsin Press.

Lazarus, R. S. (1993). Coping theory and research: Past, present, and future. *Psychosomatic Medicine, 55*(3), 234–247.

Lazarus, R. S., & Folkman, S. (1991). The concept of coping. In A. Monat & R. S. Lazarus (Eds.), *Stress and coping: An anthology* (3rd ed., pp. 189–206). New York: Columbia University Press.

Leeuw, E. de (2000). Beyond community action: Communication arrangements and policy networks [Commentary]. In B. D. Poland, L. W. Green, & I. Rootman (Eds.), *Settings for health promotion: Linking theory and practice* (pp. 287–300). Thousand Oaks, CA: Sage.

Lichtman, R. R., Taylor, S. E., & Wood, J. V. (1987). Social support and marital adjustment after breast cancer. *Journal of Psychosocial Oncology, 5*(3), 47–74.

Locke, E. A., & Latham, G. P. (1991). *A theory of goal setting and task performance.* Englewood Cliffs, NJ: Prentice Hall.

Lugg, C. A., & Boyd, W. L. (1993). Leadership for collaboration: Reducing risk and fostering resilience. *Phi Delta Kappan, 75*(3), 253–258.

Maibach, E. W., & Cotton, D. (1995). Moving people to behavior change: A staged social cognitive approach to message design. In E. Maibach & R. L. Parrot (Eds.), *Designing health messages: Approaches from communication theory and public health practice* (pp. 41–64). Thousand Oaks, CA: Sage.

Manstead, T., & Parker, D. (1995). Evaluating and extending the theory of planned behavior. *European Review of Social Psychology, 6* (pp. 69–95).

Marlatt, G. A., & Gordon, J. R. (Eds.). (1985). *Relapse prevention: Maintenance strategies in the treatment of addictive behaviors.* New York: Guilford Press.

McGrath, J. (1995). The gatekeeping process: The right combinations to unlock the gates. In E. W. Maibach & R. L. Parrot (Eds.), *Designing health messages: Approaches*

McGuire, W. J. (1985). Attitudes and attitude change. In G. Lindzey & E. Aronson (Eds.), *The handbook of social psychology: Vol. 2. Special fields and applications* (3rd ed., pp. 233–346). New York: Knopf.

McLeroy, K. R., Bibeau, D., Steckler, A., & Glanz, K. (1988). An ecological perspective on health promotion programs. *Health Education Quarterly, 15*(4), 351–377.

McLeroy, K. R., Steckler, A. B., Simons-Morton, B., Goodman, R. M., Gottlieb, N., & Burdine, J. N. (1993). Social science theory in health education: Time for a new model? *Health Education Research: Theory and Practice, 8*(3), 305–312.

Meister, J. S., Warrick, L. H., de Zapien, J. G., & Wood, A. H. (1992). Using lay health workers: Case study of a community-based prenatal intervention. *Journal of Community Health, 17*(1), 37–51.

Mermelstein, R., Cohen, S., Lichtenstein, E., Baer, J. S., & Kamarck, T. (1986). Social support and smoking cessation and maintenance. *Journal of Consulting and Clinical Psychology, 54*(4), 447–453.

Miles, M. B., & Huberman, A. M. (1984). *Qualitative data analysis: A sourcebook of new methods.* Newbury Park, CA: Sage.

Milio, N. (1981). *Promoting health through public policy.* Philadelphia: F. A. Davis.

Milio, N. (1988). Strategies for health promoting policy: A study of four national case studies. *Health Promotion, 3*(3), 307–311.

Minkler, M. (1997a). Community organizing among the elderly poor in San Francisco's Tenderloin District. In M. Minkler (Ed.), *Community organizing and community building for health* (pp. 244–258). New Brunswick, NJ: Rutgers University Press.

Minkler, M. (1997b). *Community organizing and community building for health.* New Brunswick, NJ: Rutgers University Press.

Minkler, M., & Wallerstein, N. (1997a). Improving health through community organization and community building. In K. Glanz, F. M. Lewis, & B. K. Rimer (Eds.), *Health behavior and health education: Theory, research, and practice* (2nd ed., pp. 241–269). San Francisco: Jossey-Bass.

Minkler, M., & Wallerstein, N. (1997b). Improving health through community organization and community building: A health education perspective. In M. Minkler (Ed.), *Community organizing and community building for health* (pp. 30–52). New Brunswick, NJ: Rutgers University Press.

Montaño, D. E., Kasprzyk, D., & Taplin, S. H. (1997). The theory of reasoned action and the theory of planned behavior. In K. Glanz, F. M. Lewis, & B. K. Rimer (Eds.), *Health behavior and health education: Theory, research, and practice* (2nd ed., pp. 85–112). San Francisco: Jossey-Bass.

National Cancer Institute. (1989). *Making health communication programs work.* (National Cancer Institute Pub. No. 89-1493). Washington, DC: National Institutes of Health.

Northouse, L. L. (1988). Social support in patients' and husbands' adjustment to breast cancer. *Nursing Research, 37*(2), 91–95.

Orbell, S., Hodgkins, S., & Sheeran, P. (1997). Implementation intentions and the theory of planned behavior. *Personality and Social Psychology Bulletin, 23*(9), 945–954. San Francisco: Jossey-Bass.

Parker, E. A., Schulz, A. J., Israel, B. A., & Hollis, R. (1998). Detroit's East Side Village Health Worker Partnership: Community-based lay health advisor intervention in an urban area. *Health Education and Behavior, 25*(1), 24–45.

Patrick, D. L., & Erickson, P. (1993). *Health status and health policy: Quality of life in health care evaluation and resource allocation.* New York and Oxford: Oxford University Press.

Paulussen, T., Kok, G., & Schaalma, H. P. (1994). Antecedents to adoption of classroom-based AIDS education in secondary schools. *Health Education Research, 9*(4), 485–496.

Paulussen, T., Kok, G., Schaalma, H., & Parcel, G. S. (1995). Diffusion of AIDS curricula among Dutch secondary school teachers. *Health Education Quarterly, 22*(2), 227–243.

Peter-Golden, H. (1982). Breast cancer: Varied perception of social support in the illness experience. *Social Science and Medicine, 17,* 404–411.

Petty, R. E., & Cacioppo, R. T. (1986). The elaboration likelihood model of persuasion. *Advances in Experimental Social Psychology, 19,* 124–205.

Petty, R. E., & Wegener, D. T. (1997). Attitude change: Multiple roles for persuasion variables. In D. T. Gilbert, S. T. Fiske, & G. Lindzey (Eds.), *The handbook of social psychology* (4th ed., Vol. 1, pp. 323–390). Boston: McGraw-Hill.

Pollay, R. W., Siddarth, S., Siegel, M., Haddix, A., Merrit, R. K., Giovino, G. A., & Eriksen, M. P. (1996, April). The last straw? Cigarette advertising and realized market shares among youth and adults, 1979–1993. *Journal of Marketing, 60*(2), 1–16.

Portes, A. (1998). Social capital: Its origins and applications in modern sociology. *Annual Review of Sociolology, 24,* 1–24.

Prochaska, J. O., & DiClemente, C. C. (1984). *The transtheoretical approach: Crossing traditional boundaries of therapy.* Homewood, IL: Dow Jones–Irwin.

Prochaska, J. O., DiClemente, C. C., & Norcross, J. C. (1997). In search of how people change: Applications to addictive behaviors. In G. Marlatt & G. R. Van den Bos (Eds.), *Addictive behaviors: Readings on etiology, prevention, and treatment* (pp. 671–696). Washington, DC: American Psychological Association.

Putnam, R. D. (1993). The prosperous community: Social capital and public life. *American Prospect,* No. 13, 35–42.

Putnam, R. D. (1995). Bowling alone: America's declining social capital. *Journal of Democracy, 6*(1), 65–78.

Richard, L., Potvin, L., Kishchuk, N., Prlic, H., & Green, L. W. (1996). Assessment of the integration of the ecological approach in health promotion programs. *American Journal of Health Promotion, 10*(4), 270–281.

Rogers, R. W. (1975). A protection motivation theory of fear appeals and attitude change. *Journal of Psychology, 91*(1), 93–114.

Rogers, R. W. (1983). Cognitive and physiological processes in fear-based attitude change: A revised theory of protection motivation. In J. T. Cacioppo & R. E. Petty (Eds.), *Social psychophysiology: A sourcebook* (pp. 153–176). New York: Guilford Press.

Rogers, R. W. (1985). Attitude change and information integration in fear appeals. *Psychological Reports, 56*(1), 179–182.

Rosenstock, I. M., Strecher, V. J., & Becker, M. H. (1988). Social learning theory and the health belief model. *Health Education Quarterly, 15*(2), 175–183.

Rothman, J. (1979). Three models of community organization practice, their mixing and phasing. In F. M. Cox, J. L. Erlich, J. Rothman, & J. E. Tropman (Eds.), *Strategies of community organization* (3rd ed.). Itasca, IL: F. E. Peacock.

Rudd, R. E., & Comings, J. P. (1994). Learner developed materials: An empowering product. *Health Education Quarterly, 21*(3), 313–327.

Ruiter, R., Kok, G., & Abraham, C. (1999). *Fear appeals in health education: Theory and research.* Internal report. Maastricht, Netherlands: University of Maastricht, Department of Health Education.

Sabini, J. (1992). *Social psychology.* New York: Norton.

Salovey, P., Rothman, A. J., & Rodin, J. (1998). Health behavior. In D. T. Gilbert, S. T. Fiske, & G. Lindzey (Eds.), *The handbook of social psychology* (4th ed., pp. 633–683). Boston: McGraw-Hill.

Schein, E. H. (1992). *Organizational culture and leadership* (2nd ed.). San Francisco: Jossey-Bass.

Schunk, D. H. (1998). Teaching elementary students to self-regulate practice of mathematical skills with modeling. In D. H. Schunk & B. J. Zimmerman (Eds.), *Self-regulated learning: From teaching to self-reflective practice* (pp. 137–159). New York: Guilford Press.

Schunk, D. H., & Zimmerman, B. J. (1994). *Self-regulation of learning and performance: Issues and educational applications.* Hillsdale, NJ: Erlbaum.

Shegog, R., Bartholomew, L. K., Gold R. S., Pierrel, E., Parcel, G. S., Sockrider, M. M., Czyzewski, D. I., Fernandez, M., Berlin, N., Combes, R., & Abramson, S. (1999). *Self-management education for pediatric chronic disease: A description of the Watch, Discover, Think, and Act asthma computer program.* Manuscript submitted for publication.

Simons-Morton, B. G., Greene, W. H., & Gottlieb, N. H. (1995). *Introduction to health education and health promotion* (2nd ed.). Prospect Heights, IL: Waveland Press.

Simons-Morton, D. G., Simons-Morton, B. G., Parcel, G. S., & Bunker, J. F. (1988). Influencing personal and environmental conditions for community health: A multilevel intervention model. *Family and Community Health, 11*(2), 25–35.

Skinner, C. S., Sykes, R. K., Monsees, B. S., Andriole, D. A., Arfken, C. L., & Fisher, E. B. (1998). Learn, Share, and Live: Breast cancer education for older, urban minority women. *Health Education and Behavior, 25*(1), 60–78.

Smith, D. W., Steckler, A., McCormick, L. K., & McLeroy, K. R. (1995). Lessons learned about disseminating health curricula to schools. *Journal of Health Education, 26*(1), 37–43.

Spiegel, D., Bloom, J. R., Kraemer, H. C., & Gottheil, E. (1989). Effect of psychosocial treatment on survival of patients with metastatic breast cancer. *Lancet, 2*(8668), 888–891.

Steuart, G. W. (1993). Social and behavioral change strategies. *Health Education Quarterly, 1*(Suppl.), s113–s135.

Strecher, V. J., DeVellis, B. M., Becker, M. H., & Rosenstock, I. M. (1986). The role of self-efficacy in achieving health behavior change. *Health Education Quarterly, 13*(1), 73–92.

Strecher, V. J., & Rosenstock, I. M. (1997). The health belief model. In K. Glanz, F. M. Lewis, & B. K. Rimer (Eds.), *Health behavior and health education: Theory, research, and practice* (2nd ed. pp. 41–59). San Francisco: Jossey-Bass.

Strecher, V. J., Seijts, G. H., Kok, G. J., Latham, G. P., Glasgow, R., DeVellis, B., Meertens, R. M., & Bulger, D. W. (1995). Goal setting as a strategy for health behavior change. *Health Education Quarterly, 22*(2), 190–200.

Syme, S. L. (1988). Social epidemiology and the work environment. *International Journal of Health Services, 18*(4), 635–645.

Thoresen, C. E., & Kirmil-Gray, K. (1983). Self-management psychology and the treatment of childhood asthma. *Journal of Allergy and Clinical Immunology, 72*(5, Pt. 2), 596–606.

Wallach, L., Dorfman, L., Jernigan, D., & Themba, M. (1993). *Media advocacy and public health.* Newbury Park, CA: Sage.

Wallerstein, N. B., & Sanchez-Merki, V. (1994). Freirian praxis in health education: Research results from an adolescent prevention program. *Health Education Research: Theory and Practice, 9,* 105–118.

Wallerstein, N. B., Sanchez-Merki, V., & Dow, L. (1997). Freirian praxis in health education and community organizing: A case study of an adolescent prevention program. In M. Minkler (Ed.), *Community organizing and community building for health* (pp. 195–215). New Brunswick, NJ: Rutgers University Press.

Wang, C., & Burris, M. A. (1994). Empowerment through photo novella: Portraits of participation. *Health Education Quarterly, 21*(2), 171–186.

Weiner, B. (1986). *An attributional theory of motivation and emotion.* New York: Springer.

Weinstein, N. D. (1988). The precaution adoption process. *Health Psychology, 7*(4), 355–386.

Westen, D. (1996). *Psychology: Mind, brain, and culture.* New York: Wiley.

Witte, K. (1995). Fishing for success: Using the persuasive health message framework to generate effective campaign messages. In E. Maibach & R. L. Parrot (Eds.), *Designing health messages: Approaches from communication theory and public health practice* (pp. 145–166). Thousand Oaks, CA: Sage.

Wohlfeiler, D. (1997). Community organizing and community building among gay and bisexual men: The STOP AIDS Project. In M. Minkler (Ed.), *Community organizing and community building for health* (pp. 230–243). New Brunswick, NJ: Rutgers University Press.

World Health Organization. (1986). Ottawa charter for health promotion. *Health Promotion International, 1,* iii–iv.

Zajonc, R. B. (1980). Feeling and thinking: Preferences need no inferences. *American Psychologist, 35*(2), 151–175.

Zimmerman, M. A. (1990). Taking aim on empowerment research: On the distinction between individual and psychological conception. *American Journal of Community Psychology, 18*(1), 169–177.

Zimmerman, M. A. (1995). Psychological empowerment: Issues and illustrations. *American Journal of Community Psychology, 23*(5), 581–599.

CHAPTER 5

Intervention Mapping Step 1: Preparing Matrices of Proximal Program Objectives

READER OBJECTIVES

- State desired change or program outcomes for health-related behavior and environmental conditions
- Subdivide behavior and environmental conditions into performance objectives
- Select important and changeable personal and external determinants of behavior and environmental conditions
- Differentiate the population for a health promotion program
- Create a matrix of proximal program objectives for each level of intervention planning (individual, interpersonal, organizational, community, and societal) by crossing performance objectives with determinants and writing learning and change objectives

The basic tool for Intervention Mapping is the matrix of proximal program objectives. By proximal, we mean the most immediate objectives that need to be achieved in order to accomplish the more distal health, quality-of-life, environmental and behavioral program outcomes. In this chapter, we explain how health educators use the findings from the needs assessment and other information to specify intended change in individual health-related behaviors and environmental conditions at the interpersonal, organizational, community, and societal levels. Next, performance objectives are stated for behaviors and for environmental conditions at each ecological level. These performance objectives describe exactly what the at-risk population members and the agents or influential people at each environmental level need to do in order to accomplish improvements in health outcomes. Because the number of performance objectives is potentially large, it is necessary to evaluate their relevance and changeability and to narrow the set of performance objectives to those that will have the most effect on health behavior and health status.

The matrices in this chapter are created by crossing the performance objectives with hypothetical determinants of behavior and environmental conditions. These matrices form the critical foundation for intervention conceptualization and program development, steps that are explained in Chapters 6 and 7. The matrices contain the learning and change objectives that the program will target in order to influence change in determinants and performance. This chapter describes in detail the principal components of matrices and guides the reader to use the core processes and the information from the needs assessment to create sound matrices. The final product of Step 1 of the Intervention Mapping process is a set of matrices that specifies the immediate, most proximal program objectives to be accomplished by a health education or promotion program.

PERSPECTIVES

Importance of Outcomes-Based Planning

The development of an ecologically sound health education program starts with knowing what outcomes the program is expected to achieve at the individual, interpersonal, organizational, community, and societal levels. A carefully planned needs assessment provides the health educator with a clear indication of the quality-of-life, health, behavioral, and environmental outcomes expected to be

---

The mayor's planning group had done a great job on their needs assessment. Many of the members commented that they had no idea that the problem of violence was so complex. Looking at the theories helped them to really delve into some of the root causes of violence among the youth in their neighborhoods. They were practically bubbling over with enthusiasm—and they were sure that they were ready to talk about intervention.

"Now that we know better what factors are related to violence, let's go after them."

"I could call the school district tomorrow, because surely we will want to intervene there."

"Yeah, and what about that 'Communities in Schools' group?"

"We could …"

The health educator sat quietly for a moment, getting up the courage to tell them the truth: They had just done the first phase of their planning. The process was likely to become more complex before a coherent planning framework could emerge. Finally the health educator said, "Let's back up for just a minute. There are some other things we have to do before we can talk about intervention."

Amid the moans and groans, she told the group about the building blocks of matrices.

improved as a result of a program. In addition, a needs assessment such as PRE-CEDE will identify for the planning group the predisposing, enabling, and reinforcing factors associated with the behavioral or environmental factors (Green & Kreuter, 1999; see Chapter 2). The underlying assumption in the PRECEDE model is that intervention to modify the predisposing, enabling, and reinforcing factors increases the potential of improving behavioral, environmental, and health outcomes. The realization of this potential for change depends on the accuracy and completeness of the needs assessment, the strength and appropriateness of the intervention, and the quality and completeness of the program implementation.

A good needs assessment is an essential beginning to program planning, but by itself, the needs assessment lacks the specificity needed to guide the design of intervention strategies. Traveling from the starting point of a needs assessment to the destination of a fully implemented health education program is like following a road map: planners must know where to turn and which directions to take between the starting and end points. We believe that the starting point for good program planning is knowing what outcomes the program is intended to accomplish and what specific objectives will need to be achieved to obtain these outcomes. The needs assessment provides a causal model to help planners understand the problem; similarly, the matrix of proximal program objectives in Intervention Mapping creates a causal pathway for influencing change in order to solve or prevent a problem.

The process for creating a matrix of proximal program objectives is based on the assumption that the needs assessment identified behaviors or environmental conditions that are causes of health or quality-of-life outcomes. The next assumption is that development of certain more favorable behavioral or environmental conditions will lead to better health and improved quality of life. Thus the first step to creating a causal pathway for influencing change is to specify the behavioral and environmental outcomes to be accomplished by the health promotion program.

Ecology of Cause and Intervention

An additional perspective for this chapter is the continued use of an ecological framework for the planning of interventions for a health promotion program. Causation of health problems is a web of factors that occur at multiple levels. Some of these influences work through the behavior of the at-risk individuals, such as advertising on smoking behavior of adolescents (Pierce, Choi, Gilpin, Farkas, & Berry, 1998; Pollay et al., 1996; Schooler, Feighery, & Flora, 1996), whereas others, such as air quality (Kilburn, 1998), work directly on health. These levels of causation are represented in the matrix products of this chapter. To help health educators address this complex set of causal factors, Chapters 6 and 7 guide development of interventions that can likewise occur at multiple levels. Because these levels may include needed change at the individual, interpersonal, organizational, community, or societal levels, planning groups need to identify the ecological context of the health of the at-risk population, including the ecology of the health-related behaviors. Planners need to ask, What interpersonal, organizational, community, and societal factors influence health directly? and What factors facilitate (or impede) the performance of favorable health behaviors?

Tolerance of Complexity

The next link in the causal chain is the specification of performance objectives for obtaining the behavioral and environmental outcomes. Performance objectives are statements of what a program participant will do or how an environmental condition will be modified (including who will create the change). Performance objectives are then examined in light of the determinants of behavior and environmental conditions to generate learning and change objectives. Learning objectives specify what it is that members of the at-risk population or others in the environment will need to learn to accomplish the performance objectives. Change objectives state what needs to be changed relative to external determinants to accomplish performance objectives.

The process is complex and painstaking. However, health influences are complex, and health educators cannot avoid the necessity for sophisticated thinking to create the underpinnings of interventions that will effectively deal with the complexity. In the following sections, we provide sequential procedures and tasks that enable the reader to navigate the complexity. We show how the objectives are related to findings from a needs assessment, we provide guidance in stating objectives, and we discuss both hypothetical and real examples from health education programs.

MATRIX BUILDING BLOCKS: BEHAVIORS AND ENVIRONMENTAL CONDITIONS

The first task in Step 1 of Intervention Mapping is preparing to write performance objectives by defining what health behaviors and environmental conditions need to change. One of the building blocks of the matrices of proximal program objectives is a performance objective. The development of performance objectives begins with an examination of both health-related behaviors of the at-risk group and environmental conditions. This examination results in decisions about what needs to change in order to achieve health and quality-of-life objectives.

The needs assessment should provide a clear statement of behavior and environmental conditions linked to a health problem. However, before creating a causal model for an intervention, the health educator needs to re-examine the behavior and environmental conditions in order to define them in terms of what the health education or promotion program is intended to accomplish. For example, a behavioral cause of lung cancer is smoking, but the behavioral outcome for an intervention could be either helping people to not start smoking or helping people to quit smoking (U.S. Department of Health and Human Services [U.S. DHHS], 1990, 1994). Likewise, environment can stimulate or support smoking, but an intervention would have to address a specific part of the environment, such as advertising campaigns by tobacco manufacturers (Pierce et al., 1998; Pollay et al., 1996; Schooler et al., 1996). Well-defined behavioral and environmental outcomes will lead to a better specification of performance objectives.

Identifying Health-Related Behaviors of the At-Risk Group

Many types of health-related behaviors can be the focus of the health education and promotion intervention. The needs assessment often identifies behavior related to increased risk, but intervention development requires behaviors to be restated as health-promoting behaviors. For example, one of the risk behaviors for HIV infection is having unprotected sexual intercourse. For the purpose of designing a health promotion intervention, this risk behavior can be restated into two health-promoting behaviors: using condoms when having sexual intercourse, and choosing not to have sexual intercourse when not protected. In this case, the remainder of the Intervention Mapping process would be directed to obtaining and improving the performance of these two behaviors.

When thinking of behavioral change, planners can focus on different types of behaviors. As a matter of fact, one of the difficulties in planning health education programs is confusion over what is meant by behavior. Examples of types of behavior are

- risk-taking
- health-promoting
- screening and early detection
- compliance or adherence
- self-management

RISK BEHAVIORS Epidemiologists look at risk factors as a way of understanding causes of disease and factors associated with higher prevalence and incidence of disease in different populations. For example, documented cardiovascular disease risk factors include hypertension, hyperlipidemia, lack of exercise, genetics, stress, and smoking (Labarthe, 1998; Luepker, 1998; Shekelle et al., 1981). The underlying assumption is that, if an intervention can reduce the prevalence of the risk factors, it can reduce the prevalence of the disease (depending on how closely they are linked). The difficulty in designing health education or health promotion interventions based on these risk factors is that they are not all clearly behavioral causes of the disease. There is a mixture of physiological and behavioral risks. The first task is to sort out what behavior is related to morbidity and mortality. For example, heart disease is associated with hyperlipidemia (a physiological risk), which is strongly influenced by diet (a behavioral risk) (Frank, Vaden, & Martin,

1987; Labarthe, 1998). Thus risk behaviors, as opposed to risk factors, are defined as actions, such as eating certain foods, that have been demonstrated to directly increase the risk of disease or disability.

An intervention can be approached from a population perspective, in which it is designed to reduce the prevalence of the risk behavior within a defined population, or it can be approached from an individual perspective, in which it is designed to help the individual stop (or not start) the risk behavior. Because of the addictive nature of some behaviors—smoking, for example—the goal is the elimination of the behavior, not just a reduction. For other behaviors—for example, fat intake—the goal is a reduction. However, some behaviors that contribute to fat intake, such as cooking with saturated fat, might be eliminated altogether. The desired impact of a health education program on risk behaviors is to reduce or eliminate the practice and prevalence of these behaviors.

HEALTH-PROMOTING BEHAVIORS A health-promoting behavior is, in some cases, the opposite of a risk behavior. For example, if eating high-fat food were the risk behavior, then eating low-fat food would be the health-promoting behavior. But other behaviors, particularly in the wellness movement, are regarded as improving health or quality of life without a specific link to a health risk (Shephard, 1995). Yoga and meditation are examples of wellness behaviors. In contrast, some behaviors, such as getting immunizations, wearing a bicycle helmet, wearing a seat belt, or using a condom, are health promoting because they protect against a potential risk. Increasing the practice of health-promoting behaviors can be viewed as action taking to enhance health, reduce risk, or provide protection.

Often, health education and health promotion are directed to primary prevention, that is, preventing a health problem before it occurs. However, the same principles of intervention can apply to secondary prevention, that is, reducing the consequences of a disease or slowing the progress of the disease. Secondary prevention is especially important for diseases in which early signs or symptoms are not apparent. When symptoms are not present or not easily detectable by laypeople, screening is necessary to identify individuals at high risk for the disease or to detect the disease process early so that appropriate medical treatment can be started to prevent mortality or more severe illnesses. For example, breast self-examination and mammography are used to screen for changes in the breast to detect breast cancer in the early stages, when treatment has the best chance of effectiveness (Alcoe, Wallace, & Beck, 1990; Hurley & Kaldor, 1992; Smart, Hendrick, Rutledge, & Smith, 1995). There are also screening tests for other types of cancer such as cervical, prostate, and skin cancer (Jacobs, Oram, & Bast, 1992). Blood pressure and blood cholesterol levels are examples of screening tests for elevated risk for cardiovascular disease (Abel, Darby, & Ramachandran, 1994; Labarthe, 1998; Ohkubo et al., 1997; Thompson, Pyke, & Wood, 1997). Screening tests are also used to detect infectious diseases such as STDs and HIV (U.S. Preventive Services Task Force, 1990) and genetic diseases such as Tay Sachs (Natowicz & Prence, 1996) and cystic fibrosis (Brock, 1996; Livingstone, Axton, Mennie, Gilfillan, & Brock, 1993; U.S. DHHS, 1997).

Screening and early detection range from self-administered tests to complicated medical procedures, but almost all require some behavior by the person at-risk. Participation in screening requires an individual's decision and action. Health education programs can influence individuals to make decisions to participate. In general, interventions are usually designed to motivate individuals to participate in self-administered screening or to seek out and attend screening procedures conducted by health professionals (Craun & Deffenbacher, 1987). The exact nature of the behavior is specific to the screening method and the purpose of the screening. Some screening involves a one-time behavior (i.e., going to a health care facility and having blood or other specimens taken to be examined by a laboratory or health care professional). Other screening procedures, such as breast self-examination, are repeated and require skills, reliable procedures, and long-term maintenance (Agars & McMurray, 1993). Thus, intervention strategies must match the type of behavior necessary to make the screening effective.

COMPLIANCE, OR ADHERENCE, AND SELF-MANAGEMENT BEHAVIORS Patient education, a specific type of health education, can help individuals who are receiving health care for a diagnosed health problem not only to adhere to the prescribed therapy but also to understand the disease and treatment better. With most forms of medical therapy, the patient is usually required to follow through with recommendations given by the health care provider. The extent to which the patient follows through with the recommended action is referred to as a level of compliance. Some practitioners prefer to use the term *adherence* to avoid the implication that the patient is being told what to do without any involvement in the decision. For example, if a patient were instructed to take an antibiotic medication 3 times a day for 10 days, full adherence would mean taking the right dose at the right time each day for 10 days. Studies have shown that for most recommended follow-up procedures, adherence is incomplete (DiMatteo & DiNicola, 1985; Sackett & Snow, 1979). Thus, the goal of health education interventions in this case is to improve adherence behavior.

Often the behavior required for follow-up to medical care is much more complex than simply adhering to a set of instructions, especially in the case of chronic illnesses for which management of the condition requires the patients or their families to take action at home or elsewhere outside of health care facilities. Good disease management depends on making judgments to take action based on changing physiological conditions and life situations. For example, someone with diabetes must manage the disease by balancing the intake of food, expenditure of energy, and medication (Glasgow et al., 1992). This type of behavior is referred to as self-management because monitoring, decision making, and action must be made independent of the health care provider (Clark, Janz, Dodge, & Sharpe, 1992; Clark et al., 1988; Clark & Zimmerman, 1990). The goals for self-management may include increasing the performance of the behavior as well as improving the quality of the behavior, for example, helping the patient become better at decision making and problem solving.

Stating the Health-Promoting Behaviors

Health promotion behavioral outcomes should be stated in terms of the behaviors to be accomplished as a result of the health education or promotion program. The following statements are examples of health-related behaviors:

- Reduce total fat intake to 30% of calories.
- Increase eating of low-fat foods to include 5 servings of fruits and vegetables per day.
- Use condoms correctly and consistently when having sexual intercourse.
- Practice self-examination of breasts every month at the same time of the month.
- Monitor symptoms of asthma to detect early changes in status of illness.

Later in this chapter, we present the matrices from a recently conducted project called Sun Protection is Fun (Project SPF). Funded by the National Cancer Institute, Project SPF developed and tested an intervention to prevent skin cancer by reducing preschool children's exposure to ultraviolet rays (Tripp, Hermann, Parcel, Chamberlain, & Gritz, in press). Children are the at-risk group for the project, and parents and preschool day care center staff are additional intervention because they can play a role in protecting children from sun exposure and early damage to the skin. These environmental agents also help to establish children's behavioral patterns and habits for sun protection. Because of the age of preschool children, they can take only limited action by themselves to achieve protection from the sun and to reduce the amount of exposure to ultraviolet rays. Therefore, most of the focus of Project SPF is on the behavior of others in the children's environment and on environmental change at the interpersonal and organizational levels. The health-promoting behaviors to be brought about by these changes in the child's environment were stated in this way:

- Remain indoors or in full shade during peak sun times of 11:00 a.m. to 3:00 p.m.
- Wear sunscreen with a sun protection factor (SPF) greater than 15 when outdoors

Identifying Environmental Conditions

In the needs assessment, environmental factors are identified as social or physical conditions that influence risk behavior or act as indirect causes of the health problem or cause the health problem directly. The needs assessment process should lead to an identification of environmental conditions that influence the risk behavior or the health problem and to a prioritization of conditions according to their importance and changeability (see Chapter 2). Green and Kreuter (1999) suggest that health promotion program planners concentrate attention on

Matrix Building Blocks: Behaviors and Environmental Conditions

those aspects of the environment that are more social than physical, that interact with behavior in their impact on health, and that can be changed by social action and health policy. When planners conduct an environmental analysis, they realize each level of the environment must be considered as embedded in and having reciprocal influences with the higher levels.

INTERPERSONAL ENVIRONMENT   Humans are embedded in social systems. Families are the primary influence for socialization of children and continue to have an effect on behavior throughout life. As children grow older, peer groups become more important, beginning with playmates and continuing with friends, neighbors, coworkers, and members of organizations with which they affiliate (such as churches, social clubs, and service groups). Certain individuals may hold special influence by the role they play, such as teachers, coaches, religious leaders, or health care providers.

Social support is a protective factor for health outcomes that has been studied extensively (Ganster & Victor, 1988; Heaney & Israel, 1997; House, Umberson, & Landis, 1988). The types of support that individuals may receive from their social networks include emotional support, information or advice, material support, maintenance of social identity, and social outreach (Israel, 1982; Jacobson, 1986). Social support may influence health through several pathways. There is considerable evidence that it buffers the effects of stress through the processes of cognitive appraisal of stress and coping (Hirsch & DuBois, 1992; Rhodes, Contreras, & Mangelsdorf, 1994). It may provide modeling and reinforcement for the practice of specific health behaviors (Cohen et al., 1988; Epstein & Wing, 1987), and it may also directly influence physiological health, including immune function and blood pressure (Earp & Ory, 1979; Morisky, DeMuth, Field-Fass, Green, & Levine, 1985; Uchino, Cacioppo, & Kiecolt-Glaser, 1996). The presence or absence of supports from important others within the immediate interpersonal environment of individuals may have an influence on the performance of the health behavior as well as on the health outcomes.

The CATCH program (Child and Adolescent Trial for Cardiovascular Health), a school-based cardiovascular disease prevention intervention for elementary school children, is an example of how program planning can focus on instrumental support of children's health behaviors by parents and school staff (Perry et al., 1997, 1990). Developers intended the CATCH program to influence the diet, physical activity, and tobacco-use behavior of children. The school program addressed change at the individual level for the students and change at the organizational level to modify environmental conditions in the school to be more favorable and supportive of healthful eating and physical activity. In addition, the CATCH program planners hypothesized that parental support for the children eating low-fat food and being physically active would be an important environmental factor; they therefore evaluated the additive effectiveness of a program component that addressed support from the children's parents. The focus of the family component of CATCH was not on the diet, physical activity, or smoking behavior of the parents but more directly on how they could support the healthful behavior of the children (Nader, et al., 1996).

In another example of interpersonal environment, the Watch, Discover, Think, and Act asthma program targeted the behavior of physicians in prescribing anti-inflammatory medication to children, providing an asthma action plan, and reinforcing the child and family's management efforts (Bartholomew, Gold, et al., 2000; Bartholomew, Shegog, et al., 2000). The developers of the program also focused on the self-management supportive behavior of parents, school nurses, and teachers (see Chapter 11).

ORGANIZATIONAL ENVIRONMENT Organizational environments include cultural elements such as norms, policies, practices, and facilities. These factors are often considered as enabling factors in PRECEDE model terms. For example, policies can exert strong control over behavior, as in work-site bans on smoking, which have been shown to reduce the number of cigarettes consumed by workers in a workday (Brownson, Eriksen, Davis, & Warner, 1997; Eriksen & Gottlieb, 1999). In other examples, combinations of preventive health care policies and health care facility characteristics such as service hours can determine whether workers obtain care. The availability of corporate exercise facilities and the personnel practices of management may each have an impact on physical activity of workers.

The CATCH program also provides examples of addressing environmental conditions at the organizational level. CATCH addressed the organizational practices of cafeteria food preparation and physical education teaching. In addition, CATCH addressed policies regarding tobacco use on school grounds and during school-sponsored activities. Organizational level change was needed to make it easier for children to eat healthful food, be physically active, and avoid exposure to tobacco use.

In Project SPF, the unavailability of sunscreen, the lack of shade on the playground, and the time schedule for outside play are organizational conditions that contribute either directly to increased risk of exposure or indirectly by making the protective behaviors more difficult to perform. These conditions are under the control of the center directors, who may be influenced by parents, teachers, or voluntary health agencies to take steps to decrease children's risk of skin cancer.

COMMUNITY ENVIRONMENT The community environment often contains conditions that affect the health of populations, either through behavior or directly. Examples of these conditions include work and income, the quality and quantity of housing, health care, availability of recreational resources, smoking and other health ordinances, law enforcement, judicial practices, and treatment resources for social problems such as child abuse, violence, and drug addiction. Further community environment issues deal with social capital and the capacity of the community to form and maintain problem-solving relationships (Goodman et al., 1998; Minkler & Wallerstein, 1997). Examples of supportive environments achieved by communities through health promotion projects include cleaning up toxic waste dumps in indigenous communities in Alaska, providing piped water and sanitary toilets in Malaysia, reorganizing work in Swedish auto manufacturing sites, constructing safety barriers on roads in New Zealand, painting scooter taxis yellow for visibility in Delhi, and establishing a runaway house for young people in Finland (Haglund, Finer, Tillgren, & Pettersson, 1996).

SOCIETY   The societal level focuses on legislation, enforcement, regulation, and resource allocation as well as policies, programs, and facilities of large political and geographic groups. Societal influences often function through governments, which may be at the local, state, national, or international level. For example, legislation that influences tobacco use includes minors' access laws, clean air acts, and tobacco excise taxes. These laws, along with lawsuits against tobacco companies by states and by individuals, have been pivotal to the success of the tobacco control movement (Lynch & Bonnie, 1994). State and federal agencies, including those for health, human services, education, agriculture, transportation, and food and drugs, originate regulations, policies, and programs that affect health status. Societal influences may work on individual behavior, such as the American Responds to AIDS campaign of the Centers for Disease Control (Gentry & Jorgensen, 1991), or directly on the physical environment, such as regulations for road construction in New Zealand (Haglund et al., 1996). They may also work through organizations, such as allocating resources to set up drug-free schools (Brandon, 1992; Fox, Forbing, & Anderson, 1988). Healthy Cities projects have focused on intersectoral policy development that aims to create supportive environments for health and to integrate health into the economy, culture, and life of the community (Goumans & Springett, 1997).

Stating the Health-Promoting Environmental Conditions

Intervention Mapping guides planners to reword those environmental factors in the needs assessment that require change so as to clearly state the desired environmental change outcome. For example, a lack of low-fat food options at school that contributes to high-fat diets of schoolchildren can be restated as follows: Increase the availability of low-fat foods offered in school lunch and breakfast programs to include options with less than 30% of calories from fat at every meal. Accomplishment of a change in this environmental condition would result in more low-fat food options being available in the school cafeteria and would make it easier for children to select and eat low-fat foods.

Project SPF illustrates how both behavior and environmental conditions need to be addressed to accomplish the program objectives. Young children who attend day care and preschool education programs spend an average of 6 to 8 hours a day at these centers during the time of day when exposure to the sun is likely to be the most intense and most harmful. The health-promoting environmental changes that parents and preschools need to engage in were stated by the project planning team as follows:

- Ensure that children have SPF 15+ sunscreen applied at least 30 minutes before going outside
- Ensure that SPF 15+ sunscreen is applied to children every 1.5 to 2 hours, or after swimming or profuse sweating
- Ensure that adults help dress children in protective clothing such as hats, sleeved shirts, long shorts, and sunglasses
- Direct children to play in shaded areas

An assessment of preschools identified three environmental conditions at the organizational level that either contributed directly to increased risk of exposure or contributed indirectly by making the protective behaviors more difficult to perform. These conditions were the unavailability of sunscreen, the lack of shade on the playground, and the time of day of scheduled playtime. The following environmental change outcomes at the organizational level were stated for Project SPF:

- Provide SPF 15+ sunscreen in the preschools and day care centers for staff to apply to children
- Increase the amount of shade in the play areas
- Schedule activities so children are not outside during peak sun hours

---

The mayor's group identified the major behavioral and environmental causes of the health problem and the associated quality-of-life factors. Following the lead of the health educator, two subgroups—one on at-risk youth and one on the environment—worked independently to carefully specify the changes they wanted to see as a result of the program. Now they were ready to talk about intervention—or were they? What was their next step? Here are some reactions from the group:

"Let's get going. We know what the problem is. Now let's do something about it."

"How much money do you think they will really give us? That's what we really need to know before we can decide what to do."

"Let's put together a community coalition of groups interested in this problem and ask them to come up with a program."

The health educator, carefully moving the group to the next task in matrix development, said, "Human behavior and environmental conditions that cause health problems are usually very complex. We have done a good job of specifying what needs to change. Now we have to provide enough detail about the changes to begin to develop a successful intervention. Our next step is to write performance objectives."

MATRIX BUILDING BLOCKS: PERFORMANCE OBJECTIVES

The next task in Intervention Mapping Step 1 is to write performance objectives. Once the behavioral and environmental outcomes for the program are defined, the health educator writes performance objectives for each of them. The use of performance objectives is not new, nor is it unique to health education. For example, therapeutic outcomes are sometimes stated in performance terms at the individual client level, and on an organizational level, quality assurance defines a standard of performance to maintain certain levels of service or production. In education, performance objectives usually reflect cognitive performance, the levels of which have been classified as knowledge, comprehension, application, analysis, synthesis, and evaluation (Bloom, 1956; Gagne, Briggs, & Wagner, 1992). In the area of training, participants must perform at a criterion level in order for a program to be successful. Although the term *performance objectives* may not be applied exactly the same way in each of these examples, they are used to further define program outcomes in behavioral terms.

Performance Objectives for Health-Promoting Behaviors

When first considered, health-related behavioral outcomes usually are broad conceptualizations: Stop smoking. Don't drink and drive. Exercise aerobically 20 minutes per day. Eat less than 30% of calories from fat. These injunctions do not have sufficient detail on which to base an intervention. Therefore, performance objectives are used to clarify the exact performance expected from someone affected by the intervention. To determine the performance objectives for behavior, planners ask, What do the participants of this program need to do to perform the health-related behavior or to make the environmental change?

Performance objectives enable health educators to make a transition from a health-related behavior or environmental change to a detailed description of the behavior and its components. For example, eating a low-fat diet is a health-promoting behavior, but many sub-behaviors or components make up that broader behavior. To perform the behavior, an individual would need to read labels, select low-fat food, prepare low-fat food, and avoid the use of fat additives. These sub-behaviors, specified by action words, become the performance objectives. They are used to refine, focus, and make more specific what the participants in a program are expected to do as a result of the intervention. The performance objectives also help ensure the appropriateness of the behavioral expectations of a program. For example, eating low-fat food might have a different set of performance objectives for schoolchildren than for an adult with a high risk for cardiovascular disease.

In another example, Graeff, Elder, and Booth (1993) describe a WHO intervention focused on mothers' hand washing in Guatemala. These reseachers suggest that the experts often disagree about the components of ideal performance in terms of what is really necessary to have a health impact. They described lengthy discussions of experts about how many times the hands should be rubbed, whether fingernails should be cleaned, and whether each fingernail should be washed separately. The experts' disagreements are arguments for (rather than against) good behavioral specification. Health educators have less chance of changing a behavior if they do not know precisely what it is.

In the program described by Graeff and colleagues (1993), the project team defined the ideal hand washing as a set of discrete steps that would be performed by the mothers at various times. They would wash hands after using the latrine, before and after preparing food, before eating, before giving food to an infant, after changing a diaper, before entering the home, before going to bed, and before touching the cooking or drinking water. Unfortunately, the original "performance objectives" for this project required the mother to bring an extra jug of water into her home every day and spend one hour a day washing her hands. The original objectives were impractical; they were extensively modified to include addition of an environmental change to make the entire process less consuming of both time and water (pp. 42–44).

In some fields of education, such as curriculum and instruction, there is sometimes little distinction made between learning objectives and performance objectives. Both usually are specified in cognitive or affective (rather than behavioral) terms, and the terms for these types of objectives are sometimes used interchangeably (Gronlund, 1978; Mager, 1984). Intervention Mapping makes a clear distinction. Most cognitive and affective "performance" is considered part of learning objectives, which are specified later in this chapter. Learning objectives are the combination of performance with its hypothetical determinants; performance objectives specify the detail, behavioral standards, and quality required to adequately perform the behavior. Planners can distinguish performance objectives from learning or change objectives by thinking of the performance objective as an observable subset of the behavior and a learning or change objective as what must be learned or changed in order to meet or maintain the performance objective.

We reiterate: Health-related behaviors and environmental conditions are complex. The use of performance objectives allows health educators to deal with this complexity by breaking down the behavior into component parts. They are then able to decide which parts are most essential and prioritize the objectives to focus attention on the most important parts. Health educators do not want to waste time and intervention resources on components that are not likely to make a difference in helping the target population perform the health-related behavior. Performance objectives also help program planners to sequence the behavioral learning process when the learner needs to learn one part before another and to include all necessary supports for the behavior. For example, the behavior "Use condoms correctly and consistently when having sexual intercourse" can be broken down into subcomponents, which are the performance objectives listed in Table 5.1.

Table 5.1
Performance Objectives for the Behavior of "Consistently and Correctly Using Condoms During Sexual Intercourse"

Purchase condoms
    Locate condom displays in drug or grocery store
    Choose condoms that are product tested

Carry condoms or have condoms easily available
    Carry condoms in wallet or purse for no longer than a month
    Carry or store condoms in a place that is not susceptible to extreme temperatures

Negotiate the use of a condom with a partner[a]
    State mutual goals such as prevention of pregnancy or AIDS
    State clearly the intention of using a condom as a prerequisite for intercourse
    Listen to partner's concerns
    Pose solutions to partner's concerns that reference mutual goals and personal requirements

Correctly apply condoms during use
    Use a water-soluble rather than petroleum-based lubricant
    Use a new condom for each episode of intercourse
    Follow instructions on package insert for use
    Follow instructions on package insert for disposal

Maintain use over time

[a]This performance objective uses negotiation theory as described by Fisher and Ury, 1991.

Performance Objectives for Environmental Conditions

The process for writing performance objectives for changing environmental conditions parallels the process for health behaviors. The environmental condition that needs to be modified is broken down into its component parts. For example, at the organizational level the environmental change outcome of "School lunch and breakfast provide meals that are no more than 30% of calories in total fat content" can be broken down into the following performance objectives:

- Food service directors will modify menus so that foods have 30% or fewer calories from fat.
- Food service directors will modify purchase order specifications to reduce the fat content of vender-prepared food to 30% or lower.
- Nutritionists will modify recipes to reduce the fat content by replacing fat with bouillon or water for boiling or "frying."
- Nutritionists will replace dessert recipes that call for fat with recipes that substitute fruit and grains.
- Cooks will modify cooking practices to reduce the fat content of prepared foods by chilling foods, removing the fat, and then reheating to serve.

The basic question to ask to determine performance objectives for changing environmental conditions is, What does [someone in the environment] need to do to accomplish a change in the environmental condition? This general question addresses "who" is doing the action to accomplish the change, because the agent may be different for each of the performance objectives. This question is somewhat different from the question asked about performance objectives for the health-related behavior, because the health behavior question assumes a reference to the behavior of the at-risk population. Environmental change may require people outside the at-risk population to take action to modify the environmental conditions.

Exactly who will be taking the action to accomplish the performance objectives will depend on the agent in the environment who has control over, or can influence a change in, the environmental conditions. This agent might be, for example, policy makers, lawmakers, resource controllers, or service providers. In the beginning of the planning process, it may be difficult to identify specific people to include in the performance objectives for changing an environmental condition. We suggest starting with whatever information may be available about the agent and stating the "who" in terms of general groups of people or appropriate positions of responsibility, that is, roles or agents that may be able to produce change. As work on the intervention progresses, the health educator can figure out specifically who—in terms of either roles or individuals—will be performing the change in the environmental condition.

Project SPF provides a good example. The performance objectives listed in Table 5.2 were constructed to enable change in the environmental conditions. At the interpersonal level of the environment, the focus was primarily on changing the behavior of the parents and preschool staff to protect children from sun exposure. The sun-protective behaviors of parents and preschool staff were fairly simple. However, the stating of the performance objectives added specificity that enabled the program planners to more effectively communicate the essential components that should be addressed by the intervention.

Core Processes for Writing Performance Objectives

How to break down a health-related behavior or an environmental condition into subparts is not always apparent and may require additional thinking and information. The core processes presented in Chapter 3 serve as guides for writing performance objectives as applied in the following steps.

The starting place is to formulate a question. For health-related behavior, the question is, What do the participants of this program need to do to perform the health-related behavior? For environmental conditions, the question is, What does [someone in the environment] need to do to accomplish the environmental condition change? The answers to these questions form a provisional list of performance objectives. Often the initial list is a logical sequence of smaller steps that are necessary to perform the behavior or achieve the environmental condition.

Table 5.2
Environmental Conditions and Performance Objectives for Project SPF

INTERPERSONAL ENVIRONMENT

Apply SPF 15+ sunscreen to children before exposure to the sun
    Parents and preschool staff apply sunscreen at least 30 minutes before going outside
    Parents and preschool staff spread sunscreen evenly
    Parents and preschool staff cover all exposed areas, head to toe

Reapply SPF 15+ sunscreen to children when original application is no longer effective
    Parents and preschool staff carry sunscreen on outdoor outings
    Parents and preschool staff reapply sunscreen if children have more than 2 hours continued exposure to sun
    Parents and preschool staff reapply sunscreen after children have been swimming or sweating profusely

Dress children in protective clothing: hats, sleeved shirts, long shorts, and sunglasses
    Parents and preschool staff ensure that child has protective clothing at day care
    Parents and preschool staff ensure that child wears protective clothing before going outside
    Parents and preschool staff ensure that child keeps wearing protective clothing when outside

Direct children to play in the shade
    Parents and preschool staff locate shaded areas
    Parents and preschool staff plan activities for shaded areas

Reduce unnecessary sun exposure
    Parents and preschool staff limit time children spend in the sun
    Parents and preschool staff avoid peak sun hours

ORGANIZATIONAL ENVIRONMENT

Provide SPF 15+ sunscreen in the day care centers for staff to apply to children
    Preschool director purchases or obtains sunscreen with an SPF 15+
    Preschool teachers modify daily schedules to allow time to apply sunscreen to children

Increase the amount of shade in the play areas
    Preschool staff assesses the adequacy of the current natural and structural shaded areas and determines ways to increase shade
    Preschool director assesses available resources for accomplishing changes to increase shade
    Preschool director and/or governing board seeks additional resources to accomplish changes to increase shade
    Preschool director determines structures to implement based on ranking of effectiveness and feasibility
    Preschool director seeks feedback from teachers and staff
    Preschool director garners administrative approval for proposed changes

Schedule activities so children are not outside during peak sun hours
    Preschool teachers determine which outdoor activities fall within peak sun hours
    Preschool teachers modify schedules to keep children indoors during peak sun hours
    Preschool director approves and communicates the modified schedule

Next, the planner reviews the research and practice literature to determine whether the performance objectives on the provisional list are consistent with what is reported in the literature as essential subparts of the behavior or environmental condition. The review results in revisions, deletions, or additions to the provisional list.

Sometimes theory provides a rationale for performance objectives. For instance, a number of theories suggest that the self-control or self-regulatory process underlies behavior change (Bandura, 1986). In that case, the subprocesses of self-control, self-monitoring, comparison to a personal standard, and self-evaluation and reward would become performance objectives as they relate to a specific behavior. Often these processes are extended to include goal setting, monitoring and appraisal, problem identification, solution identification, action, and evaluation (Clark & Zimmerman, 1990; Janis & Mann, 1977; Lazarus, 1993). Health educators may find it useful to consider the self-regulatory process when designating health-promoting behaviors for the self-management of chronic disease. For example, in a pediatric asthma self-management program, Bartholomew and colleagues (Bartholomew, Gold, et al., 2000; Bartholomew, Shegog, et al., 2000) conceptualized both asthma-specific behaviors (e.g., taking control medications) and self-regulatory behaviors (e.g., monitoring for symptoms of asthma) in their performance objectives (see Chapter 11). Other theories (Marlatt & Gordon, 1985) would suggest a last performance objective for many behaviors: maintenance of the healthy behavior.

Finally, the planner will review the list of performance objectives and reduce the list to essential objectives needed to perform the behavior or achieve the environmental condition. This final step is important because each performance objective is the basis for further work. Each will be linked with determinants to form learning and change objectives. Nonessential (interesting but not necessary) performance objectives will expand the subsequent planning and potentially diffuse the focus of the intervention.

Validating Performance Objectives

To validate performance objectives, the planner obtains additional information by questioning and observing both members of the intervention groups and the service providers. The Cystic Fibrosis Family Education Program illustrates the process of asking service providers to validate performance objectives (Bartholomew et al., 1993). In this project, program planners sent the draft of performance objectives for cystic fibrosis (CF) self-management to a panel of five physicians who specialize in the treatment of CF and five behavioral scientists experienced at working with CF patients. The panel was asked to rate the importance of each performance objective in contributing to the health and quality of life of a child with CF. Following a revision of the objectives based on the experts' ratings and comments, the performance objectives were sent to all the directors of CF treatment centers in the United States. About 50% of the directors returned the rating questionnaire, which was sufficient to enable the program planners to revise the performance objectives. Although it did take some time and resources to conduct the validation, the program planners could go forward with the intervention development process with a high level of confidence that their performance objectives were in line and consistent with a wide consensus regarding CF care.

Another source for identification or validation of performance objectives is to obtain a review and feedback from representatives of the community. Through focus groups or interviews, potential program participants can be asked if the performance objectives fit with their views of how they would go about performing the health-related behaviors. Getting feedback from individuals who have had experience with the health behavior or the environmental condition can also be very helpful. For example, in planning a smoking cessation program, talking with both successful quitters and those who have had difficulty can give the planner ideas of how to construct performance objectives.

An often overlooked, but in some cases essential, source of information about performance objectives is direct observation of the health behavior or environmental condition. For some health problems, there may be a limited amount of information, experience, or documentation of how the related health behavior is performed or how environmental conditions break down into component parts. Observation of performance in natural settings as well as in simulated settings can be very helpful. For example, program planners developing a nutrition improvement program for schoolchildren can spend time in the school cafeteria observing how children select food, trade food, modify food, and eat or don't eat food. Observations may be done by program planners or by participant observers who are interviewed by or report on their experiences to the program planners.

MATRIX BUILDING BLOCKS: PERSONAL AND EXTERNAL DETERMINANTS

The third task in Intervention Mapping Step 1 is to select important and changeable determinants of the health behavior and environmental conditions. Determinants are those factors that have been found to be associated with the performance of the behavior or environmental change and that can be hypothesized to mediate the behavior or change. The needs assessment, completed before starting the Intervention Mapping process, may provide some information on determinants, but more refinement is usually necessary. The writing of the performance objectives adds specificity to the health behaviors and environmental conditions and may help narrow or expand the list of possible determinants. The grouping of determinants may vary, depending on what planning model or theoretical framework is being applied. Green and Kreuter (1999) organize determinants into predisposing, enabling, and reinforcing factors. However, for Intervention Mapping, we suggest a simple grouping into two categories: personal determinants and external determinants.

A matrix of proximal program objectives at a certain ecological level, then, is created by entering the performance objectives into the left column of the matrix and entering the personal and external determinants across the top of the matrix. Because there are separate matrices for each selected level, additional decisions will be necessary to assign determinants to each matrix. Determinants may be duplicated in more than one matrix. The basic assumption is that if a determinant can be considered an important influence for accomplishing one or more of the performance objectives, it should be included in the matrix.

Those factors that rest within individuals and are subject to their direct control or influence are referred to as personal determinants. These factors can be changed or influenced by interventions that involve individual learning. Personal determinants usually include cognitive factors such as knowledge, attitudes, beliefs, values, self-efficacy, expectations, and capabilities such as skills.

Those factors that rest outside the individual and influence health behavior or environmental conditions are referred to as external determinants. These factors may be social influences such as norms, social support, and reinforcement or structural influences such as access to resources, policies, and organizational climate. The individual is not able to directly control these factors; therefore, change in these determinants is not likely to be accomplished by an individual learning process.

The educational diagnosis of the needs assessment should provide a good starting list of determinants in answer to the questions, Why would a person perform a certain behavior? Why would a certain environmental agent make an environmental change? To refine or add to this provisional list, the health educator can follow the core processes outlined in Chapter 3. In reviewing the literature, the planner begins with studies regarding the issue at hand. Next is the review of theoretical constructs that have been used to explain the health behavior or environmental change of interest or related behaviors or conditions. Finally, a review of the literature on general theories that include some of the identified determinants as constructs within those theories is undertaken. For example, if the review of the literature identified self-efficacy as a possible determinant of the behavior, then it would be useful to go to the literature on social cognitive theory for which self-efficacy is a central construct (Bandura, 1986). A review of the general theory may suggest other constructs that might be considered as important determinants of the health behavior.

The needs assessment and the literature reviews provide the planner with informed or hypothesized relationships of determinants to the health behavior or environmental conditions. Determinants on the provisional list should be well-supported by the literature, and only those with the strongest relation to the behaviors should be retained. Planners often need to collect data from the at-risk groups and environmental agents to identify additional determinants and to understand how determinants manifest in a particular group.

Qualitative methods, such as focus groups or interviews, can be helpful in generating new ideas for determinants or in checking out some of the findings from the research literature. Quantitative data collection, using questionnaires that measure the determinants and the health behavior and environmental conditions of interest, can be especially helpful in judging the strength of the association between determinants and behavior or environmental conditions. With both types of data collection, planners can obtain some estimate of the presence or absence of the determinant as well as its importance for influencing change. For example, in designing an AIDS prevention program for adolescents, knowledge about the seriousness of AIDS may at first be viewed as an important determinant of risk-reduction behavior. However, pilot data collection may show that adolescents know about AIDS, and that it is therefore unlikely that an intervention to increase knowledge about AIDS will have much of an effect on behavior. Another way to judge whether a determinant is important is to measure the determinant in subgroups of the population: those who practice the behavior and those who do not. For example, if children who eat five servings of fruits and vegetables daily have a high self-efficacy for the behavior and those who eat only two servings of fruits and vegetables daily have a low self-efficacy for the behavior, then self-efficacy is likely to be judged as an important determinant.

Eventually, the list of determinants must be refined. A long list of determinants is not practical for program development. Determinants that have no logical or theoretical inter-relatedness may lead to a program that is too scattered and lacks a focus, wasting precious energy and resources. Therefore, careful analysis of the determinants at this stage improves planning results at later stages. To conduct this analysis, planners can start by rating each determinant in terms of *importance* (i.e., strength of association with the behavior or environmental condition) and *changeability* (i.e., how likely it is that health education or promotion intervention is going to influence a change in the determinant). As much as possible, the basis for rating importance and changeability should be based on evidence from the research literature. Occasionally a proposed determinant will not be adequately discussed in the literature, and the planner will need to collect data from the at-risk group and from others in the field. In addition, decisions to retain or delete determinants may be based entirely on a theoretical or conceptual basis when data are not available. For example, the evidence may be strong for one determinant such as self-efficacy, but there may be little evidence in the literature to support the importance of a related factor such as outcome expectations. However, the theoretical literature suggests that these two constructs are inter-related, and for some behaviors it may be important to address both with intervention strategies (Bandura, 1986, 1997).

MATRIX BUILDING BLOCKS: LEARNING AND CHANGE OBJECTIVES

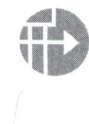

The fourth task in Intervention Mapping Step 1 is to create the matrices. Related to this task are the processes of selecting intervention levels and differentiating the population. Performance objectives and hypothetical determinants are the building blocks of matrices. Matrices are simple tables, formed by entering the performance objectives on the left side of the matrix and determinants along the top (see the matrices for Project SPF in Tables 5.3 and 5.4). Learning and change objectives are entered into the cells formed at the intersection of each performance objective and each determinant. Conceptually, a matrix of proximal program objectives represents the pathways for the most immediate changes in motivation and capability to influence health behavior and environmental conditions. Thus, each element of the matrix is inter-related, and collectively the elements are a causal model for the change process.

Selecting Intervention Levels

A separate matrix is constructed for each level of intervention for which performance objectives have been written. The final number of matrices of proximal program objectives are different for each program and are influenced by the complexity of the problem, the span of the program across levels, and the diversity of the population. To select intervention levels, program planners ask, At what levels of intervention is it necessary to attain the performance objectives? For example, Project SPF was developed for the organizational setting of preschools, and the project team identified only a few performance objectives for children (i.e., at the individual level). Most of the emphasis was on parents, teachers, and administrators to create environmental changes to reduce children's exposure to the sun. Therefore, the intervention also addressed interpersonal and organizational levels, and matrices were created for the individual, interpersonal, and organizational levels. Had the needs assessment identified important community or governmental factors influencing young children's sun exposure, then these levels would also have been reflected in the performance objectives.

Differentiating the Intervention Population

Planners may also need to create separate matrices for subgroups at any level of intervention (most often at the individual or at-risk group level). To differentiate a population means to describe two or more subgroups in which membership affects determinants of the health-related behavior, environmental condition, or performance objectives. Differentiating a population often occurs simultaneously with writing performance objectives or exploring determinants because of the question that guides differentiation: Are either performance objectives or determinants substantially different for subgroups?

The rationale for differentiating a population is the basic understanding that populations are made up of individuals and groups with different characteristics and needs, which must be considered in relation to a health problem and to a health promotion program. The greater these differences, the less likely that a single intervention focus will fit everyone in the intervention population. Differentiating the group leads to separate matrices for the proximal program objectives so that a parallel planning process can be undertaken.

Table 5.3
Matrix for Children (At-Risk Group) in Project SPF (Sample Cells)

PERFORMANCE OBJECTIVES FOR THE CHILD	PERSONAL DETERMINANTS			EXTERNAL DETERMINANTS			
	ATTITUDES	SKILLS AND SELF-EFFICACY	KNOWLEDGE	OUTCOME EXPECTATIONS	CUES	REINFORCEMENT	NORMS
Cooperate with sun protection practices by parent or pre-school staff	Expresses positive feeling toward being protected from the sun			Describes how cooperating will keep skin healthy	Parents and day care teachers provide cues for cooperating with sunscreen application		Preschool director posts pictures and guidelines for sun protection Children in the school talk to each other, parents, and teachers about sun protection
Stand still for application	Expresses positive attitude toward being a helper		Tells about how standing still allows sunscreen to be put on evenly			Parents and day care teachers praise the child for standing still and getting good coverage of sunscreen	
Dress in covering clothes for playing outside						Parents and day care teachers praise the child for dressing in covering clothes	
Leave on clothes and hat	Feels positive about protective clothes Likes sun hat			Expects to be safe from the sun and healthy when wearing protective clothing	Hat and clothes hang by preschool door and by door at home	Parents and day care teachers praise the child for leaving on hat and covering clothes while in the sun	Family and playmates wear protective clothing

(handwritten note in KNOWLEDGE column: "learning & change objectives")

PERFORMANCE OBJECTIVES FOR THE CHILD	PERSONAL DETERMINANTS				EXTERNAL DETERMINANTS		
	ATTITUDES	SKILLS AND SELF-EFFICACY	KNOWLEDGE	OUTCOME EXPECTATIONS	CUES	REINFORCEMENT	NORMS
Remind parent or preschool staff to practice sun protection on behalf of the child						Parents and preschool staff praise the child for reminding adults about sunscreen	
Tell adult that child can't go outside without sunscreen		Demonstrates telling an adult about the need for sunscreen Expresses confidence about ability to tell an adult about sunscreen		Describes expectation that an adult will help with sunscreen if reminded Describes expectation that even coverage by an adult will help every part of the skin stay healthy	Parents and teacher place sun protection preparation station by door	Parents and prescool staff praise the child for standing still and getting good coverage of sunscreen	Teachers talk about how good it is for children to remind parents about health issues in general and sunscreen in particular
Bring sunscreen to adult		Demonstrates bringing-sunscreen to adult		States that an adult will help with sunscreen if reminded States that even coverage by an adult will help every part of the skin stay healthy	Parents and teacher place sun protection preparation station by door	Parents and day care teachers praise the child for bringing sunscreen to adult as part of preparation for playing outside	
Come to adult for reapplication					Parent and teacher place sun protection preparation kit in tote bag	Parents and day care teachers praise the child for coming when called for sunscreen	

Table 5.4
Matrix for Organizational Environmental Change in Project SPF (Sample Cells)

PERFORMANCE OBJECTIVES FOR THE PRESCHOOL DIRECTOR	PERSONAL DETERMINANTS					EXTERNAL DETERMINANTS	
	PERCEIVED NORMS	ATTITUDES	SKILLS AND SELF-EFFICACY	KNOWLEDGE	OUTCOME EXPECTATIONS AND PERCEIVED SUSCEPTIBILITY	CLIMATE AND MANAGEMENT SUPPORT	REINFORCEMENT
Provide shade in outdoor areas used by preschoolers	Recognizes sun protection and shade adequacy as concerns for preschool administration	Describes ensuring shade as positive			Describes children as susceptible to skin cancer caused by by lack of shade. Argues that increasing shade will decrease risk	Management expresses concern for need for shade	Management and parents notice staff providing shade and praise them
Assess adequacy of current natural and structural areas and determine ways to increase shade	Recognizes that peers are taking action to assess shade		Demonstrates ability to assess shade. Expresses confidence in ability to assess shade			Management makes time and resources available to conduct assessments	
Assess available resources for accomplishing changes to increase shade	Talks about other preschool administrators as seeking resources for sun protection			States cost of change in terms of money, time, and personnel		Management shares information on current resources with director	Management and parents provide help for seeking additional funding

PERFORMANCE OBJECTIVES FOR THE PRESCHOOL DIRECTOR	PERSONAL DETERMINANTS					EXTERNAL DETERMINANTS	
	PERCEIVED NORMS	ATTITUDES	SKILLS AND SELF-EFFICACY	KNOWLEDGE	OUTCOME EXPECTATIONS AND PERCEIVED SUSCEPTIBILITY	CLIMATE AND MANAGEMENT SUPPORT	REINFORCEMENT
Obtain additional resources to accomplish changes to increase shade			Demonstrates ability to contact community organizations about funding	Identifies sources for seeking funds		Director and management maintain open communication. Management listens to suggestions from director and staff for use of resources	
Seek construction consultation and determine structures to implement based on ranking of effectiveness and feasibility			Expresses confidence in ability to rank structural changes	Identifies features that make options for shade more effective and feasible			
Seek feedback from teachers and staff						Staff members express support for plans to increase shade	
Garner administrative approval for proposed changes			Expresses confidence in ability to discuss changes with management			Management expresses support for plans to increase shade	

Some of the variables that may be important to consider in the differentiation of a population are the ones that were mentioned in the needs assessment. They include age and gender, geographic location, socioeconomic status, education, and race/ethnicity. In addition, using stage theories and models such as child development, adult development, stages of change models (DiClemente & Prochaska, 1998; Prochaska & DiClemente, 1984), and stages of organizational change (Goodman & Steckler, 1989; Scheirer, Allen, & Rauch, 1987; Trice, Beyer, & Hunt, 1978; Zaltman & Duncan, 1977) to differentiate populations will, in many cases, enhance a planner's ability to develop learning and change objectives that successfully define the program change for a group.

Differentiation by developmental stage offers a good example. To formulate performance objectives for the Cystic Fibrosis Family Education Program, planners asked, What should the child with cystic fibrosis be able to do to manage CF? (Bartholomew et al., 1991, 1993). Because the ages of children in the CF population spanned the range of 4 through 18 years, the planners asked how the performance objectives would be different for the developmental stages represented by preschoolers ages 4 through 6, school-age children ages 7 through 11, and adolescents ages 12 through 18. Having different objectives for different age groups was important because the behavioral, cognitive, emotional, and social capabilities of children at these various stages of development are so different that the children could not be expected to carry out similar activities to manage their chronic illness (Eiser, Patterson, & Tripp, 1984; Johnson et al., 1982).

Another reason to differentiate a population is that determinants, the variables that lead to learning and performing behaviors or to making environmental changes, may be different for subgroups even when the performance objectives are the same. For example, peer norms may strongly influence a smoker in the precontemplation stage of change for cessation, whereas lack of skills for quitting might have a higher impact on the behavior of a smoker in the preparation, action, or maintenance stages of change. Furthermore, if the determinants are different, then the theoretical methods chosen to influence the determinants may be different. For example, some research suggests that determinants of condom use among high school students vary according to experience with sexual intercourse using condoms (Schaalma, Kok, Poelman, & Reinders, 1994). Young men who had previous experience with condoms had more negative attitudes about the effects of condoms on pleasure. Self-efficacy for buying and having condoms was higher, but self-efficacy for negotiating condom use with a partner was lower. Experience with condom use was correlated with age and having a steady relationship, and when people had a steady relationship, intention to use condoms was lower. Based on this knowledge of determinant difference related to experience, program planners might choose to develop different matrices of proximal objectives and include program strategies and messages for these different intervention groups.

Both performance objectives and determinants may be different for subgroups. In Project PANDA, an intervention to help pregnant women who had stopped smoking refrain from returning to smoking after the delivery of the baby, the planners differentiated the population of women by stage of change: precontemplators, contemplators, and action and maintenance stages (see Chapter 13). The planners hypothesized that the women, although they had stopped smoking, were not all in the action stage of change. There was considerable evidence that most of the women during pregnancy had not used the processes of change that would enable them to remain nonsmokers. Therefore, performance objectives and determinants were defined for each group according to stage of change. For example, precontemplators needed to move to contemplation of remaining smoke-free, and to do this they had to shift their decisional balance to being more negative about smoking. Those women in the action stage needed to apply processes to remain in action, for example, stimulus control, or removing items from their environments that stimulate smoking. The PANDA example also illustrates the point that the development of separate matrices does not imply the need for separate programs, but does imply the need for program methods to address the different learning and change objectives from each of the matrices.

Similar to differentiation, segmentation refers to grouping the population by variables (such as preferred communication network) that will influence the effectiveness of the message (Lefebvre, 1992; Lefebvre & Flora, 1988; Lefebvre, Lurie, Goodman, Weinberg, & Loughrey, 1995; Lefebvre & Rochlin, 1997; Leviton, Mrazek, & Stoto, 1996; Ling, Franklin, Lindsteadt, & Gearon, 1992). The variables used by marketers and communicators to segment a population in service of message development may imply underlying differences in determinants, but these differences may not be explained as they are in Intervention Mapping.

Differentiation is part of the basis for tailoring, a technique of using computer technology to individualize intervention messages based on certain measured characteristics of the population (Campbell et al., 1994; Kreuter & Strecher, 1996; Skinner, Strecher, & Hospers, 1994; Strecher et al., 1994). Tailoring may be done on the basis of differences in behaviors or determinants, the basis of differentiation. But tailoring may also be done at a later stage of program development on characteristics that did not lead to differentiation and the creation of different matrices. For example, materials may be tailored on ethnicity or gender to increase identification with role models in communicated messages. Tailoring and segmentation are very important for development of intervention strategies and programs, but they do not imply the need for separate matrices in Step 1 of Intervention Mapping. They can be done later and are discussed again in Step 3 (Chapter 7).

In summary, differentiating the population leads to separate matrices of proximal program objectives for each group. The matrices are used to guide program planning to design interventions appropriate for each subgroup. The result may be a separate program for each group or a single program with multiple components, methods, or strategies that can accommodate differences among groups.

Constructing Matrices and Writing Learning and Change Objectives

At this point, the planner has made a preliminary decision about the number of matrices for the project, based on population differentiation and levels of environmental change. The planner enters the performance objectives down the left side of a matrix and the determinants across the top. The next task is to assess each cell of the matrix to judge whether the determinant is likely to influence accomplishment of the performance objective. It is unlikely that each of the determinants will be an important influence for every performance objective. Because learning or change objectives are needed for those cells in which the determinant is likely to influence accomplishment of the performance objective, this task can be a review and elimination process. One way that the planner accomplishes this task is to look at each cell, decide whether change in a particular determinant is necessary for the performance objective, put an X through unimportant cells, and then write learning and change objectives for the cells that have not been eliminated.

Learning objectives are written for the personal determinants and change objectives for the external determinants. The basic question that leads to formation of a learning objective is, What do the participants in the program need to learn (related to the determinant) to do the performance objective? For example, Table 5.5 shows a cell in which the performance objective (PO) "purchase condoms" is paired with the determinant of "knowledge." The question used to address this cell can be worded as, What do the participants in the program need to learn related to knowledge to be able to purchase a condom? Answers to this question lead to the following learning objectives (LO):

PO: Purchase condoms

LO: List places where condoms can be purchased or obtained free

LO: Compare different types of condoms and features to improve effectiveness

LO: Explain how to buy or obtain a condom

These learning objectives become the learning steps toward increasing knowledge to purchase condoms. In another example that uses the same performance objective, a focus on the cell connected with the determinant of self-efficacy leads to the question, What do the participants need to learn related to self-efficacy to be able to purchase condoms? This question yields the following learning objectives:

PO: Purchase condoms

LO: Express confidence in ability to go into a store and buy a condom

LO: Express confidence in ability to deal with embarrassment when buying a condom

These examples show that learning objectives are stated with strong verbs. Words to help with this task are included in Table 5.6. Learning objectives begin with a verb that defines the action. The action is followed by a context or condition in which the behavior is likely to occur, and is completed by restating the behavior from the performance objective. The purpose of stating learning objectives in this manner is to make as specific as possible what learning outcome needs to be achieved to accomplish the learning objective. Planners who write learning objectives with an action verb, context, and behavior have a clear direction to the next steps in the Intervention Mapping process: selecting intervention methods and translating methods into learning strategies.

Change objectives define what needs to be changed in determinants that are external to the individual and needed to accomplish the performance objective. For example, a planning group addressing smoking prevention in adolescents has identified from the research literature that peer norms are an important external determinant of smoking behavior. The behavioral outcome for the program is "choosing not to smoke." One of the performance objectives for choosing not to smoke is "resist peer pressure to smoke a cigarette." When the external determinant of peer norms is crossed with the performance objective, the following examples of change objectives (CO) can be formulated and then used to guide the design of intervention methods and strategies:

PO: Resist peer pressure to smoke a cigarette

CO: Peers demonstrate resisting pressure to smoke

CO: Peers desist in pressuring others to smoke

Project SPF can be used here to illustrate the writing of change objectives for external determinants at the interpersonal level of environmental change. One of the environmental outcomes is that staff will apply sunscreen to children in the preschools. Here is a sample performance objective crossed with the external determinant "cues" to create change objectives:

PO: Teachers will apply sunscreen to children at least 30 minutes before going outside

CO: Child asks for sunscreen

CO: Fellow teachers remind teacher to apply sunscreen to children

CO: Teachers place sun protection supplies by the classroom door

Clarifying External Determinants and Environmental Conditions

Neither external determinants nor environmental conditions are under the control of the individual. They are controlled by external agents, for instance, peers for social support, teachers for reinforcement, managers for organizational climate, decision makers for policies, gatekeepers for access to resources. As a result, change objectives are formulated by referring to an external agent who will act: peers will give support, teachers will reinforce, and managers will

Table 5.5
Matrix of Personal Determinants for the Behavior of "Consistently and Correctly Using Condoms During Sexual Intercourse" (Sample Cells)

PERFORMANCE OBJECTIVES FOR THE AT-RISK GROUP	KNOWLEDGE	SKILLS AND SELF-EFFICACY	OUTCOME EXPECTATIONS	PERCEIVED NORMS
Puchase condoms	Explains how to buy or obtain a condom	Reflects confidence in ability to go into a store and buy a condom		Explains that peers go into stores and buy condoms
Locate condom display in drug or grocery store	Lists places where condoms can be purchased or obtained free	Expresses confidence in ability to deal with embarrassment when buying a condom		
Choose condoms that are product tested	Compares different types of condoms and features to improve effectiveness			
Carry condoms or have condoms easily available				States that peers carry condoms in purses and wallets
Carry condoms in wallet or purse for no longer than a month	Describes how long condoms can be kept without increasing risk of breakage			
Carry or store condoms in a place that maintains correct temperature	States safe temperatures for storing condoms			

[a] This performance objective uses negotiation theory as described by Fisher and Ury, 1991.

PERFORMANCE OBJECTIVES FOR THE AT-RISK GROUP	KNOWLEDGE	SKILLS AND SELF-EFFICACY	OUTCOME EXPECTATIONS	PERCEIVED NORMS
Negotiate the use of a condom with partner[a]	Lists the steps of successful negotiation		Describes a personal belief that negotiation will lead to positive experience in which both partners are satisfied	Explains that peers talk to their partners about condom use
State mutual goals such as prevention of pregnancy or AIDS		Summarizes mutual goals as would be said to a partner		
State clearly the intention of using a condom as a prerequisite for intercourse		Advocates clear intention to not have sex without a condom	States a belief that negotiation will result in condom use	
Listen to partner's concerns		Demonstrates discussing partner's concerns	Describes how condom use protects against STDs and HIV	
Pose solutions to partner's concerns that reference mutual goals and personal requirements		Expresses confidence in ability to do each step of negotiation		

[a]This performance objective uses negotiation theory as described by Fisher and Ury, 1991.

Table 5.6
Strong Verbs for Writing Learning Objectives

accept	cooperate	install	rank
adopt	check	interview	recall
advocate	defend	judge	recognize
analyze	define	justify	reflect
arrange	demonstrate	label	remove
approve	describe	list	research
appraise	develop	locate	resolve
bargain	differentiate	manipulate	review
calculate	discriminate	modify	select
care	draw	name	sort
change	evaluate	operate	specify
choose	execute	organize	state
classify	explain	outline	study
categorize	express	persuade	take
challenge	fill out	plan	tell
chart	forecast	prepare	translate
compare	formulate	prescribe	use
conduct	generate	produce	write
construct	identify	purchase	
contrast	inform	question	

Note. From *Planning Programs for Adult Learners: A Practical Guide for Educators, Trainees, and Staff Developers*, by R. Caffarella, 1985, San Francisco: Jossey-Bass.

support the innovation. There is a logical relation between external determinants and environmental conditions on the one hand and between change objectives and performance objectives for environmental conditions on the other hand. If the analysis of the environment is done very carefully and exhaustively, not many external determinants are left for the *individual's* behavior because they are part of the specified *environmental* change and performance objectives. But if the environmental analysis is insufficient (in hindsight), some very relevant external determinants may show up after the fact.

The earlier example about school lunches identified "Availability of low-fat alternatives in the schools" as an environmental factor, with a performance objective of "Food service directors will modify menus to include more low-fat food." As a result, the planning team members who are creating this matrix did not need the external determinant "availability" for the individual student's behavior. However, if they had not identified availability as an environmental condition, they might have perceived later that availability is indeed a relevant external determinant of students' food choices. Their change objective would then be "Food service directors will modify menus to include more low-fat food."

The school lunch example illustrates the importance of making judgments in using Intervention Mapping as a planning tool. In some cases, leaving an external determinant as a determinant and using change objectives as the proximal objectives will fit well with planning the program. In other cases, the external determinant is such a strong environmental influence that it makes sense to elevate it to an environmental condition and address it in greater detail with performance objects and related determinants. Intervention Mapping does not offer a cookbook approach; planning groups need to continuously make judgments about where external determinants fit best in the matrix structure.

One consideration planners can use in deciding where to place an external determinant is to look at the intervention's main emphasis. In other words, can the change objective be taken care of in the program (e.g., the food service director as one of the implementers), or does part of the program need to be directed at an environmental condition (e.g., the food service director as an environmental agent)? Notice that in both cases the planning team has to follow the Intervention Mapping process of analyzing determinants of the behavior, selecting methods and strategies, and developing an intervention, such as training. The difference is that in the first case, the team does this process as part of anticipation of implementation (Chapter 8), and in the second case they do it with the intervention program component that targets environmental conditions.

Another example can be illustrated by the use of the external determinant of reinforcement. In the asthma self-management program, the planning team identified reinforcement as an external determinant for the child's performance objectives. The question they asked themselves was, Should we address reinforcement in the intervention component for children, or should we create a program component for an environmental agent who will provide the reinforcement? The team could, for instance, have decided to develop a computer program that would reinforce the child after successful self-management behavior. In that case, they could have taken care of the change objective in the computer program. They could also have decided to have the asthma specialist give the reinforcement to the child. In that case, because they knew how difficult it is to change specialists' behavior, they might have wanted to direct a substantial part of their intervention to this environmental agent. Therefore, they would have needed to formulate specific performance objectives, define personal and external determinants, and choose specific learning and change objectives. They would have needed to include the specialist as an environmental factor and develop a matrix.

When health educators treat a change objective as something that can be handled through the at-risk groups as a small part of the program, they leave the change objective where it is: in the cell that crosses performance objective with external determinant. When they decide the change objective is a bigger issue, they add a new item to the list of environmental conditions: The external determinant now becomes an environmental condition. Then the planners add new performance objectives, determinants, and change objectives. The planners, of course, need to think about personal and external determinants of these new performance objectives, which may lead to a repetition of this whole process at a higher level. For instance, food service directors may be seriously restricted by regulations or specialists may be seriously restricted by time. This shift to higher levels, however, soon reaches a point at which the determinants are outside the scope of the health educators to plan and execute appropriate programs.

External determinants may present another challenge. Sometimes individuals can actually do something about external determinants. When the social norm is negative, planners might want to change the social norm, but they could also try to increase the individual's resistance to that norm (Evans et al., 1978). When physicians do not take enough time to explain expected treatment behaviors to patients, for example, health educators might want to change the physician's behavior, but they could also try to prepare the patients to ask certain questions. When the external determinants are very difficult to change, a health educator's only alternative may be an indirect approach through personal determinants and learning objectives of the individual or the agent. An example of this situation is tobacco advertising. The local group planning a tobacco prevention program for adolescents may not be able to get the tobacco companies to alter their marketing to young people; the group can, however, create learning objectives for adolescents to resist the messages of tobacco advertising (U.S. DHHS, 1994). A word of caution is in order: Program planners must be careful not to place individuals in situations that make them responsible for environmental conditions that are not in their control, and not to raise unrealistic expectations that individuals can influence these conditions without interventions occurring at other levels of the environment.

SUMMARY

Matrices provide clear statements of what factors need to be changed by a program. Once matrices of proximal program objectives are complete, they serve as maps for both the development of intervention components and the planning of program evaluation. In Intervention Mapping Step 2, matrices are used to guide the choice of theoretical change methods. The process of finding theoretical methods depends on the columns of learning and change objectives that are listed under the heading "determinants." The matrices also help with the planning of practical strategies to deliver the methods. The creation of strategies is aided by a study of learning and change objectives in the rows of the matrices that are listed under the heading "performance objectives." Strategies are matched to performance objectives.

Tasks for Intervention Mapping Step 1:
Preparing Matrices of Proximal Program Objectives

- State expected changes in behavior and environment
- Specify performance objectives
- Specify determinants
- Create matrices of proximal program objectives, and write learning and change objectives (if necessary, differentiate the population and specify levels of change)

REFERENCES

Abel, E., Darby, A. L., & Ramachandran, R. (1994). Managing hypertension among veterans in an outpatient screening program. *Journal of the American Academy of Nurse Practitioners, 6*(9), 413–419.

Agars, J., & McMurray, A. (1993). An evaluation of comparative strategies for teaching breast self-examination. *Journal of Advanced Nursing, 18*(10), 1595–1603.

Alcoe, S. Y., Wallace, D. G., & Beck, B. M. (1990). Ten years later: An update of the case for teaching breast self-examination. *Canadian Journal of Public Health, 81*(6), 447–449.

Bandura, A. (1986). *Social foundations of thought and action: A social cognitive theory.* Englewood Cliffs, NJ: Prentice Hall.

Bandura, A. (1997). *Self-efficacy: The exercise of control.* New York: Freeman.

Bartholomew, L. K., Gold, R. S., Parcel, G. S., Czyzewski, D. I., Sockrider, M. M., Fernandez, M., Shegog, R., & Swank, P. R. (2000). Watch, Discover, Think, and Act: Evaluation of computer-assisted instruction to improve asthma self-management in inner-city children. *Patient Education and Counseling, 39*(2–3), 269–280.

Bartholomew, L. K., Parcel, G. S., Seilheimer, D. K., Czyzewski, D., Spinelli, S. H., & Congdon, B. (1991). Development of a health education program to promote the self-management of cystic fibrosis. *Health Education Quarterly, 18*(4), 429–443.

Bartholomew, L. K., Shegog, R., Parcel, G. S., Gold, R. S., Fernandez, M., Czyzewski, D. I., Sockrider, M. M., & Berlin, N. (2000). Watch, Discover, Think, and Act: A model for patient education program development. *Patient Education and Counseling, 39*(2–3), 253–268.

Bartholomew, L. K., Sockrider, M. M., Seilheimer, D. K., Czyzewski, D. I., Parcel, G. S., & Spinelli, S. H. (1993). Performance objectives for the self-management of cystic fibrosis. *Patient Education and Counseling, 22*(1), 15–25.

Bloom, S. S. (1956). *Taxonomy of education objectives: Handbook I. Cognitive domain.* New York: McKay.

Brandon, P. R. (1992). State-level evaluations of school programs funded under the Drug-Free Schools and Communities Act. *Journal of Drug Education, 22*(1), 25–36.

Brock, D. J. (1996). Population screening for cystic fibrosis. *Current Opinion in Pediatrics, 8*(6), 635–638.

Brownson, R. C., Eriksen, M. P., Davis, R. M., & Warner, K. E. (1997). Environmental tobacco smoke: Health effects and policies to reduce exposure. *Annual Reviews of Public Health, 18,* 163–185.

Caffarella, R. (1985). *Planning programs for adult learners: A practical guide for educators, trainees, and staff developers.* San Francisco: Jossey-Bass.

Campbell, M. K., DeVellis, B. M., Strecher, V. J., Ammerman, A. S., DeVellis, R. F., & Sandler, R. S. (1994). Improving dietary behavior: The effectiveness of tailored messages in primary care settings. *American Journal of Public Health, 84*(5), 783–787.

Clark, N. M., Janz, N. K., Dodge, J. A., & Sharpe, P. A. (1992). Self regulation of health behavior: The "Take PRIDE" program. *Health Education Quarterly, 19*(3), 341–354.

Clark, N. M., Rakowski, W., Wheeler, J. R., Ostrander, L. D., Oden, S., & Keteyian, S. (1988). Development of self-management education for elderly heart patients. *Gerontologist, 28*(4), 491–494.

Clark, N. M., & Zimmerman, B. J. (1990). A social cognitive view of self-regulated learning about health. *Health Education Research: Theory and Practice, 5*(3), 371–379.

Cohen, S., Lichtenstein, E., Kingsolver, K., Mermelstein, R., Baer, J. S., & Kamarck, T. W. (1988). Social support interventions for smoking cessation. In B. H. Gottlieb (Ed.), *Marshaling social support: Formats, processes, and effects* (pp. 211–240). Newbury Park, CA: Sage.

Craun, A. M., & Deffenbacher, J. L. (1987). The effects of information, behavioral rehearsal, and prompting on breast self-exams. *Journal of Behavioral Medicine, 10*(4), 351–365.

DiClemente, C., & Prochaska, J. (1998). Toward a comprehensive transtheoretical model of change. In W. Miller & N. Heather (Eds.), *Treating addictive behaviors* (pp. 3–24). New York: Plenum Press.

DiMatteo, M. R., & DiNicola, D. D. (1985). *Achieving patient compliance: The psychology of the medical practitioner's role.* New York: Pergamon Press.

Earp, J. A., & Ory, M. G. (1979). The effects of social support and health professionals' home visits on patient adherence to hypertension regimens. *Preventive Medicine, 8,* 155–165.

Eiser, C., Patterson, D., & Tripp, J. H. (1984). Illness experience and children's concepts of health and illness. *Child: Care, Health, and Development, 10*(3), 157–162.

Epstein, L. H., & Wing, R. R. (1987). Behavioral treatment of childhood obesity. *Psychological Bulletin, 101*(3), 331–342.

Eriksen, M. P., & Gottlieb, N. H. (1999). A review of the health impact of smoking control at the workplace. *American Journal of Health Promotion, 13*(3), 83–104.

Evans, R. I., Rozelle, R. M., Mittlemark, M. B., Hansen, W. B., Bane, A. L., & Havis, J. (1978). Deterring the onset of smoking in children: Knowledge of immediate physiological effects and coping with peer pressure, media pressure, and parental modeling. *Journal of Applied Social Psychology, 8*(2), 126–135.

Fisher, R., & Ury, W. (with Patton, B.). (1991). *Getting to yes: Negotiating agreement without giving in.* New York: Penguin Books.

Fox, C. L., Forbing, S. E., & Anderson, P. S. (1988). A comprehensive approach to drug-free schools and communities. *Journal of School Health, 58*(9), 365–369.

Frank, G. C., Vaden, A., & Martin, J. (1987). School health programs: Child nutrition programs. *Journal of School Health, 57*(10), 451–460.

Gagne, R. M., Briggs, L. J., & Wagner, W. W. (1992). *Principles of instructional design.* Orlando, FL: Harcourt Brace Jovanovich.

Ganster, D. C., & Victor, B. (1988). The impact of social support on mental and physical health. *British Journal of Medical Psychology, 61*(Pt. 1), 17–36.

Gentry, E. M., & Jorgensen, C. M. (1991). Monitoring the exposure of "America Responds to AIDS" PSA campaign. *Public Health Reports, 106*(6), 651–655.

Glasgow, R. E., Toobert, D. J., Hampson, S. E., Brown, J. E., Lewinson, P. M., & Donnelly, J. (1992). Improving self-care among older patients with type II diabetes: The "Sixty Something . . ." study. *Patient Education and Counseling, 19*(1), 61–74.

Goodman, R. M., Speers, M. A., McLeroy, K., Fawcett, S., Kegler, M., Parker, E., Smith, S., & Sterling, T. (1998). Identifying and defining the dimensions of community capacity to provide a basis for measurement. *Health Education and Behavior, 25*(3), 258–278.

Goodman, R. M., & Steckler, A. (1989). A model for the institutionalization of health promotion programs. *Family and Community Health, 11*(4), 63–78.

Goumans, M., & Springett, J. (1997). From projects to policy: "Healthy Cities" as a mechanism for policy change for health? *Health Promotion International, 12*(24), 311–322.

Graeff, J. A., Elder, J. P., & Booth, E. M. (1993). *Communication for health and behavior change: A developing country perspective.* San Francisco: Jossey-Bass.

Green, L. W., & Kreuter, M. W. (1999). *Health promotion planning: An educational and ecological approach* (3rd ed.). Mountain View, CA: Mayfield.

Gronlund, E. E. (1978). *Stating objectives for classroom instruction* (2nd ed.). New York: Macmillan.

Haglund, B. J. A., Finer, D., Tillgren, P., & Pettersson, B. (1996). *Creating supportive environments for health.* Geneva, Switzerland: World Health Organization.

Heaney, C. A., & Israel, B. A. (1997). Social networks and social support. In K. Glanz, F. M. Lewis, & B. K. Rimer (Eds.), *Health behavior and health education: Theory, research, and practice* (2nd ed., pp. 179–205). San Francisco: Jossey-Bass.

Hirsch, B. J., & DuBois, D. L. (1992). The relation of peer social support and psychological symptomatology during the transition to junior high school: A two-year longitudinal analysis. *American Journal of Community Psychology, 20*(3), 333–347.

House, J. S., Umberson, D., & Landis, K. R. (1988). Structures and processes of social support. *Annual Review of Sociology, 14,* 293–318.

Hurley, S. F., & Kaldor, J. M. (1992). The benefits and risks of mammographic screening for breast cancer. *Epidemiologic Reviews, 14,* 101–130.

Israel, B. A. (1982). Social networks and health status: Linking theory, research, and practice. *Patient Counselling and Health Education, 4*(2), 65–79.

Jacobs, I. J., Oram, D. H., & Bast, R. C., Jr. (1992). Strategies for improving the specificity of screening for ovarian cancer with tumor-associated antigens CA 125, CA 15-3, and TAG 72.3. *Obstetrics and Gynecology, 80*(3, Pt. 1), 396–399.

Jacobson, D. E. (1986). Types and timing of social support. *Journal of Health and Social Behavior, 27*(3), 250–264.

Janis, I. L., & Mann, L. (1977). *Decision making: A psychological analysis of conflict, choice, and commitment.* New York: Free Press.

Johnson, S. B., Pollak, R. T., Silverstein, J. H., Rosenbloom, A. L., Spillar, R., McCallum, M., & Harkavy, J. (1982). Cognitive and behavioral knowledge about insulin-dependent diabetes among children and parents. *Pediatrics, 69*(6), 708–713.

Kilburn, K. H. (1998). Pulmonary responses to gases and particles. In R. B. Wallace (Ed.), *Maxcy-Rosenau-Last Public health and preventive medicine* (14th ed., pp. 577–591). Stamford, CT: Appleton & Lange.

Kreuter, M. W., & Strecher, V. J. (1996). Do tailored behavior change messages enhance the effectiveness of health risk appraisals? Results from a randomized trial. *Health Education Research: Theory and Practice, 11*(1), 97–105.

Labarthe, D. R. (1998). *Epidemiology and prevention of cardiovascular diseases: A global challenge.* Gaithersburg, MD: Aspen.

Lazarus, R. S. (1993). Coping theory and research: Past, present, and future. *Psychosomatic Medicine, 55*(3), 234–247.

Lefebvre, R. C. (1992). The social marketing imbroglio in health promotion. *Health Promotion International, 7*(1), 61–64.

Lefebvre, R. C., & Flora, J. A. (1988). Social marketing and public health intervention. *Health Education Quarterly, 15*(3), 299–315.

Lefebvre, R. C., Lurie, D., Goodman, L. S., Weinberg, L., & Loughrey, K. (1995). Social marketing and nutrition education: Inappropriate or misunderstood? *Journal of Nutrition Education, 27*(3), 146–150.

Lefebvre, R. C., & Rochlin, L. (1997). Social marketing. In K. Glanz, F. M. Lewis, & B. K. Rimer (Eds.), *Health behavior and health education: Theory, research, and practice* (2nd ed., pp. 384–402). San Francisco: Jossey-Bass.

Leviton, L., Mrazek, P., & Stoto, M. (1996). Social marketing to adolescents and minority populations. *Social Marketing Quarterly, 3,* 6–23.

Ling, J. C., Franklin, B. A. K., Lindsteadt, J. F., & Gearon, S. A. N. (1992). Social marketing: Its place in public health. *Annual Review of Public Health, 13,* 341–362.

Livingstone, J., Axton, R. A., Mennie, M., Gilfillan, A., & Brock, D. J. H. (1993). A preliminary trial of couple screening for cystic fibrosis: Designing an appropriate information leaflet. *Clinical Genetics, 43*(2), 57–62.

Luepker, R. V. (1998). Heart disease. In R. B. Wallace (Ed.), *Maxcy-Rosenau-Last public health and preventive medicine* (14th ed.). Stamford, CT: Appleton & Lange.

Lynch, B. S., & Bonnie, R. J. (Eds.) (with Committee on Preventing Nicotine Addiction in Children and Youths, Institute of Medicine). (1994). *Growing up tobacco free: Preventing nicotine addiction in children and youths.* Washington, DC: National Academy Press.

Mager, R. F. (1984). *Preparing instructional objectives* (rev. 2nd ed.). Belmont, CA: Lake Publishing.

Marlatt, G. A., & Gordon, J. R. (1985). *Relapse prevention: Maintenance strategies in the treatment of addictive behaviors.* New York: Guilford.

Minkler, M., & Wallerstein, N. (1997). Improving health through community organization and community building: A health education perspective. In M. Minkler (Ed.), *Community organizing and community building for health.* San Francisco: Jossey-Bass.

Morisky, D. E., DeMuth, N. M., Field-Fass, M., Green, L. W., & Levine, D. M. (1985). Evaluation of family health education to build social support for long-term control of high blood pressure. *Health Education Quarterly, 12*(1), 35–50.

Nader, P. R., Sellers, D. E., Johnson, C. C., Perry, C. L., Stone, E. J., Cook, K. C., Bebchuk, J., & Luepker, R. V. (1996). The effect of adult participation in a school-based family intervention to improve children's diet and physical activity: The Child and Adolescent Trial for Cardiovascular Health. *Preventive Medicine, 25*(4), 455–464.

Natowicz, M. R., & Prence, E. M. (1996). Heterozygote screening for Tay-Sachs. *Current Opinion in Pediatrics, 8*(6), 625–629.

Ohkubo, T., Imai, Y., Tsuji, I., Nagai, K., Watanabe, N., Minami, N., Itoh, O., Bando, T., Sakuma, M., Fukao, A., Satoh, H., Hisamichi, S., & Abe, K. (1997). Prediction of mortality by ambulatory blood pressure monitoring versus screening blood pressure measurements: A pilot study in Ohasama. *Journal of Hypertension, 15*(4), 357–364.

Perry, C. L., Sellers, D. E., Johnson, C., Pedersen, S., Bachman, K. J., Parcel, G. S., Stone, E. J., Luepker, R. V., Wu, M., Nader, P. R., & Cook, K. (1997). The Child and Adolescent Trial for Cardiovascular Health (CATCH): Intervention, implementation, and feasibility for elementary schools in the United States. *Health Education and Behavior, 24*(6), 716–735.

Perry, C. L., Stone, E. J., Parcel, G. S., Ellison, R. C., Nader, P. R., Webber, L. S., & Luepker, R. V. (1990). School-based cardiovascular health promotion: The Child and Adolescent Trial for Cardiovascular Health (CATCH). *Journal of School Health, 60*(8), 406–413.

Pierce, J. P., Choi, W. S., Gilpin, E. A., Farkas, A. J., & Berry, C. C. (1998). Tobacco industry promotion of cigarettes and adolescent smoking. *Journal of the American Medical Association, 279*(7), 511–515.

Pollay, R. W., Siddarth, S., Siegel, M., Haddix, A., Merritt, R. K., Giovino, G. A., & Eriksen, M. P. (1996, April). The last straw? Cigarette advertising and realized market shares among youths and adults, 1979–1993. *Journal of Marketing, 60*(2), 1–16.

Prochaska, J. O., & DiClemente, C. C. (1984). *The transtheoretical approach: Crossing traditional boundaries of therapy.* Homeward, IL: Dow Jones–Irwin.

Rhodes, J. E., Contreras, J. M., & Mangelsdorf, S. C. (1994). Natural mentor relationships among Latina adolescent mothers: Psychological adjustment, moderating processes, and the role of early parental acceptance. *American Journal of Community Psychology, 22*(2), 211–227.

Sackett, D. L., & Snow, J. C. (1979). The magnitude of compliance and noncompliance. In R. B. Haynes, D. W. Taylor, & D. L. Sackett (Eds.), *Compliance in health care* (pp. 11–22). Baltimore, MD: Johns Hopkins University Press.

Schaalma, H., Kok, G., Poelman, J., & Reinders, J. (1994). The development of AIDS education for Dutch secondary schools: A systematic approach based on research, theories, and cooperation. In D. R. Rutter (Ed.), *The social psychology of health and safety: European perspectives* (pp. 175–194). Aldershot, UK: Avebury.

Scheirer, M. A., Allen, B. F., & Rauch, H. J. (1987). The adoption and implementation of the fluoride mouthrinse program: Descriptive results from school districts. *Journal of Public Health Dentistry, 47*(2), 98–107.

Schooler, C., Feighery, E., & Flora, J. A. (1996). Seventh graders' self-reported exposure to cigarette marketing and its relationship to their smoking behavior. *American Journal of Public Health, 86*(9), 1216–1221.

Shekelle, R. B., Shryock, A. M., Paul, O., Lepper, M., Stamler, J., Liu, S., & Raynor, W. J., Jr. (1981). Diet, serum cholesterol, and death from coronary heart disease: The Western Electric study. *New England Journal of Medicine, 304*(2), 65–70.

Shephard, R. J. (1995). Physical activity, health, and well-being at different life stages. *Research Quarterly for Exercise and Sport, 66*(4), 298–302.

Skinner, C. S., Strecher, V. J., & Hospers, H. (1994). Physicians' recommendations for mammography: Do tailored messages make a difference? *American Journal of Public Health, 84*(1), 43–49.

Smart, C. R., Hendrick, R. E., Rutledge, J. H., & Smith, R. A. (1995). Benefit of mammography screening in women ages 40 to 49 years: Current evidence from randomized controlled trials. *Cancer, 75*(11), 1619–1626.

Strecher, V. J., Kreuter, M., Den Boer, D. J., Kobrin, S., Hospers, H. J., & Skinner, C. S. (1994). The effects of computer-tailored smoking cessation messages in family practice settings. *Journal of Family Practice, 39*(3), 262–270.

Thompson, S. G., Pyke, S. D., & Wood, D. A. (1997). Using a coronary risk score for screening and intervention in general practice: British Family Heart Study. *Journal of Cardiovascular Risk, 3*(3), 301–306.

Trice, H. M., Beyer, J. M., & Hunt, R. E. (1978). Evaluating implementation of a job-based alcoholism policy. *Journal of Studies on Alcohol, 39*(3), 448–465.

Tripp, M. K., Hermann, N. B., Parcel, G. S., Chamberlain, R. M., & Gritz, E. R. (1999). *Development of a skin cancer prevention program for preschools using the Intervention Mapping process.*

Uchino, B. N., Cacioppo, J. T., & Kiecolt-Glaser, J. K. (1996). The relationship between social support and physiological processes: A review with emphasis on underlying mechanisms and implications for health. *Psychological Bulletin, 119*(3), 488–531.

U.S. Department of Health and Human Services. (1990). *The health benefits of smoking cessation: A report of the Surgeon General* (DHHS Publication No. CDC 90-8416). Rockville, MD: Center for Chronic Disease Prevention and Health Promotion, Office on Smoking and Health.

U.S. Department of Health and Human Services. (1994). *Preventing tobacco use among young people: A report of the Surgeon General.* Washington, DC: Government Printing Office.

U.S. Department of Health and Human Services. (1997). Genetic screening for cystic fibrosis. *NIH Consensus Statement, 15*(4), 1–37.

U.S. Preventive Services Task Force. (1990). Screening for sexually transmitted diseases. *American Family Physician, 42*(3), 691–702.

Zaltman, G., & Duncan, R. (1977). *Strategies for planned change.* New York: Wiley.

CHAPTER 6

Intervention Mapping Step 2: Selecting Theory-Based Intervention Methods and Practical Strategies

READER OBJECTIVES

- Distinguish between theoretical methods and practical strategies and ensure that all program components contain methods
- Use the core processes to identify theoretical methods that can influence change in determinants
- Identify the conditions under which a given theoretical method is most likely to be effective
- Match theoretical methods to the proximal program objectives
- Select or design practical strategies for delivering the methods to intervention groups at each environmental level

A theoretical method is a general technique or process for influencing changes in the determinants of behaviors and environmental conditions. A practical strategy is a specific technique for the application of theoretical methods in ways that fit the intervention population and the context in which the intervention will be conducted. For example, a proximal program objective for an intervention might be to increase adolescents' self-efficacy to resist social pressure to use drugs. For the learning objective of increasing self-efficacy, theoretical methods might include modeling, skill training, guided practice with feedback, and reinforcement. One strategy for modeling could be a videotaped step-by-step demonstration by adolescents of how to resist peer pressure in situations they commonly encounter.

Methods and strategies form a continuum that extends from abstract theoretical methods, through practical strategies, to organized programs with specified scope, sequence, and support materials. For instance, "skills training" is a theoretical method; a step-by-step instruction from a videotape with guided practice would be a practical strategy to deliver the skills training; and a program would include descriptions of when and how the training would be delivered and supported.

The difference between theoretical methods and practical strategies can be confusing. Modeling is more a method than a strategy, role-model stories are both a method and a strategy, and demonstrations are more a strategy than a method. The point is that methods should always be considered, and strategies should never be devoid of the effective component—the method. Yet, it is easy to overlook methods because health educators most often think in terms of concrete program components—a videotape, a brochure.

In this chapter we show how to choose methods from theory and the literature. These methods will be the basis of intervention components to change proximal program objectives. The planner's challenge is to cover all of the objectives while creatively translating methods to strategies. Planners use methods and strategies from all intervention levels (individual, interpersonal, organizational, community, and societal) to match determinants. An intervention at higher system levels may have direct or mediated influence on lower (embedded) levels and may be the intervention of choice to change individual behaviors. For example, a media campaign may influence individuals to change their behavior directly or may influence a change in public or organizational policy, which then influences individuals. Interventions at levels beyond the individual may also operate directly to change characteristics of that system (i.e., family, organization, community) itself.

We focus first on general methods that can be used with a wide variety of determinants, then on methods for determinants that are related to individual behavior change; we apply these methods both to the individual whose health is at risk and to the agents who control aspects of the environment related to health. Finally, we discuss intervention methods more specifically appropriate for groups, organizations, communities, and public policy. We also discuss the importance of power, types of power, and how power can be influenced to effect health-promoting changes at each of the ecological levels. We describe only a sample of methods that can be used to reach learning and change objectives, grouped by determinants, and refer the reader to social science textbooks, particularly those with explicit applications to health education (Bracht & Kingsbury, 1990; Glanz, Lewis, & Rimer, 1997; Maibach & Parrott, 1995; McGuire, 1985).

PERSPECTIVES

The Case of the Missing Methods

The causal chain from objectives to methods to strategies is not often reported in the health education literature. Most publications on health education interventions, often evaluation studies, lack clear information about what the authors actually expected to cause a change. They do talk about the strategy and the program, a tailored letter to encourage mammography or a videotape to teach breast self-exam, for example. But they may not be explicit about what methods are used in the letter or how the videotape actually teaches or motivates the screening behavior. Tailoring can be considered a general method, but there must be specific methods in the letter that would hypothetically "cause" a woman to obtain a mammogram. Did the researchers use persuasion, modeling with vicarious reinforcement, cue to action, or some other method? In another example, researchers might write that they used nonsmoking contracts to stimulate resistance to smoking but they don't mention the theoretical method of commitment on which the strategy was based. All program components must contain methods as well as strategies.

One source of confusion about methods may be that the same concept, such as modeling or reinforcement, can be used to describe both determinants and methods. The double use of these concepts is actually an interesting part of theories, because it means that the theory explains both behavior and behavior change. One way to look at methods is to see them as determinants of behavior change. The difference for health promoters is that modeling as a determinant refers to what happens in the actual situation, whereas modeling as a method will be part of a well-designed program. For instance, with respect to condom use, modeling that occurs in the television shows and movies seen by adolescents may be negative, whereas health educators may use positive role models in their program to compensate for negative media role models (Kok, Schaalma, DeVries, Parcel, & Paulussen, 1996).

Methods at the Different Ecological Levels of Intervention

There are two basic differences between descriptions in the literature of individual-level methods and descriptions in the literature of methods at the higher levels. One difference is that theories at the individual level are more likely to be process theories (i.e., closer to what we call methods) whereas theories at the higher levels are more likely to be implementation theories (i.e., closer to what we call strategies) (Goodman, Steckler, & Kegler, 1997; Porras & Robertson, 1987).

The second difference is in the way knowledge is garnered regarding the application of different types of theories to health education. In individual behavior change, there has been a somewhat deductive approach—extracting behavioral science theoretical change constructs and then applying them to health. This approach to theory application is not theory testing; it is still a theory-of-the-problem approach, but it is not, in its philosophy, too dissimilar from theory testing. On the other hand, social change activities—people doing things such as community organization and coalition building—have been reported in the literature. This is not a process of applying a construct in a community, and sometimes it is not possible to determine whether these activities are methods or strategies and whether there are theoretical constructs involved in the applications. Possibly this approach to intervention is more inductive—intervening with a strategy without naming the method. Where possible in this chapter we label the methods inherent in community-oriented strategies. However, we do not force the upper ecological levels into theoretical constructs when none seem available. If mostly strategies are reported in the literature, then we report strategies. Sometimes we speculate about methods, or label something as a method. Health educators should consider what method is used in a social change strategy so they can be clear what aspect of an intervention is expected to produce what change.

IDENTIFYING METHODS

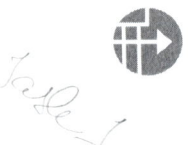

The first task in Intervention Mapping Step 2 is to brainstorm methods.

Work Style

People have different work styles; work groups do too. In selecting methods and strategies, health educators may take any of several routes based on their experience with theory and practice. Some will move carefully from objectives to methods and then to strategies. Others will move from objectives to strategies and then back to the underlying method. Still others will brainstorm methods and strategies simultaneously. For example, one health educator may think of commitment as a theoretical method for increasing self-efficacy of adolescents to remain nonsmokers. He or she would then brainstorm about practical strategies to actually apply that method. Another health educator may think of a nonsmoking contract as a strategy for improving self-efficacy, and then find out from the literature that the underlying theoretical method is commitment. During that process the health educator might also find alternatives to a nonsmoking contract that may have the same or even better results. What is essential in these different routes is that methods are identified, and the parameters of the methods—the conditions under which the methods are shown to be effective—are kept in mind during the translation from method to strategy (and to program). For example, the health educator who likes the idea of a nonsmoking contract should be aware that commitment is only effective as a method for increasing self-efficacy when the act of commitment has been made public. Therefore, contracts that individuals make themselves in private settings may have positive effects as reminders, but they do not have the strong effect of public commitment.

Core Processes

Two of the core processes from Chapter 3 are essential in identifying and selecting methods for objectives: reviewing existing empirical evidence in the literature and reviewing theories of change. With the issue or topic approach to finding and using theory, the health educator goes back to the literature on the problem. If the problem is drug abuse, for example, the health educator discovers what methods others have used to influence resistance to social pressure. Unfortunately, much of

The mayor's work group at this point is deliberating not on *where* to go from here but on *how* to go from here. The one member who had used Intervention Mapping previously was quite comfortable continuing in a somewhat linear process: "Okay, now we just group the learning and change objectives at each ecological level by determinants. Then we discuss what methods could change that group of objectives. You see, the whole process at this point is driven by the determinants."

"What?" asked another member. "I thought we had already dealt with the determinants. Now we are back at the matrices with the learning and change objectives?"

"Yes. That's right. The determinant part of the matrix—the determinant grouping—guides this process."

Many members of the mayor's group groaned, and one spoke up: "I am so tired of tables. I just cannot think this way anymore. Isn't there any other way of doing this? I have so many ideas about this program, and I've managed to keep my enthusiasm through this entire Intervention Mapping process to this point. But to tell the truth, if I have to do one more table, I might lose all my creative program ideas."

"I feel the same way," said another member. "And on top of that, I don't understand the difference between a method and a strategy. It seems to me that this is just one more set of unnecessary vocabulary words that get in the way of really being creative about a program. Furthermore, throughout the planning process, I have been asked to 'hold on to my program ideas.' When do I get to stop 'holding on'? Is that now?"

The mayor's health educator listened to these comments and recommended that the group close their Intervention Mapping notes and put away their matrices. The educator structured the next hour as a brainstorming session. Brainstorming had worked well for this group in the past, and they liked generating ideas without censure or correction. The health educator drew a line down the board and labeled one side "Methods" and the other side "Strategies." The group looked at one determinant at a time with its set of learning objectives and thought about what method would effect those objectives. Each time someone came up with an idea, the group decided whether the suggestion was a theoretical way to change the determinant, that is, a method, or a programmatic idea about how to apply the methods, that is, a strategy. The health educator recorded the ideas in the appropriate columns.

Table 6.1 is the group's initial attempt to generate methods for the determinant "hope for the future."

the literature is vague about methods and more forthcoming about practical strategies. The health educator can then use the construct approach, with the learning objective "resist social pressure to use drugs," and find theoretical methods specifically on resisting social pressure to use drugs, on resisting social pressure to other risk behaviors such as smoking, and on resisting social pressure in general. The health educator may find that this literature cites theories on conformity and nonconformity and on social comparison. The health educator may

Table 6.1
Mayor's Task Group Methods and Strategies
for the Determinant "Perception of Hope for the Future"

METHODS	STRATEGIES
Modeling	Getting role models with good jobs from the neighborhood
	Making a videotape of the models
	Having the models talk at school
	Having the models form groups that could talk to kids who are out of school
Skill training for study skills	Using the same group of role models as training mentors
Skill training for finding job training and school programs and for obtaining GEDs	
Skill training for problem solving	
Modeling of people from the youth population who are working toward a good job	Training the program people to deal better with the out-of-school group
Vicarious reinforcement	Using billboards with short role model stories of our program successes

also use the general theories approach to explore those theories that address behavior change in general (e.g., social cognitive theory) and what they have to offer about accomplishing this particular objective.

There may be several methods for one objective as well as one method for multiple objectives. In cases in which available information is extremely sparse, such as the reduction of fear for social contact with people with AIDS, planners may have to develop more insight on appropriate methods through a third core process: additional research with the intervention group (Dijker, Kok, & Koomen, 1995). See Figure 6.1 for a checklist that can be used to apply the core processes to picking methods.

TRANSLATING THEORETICAL METHODS TO PRACTICAL STRATEGIES

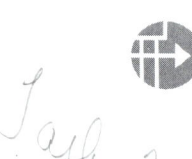

The second task in Intervention Mapping Step 2 is to translate methods into practical strategies. A method is a theoretically and empirically derived general statement about the association between an intervention action and a change in a type of determinant. For instance, modeling is a method for changing self-efficacy. A strategy is the translation of a theoretical method into a practical strategy. Modeling for self-efficacy may, for instance, be organized by real models, by videotaped models, by role-model stories, or by role plays. For every method, strategies will vary, depending on the situation and the intended program imple-

> - ☐ Organize a complete list of learning and change objectives by determinants (the matrix columns).
> - ☐ Brainstorm a provisional list of methods that may be helpful to influence each determinant, taking into consideration the list of objectives that go with the determinant.
> - ☐ Use the issue or topic approach. Go to the literature related to the specific problem, for example, drug abuse, to identify evidence to support, refute, or add to the list of methods.
> - ☐ Use the construct-related approach. Review the list of methods, determinants, and objectives, and follow these constructs into the literature on general and specific theories of behavior and environmental change. Also use the constructs on the brainstormed lists of methods. Be aware of gathering information on the specific conditions that are needed for the method to be effective. Add or delete methods from the list.
> - ☐ Use the general theories approach. Review the list of methods to see if there is a general pattern that would fit a general change theory. Review the theoretical literature, and based on the general theory, add or delete methods from the list. Also review familiar theories that might shed light on changing the determinants.
> - ☐ In cases with little empirical evidence, collect additional data on appropriate methods through qualitative or quantitative research. For example, conduct a small-scale study to find out if it is possible to give adequate individual feedback to the intended population.

FIGURE 6.1 Methods Checklist

menters and end users. For instance, in school programs videotaped models may be practical, whereas in street counseling they may not be. The case studies in Chapters 10 through 13 give examples of the links between objectives, methods, strategies, and programs.

However, the dilemma that this task presents for most health educators is how to think of creative strategies. Many people find themselves stymied by having looked at boxes and arrows for too long. We suggest that health educators close the book at this point and discuss all the ideas that have been bubbling up.

It is important at this time for health educators to revisit the intervention population and the proposed program setting, because strategies will depend greatly on to whom and where the program is being delivered. For example, the Cystic Fibrosis Family Education Program included many social cognitive theory methods, so it would have been logical for the planning team to think of strategies that included a lot of interaction, such as group sessions and role plays for modeling. However, the team knew from having met with parents and adolescents during the needs assessment that they could reach only about 25% of the parent intervention group and almost none of their adolescents in a group setting. They therefore used strategies such as role-model stories in newsletters, and they integrated delivery into the clinical encounter (Bartholomew et al., 1993). These types of strategy decisions, based on formative work, are very important. In Chapter 10, for example, chapter authors Herman Schaalma and Gerjo Kok describe trying to operationalize modeling with role plays in vocational schools. The teachers, however, had a different idea. They were so uncomfortable with organizing and moderating role plays that Schaalma and Kok knew they had to resort to another strategy.

An Example of Methods and Strategies

El-Basel, Ivanoff, Schilling, Borne, and Gilbert (1997) carefully described an HIV prevention program for women in jail. Their behavioral targets were the reduction of unsafe sex through condom use and abstinence and the reduction of needle sharing. Their program focused on the following determinants: knowledge about HIV and STD risks, perceived vulnerability to HIV and STDs, cognitive-behavioral and technical skills tailored to cultural and social factors, motivation to use condoms (i.e., attitudes, barriers, pros and cons, and access), social support, and formal and informal help-seeking skills. Theoretical methods were derived from various theories, particularly social cognitive and relapse prevention theories. The methods and strategies are presented in Table 6.2. In addition to the specific methods listed in the table, the researchers used three general methods: relevance (i.e., adaptation of the program to knowledge, beliefs, circumstances, and prior experiences of the intervention population based on focus groups and surveys), active learning facilitated by professional group workers, and repetition by trained peer educators (booster sessions).

The program methods were applied in an organized group intervention that consisted of eight weekly sessions of 1½ hours each. A facilitator and a cofacilitator used a standardized protocol to lead the groups of ten women. Group members were given a workbook of exercises that could be completed with minimal literacy. Group facilitators were experienced in working with drug users, were credible and comfortable with the group, and valued group work and skills training approaches.

Within this program, various strategies were used to apply the methods. For instance, skills training and guided practice were delivered through discussions and homework exercises. Facilitators reviewed common triggers (i.e., places, people, moods, and substance use), and group members learned to identify high-risk situations that served as personal triggers for engaging in risky behaviors. Participants discussed how these triggers influence their decisions to have unsafe sex and to use drugs. Using member examples, facilitators emphasized the powerful, multilayered connections between drug use (particularly crack) and having unsafe sex. Through awareness exercises in and outside the group, each member identified her own list of triggers. As participants shared their lists of triggers, facilitators and other members helped identify potential steps to minimize, avoid, or counteract the influence of these triggers.

Negotiation and assertiveness skills were taught within the context of risk appraisal. The women assessed the possible adverse outcomes of being assertive and identified avenues of escape from partners who might respond abusively.

They learned four steps to negotiate safer sex when partners are not interested in using condoms: (a) State what you want; (b) explain, without blame or accusation, why you want it; (c) indicate understanding of the other's position; (d) attain a solution to the problem without compromising your needs. Members then practiced refusing unsafe sex in situations in which negotiation fails. Instructors encouraged direct refusal of unsafe sex in situations in which the women are confident that partners will cooperate, and indirect refusal when partners are unresponsive or threatening. The program relied on videotaped stimulus vignettes for teaching these and other skills. Participants evaluated the effectiveness of the assertions, negotiations, and refusals used in the stimulus

Table 6.2
HIV Prevention Program Methods and Strategies

DETERMINANTS	METHODS	STRATEGIES
Knowledge	Information	Demonstrations Workbook Group sessions
Confrontations with risks	Modeling	Personal risk appraisal
Risk perception Skills for identifying high-risk situations	Confrontations with risks Modeling Personal risk appraisal Skill training, with guided practice and feedback	Discussions and homework, including practice on identifying triggers from participants' own examples Facilitator presentation of examples Awareness exercises
Skills for coping, problem solving, help seeking, and negotiation	Modeling Skill training with guided practice and feedback	Group teaching of the skills by facilitators Practice by group members Identification by group members of possible negative outcomes and how to handle them Videotaped stimulus vignettes with evaluation by participants Skill practice in role plays with feedback Booster sessions in the community
Attitudes	Decisional balance Identification of barriers for condom use	Discussion in groups Videotaped stimulus vignettes
Social support	Modeling Guided practice Social comparison	Mobilization through network and contact identification

Note. This table is based on "Skills Building and Social Support Enhancement to Reduce HIV Risk Among Woman in Jail," by N. El-Basel, A. Ivanoff, R. F. Schilling, D. Borne, and L. Gilbert, 1997, *Criminal Justice and Behavior, 24*, 205–223.

vignettes and generated alternative responses. Participants then practiced these skills in multiple role plays. Facilitators provided constructive feedback and support throughout the training.

Prior to the participants' release from prison, counselors met with participants individually to review triggers for risk behavior, plans for reducing risk behaviors, resources contacted on the outside, and steps they would take during the first few days after release to carry out their plans. Individual booster sessions delivered by counselors in the community took place during the first two months after release. During booster sessions, problem-solving goals and objectives were linked with concrete action plans, and role play was used to access skills and to practice plans.

Ensuring Effectiveness of Methods

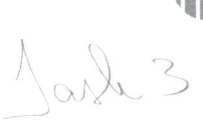

The third task in Intervention Mapping Step 2 is to organize methods and strategies by groups of learning objectives at each ecological level, and check that methods are properly operationalized. When theoretical methods are applied, it is essential to understand the parameters under which effectiveness of the method has been shown. As we review the change-process theories, we note the parameters that need to be fulfilled for the method to be effective. For instance, active learning can be an effective method for many learning objectives, but only when the participants have sufficient time, information, and skills to be able to learn from their experiences (Bandura, 1986). In another example, modeling can be effective when the viewer pays attention, remembers, has certain skills, and is reinforced. In structured modeling strategies such as videotaped modeling, those parameters can be guarded quite easily. In unstructured situations, such as role plays, those parameters have to be guarded rather carefully by the facilitator. For example, the role of the smoker in smoking prevention role plays may be an attractive role for some students and is therefore often played by the teacher or a trained peer educator.

BASIC METHODS

Before planners can be concerned about changing specific determinants or learning and change objectives, certain initial states must be reached. The members of the intervention group, for example, must pay attention to the message and must process it centrally. This section addresses these basic requirements of health education and promotion (Table 6.3).

Successful Communication

McGuire's (1985) persuasion communication model stresses the importance of successful communication before any other method can be used. A program cannot have any effect if the population is not exposed, does not pay attention to the

Table 6.3
Summary of Basic Methods

METHODS	CONSIDERATIONS FOR USE
Attention and comprehension	Requires relevance and message not too discrepant from target group's experience; can be further stimulated by surprise and repetition
Active learning	Requires time, information, and skills
Tailoring	Must concern factors related to behavior change (e.g., stage) or to relevance (e.g., culture, socioeconomic status)
Individualization	Depends on personal communication that responds to a learner's needs
Feedback	Must be individual, follow the desired behavior closely in time, and be specific
Reinforcement	Must be individual and follow the desired behavior closely in time
Facilitation	Usually requires changes in the environment

program, or does not understand the message. Any program that includes methods for changing determinants and behavior should also include methods to achieve successful communication. The elaboration likelihood model suggests that people only process the message seriously, via the central route, when they are motivated and able to do so (Petty & Cacioppo, 1986). Careful thinking about the message is stimulated by messages that are personally relevant, surprising, and repeated. Susser, Valencia, and Torres (1994), for instance, developed Sex, Games, and Videotapes—an HIV prevention program for homeless mentally ill men in a New York shelter—around playing competitive games, storytelling, and watching videos, which are common pastimes in a homeless shelter.

Anticipation of interaction over the message and direct instructions to process the message carefully can help centralize the processing (Petty & Wegener, 1997). When the intervention group has the time and the behavioral capability, active learning can be used to promote central information processing. However, even with high involvement, messages that are too discrepant from the receivers' positions will not have much effect (McGuire, 1985).

Relevance, Tailoring, and Individualization

Relevance, tailoring, and individualization have all been shown to be effective basic methods in health education interventions. Adapting the program to the knowledge, beliefs, circumstances, and prior experience of the learner, as assessed by pretesting or other means, can create relevance (Mullen, Green, & Persinger, 1985; Mullen, Mains, & Velez, 1992). Computer programs enable one to tailor interventions to measured characteristics of the individual, such as stage of change, beliefs, attitude, and self-efficacy (Brug, Glanz, Van Assema, Kok, & van

Breukelen, 1998; Brug, Van Assema, Kok, Lenderink, & Glanz, 1994; Campbell et al., 1994; Skinner, Strecher, & Hospers, 1994; Strecher, 1999; Strecher et al., 1994).

Tailoring will be effective only when there is a clear link between characteristics of the person and the messages that are supposed to address those characteristics (Brug et al., 1998). Witte (1995) points out that tailoring the message to salient beliefs of the intervention group would increase people's motivation and ability to process the message carefully, thereby increasing the chance of persistent changes in attitudes and behavior. Salovey, Rothman, and Rodin (1997) stress the importance of tailoring interventions to laypeople's beliefs about illness, such as causes, consequences, duration, and cure. Witte (1995) proposes a protocol for defining types of important beliefs from a health communication perspective. She suggests that an intervention developer must know a group's current beliefs to determine which beliefs have to be changed (e.g., condoms are inconvenient); which beliefs can be reinforced (e.g., family values); what new beliefs should be introduced (e.g., personal susceptibility to HIV infection); and what cues should be addressed (e.g., cultural values).

The concept of tailoring also works for organizational change. For example, organizations adopting innovations move through a sequence of stages in the process of change. These stages have been described as sensing of unsatisfied demands, searching for possible responses, evaluating alternatives, initiating the program, implementing the program, and then institutionalizing it (Beyer & Trice, 1978; R. M. Goodman et al., 1997). To help an organization move through these stages requires addressing different personnel and their specific determinants at different stages and then tailoring messages to match. For example, in the adoption of a tobacco prevention program, both administrators and teachers are important in developing awareness of a problem, whereas administrators are key to adoption and teachers are key to implementation (R. M. Goodman et al., 1997; Parcel, Simons-Morton, & Kolbe, 1988). Similarly, coalitions move through stages. In Butterfoss, Goodman, and Wandersman's (1993) conceptualization, these stages are formation, implementation, maintenance, and the accomplishment of goals or outcomes. Technical assistance and consultation on organizational structure and processes must match the coalition's stage and context.

Individualization is the provision of opportunities for learners to have personal questions answered or instructions paced according to their individual progress (Mullen et al., 1985; Mullen et al., 1992). It may also include the ability to offer instruction that is geared to specific needs and disease characteristics. The Watch, Discover, Think, and Act asthma computer application individualizes instruction to each child's asthma triggers and symptoms based on information the child enters into the computer program (Bartholomew, Gold, et al., 2000; Bartholomew, Shegog, et al., 2000).

Both individualization and tailoring are related to the concept of cultural competence, which is discussed further in Chapter 7. Both program methods and strategies not only must be acceptable to the intervention groups, but they must embody cultural fit to foster empowerment and program effectiveness. Development of a culturally competent program requires participation of the community as program planners. The Pathways to Early Cancer Detection in Four Ethnic Groups project, for example, developed specific interventions for early cancer detection for Latinos, Vietnamese women, and a multiethnic indigent population who used emergency rooms for health care. Although the goals and objectives and the theoretical base of the interventions were similar, there were some specific differences in the mode of intervention (e.g., mass media vs. interpersonal communication), use of role models and lay health workers, staffing patterns, content of messages, and the language, idiom, and designs of the print material for specific populations (Pasick, D'Onofrio, & Hiatt, 1996).

Feedback and Reinforcement

Feedback and reinforcement have also been shown to be effective methods for changes in various determinants and behavior (Bandura, 1986; Mullen et al., 1985; Mullen et al., 1992). Feedback is information given to the learner regarding the extent to which learning or performance is being accomplished (e.g., reduction in fat intake, increase in aerobic exercise) or the extent to which change is having an impact (e.g., blood pressure, physical condition, weight). Feedback functions as a method for awareness regarding learning and performance, but it can also function to raise awareness regarding risk (Prochaska, DiClemente, & Norcross, 1997).

Reinforcement is any component of the intervention that is designed to reward the behavior after the behavior has been enacted. Positive reinforcement is the application of something pleasant that increases the frequency of a behavior, whereas negative reinforcement is the removal of something aversive, which is experienced as positive and increases the frequency of the behavior. Punishment, the onset of an aversive stimulus or the removal of a pleasant stimulus, is something that discourages the behavior. Bandura (1986) also distinguishes among directly applied reinforcement rewards and punishments (e.g., social reinforcement such as praise from a doctor to patient), vicarious reinforcement (reinforcement of another who is functioning as a model for the behavior), and self-reinforcement (giving oneself a reward).

Facilitation

All learning has to be complemented by the provision of means for the learner to take action or means to reduce barriers to action (Bandura, 1986; Mullen et al., 1985; Mullen et al., 1992). Facilitation often means a change in the environment. For instance, a program that targets improvement in drug users' self-efficacy for using clean needles must also facilitate clean needles being easily accessible. People with higher self-efficacy will put more effort and strategy-development into their intended health behavior, but the balance between their real skills and the real barriers ultimately mediates what the effect will be.

METHODS FOR PERSONAL DETERMINANTS

This section contains theoretical methods grouped by determinants for which they can be effective in creating change. These methods are geared to changing personal determinants (e.g., attitude, skills) of the at-risk individuals and environmental agents. We start with methods at the individual level and then move to more or less similar methods for the same determinant for agents at higher environmental levels. For instance, attitude change of an individual could be facilitated by persuasive communication. Attitude change of a politician who serves as a gatekeeper for policy change could also be facilitated by persuasive communication. However, the content and the source of the messages would be quite different.

We combine comparable determinants when they appear in more than one theory, for example, attitudes and outcome expectations. The various determinants are not independent of each other; we start with a knowledge determinant as the basis for many other determinants, such as risk perception, attitude, and skills. Risk perception in turn is a specific part of attitude. Methods described for one determinant can be used for other determinants as well.

Methods to Influence Knowledge

Knowledge is necessary but not sufficient for most other determinants, such as risk perceptions, behavioral beliefs, perceived norms, or skills. Many methods for other determinants will also change knowledge. Conventional wisdom long held that giving people information could change behavior and thereby solve health and social problems. However, knowledge does not generally lead directly to behavior change; nor is ensuring that the members of the population attain knowledge necessarily an easy task. Information processing theory (IPT; really a framework that has been adopted by many cognitive psychologists) provides several concepts that suggest methods for successfully conveying information. Table 6.4 provides an overview of the methods and parameters for knowledge.

CHUNKING, ADVANCE ORGANIZERS, AND IMAGES IPT is concerned with how information is perceived, stored, and retrieved. Drawing from the gestalt school of psychology (Koffka, 1933), IPT suggests that information is perceived by the senses in the context of what people already know. People perceive information actively to make sense of incomplete stimuli. For instance, someone who sees only eyes and a forehead will tend to perceive a face in order to complete the recognized pattern in the act of perception. Theorists suggest that people then use a "work space" referred to as short-term memory in order to encode information for long-term storage, retrieve information from long-term storage, and work on information in order to solve problems. Attention in IPT is the allocation of short-term memory to a task. Working memory is a small space, and its effectiveness can be increased by a method called chunking. A chunk is a stimulus pattern

Table 6.4
Summary of Methods to Increase Knowledge

METHODS	CONSIDERATIONS FOR USE
Chunking	Requires that labels or acronyms be assigned to material to aid memory
Advance organizers	Requires concrete examples in front of what is to be learned
Images	Must use familiar physical or verbal images as analogies to a less familiar process
Tailoring	Can tailor information to concepts that the learner already has
Discussion	Requires listening to the learner to ensure that the correct schemas are activated
Active learning	Can stimulate elaboration by encouraging the learner to add something to the information to be remembered
Cues	Must ensure that the same cues are present at the time of learning and the time of retrieval

that may be made up of parts but is perceived as a whole, for example, FBI (Federal Bureau of Investigation) or ER (emergency room). A use of chunking as a method might be to assign an acronym or a summary slogan to a process so that the entire process can be encoded into memory. For example, children in the asthma self-management program learned a rap song with Watch, Discover, Think, and Act for the stages of self-management. Other slogans are Stop, Drop, and Roll for burn prevention, Slip, Slap, and Slop for using hats and sunscreen, and Stop, Look, and Listen for traffic safety.

IPT also presents some ideas about how knowledge is stored in long-term memory. Long-term memory comprises information about events, concepts, and procedures, or how to do something. The storage is described as a network of nodes (cognitive units of concepts and propositions) with links between the nodes that enable activation of a single node to spread to linked nodes (Anderson, 1983). Other theorists describe schemas that have both passive and active qualities. In other words, schemas contain related information that people can activate passively, by perceiving an object, or actively, by consciously thinking of a group of concepts in order to compare a new perception with an existing category (Rumelhart, 1980).

The idea of schemas suggests that a health message will be better understood if it activates existing schemas—if, in other words, the receiver has a handy place to store the information and some conscious ideas regarding where the information is stored. An important method is called an advance organizer—overview material with familiar, concrete examples that enables a learner to activate relevant schemas so that new material can be associated (Derry, 1984; Mayer, 1984).

Another method is the use of imagery—the encoding of pictures with concepts to be stored in long-term memory (Glover, Ronning, & Bruning, 1990).

Hamilton and Ghatala (1994) relate the ancient Greek method of loci, in which orators mentally attached parts of long speeches to landmarks on well-known travel routes (p. 86). One might imagine a patient educator helping a learner memorize a long self-care process by attaching the steps in the procedure to landmarks on a familiar daily route. In another example, a novel visual image of a frying egg has been attached to the verbal message "your brain on drugs" in the America Against Drugs Campaign. Verbal images or analogies are also helpful for encoding information to long-term memory. If material is too foreign or discrepant it will not be learned. Therefore, analogies to more common events, concepts, or processes may be a helpful method, especially if learners can be guided to create their own analogies (Hamilton & Ghatala).

Pre-existing schema that contradict an informational message certainly may interfere with the encoding of the message for long-term memory. For example, a child who knows ivy as a plant may activate an entirely wrong schema when told in the hospital about an IV (intravenous administration of medication). In cultures in which the etiology of certain diseases is thought to be an imbalance in temperatures, an explanation of immunizations may not readily activate an appropriate schema, making it difficult to process information about immunizations.

ELABORATION AND CUES   Getting information into long-term memory is only the first part of learning. Usually, the learner must also get the information back out—retrieval. Retrieving information from memory is easier when the memory is a strong one. Strong memories are made when encoding is effortful. Effort requires the learner to add to the meaning of the material, to elaborate on it. Elaboration is particularly effective if it helps tie the information together. Rehearsal of information is more effective in promoting remembering when it is elaborative rehearsal—when something is added to the information being learned. For example, a leader who is working on more effective group management and who wants to remember three new skills for the next meeting could simply rehearse the concepts of summarizing, gatekeeping, and connecting. However, once he or she is in the meeting, these abstract concepts may be hard to retrieve. Elaborating the concepts with images may help. The leader might put the visual image of a gate for gatekeeping—letting people and their ideas into the conversation. Adding to the image of the gate, the leader puts all the sheep (ideas) into the corral, summarizing and then pairing (or connecting) them up two by two. Although it seems counterintuitive to have to learn more in order to remember, the method of elaboration does create stronger memories.

Providing cues is another method for getting information out of memory. For a cue to be effective, it should be present at the time of encoding and at the time of retrieval. Providing cues has many implications for health educators. For example, for teens who are learning to negotiate condom use, the cues present during learning and practice—such as what the partner says and the situation or setting—should be as similar as possible to what teens will actually encounter when they try to retrieve and apply the steps of negotiation.

Methods to Change Risk Perception, Awareness, and Health Beliefs

Table 6.5 summarizes methods that can be used to improve people's risk perceptions and their awareness of the problem.

UNREALISTIC OPTIMISM People often underestimate their risk, a condition that risk perception theories call unrealistic optimism (Brug et al., 1994; Van der Pligt, Otten, Richard, & Van der Velde, 1993). The main reasons for unrealistic optimism are that people underestimate what techniques others undertake to protect themselves and that they have stereotypes of people who run high risks (see Salovey et al., 1997). To illustrate, adolescents may refrain from condom use because they think that other adolescents do not use condoms to protect themselves, that other adolescents have multiple partners whereas they have regular partners, and that only adolescents who often change partners are at risk for contracting HIV. Health education should assist in making clear each person's risks, preferably through undeniable feedback, and should also indicate that risk is a matter of risk behavior rather than what risk groups the person belongs to. Strecher and Rosenstock (1997) suggest the following methods for changing the risk perception variables of the health belief model:

- Define the risk levels of the populations at risk
- Personalize risk based on a person's behavior
- Make perceived susceptibility more consistent with individual's actual risk
- Specify consequences of the risk and the condition

Table 6.5
Summary of Methods to Change Awareness and Risk Perception

METHODS	CONSIDERATIONS FOR USE
Information about personal risk	Should be presented as individual, undeniable, on same dimension, congruent with actual risk, and cumulative rather than for one occasion; should be presented with qualitative and quantitative examples
Loss frame or gain frame	More effective to use loss frame for detection behaviors and gain frame for prevention behaviors
Re-evaluation, self-evaluation, and consciousness raising	Can use feedback and confrontation; however, raising awareness must be quickly followed by increase in problem-solving ability and self-efficacy
Dramatic relief	Probably should be done in counseling context so that emotions can be aroused and subsequently relieved
Fear arousal	Requires high self-efficacy expectations rather than high outcome expectations alone

Holtgrave, Tinsley, and Kay (1995) suggest various methods to effectively communicate risks. Health educators can, for example, compare risks on the same dimension or compare risks with similar dimensional profiles, such as dread, control, catastrophic potential, equity, and novelty. For example, people become angry when a risk over which they have no control, say, air pollution, is compared to a risk over which they do have control, say, smoking. Health educators can give cumulative risk information and can emphasize cumulative probabilities instead of single incident probabilities. Holtgrave and colleagues suggest that health educators avoid giving the probability of getting infected with HIV in one unprotected sexual encounter; instead, the message should be "Think of those times that you are likely to have sex in the next 2 years. . . . Unsafe sex will catch up with you, and you will become HIV infected." Health educators can provide both qualitative and quantitative expressions of risks; they can say both "90% chance" and "extremely likely." Finally, health educators can choose success framing of the message instead of failure framing when the message relates to the effectiveness of a health behavior. For example, they can state that "condom use is 95% effective," rather than "the failure rate is only 5%."

Currently, work is being done to apply economic theory to the specification of risk. Allegrante and Roizen (1998) are calculating biological age of coronary bypass patients based on unmodified risk factors. They are counseling patients to compare biological with chronological age as a way of making risk concrete.

AWARENESS Awareness is often described as the first step in the change process. In the theories of self-regulation and coping, the first step in an intervention is some form of need recognition or problem appraisal (see Chapter 4). However, these theories do not provide clear methods for stimulating need recognition. Often, self-regulatory and coping theories are applied in situations in which people have a disease, such as asthma, cystic fibrosis, or AIDS (Lerman & Glanz, 1997). Individuals are taught appraisal skills to detect a disease or a self-management related problem and then are taught other skills to solve the problem (Bartholomew et al., 1993). Without these additional problem-solving skills to raise self-efficacy, avoidance may ensue. For people who are not motivated to perform appraisal, health educators may apply risk information, confrontation, and fear arousal methods.

In organizational change theories, sensing of unsatisfied demands, or diagnosis, is the first step, comparable to awareness or need recognition (see Chapter 4). Organizational theories do not suggest clear methods for change; instead, they focus on procedures to carry out the change. Diagnosis is typically done with surveys that concern norms, beliefs, values, and behavior of organizational members. Often an outside consultant is hired to do the diagnosis and confront the organization with the results (Goodman et al., 1997). Again, the diagnosis is the first step, followed by evaluation and action.

People are often not aware of the negative outcomes of their behavior. The transtheoretical model of stages of change suggests that cognitive and affective methods raise awareness of negative outcomes, thereby moving people from precontemplation to contemplation (see Chapter 4; Prochaska et al., 1997). Consciousness raising involves increased awareness about a risk behavior as a cause of a particular health problem, about the consequences of the risk behavior, and about possible health-promoting behaviors. Intervention methods that can cause consciousness raising include feedback, confrontations, and interpretations. Dramatic relief initially produces increased emotional experiences followed by reduced affect if appropriate action is taken. Psychodrama, role playing, grieving, and personal testimonies are examples of strategies for operationalizing dramatic relief. Maibach and Cotton (1995) stress that messages to promote awareness should focus on self-evaluation related to risk and re-evaluation of outcome expectations rather than on action. Messages could include personalization by reminding someone of recent episodes of the risk behavior and potential consequences of the person's risk behavior on significant others (Maibach & Cotton). At a higher ecological level, mass media gatekeepers must also become aware of an issue as a necessary condition for featuring health-promotion issues (McGrath, 1995).

FEAR Often people suggest the use of fear arousal as a method to raise awareness of risk behavior and to change the risk behavior into health-promoting behavior. Using fear is intuitively appealing, and research on fear-arousing communication has a long tradition in social psychology and public education (Hale & Dillard, 1995; Maibach & Parrott, 1995; McGuire, 1985). In their extensive review, Eagly and Chaiken (1993) summarize the inconclusive state of the art with respect to fear arousal. Most relevant theories and the available empirical data suggest that fear, as a result of subjective appraisals of personal susceptibility and severity, motivates an individual to action. However, the type of action is dependent on both outcome expectations and self-efficacy expectations. For instance, smokers may become afraid of cancer when they recognize their own susceptibility to cancer and the severity of the disease. Their fear may motivate them to stop smoking, but only when they are convinced that quitting is really effective in preventing cancer (outcome expectation) and when they feel confident that they are able to quit (self-efficacy). In this particular example, low self-efficacy may be the most important barrier to quitting for most smokers.

What happens when people are afraid but they are not convinced of the effectiveness of the alternative behavior or of their own self-efficacy? Most data suggest that under those conditions the resulting behavior may be defensive, more avoidance oriented than action oriented (avoidance of the antismoking message, that is). Smokers may deny the risks of cancer, and extremely fear-arousing messages may result in more smoking. What does this response mean for the use of fear-arousing communication as a method? At the moment, understanding of the underlying process of fear arousal is still insufficient to make definitive statements, but there seem to be two important methodological points (Eagly & Chaiken, 1993; Ruiter, Kok, & Abraham, 1999): First, fear is a motivator to behavior change, that is, no fear, no action; second, fear motivates health-promoting behavior, but probably only if the individual has high outcome expectations and high self-efficacy expectations.

In cases in which people are not aware of their risk, as in precontemplation, some fear arousal may be effective. In situations in which people are aware of their risk but lack self-efficacy for health-promoting alternative behavior, messages should focus on improving self-efficacy. A word of caution: Precontemplation may, for some people, be the result of denial, and in that case, those precontemplators will not react positively to fear-arousing messages.

NEGATIVE AND POSITIVE APPEALS Monahan (1995) analyzes the effects of negative and positive appeals and concludes that, to be effective, emotional appeals in a message should be congruent with existing feelings of the target. In line with that conclusion, Salovey and colleagues (1997) report that messages with a loss frame are more effective with detection behaviors, whereas messages with a gain frame are more effective with preventive behaviors. For example, early detection of cancer by getting a Pap smear every year can save your life (loss frame). Being physically active helps you feel better and less stressed (gain frame).

Methods to Change Attitudes

Table 6.6 lists some of the methods that can be used to change people's health-related attitudes. Attitudes are a positive or negative reaction to something, but can include more specific constructs of beliefs, outcome expectations, assessment of advantages and disadvantages, perceived benefits and barriers, self-evaluation, and motivation to act. Social psychology has devoted much attention to addressing the problem of changing health-related attitudes, and we present here a very brief summary of this work (for a more in-depth review, see McGuire, 1985; Eagly & Chaiken, 1993; and Petty & Wegener, 1997).

RE-EVALUATION Evaluation is the second stage in self-regulation, in which a person compares current performance to a personal standard. We treat variables related to self-presentation—such as self-evaluation (I am satisfied with my performance), personal moral norm (I feel I should do X), and anticipated regret (How would you feel after you did X?)—as part of this group of attitudinal variables. Other authors see those variables as a separate cluster (Abraham, Sheeran, & Johnston, 1998). Self-evaluations may be activated by setting goals and giving feedback (Bandura, 1986). Personal moral norms may be enhanced by counseling or small group discussions on values and moral norms (Godin, Savard, Kok, Fortin, & Boyer, 1996). Anticipated regret may be enhanced literally by asking people to imagine how they would feel after a risk behavior, for instance, having had unsafe sex (Richard, Van der Pligt, & De Vries, 1995).

Prochaska and colleagues (1997) mention methods for bringing precontemplators to contemplation and preparation. In self–re-evaluation, a person combines cognitive and affective assessments of self-image with and without a

Table 6.6
Summary of Methods to Change Attitudes

METHODS	CONSIDERATIONS FOR USE
Belief selection	Requires investigation of the current beliefs of the individual before choosing the belief on which to intervene
Self–re-evaluation	Better to stimulate both cognitive and affective appraisal of self-image
Environmental re-evaluation	Better to stimulate both cognitive and affective appraisal and to improve appraisal and empathy skills
Shifting perspective	Must begin with the perspective of the learner
Arguments	Requires arguments new to the individual
Direct experience	Must ensure that the individual's experience with the behavior has rewarding outcomes or that the individual can cope with and reframe negative outcomes
Modeling	Must ensure that the model is reinforced
Persuasive communication	Requires consideration of the source, message, channel, and receiver
Anticipated regret	Must stimulate imagery

particular unhealthy habit (for example, as a sedentary person and as an active person). Clarifying values, having healthy role models, and using mental imagery are methods that can move people to more realistically evaluate their current behavior. Environmental re-evaluation combines both affective and cognitive assessments of how the presence or absence of a personal habit affects a person's social environment. For example, a father might assess the effect of his smoking on his children. Such re-evaluation can also include people's awareness that they can serve as positive or negative role models for others. A method such as empathy training may lead to such assessments. In Project PANDA, Mullen and colleagues targeted interventions to the new fathers' assessment of their potential impact on their children to enlist fathers in preparing smoke-free environments and helping mothers stay off cigarettes (see Chapter 13).

Holtgrave and colleagues (1995) stress the importance of understanding a person's decision-making perspective. When health education tries to shift the individual's perspective to a more health-promoting one or tries to change the decisional balance, it must be within the perspective of the learner. Accordingly, health promotion messages should also fit with the learner's time frame, which is often short term.

Strecher and Rosenstock (1997) suggest methods for changing the perception of benefits and barriers (in the health belief model). They suggest defining the specific action to take in terms of how, where, and when, and clarifying the positive effects to be expected. They also suggest reassurance, correction of misinformation, and provision of incentives and assistance as methods for reducing perceived barriers.

The strategy of gaps analysis has been used in organizational development to compare the current situation within the organization to values espoused by the organization or to a vision of the preferred future. For example, surveys of organization members to determine the existing cultural norms and practices are conducted and the findings discussed in relation to the culture desired by the members. This strategy provides the motivation and direction for intervention (Allen & Bellingham, 1994; Cummings & Worley, 1993).

PERSUASION   One of the most widely used intervention methods for attitude change is the presentation of arguments in a persuasive message. The elaboration likelihood model predicts that high-quality arguments are effective only when the receivers process the message via the central route, not when they use the peripheral route (see Chapter 4). Because attitude change through the central route is more persistent, more resistant to change, and more related to behavior, health promoters would like to promote central information processing. A higher number of arguments does not ensure quality; in fact, it may be negatively related. More arguments may be convincing for people who process the information via the peripheral route, but will be less convincing for people who process via the central route. Quality of arguments, that is, effectiveness after careful processing, is determined by a number of variables (Petty & Wegener, 1997). These variables include the following characteristics:

- Expectancy value: People like outcomes that are likely and desirable and avoid outcomes that are likely and undesirable.
- Causal explanations: A causal explanation will convince receivers of the likelihood of the outcome.
- Functionality: Arguments that match the way people look at the world are more convincing.
- Importance: Relevance of outcomes determines effectiveness of the argument.
- Novelty: An unfamiliar or unique argument has more impact than a familiar argument.

Persuasive arguments may be used at the individual level to encourage people to adopt healthful behaviors and may be used for agents at higher ecological levels. For example, viewing a television broadcast that concerns the health outcomes to children from environmental tobacco smoke and the benefits of protecting children from smoke may influence a mother to declare her home smoke free. Seeing other legislators receive media attention for promoting healthful policy may lead legislators to vote for health legislation. Both outcome expectations and expectancies must be high. For example, a city council must be persuaded both that fluoridation prevents dental caries and that the prevention of dental caries is something to be valued because of its effect on children's health. A persuasive argument about the extent of dental disease in children in the community and the outcome to their overall health that uses facts and personalized models might influence the council to accept both beliefs and to change its voting.

DIRECT EXPERIENCE   Maibach and Cotton (1995) cite direct experience as a method for changing outcome expectations. Modeling is also powerful, especially if it is clear that the model's behavior resulted in a lower risk and in positive health or other attributes. One caution is advisable when using direct experience (enactment) as a method. Although outcome expectations may be enhanced, they also may be lowered in the presence of unpleasant results of the behavior, such as discomfort during a mammogram or decreased sensation during condom use.

Methods for Changing Social Influence

The influence of the social environment, including perceived social influence and subjective norms, is an important determinant of many behaviors, and as such will be found in many learning and change objectives. One theory that tries to explain social influence is Ajzen's (1988) theory of planned behavior (TPB; see Chapter 4). TPB states that behavior is determined by intention and that intention is determined by attitudes, subjective social norms, and self-efficacy. Social influence in this theory is seen as social expectations, and the theory does not cover social influence in the form of modeling. Social influence through modeling is a central construct in social cognitive theory, which explicates intervention methods that change the social environment as well as the perceived social influence (Bandura, 1986). Table 6.7 presents methods for changing these social influences.

SUBJECTIVE NORMS   TPB states that the subjective social norm is a combination of normative beliefs about what reference persons expect someone to do and to what degree that person desires to comply. The relative impact of the subjective social norm is indicated by the weight of the norm in the prediction of intention

Table 6.7
Summary of Methods to Change Social Influence

METHODS	CONSIDERATIONS FOR USE
Visible expectations	Requires the positive expectations to be available in the environment
Resistance to social pressure	Requires skill building for refusal skills; also important are commitment to earlier intention, relating intended behavior to values, and psychological inoculation against pressure
Shifting focus	Must shift focus to a new reason for performing the behavior
Modeling and vicarious reinforcement	Requires attention, remembrance, and skills
Mobilizing social support	Must combine caring, trust, openness, and acceptance as well as support for behavioral change

and behavior. Following the theory, health educators have three ways to influence social expectations. The first is influencing normative beliefs by making peer expectations visible. The second is influencing motivation to comply by building resistance to social pressure to engage in risk behavior or increasing motivation to comply with positive social pressure. Finally, if health educators are unable to shift either the norm or the motivation to comply, they can hide the behavior or shift attention from the behavior.

For example, a planning team has found that young women do not want to ask their partners to use a condom for AIDS prevention because they expect the partners to react negatively. An approach of the first type would be to mobilize peers to talk about safe sex to make the norms for using condoms more visible. This approach assumes that positive peer experiences are available for discussion in the environment—both that boys are willing to wear condoms and that girls agree to ask the boys to wear them. The second type of approach would be to build resistance to social pressure, which in this case might mean that girls learn effective refusal skills when their partners do not want to use a condom. The last type of approach, hiding or shifting attention from the behavior, might be translated into methods and strategies in which girls are taught to shift attention from the reason for using a condom—to prevent HIV infection—by telling their partners that the reason they want to use a condom is pregnancy prevention.

Methods for changing social influences and methods for self-efficacy improvement are sometimes the same when they both relate to self-efficacy and skills. Resistance to social pressure, for instance, can be seen as a skill. How can health educators teach people to resist social pressure? A summary of the literature suggests five methods: training refusal skills; modeling resistance; commitment to earlier intention and behavior; relating intended behavior to values; and psychological inoculation against pressure (McGuire, 1985).

SOCIAL SUPPORT Prochaska et al. (1997) describe a process of change related to mobilizing social support (helping relationships that combine caring, trust, openness, and acceptance as well as support for the behavioral change). These helping relationships can be encouraged in numerous ways, such as rapport building, therapeutic alliances, counselor calls, and buddy systems. The California Department of Mental Health conducted a media campaign titled "Good Friends Make Good Medicine," which was designed to increase awareness of the importance of social support and to suggest specific actions that individuals could take to strengthen their support networks (Hersey, Kibanoff, Lam, & Taylor, 1984).

MODELING Another theory that explains social influence is Bandura's (1986) social cognitive theory (SCT; see Chapter 4). SCT states that outcome expectations, the perceived behavior of others, and self-efficacy expectations are the main determinants for behavior, whereas reinforcement and vicarious learning (modeling) are methods for change. Outcome expectations can be presented verbally and developed through reinforcement. For example, parents tell a child what they expect, and the child also learns by parents' reactions (e.g., praise or punishment) what behaviors are desired. Modeling with vicarious reinforcement is also a method for changing outcome expectations (Bandura, 1986). By observing other people, an individual learns that some behavior is reinforced and other behavior is not. A person may also learn new behaviors and skills.

Modeling can be effective only when certain criteria have been met. Those criteria are

- attention to and perception of the relevant aspects of the modeled activity
- remembrance of the modeled information, for instance, through rehearsal
- skills for translating the modeled information into adequate action, for instance, through feedback
- expectation of positive reinforcement of the modeled activity
- models who are similar to the intended population groups, who represent a coping rather than a mastery model, and who are reinforced for the behavior

Expectations that others have of behavior motivate the behavior of agents, including organizational managers and policy makers. The expectations that are conveyed might concern allocation of resources for health promotion programs, development of regulations that facilitate healthful choices by the public, or enforcement of laws. Community development methods could include having significant others (managers, supervisors, opinion leaders, and constituents) clearly communicate their beliefs and participate in a coalition in which shared goals are developed through small group discussion. Social action methods could include holding legislative briefing sessions to set agendas and using newspaper and television coverage to convey community concerns or demands.

Methods to Influence Skills, Capability, and Self-Efficacy

Self-efficacy is often a crucial determinant in health behavior change. When people are motivated, the remaining question is whether they are able, and feel confident, to change their behavior. Self-efficacy is a determinant for the precursors of behavior—intention, preparation to act, and decision to act. But it also directly influences behavior and maintenance of behavior change. Self-efficacy and related concepts are all personal, but there is a distinction between perceptions (e.g., perceived skills) and reality (e.g., real skills). Even with sufficient real skills, people may not try a new behavior when their perceived skills are low, and people with high perceived skills may fail because of insufficient real skills. Methods to improve self-efficacy are therefore often methods that also improve real skills. Table 6.8 presents skill- and efficacy-enhancing methods and their parameters.

SKILL BUILDING   Social cognitive theory (Bandura, 1986) provides health educators with systematic methods for skills training. These methods include division of the skills into subskills; instruction; modeling; guided enactment and

Table 6.8
Summary of Methods for Skills, Capability, and Self-Efficacy

METHODS	CONSIDERATIONS FOR USE
Modeling	Requires attention, remembrance, skills, reinforcement
Guided practice	Must include subskill demonstration, instruction, and enactment with feedback
Enactment	Depends on skills and feedback; should be a mastery experience
Verbal persuasion	Requires credible source, method, and channel
Physiological and affective state management	Must carefully interpret anxiety
Reattribution training	Requires counseling unstable and external attributions for failure
Goal setting	Requires commitment to the goal and a goal that is difficult but available within the individual's skill level
Planning coping responses	Must include identification of high-risk situations and practice of coping response

feedback in simple situations; and guided enactment and feedback in complex situations. It is easy to think of behaviors that obviously have skills as an important determinant, such as psychomotor skills for taking blood pressure. Social skills may be less obvious, and they are often more complex and difficult to teach. Several types of behavioral reactions to social pressure have been described by Evans and colleagues and include simple rejection ("just say no," which is the least effective reaction), repeated rejection, postponement, making excuses, avoiding the issue, and counterpose (Evans, Getz, & Raines, 1991; Evans et al., 1978). To develop skills for any one of these reactions, the method would require division of the reaction into subskills; instruction; modeling of each subskill; learner enactment and feedback.

EXPERIENCE AND ATTRIBUTION There is also a method to improve self-efficacy related to the most basic sources of self-efficacy expectations (Bandura, 1986): experience and attributions. Experience with the health-promoting behavior, successes as well as failures, is a most potent source of self-efficacy expectations. However, the effects of experience on self-efficacy are mediated by the attributions that people make about their successes and failures (Kok et al., 1992; Weiner, 1986; see Chapter 4). Theoretically, three attributional dimensions have been distinguished: locus (internal-external), stability (stable-unstable), and controllability (controllable-uncontrollable). Weiner's model suggests that expectancy of success, or self-efficacy, is determined by the perceived stability of the causes for success and failure. A person attributing a success to a stable cause (e.g., ability) will have a higher expectancy of success when having to perform the task again compared to somebody who attributes a success on the same task to an unstable cause (e.g., luck). After failure, these effects are reversed (Hospers, Kok, & Strecher, 1990).

Different attributions in terms of locus and controllability affect the emotional reaction to success and failure, which may in turn be motivating or debilitating for people's self-efficacy. Health educators may improve self-efficacy by the method of reattribution training: changing people's attributions for success and failure. In practice, the focus is usually on attributions for failures, such as returning to smoking, gaining weight, stopping exercise, or discontinuing medicines. What kind of attribution for these lapses is the best predictor of high self-efficacy? For failure, attributions that are stable and uncontrollable result in low self-efficacy, whereas attributions that are unstable and controllable will result in higher self-efficacy. For instance, people who try to lose weight may think that their failure is the result of genetic predisposition, a stable and uncontrollable attribution. In order to improve self-efficacy, these people need to learn that there is a relation between the amount of food they eat, their exercise behavior, and their weight, reflecting an unstable and controllable attribution.

Bandura (1997) summarized the methods for self-efficacy enhancement based on the four sources of self-efficacy formation:

- Provision of enactive mastery experiences (with feedback) that serve as indicators of capability (provided people make the "right" attributions)
- Provision of vicarious experiences (modeling) that alter efficacy expectations through transmission of competencies and comparison with the attainment of others
- Verbal persuasion and allied types of social influences that convince the person, agent, or group that they possess certain capabilities
- Enhancement or reduction of physiological and affective states (e.g., anxiety) from which people partly judge capability, strength, and vulnerability to dysfunction

All SCT interventions are based on reinforcement and active learning (Bandura, 1997). Strecher and Rosenstock (1997) suggest methods for self-efficacy improvement that are largely based on SCT: provide training and guidance, use progressive goal setting, give verbal reinforcement, demonstrate desired behaviors, and reduce anxiety. Maibach and Parrot (1995) would add the identification of barriers and planning of solutions. Most theories agree that self-efficacy expectations in combination with outcome expectations have a causal relation with intentions and behavior. However, intentions are not always translated into actual behavior because there may be strong situational influences (Salovey et al., 1997). To combat this problem, interventions should be based on information about self-efficacy that is related as closely as possible to the actual situation.

Prochaska and colleagues (1997) mention various processes of and methods for change that are related to self-efficacy improvement and skills training: self-liberation, counterconditioning, contingency management, stimulus control, and social liberation. Self-liberation is both the belief that one can change and the commitment to act on that belief. Public commitment, public testimonies, and multiple rather than single choices may enhance persistence. Counterconditioning requires the learning of healthy behaviors that can substitute for problem behaviors. Relaxation, assertion, desensitization, nicotine replacement, and positive self-statements are strategies for finding safer substitutions. Contingency management provides consequences, mostly rewards, comparable to self-reinforcement, for taking steps in a particular direction. Contingency contracts, overt and covert reinforcements, and group recognition are procedures for reinforcement when contingencies are met. Stimulus control removes cues (avoidance and environmental re-engineering) for unhealthy habits and adds prompts for healthier alternatives. Social liberation requires an increase in social opportunities or alternatives. Advocacy, empowerment procedures, and appropriate policies can be used to help people change.

The efficacy construct is also applicable to groups, communities, and societies. As we discussed in Chapter 4, collective efficacy refers to the group's shared belief in its capacity to organize and carry out actions required to produce goals. The most effective way to increase collective efficacy is through successful performance.

GOAL SETTING AND FEEDBACK Another method that can be used for motivating people to change behavior and help them maintain that behavior is goal setting and feedback (Locke & Latham, 1991; Strecher et al., 1995). Setting challenging but feasible goals has a beneficial effect on effort, persistence, and concentration and thus will encourage people to try harder and for a longer period of time, with less distraction from the task at hand. In general, the higher the goal, the better people perform, even when the goal is very high. If the goal a person is committed to is not achieved, dissatisfaction will occur, leading to greater subsequent effort, concentration, and persistence. Goal setting is therefore also a useful method in relapse prevention.

The three necessary conditions for the use of goal setting are commitment to the goal, a fit between abilities of the individual (and his or her self-efficacy) and complexity of the task, and the access to natural or organized feedback. One way for the intervention to stay within the last two conditions is having members of the community and the health educator participate mutually in setting the goal.

Gollwitzer (1993) presents a series of studies on goal intentions and implementation intentions. Goal intentions (I intend to pursue X) result in a commitment to realize a wish or desire. Implementation intentions (I intend to initiate behavior X when conditions Y are met) connect a certain goal-directed behavior with an anticipated situation. The purpose of an implementation intention is to lay down a specific plan to promote the initiation and efficient execution of goal-directed activity. Gollwitzer shows that by forming implementation intentions, people pass the control of the behavior over to the environment. Situations and means are turned into cues to action that are hard to forget, ignore, or miss. It appears that forming an implementation intention is a conscious mental act that has automatic consequences.

To help people realize their intentions, an important method is to facilitate the forming of implementation intentions: to get people to stipulate when, where, and how they intend to achieve their goals. Such commitments specify the situational contexts and means that are to be used, and they spell out the behaviors that are to be initiated once these contexts and means are encountered (see also the next paragraph on relapse prevention). Abraham and colleagues (1998) give an example of the use of implementation intentions in health education. A smoker who has regularly smoked with friends while drinking alcohol may find that, although successfully resisting smoking during the day, he or she experiences very strong desires for a cigarette while drinking and, seemingly without thinking, asks friends for a cigarette. A clear understanding of why this craving happens, self-monitoring of such automatic desires, and conscious initiation of alternative, cognitively rehearsed implementation intentions (e.g., declaring craving and asking for social support as soon as the desire is felt) may, through practice, disrupt this automatic, context-prompted behavior.

Self-efficacy expectations and perceived skills are relevant not only for new behavior but also for the maintenance of behavior changes. Relapse prevention theory describes the process of lapses, attributions, self-efficacy estimations, and successes and failures in maintaining the behavior change. The major distinction between success and failure is the presence or absence of a coping response for high-risk situations (Dimeff & Marlatt, 1998; Marlatt, 1985; Shiffman, 1984). High-risk situations are those situations that invite or pressure people to take up their risk behavior again. For instance, a worker who has quit smoking goes to the coffee shop where colleagues are smoking. People who have an adequate coping response will be more likely to maintain their health-promoting behavior and may develop an even higher estimation of self-efficacy. However, people who do not have an adequate coping response to a high-risk situation may lapse into their earlier risk behavior and experience a sense of failure. They may attribute this failure to stable and uncontrollable causes and, as a result, develop lower self-efficacy and a higher chance of complete relapse.

How can health educators help people prevent relapse? The theory suggests a series of primarily face-to-face or group methods that involve helping the person at risk identify high-risk situations, plan coping responses, and practice the responses until they become automatic. It also suggests reattribution training for incidental lapses so that the at-risk person can interpret these lapses as opportunities for learning.

METHODS AND STRATEGIES TO CHANGE EXTERNAL DETERMINANTS

This section presents methods and strategies to change external determinants, such as norms and resources, at the interpersonal, organizational, community, and societal levels. In Chapter 5, external determinants of behavior were described as those factors outside the individual that influence either health behavior or environmental conditions. These factors include social influences, such as norms, social support, and reinforcement, and structural influences, such as access to resources, organizational climate, and policies. Barriers to performing a health behavior are often structural, such as lack of health insurance, inconvenient clinic hours, lack of transportation, high-fat cafeteria foods, high cost of healthful foods, intense advertising of cigarettes and alcohol, and unsafe neighborhoods for jogging or walking.

In the previous section, methods presented included ways to help individuals influence external determinants, such as resisting or coping with norms or barriers, and ways to influence the decision makers who control the resources. We also talked about how the methods directed toward determinants of individual behavior could influence individual agents or gatekeepers at any environmental level. So, to some extent we have already begun to discuss methods and strategies for influencing health through these higher ecological levels.

However, we realize that this perspective does not fully capture the process of collective action. In dealing with these gatekeeper behaviors, we have not emphasized how these behaviors occur as part of a collective, such as a legislature, work site, or social network, or how these collectives are systems in their own right with their own regulatory processes. In a collective, the whole is more than the sum of the parts. Clearly, a single legislator's vote does not lead to passage of a law. Law making is a complex process and much goes on behind the scenes. For example, in the United States, a powerful Speaker of the House sometimes assigns the bills to committees in which they will die; key committee chairs schedule hostile hearings; senators make compromise deals in the construction of bills; opposition party members add fatal amendments; and political party leaders bring their legislators' votes in line.

In the remainder of the chapter we describe organizational, community, and social change methods that rely on the power and authority vested in organizations, associations of citizens, and government. We examine the methods and strategies at these higher ecological levels used to target collective action at each level that may have an effect on that level or embedded levels (e.g., the legislature passes a law limiting minors' access to cigarettes; the company goes tobacco free; a social network supports a first-time mother). These actions may influence the population for risk reduction both directly, as in these examples, or indirectly, as in the legislature's passing a law that companies must reduce emissions of pollutants or a law that manufacturers must produce cars that use only lead-free gas. When health educators seek to address these upper ecological levels, they often find general methods for community organization and organizational development, but less specificity on how to actually engage in the process. We attempt to open this black box through a careful review of methods and strategies combined with our earlier discussion of the use of individual-level determinants for persons in specific roles within social systems, for example, a legislator, school principal, or union official.

Figure 6.2 provides an overview of the process by which methods and strategies influence collectivities to provide the products that are external determinants of individual behavior. The products can also be considered as ends in themselves, that is, the particular system has healthful characteristics, in which case the end target of health of the population would not be considered. However, in general, the assumption is made, either explicitly or implicitly, that the end result is population health.

Looking at Healthful Environments as Outcomes

Another way of looking at the environment is not as a determinant but as a desired outcome, irrespective of individual health outcomes. For example, a healthy city could be characterized as one that has health-promoting policy across all sectors: a large green belt, low population density, recreation facilities, and low unemployment (Haglund, Finer, Tillgren, & Pettersson, 1996; Nutbeam & Harris, 1995). A healthy organization would have healthful policies, a health-promoting culture, commitments to self-knowledge and development, respect for individual differences, jobs that foster responsibility and autonomy, safe and healthy working environments, and equitable salaries and promotion opportunities (National Health Strategy, 1993; Rosen, 1992). A healthy school would have a coherent sequential health and physical education curriculum, teacher training, an ethos that supports student and staff well-being, health-promoting policies and practices including those of nutrition and food services, comprehensive health services, counseling, social services, and school-community partnerships (Allensworth, Lawson, Nicholson, & Wyche, 1997; Rowling, 1996). Achieving

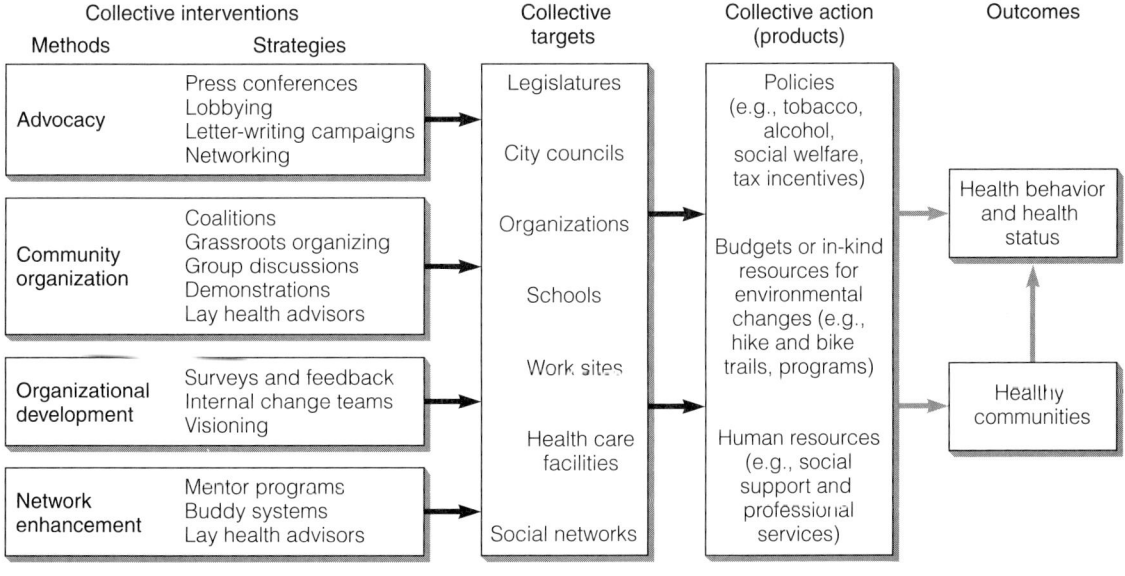

FIGURE 6.2 Overview of Intervention Process at Higher Ecological Levels

these healthful community characteristics involves methods of organizational and social change and, as mentioned earlier, the use of power.

Understanding Power

Understanding *power*—the probability that an individual or group will determine what another individual or group will do even if it is contrary to the latter's interests—is a crucial concept in order to influence collective action (Orum, 1988). Weber (1947) recognizes three sources of power: authority, charisma, and legitimacy. Each of these levels has different power structures and methods for the delivery of social influence. In small groups, social influence occurs through interaction and through leadership. The leadership might be shared by members of the group, as in a self-help group; given over voluntarily to an individual leader by the group, as in a work group; or vested in an individual from a higher authority, as in a discussion group led by a church deacon. At the organization level, the power of authority comes through the organizational hierarchical structure—who is above whom in the organizational chart. Informal power arises from an individual's charisma, from other peoples' satisfaction with a person's previous leadership activities, or from legitimacy, for example, "He's been elected, so I say we do it."

At the community and societal levels, power is "the social capacity to make binding decisions that have major consequences over the directions in which a society moves" (Orum, 1988, p. 402). The role played by power differs in the three types of social change defined by Rothman (1987). In locality development, the democratic town hall process distributes power equally; in social planning, the power rests with experts; and in social action, power is wrested from the official power structure by the people. Formal leadership in a community rests with elected and appointed officials to whom community members have given authority to govern. This authority is distributed to the government agencies that carry out federal, state, and local programs. Private organizations, because of their economic power (providing jobs and products), may be even more influential to a community.

Minkler and Wallerstein (1997) have distinguished between power with and power over, using a feminist perspective that views power as a limitless resource. They suggest that community building and capacity building are models of power with, whereas empowerment-oriented social action is a model of challenging power over. These two types of community organization lead to community competence, leadership development, and critical awareness.

Power provides a new dimension to the social influence mechanisms for changing personal determinants that we discussed in this chapter. Power is key to creating change at the higher environmental levels. In planning interventions at higher ecological levels, the health educator can bring power to play in two ways. It is critical both to choose the agent who has the power to carry out the desired change and to choose the change method that is most effective given the position of the agent and the form of power the person holds.

Shifting Social Norms

Methods and Strategies to Change External Determinants

Social norms, that is, expectations of behavior that others in the social group hold for a person, are a property of a community. Norms are the external determinant that is the basis for perceived social influence, the individual-level variable we discussed earlier. Norms are transmitted to individuals through the process of socialization. Socialization occurs primarily in childhood through the family and then is continued through institutions, such as churches, voluntary associations such as Boy Scouts, and schools (Smelser, 1988). Table 6.9 summarizes methods and strategies to change social norms.

Mass media portrayals of role models and reinforcement have been used to shift social norms. Enter-education, or edu-tainment, combines education and entertainment to transmit social norms and culture (Bouman, Maas, & Kok, 1998; Steckler et al., 1995). In various formats, including soap operas, popular music, films, and comic books, popular characters have modeled health behaviors. For example, in Nigeria, family planning was introduced in a popular television series in which characters began to use family planning and were reinforced or were socially punished for resisting adoption. Evaluation showed that family planning clinic visits increased threefold, and about half the new clients mentioned the television show as a referral source (see Rogers, 1995, pp. 344–345).

Behavioral journalism uses mass media role model stories of community members and advice from experts to increase adoption of behaviors. News stories, talk shows, feature stories in newspapers, and cartoon-style newsletters have been used as media vehicles. The media materials use models who are perceived as attractive and similar to members of the at-risk population, and these models give their reasons for adopting the new behavior, demonstrate skills used or acquired in adopting the behavior, and state the perceived reinforcing outcomes they received. Potential models are interviewed with questions designed to elicit this information in their own words. The distribution of role-model stories in a campaign may address different stages of change. Behavioral journalism has also been combined with use of a community network of volunteers who cue people to watch the television documentary stories. Community volunteers also model for their contacts by stating intentions or demonstrating the targeted behaviors.

Table 6.9
Summary of Methods to Change Social Norms

METHODS	CONSIDERATIONS FOR USE
Mass media portrayals	Must consider source and channel
Behavioral journalism	Requires role models from the community and elicitation interviews to describe the behavior and the positive outcome
Mobilizing social networks	Requires presence of a network that can potentially support health behavior
Mobilizing organizations	Must have willingness to engage in complex change process (described in 5 steps)

These methods increase the visibility of behaviors of opinion leaders and early adopters, increasing the speed of adoption of the behaviors within the population (McAlister, 1991; Pulley, McAlister, Kay, & O'Reilly, 1996; Ramirez et al., 1999).

Mobilizing social networks is a method that can also be used to influence social norms. For example, in a natural helper model intervention, Kelly and colleagues (1992) trained respected and popular patrons of gay bars to adopt protective sexual practices and persuade acquaintances to follow their example. This intervention led not only to a change in individual behavior but to increased norms supportive of protective behavior.

Norms within organizations usually relate to how work is carried out. In addition, however, norms for health-related behavior also exist within work sites. Norms related to health can be changed by the following process:

- Assess what the existing norms are (typically done using surveys)
- Examine the supportive factors (these factors include modeling, training, rewards and recognition, communication, orientation, resource allocation, and commitment)
- Identify strengths and opportunities for improvement
- Work with small groups of employees and managers to develop a vision of what the norms could be
- Analyze the gaps between what exists and what would be possible
- Use action planning to identify leverage points, to change the organization's supportive factors and norms, and to choose strategies
- Use periodic monitoring and feedback to determine if the methods and strategies are effective at changing the norms

Strategies might include leader role modeling and coaching, reinforcement for healthful behaviors and supportive teamwork, changes in the budget to include health promotion, the design of a health-promoting environment, or the addition of health and well-being to corporate mission statements.

Increasing Social Support and Social Capital

Social networks link individuals together and are the basis for community. Methods and strategies to change social networks to increase social support and social capital are presented in Table 6.10. The function of social networks is determined by both structure (such as size and pattern of linkages) and interaction (such as the nature of relationships and the benefits individuals receive from them). This section includes methods and strategies directed to the characteristics of both social network structure and social network interaction. It also includes methods and strategies at the interpersonal and organizational levels, at which the benefit is social support, and at the societal level, at which the benefit is social capital (R. M. Goodman et al., 1997).

Table 6.10
Summary of Methods to Change Social Networks

METHODS	CONSIDERATIONS FOR USE
Social support	
Training network members to provide support	Must include decisions about the type of support needed and must intensively train social skills such as empathy and information giving
Increasing reciprocity	Could use organized cooperatives for services such as baby-sitting and transportation
Creating new linkages	Benefits from consideration of activities for stimulating both within-network and out-of-network ties
Social capital	
Linking individuals to community organizations and organizations to each other	Requires democratic management and cooperative decision making

SOCIAL SUPPORT   It is possible to enhance a social network to improve its delivery of cognitive, affective, and tangible social support (Heaney & Israel, 1997). Because different characteristics are associated with different forms of support, planning should include decisions about the type of support needed by network members in a particular context. Small, intense, dense, and geographically close networks are best for providing affective support and appraisal support, whereas larger, more diffuse, less intense, and less homogeneous networks facilitate social outreach and informational support (Gottlieb & McLeroy, 1994; Heaney & Israel).

Network members can be trained to provide support more effectively. Behaviors addressed in such skills training include how to contact social network members in person, by telephone, and by letter. Training also can include how to listen, express empathy and concern, provide information and suggestions, and offer help with tangible needs.

Strategies to increase density can include activities to bring network members together to get to know one another, persuasion and encouragement for networks to reach out to incorporate new members, and incorporation of information from network members who hold membership in other networks. To increase reciprocity, strategies can include exchange structures such as baby-sitting or housecleaning exchanges. New network linkages can be developed through mentor programs, buddy systems, and self-help groups. Norms and incentives for volunteerism and for supporting coworkers, neighbors, and parishioners strengthen social networks. A cultural value on cooperation fosters social support in contrast to the value of radical individualism.

The use of natural helpers or lay health advisors has been a strategy to enhance social support networks, particularly around health issues. Natural helpers are community members to whom other persons turn and who agree to become a link between the community and the formal service delivery system. Their role is to recruit, train, and support community members to offer social support to members of their networks, to negotiate with professionals for support from the health care system, and to mobilize community resources to sustain support for the health care system (Eng, Parker, & Harlan, 1997; Eng & Smith, 1995).

Earp and colleagues (1997) have described the recruitment and training program for the lay health advisors in the North Carolina Breast Cancer Screening Program. The project recruited women from the communities who were respected, caring leaders with an interest in helping others. These women were able to maintain close, supportive, and reciprocal relationships, were comfortable and effective accessing the health care system, and had an interest in women's health and social issues. Training focused on ability to provide informational and instrumental support related to breast cancer screening including knowledge of services, how to make appointments, and how to access funding sources for screening. The program also taught women how to provide emotional and appraisal support to move other women through the stages of change for breast cancer screening. They also worked on skills needed to carry out basic behaviors required in their role, including working with women one-on-one, making group presentations, developing an agenda, and running a productive meeting.

At the government and society level, legislation can be enacted to support social networks. Examples of legislation are family leave acts, policies to promote volunteerism, and funding for child and elder care programs (Gottlieb & McLeroy, 1994). Methods for policy change will be described later in this chapter.

SOCIAL CAPITAL As we mentioned in Chapter 4, social capital is also a function of social networks. Social capital at the community level involves trust, cooperation, civic engagement, and reciprocity (Green & Kreuter, 1999). Interventions to increase social capital can occur at the community level and include community development and participatory problem solving, which are discussed in the following section. In this section, we emphasize the importance of linking persons to community organizations, such as churches, social clubs, schools, political groups, and work settings, in which they can engage in voluntary association with others to address issues of community concern. For residents to have loose ties outside their primary networks to bring in new information and resources is also important, and these ties can be fostered by interorganizational meetings and coalitions (Goodman et al., 1997). For example, statewide meetings of church associations, nonprofit health agency volunteers, political conventions, and joint neighborhood association meetings allow the opportunity for residents to connect with others with similar concerns and interests, to learn about their activities, and to team up to work together. Democratic management in which "members share information and power, utilize cooperative decision-making processes, and are involved in the design, implementation, and control of efforts toward mutually defined goals" is essential (Israel, Checkoway, Schulz, & Zimmerman, 1994, p. 152).

The Mpowerment Project, a community-level HIV prevention intervention, was structured with a core decision-making group of 12 to 15 young (age 18 to 29) gay men, a community advisory board of men and women from the AIDS, gay and lesbian, public health, and university communities, and a part-time staff of four young gay men (Kegeles, Hays, & Coates, 1996). An outreach team conducted peer outreach, both formally through visiting locations frequented by young gay men and informally to their friends in casual conversation. Outreach included the recruitment of men for the project's educational and social activities and informal discussions promoting safer sex. The project is an excellent example of the use of social networks for diffusion of health behavior, shifting of norms, and community capacity building through decision-making control and participation.

Enhancing Access to Resources

From the standpoint of health promotion, important organizational and community resources include healthful food, facilities for physical activity, health care, clean air and water, transportation, and education. In this section, we examine methods for obtaining resources at a higher ecological level than that of the individual or small group. We present methods from organizational development, community organization, and politics that can be used to obtain resources for health promotion and to establish programs and policies. Table 6.11 presents methods and strategies for enhancing access to resources.

Table 6.11
Summary of Methods to Change Access to Resources

METHODS	CONSIDERATIONS FOR USE
Organizational change	Requires attention to stages of organizational change
Organizational and community-wide partnerships	Requires attention to stages of partnership development
Community building	Must start where the community is and encourage community to identify issues
Challenging power over	Requires collaboration across various agendas and acquisition of legislative representation
Conscientization	Requires being with the people in the community
Advocacy	Must match advocacy group's style and tactics with the issue and the community
Media advocacy	Requires both getting media to accept a story and shifting how responsibility for the problem is handled in the story
Policy advocacy	Must match the model by which the issue is getting on the agendas

ORGANIZATIONAL CHANGE Kurt Lewin (1947) proposed that organizations were in a state of "quasi-stationary equilibrium," in which two sets of forces—those driving for change and those striving for the status quo—were approximately equal. For change to occur, the forces driving for change could increase, or the forces maintaining the status quo could decrease, or both could occur. Lewin advised that decreasing the status quo forces was less disruptive and more effective than increasing forces for change. He saw the change process as having three phases: unfreezing, moving, and refreezing. Unfreezing reduces the forces that maintain the organization's current behavior, often by providing information that shows that behaviors or conditions desired by organizational members are different from those they currently exhibit. During the moving phase, changes in organizational structures and processes lead to new behaviors, values, and attitudes. In refreezing, organizational norms, policies, and structures are put into place that support the new state of equilibrium (Cummings & Worley, 1993; Lewin).

Table 6.12 presents an expansion of Lewin's three phases of change to five stages, as described by Brager and Holloway (1978). Stages include initial assessment, preinitiation, initiation, implementation, and institutionalization. This model provides a set of strategies or steps for moving an organization through a change process. Table 6.12 also includes some of the motivational and political concerns during change (Cummings & Worley, 1993). In one example, a university health educator used these five stages as a basis for helping a voluntary health agency adopt a health promotion program to be offered by the agency to work sites (Simons-Morton, Greene, & Gottlieb, 1995).

INTERORGANIZATIONAL AND COMMUNITY-WIDE PARTNERSHIPS Partnerships among organizations fall along a continuum, from lesser to greater complexity of purposes, intensity of linkages, and formality of agreements. Points on the continuum are described as networking, cooperation, coordination, and collaboration (see Chapter 4; Daka-Mulwanda, Thornburg, Filbert, & Klein, 1995; Habana-Hafner & Reed, 1989). In starting a partnership, an important first step is to determine what type of organizational arrangement is both feasible and appropriate to accomplish the goals that have been set. To accomplish their goals, coalitions must move through a series of stages (Butterfoss et al., 1993; Texas Department of Health Coalition Task Force, 1996). Table 6.13 presents the terminology often used in practice to highlight the stages—forming, storming, norming, and performing—and identifies the tasks to be accomplished at each stage. Intervention methods to facilitate communities to move through these steps include training, modeling, mentoring, and resource brokering.

The community development process used by the Health Care Forum expands on the process of community partnerships (Johnson, Grossman, & Cassidy, 1996). This model, applied extensively in the Healthy Communities movement in the United States, is typically professionally driven and involves the entire community, including those citizens in the mainstream of power. However, the methods and strategies can be applied to more narrowly focused partner-

Table 6.12
Stages and Tasks for Planned Organizational Change

STAGE	TASKS	CRITICAL ELEMENTS
Initial assessment	Problem assessment and selection of change goals Force field analysis of driving and restraining forces Choices of tactics for change	
Preinitiation	Choice of a change agent with credibility and legitimacy Increased awareness within the organization of the need for change through evaluations and formal and informal discussion	Motivating change and developing political support
Initiation	Selection of top-down or bottom-up change strategies Specification of any policies or procedures in the change	Attention to the politics of change
Implementation	Choice of formal and informal communication channels for the change Development of administrative procedures for the change Analysis of driving and restraining forces for implementation Monitoring of change process	Attention to the politics of change Skill training for employees to learn technical and social skills needed for the change
Institutionalization	Inclusion of change in strategic plans and in organization goals and objectives Written job descriptions Hiring of permanent staff Stable source of funding	Reinforcement of changed behavior using monetary, social, and intrinsic rewards

Note. Adapted from *Changing Human Service Organizations: Politics and Practice,* by G. A. Brager and S. Holloway, 1978, New York: Free Press, as presented in *Introduction to Health Education and Health Promotion* (2nd ed., p. 333), by B. G. Simons-Morton, W. H. Greene, and N. H. Gottlieb, 1995, Prospect Heights, IL: Waveland Press.

ships, including, for example, special interest coalitions or neighborhood groups. The model consists of a metaprocess called Organizing the Effort and six additional processes titled Convening the Community, Creating a Shared Vision, Assessing Current Realities and Trends, Action Planning, Doing the Job, and Monitoring and Adjusting.

Organizing the Effort lays a foundation for partnership and includes the mechanisms that must be developed to enable the stakeholders and staff to work together across community sectors and to develop trust and commitment among

Table 6.13
Tasks for Each Stage of Coalition Development

COALITION STAGE	TASKS
Forming: Establishing a coalition to address a need identified by some groups within the community	Identify an issue to champion
	Determine whether a coalition is the most appropriate strategy to address the issue
	Determine if there is another group adequately addressing the issue
	Research the issue
	Determine the type of coalition that is most appropriate to the issue
	Identify stakeholders—groups or individuals who affect or are affected by the problem
	Prepare a sales pitch, identify people to be contacted, and contact them
	Hold the first meeting
Storming: Early phase in which diverse members come together to define the processes and work of the coalition	Provide opportunities for members to get to know each other by talking about their beliefs, assumptions, and values and what motivates them to work for their community
	Develop a shared understanding of the problem
	Acknowledge the assets and commitment each member brings to the coalition
	Acknowledge the needs that each member brings to the coalition
	Teach participants process skills, including shared group leadership
	Decide ground rules together, including how to respect and value different points of view and diversity in experiences, how decisions will be made, who will speak to the media, what should be confidential, how information will be distributed, and the role of representatives
	Use communication tools, including shared meeting notices, agendas, and minutes and participant contact information
	Use a neutral meeting place that is conducive to face-to-face interactions
Norming: Solidification of structure and governance	Develop a formal infrastructure for the coalition, perhaps including formal vision and mission statement, bylaws, articles of incorporation, evaluation reports
	Formulate goals, objectives, and an action plan using work groups
Performing: Full-fledged implementation of work in the community	Implement the action plan, monitoring specific dates for completion of projects
	Involve additional members
	Promote coalition activities through media
	Maintain the coalition through meetings and communication with members, obtaining necessary resources, orientation of new members, and entertaining new ideas
	Evaluate performance

Note. Adapted from *Coalition Building: A Healthy Community Is Everyone's Business,* by Texas Department of Health Coalition Task Force, 1996, Austin, TX: Texas Department of Health (1100 West 49th Street, Austin, TX 78756); and from "Developing Multisector Collaboration," by M. Axner and B. Berkowitz, August 18, 1999, in *Community Tool Box* [On-line], chap. 18, sec. 11, available: http://ctb.lsi.ukans.edu

partners. This metaprocess lays out tasks for the facilitator or organizer to accomplish so that the work of the partnership can be carried out.

After organizing the effort, the facilitator convenes the community to begin identification of leadership, that is, to find the individuals who will catalyze the collaboration process. Those leaders then define the purpose and scope of the project and determine who the potential stakeholder groups are. It is important that the partnership include representatives of diverse demographic groups within the community and that all sectors necessary to project success are included. Stakeholders are then invited to participate, and efforts to gain trust and credibility within the group are begun. At this stage, openness and discussion of the benefits of collaboration are essential.

Next, Creating a Shared Vision is carried out through a facilitated event in which all partners participate. Individuals describe their vision of the future of their community, and the facilitator encourages consensus to develop the shared vision. The partnership publicizes the vision, validates it with other members of the community, uses it as a touchstone in its deliberations, and updates it as necessary.

Assessing Current Realities and Trends involves the assessment of both assets and needs within the community. We have discussed this process in detail in Chapter 2. The partnership needs to plan the assessment—including the purpose and scope, resources required, and types of data to be collected—identify priorities from the data, and report key findings to appropriate audiences. Action plans are then developed that lay out the goals and objectives of the partnership and the specific strategies and methods it will use to address them. In developing a plan, there must be clear logic between the activities and the expected outcomes. Both short-term "small wins" and longer term actions should be included, and persons responsible, resources needed, and a timeline should be provided for each action. Ownership in the plan should be fostered through broad discussion and through assignment of realistic roles and responsibilities. Formal commitments should be made, and the plan distributed to current and potential collaborators.

For action plan implementation, or Doing the Job, human and fiscal resources need to be in place, including confirmation by the stakeholders of their role in the plan. More partners typically need to be recruited, and support obtained from leaders and organizations who have not participated in the partnership's action planning process. As the implementation begins, coordination and monitoring are key. The partnership should capitalize on opportunities for building synergy across elements of the plan and on working for both short- and long-term objectives. Partners should be alert for changes in the community context that might require a shift in actions, which allows for fine-tuning of the plan or, for major changes, revision of the plan.

The partners then monitor and adjust by establishing a monitoring system, carrying out an evaluation, and using the results to provide feedback to the stakeholders.

COMMUNITY BUILDING As we discussed in Chapter 4, newer community organization approaches are described by Minkler and Wallerstein (1997) and by Walter (1997) as community building, and they flow from a strengths-based model. Within this model (as well as others), grassroots organizing is the process of people coming together to assert their needs (Pilisuk, McAllister, & Rothman, 1997).

Important methods for health educators engaged in this process are participation and relevance, that is, starting where the people are; issue identification, which must be a community effort rather than one imposed by the health educator; network assessment and mapping of community assets, that is, mapping the networks of social ties in which community members are embedded (Heitzmann & Kaplan, 1988; McCallister & Fischer, 1978) as well as other types of community assets (Kretzmann & McKnight, 1993); and culturally competent practice, whereby the practitioner can actually hear the real community discourse (Ladson-Billings, 1995).

CHALLENGING POWER OVER Social action organizing, according to Rothman (1979), has as its goal the shifting of power relationships and resources from the haves to the have-nots. Social action as a method achieves change by the crystallization of issues and by organizing people to take action. Historical examples of this type of community organization practice have included Alinsky method organizing, the civil rights movement, the United Farm Workers movement, Community Action Programs, and the work of the Students for a Democratic Society, the Student Non-Violent Coordinating Committee, the Black Panthers, the Brown Berets, and *La Raza Unida* (Fisher, 1997). Methods include boycotts, demonstrations, and strikes.

Fisher and Kling (1991) see contemporary community-based social action as blending social action with community development and social planning. Strategies used include coalition building across constituency groups and integrating community politics more closely with electoral activity (Fisher, 1997). These theorists believe that policy advocacy is not sufficient, that groups must win and hold power through elected office. Fisher develops the argument that a major focus must be on challenging the ideology of privatization and free enterprise that serves the needs of international capital rather than the needs of low and moderate income people. This challenge should be mounted through legislation to protect public sector services and public life. Finally, community organizers must bring together people across different agendas and different cultural and identity-based groups to organize around common grievances with a commitment to "human solidarity, mutual responsibility, and social justice" (p. 65).

CONSCIENTIZATION Critical consciousness, or conscientization, links individual and community-level empowerment and is a key method for strengths-based community organization. The method by which critical consciousness emerges was described by Paulo Freire, a Brazilian educator, in the context of developing literacy in his country. Educators began the process by being with the people in a local community, by discovering the way they talked about daily life, that is, the words and phrases they used, and by observing the way life was lived. Generative words were then selected for their social meaning and also to represent all phonemes in the language. The educators continued to divide and reintegrate these codes, or representations of the life of the people, to develop the program content of their interventions. These codes, which might be pictures, songs, or words, were next discussed by program participants—through a questioning process, in cultural circles, or in learning groups—in terms of the participants' lives and the root causes of the conditions of their lives. This reflection on root causes gave rise to a political and social understanding that was accompanied by action to transform this reality. Literacy was an instrument of this struggle. The final step of conscientization was the understanding that oppressive reality is a process that can be overcome. This understanding results in praxis, the unity between a person's understanding and actions (Freire, 1973; Gadotti, 1994).

The Freirian method has been applied in health education in such areas as women's health; tobacco, drug, and alcohol prevention; sexuality; environmental health; occupational health; and health of the elderly (Goodman, 1998; McFarlane, Fehir, & De Madres a Madres,1994; Minkler, 1997; Rudd & Comings, 1994; Wallerstein & Sanchez-Merki, 1994; Wang & Burris, 1994; Wang, Yi, Tao, & Carovano, 1998). The codes for discussion varied among these projects. For example, Wang and colleagues used photographs taken by rural Chinese women of their everyday activities. Photonovels for environmental health ("A Working Neighborhood: What Does It Take?"), smoking prevention ("Decisions, Decisions"), and occupational health ("Workers Take Action: Fighting Asbestos in the Building Trades") were developed by participants in the three programs described by Rudd and Comings through dialogue about the issues to explore root causes, development of a story line, and design and production of the books. Triggers for discussion in the Adolescent Social Action Program were stories that students would listen to from hospital patients and jail residents who had problems related to drug and alcohol abuse, violence, unsafe sex, and other risky behaviors. Other triggers included role plays, student life stories, videotapes, collages, and photographs (Wallerstein, Sanchez-Merki, & Dow, 1997). Codes developed by Cherokee parents were short paragraphs describing the gap between what was needed and what was being done to help people in such diverse areas as healthy sexual decision making, culturally sensitive programming for Indian youth, teen pregnancy, and cultural traditions as guidelines for living (Goodman, 1998).

These projects all rely on participatory analysis using critical reflection and dialogue. Questions to encourage a critical stance, described by Shaffer (1993) and used by Wang and colleagues (1998), include "What do you see here? What's really happening here? How does this relate to our lives? Why does this problem or this strength exist? What can we do about this?" (Wang et al., p. 80). Issues, themes, and theories emerge that inform action.

The cycle of reflection-action-reflection continues. The rural Chinese women presented their concerns to provincial policy makers (Wang et al., 1998); adolescents have been involved in peer education, participating in a statewide youth leadership group for policy development, and carrying out service projects (Wallerstein et al., 1997); and low-income elderly hotel residents have formed building tenants' associations, achieved better living conditions, and received compensation for lack of services (Minkler, 1997). However, a sustained effort is required for action and advocacy to be demonstrated. The completion of the photonovels for environmental health, smoking prevention, and occupational health was the major outcome of the interventions. The photonovels were disseminated to other groups, who found them to be credible and used them to increase their intention to act. However, the participants who developed them did not engage in active advocacy (Rudd & Comings, 1994).

ADVOCACY   Advocacy has been defined as "the set of skills used to create a shift in public opinion and mobilize the necessary resources and forces to support an issue, policy, or constituency" (Wallach, Dorfman, Jernigan, & Themba, 1993, p. 27). Advocacy ensures that the rights of disenfranchised individuals are protected, that institutions work the way they should, and that legislation and policy reflect the interest of the people. It addresses attitudes and policies at all levels—from organizational, through community and state, to the national arena. In public health advocacy, efforts are made to change community conditions, often pitting consumers against large industry and citizens against city hall. Community activism is rooted in democratic principles and practices, and though often viewed as synonymous with social action, it includes cooperation as well as confrontation. Examples of advocacy groups include local and national groups participating in social movements—such as those for the environment, environmental justice, and tobacco control—and citizen groups that have come together to support issues of importance in their communities. Advocacy groups have different tactics. For example, some are confrontational, such as ACT UP (an AIDS awareness activist group); others are research based, such as the League of Women Voters (Altman, Balcazar, Fawcett, Seekins, & Young, 1994; Wallack et al., 1993).

It is important that tactics and activities be chosen that fit the issue and the community. Groups must decide how they intend to accomplish goals, and those activities will likely change over time in response to reactions to actions taken and to shifting external forces. Altman and colleagues (1994) list the following approaches to advocacy: coalition building, community development, coordination, education, networking, public awareness, and policy or legislative change (p. 53).

Strategies are the specific actions to be undertaken by the group. Altman and colleagues (1994) provide six principles to enhance tactical efforts (Table 6.14). These principles should underlie action, regardless of whether the action flows from a social action, community development, or social planning perspective. Another basic element is framing the issue, which we discuss more fully in the section titled "Media Advocacy." The issue must be framed in terms put forward by the advocacy group. For example, the tobacco industry might say "Smoking is a matter of personal choice," whereas a public health advocacy group would say "People smoke because they are addicted"; the tobacco industry would say "Smoking bans discriminate against smokers," whereas the advocacy group would say "Nonsmokers have the right to breathe clean air" (Altman et al., 1994, p. 61).

Altman and colleagues (1994) divide advocacy strategies into three categories: research and investigation, encouragement and education, and direct action. Research and investigation includes conducting studies of the issue to understand it as fully as possible, gathering data on public opinion, obtaining

Table 6.14
Principles Underlying Effective Tactics

PRINCIPLE	WHAT TO DO
Presence	Remind people of the issue by doing something about it frequently
Generosity	Praise others for their strengths and actions, to gain goodwill, and to reinforce their actions
Shaping	Reward small steps of those who change toward your goals
Escalation	Continue to mobilize more people and increase the intensity of the tactics if the first efforts are unsuccessful
Accuracy and honesty	Be scrupulously accurate to maintain credibility and to keep opponents from successfully arguing against the issues raised
Consistency	Distribute praise and criticism fairly; if one group is criticized for its position, other groups should be treated the same way

Note. Adapted from *Public Health Advocacy: Creating Community Change to Improve Health* (p. 60), by D. G. Altman, F. E. Balcazar, S. B. Fawcett, T. M. Seekins, and J. Q. Young, 1994, Palo Alto, CA: Stanford Center for Research in Disease Prevention.

information about the opposition and its strategies and tactics, and acting as a watchdog of target organizations. The advocacy group can also request accountability by formally asking responsible parties the reasons behind a decision of concern to them, by documenting complaints with evidence, by organizing consumer service audits, and by demonstrating the financial benefits of acting on their issue.

Strategies for encouragement and education include giving personal compliments and public support to reinforce other people's actions, arranging celebrations and publicizing them, developing a detailed proposal for addressing the problem being focused on, and establishing contact with the opposition organization even to the extent of influencing its decision-making processes. Also suggested are preparing fact sheets on the advocacy group and the issue to maintain consistency and continuity in public relations, offering public education through mass media and presentations to community groups, and countering attacks by explaining the group's point of view.

Interventionists use direct action strategies to make the group's presence felt, mobilize public support, and use the system (Altman et al., 1994). Strategies to make the group's presence felt include postponing action until the issue has matured, establishing alternative programs or finding another source to provide the service, establishing lines of communications with the opponent's traditional allies, criticizing unfavorable actions first privately and then publicly if there are no results, expressing opposition publicly, reminding those responsible, making complaints (first informally, then formally), and lobbying decision makers. Ways to mobilize public support include sponsoring a conference or public hearing; conducting a letter-writing campaign, a petition drive, or a ballot drive; registering voters; and organizing public demonstrations. For using the system, the advocacy group might file a formal complaint; seek enforcement of existing laws and policies; lobby for new laws, policies, or regulations; use other resources such as a negotiator, mediator, or fact-finder to work with opponents; and initiate legal action if that proves to be the only way to address the issue. Altman and colleagues also describe getting serious, which includes the strategies of arranging a media exposé, overwhelming an unworkable system (for example, by having unmanageable requests for service), organizing a boycott, and using passive resistance.

Advocacy can lead to counteradvocacy by opponent groups. They may deflect the issue or shift the focus of attention away from the responsible party. Delay techniques, denial, and discounting the importance of the problem or of the advocacy group's legitimacy are also countering strategies. Deception, dividing the advocacy group by co-opting leaders or by splitting moderate and militant members, appeasing the group with short-term benefits, discrediting the advocacy group, and destroying the group are all designed to silence the advocates. If those tactics don't work, opponents may make a deal that falls short of the advocates' goals. Altman and colleagues (1994) suggest how to turn negatives into positives in response to the opposition's tactics. They suggest going public with the opponent's tactics, framing the debate on the advocate's terms, keeping the opponent off balance by being unpredictable, and knowing when to negotiate. A list of 20 rules of etiquette, drawn from the experiences of a number of advocates and summarized by Altman and his co-authors, provides guidelines for advocacy (Table 6.15).

MEDIA ADVOCACY Wallach and his colleagues (1993) have developed the approach of media advocacy, a set of strategies for using the media to promote public health. They recognize that the mass media, particularly television, provide the forum for the surfacing and discussion of issues, setting the agenda for policy makers and the public. Media advocacy seeks to influence the selection of topics by the media and the way they are presented in order to set and achieve a public health agenda.

Media advocacy is based on three steps: setting the agenda, shaping the debate, and advancing the policy. In setting the agenda, the goal is to get the media to select the story. Shaping the debate involves shifting the view of health from the individual to the societal level and dealing with the complexity of health and social problems so that the debate is defined by a public health perspective. Advancing the policy includes making sure the content reaches the key decision makers. This latter step is congruent with the Intervention Mapping approach of focusing on agents at each of the environmental levels involved in the health problem.

Health educators must understand the various access points of each of the major media outlets. For television, these access points are news, public affairs, entertainment, editorials, paid advertising, and public service advertising; for newspapers, the access points are the front page, sports, lifestyle, arts, comics, business, editorials, letters to the editors, and paid advertising. The media advocate needs to understand where and how to place the particular issue within the

Table 6.15
Guidelines for Effective Advocacy: Rules of Etiquette

1. Accentuate the positive.
2. Plan for small wins.
3. Begin by assuming the best of others.
4. Do your homework and document your findings.
5. Take the high ground.
6. Reframe opponents' definitions of the issue.
7. Keep it simple.
8. Be passionate and persistent.
9. Be willing to compromise.
10. Be opportunistic and creative.
11. Don't be intimidated.
12. Maintain focus on the issues.
13. Make it local and keep it relevant.
14. Be broadly based and nonpartisan from the beginning.
15. Develop an independent public identity.
16. Try to stay within the experiences of individuals in your group.
17. Whenever possible, go outside the experience of your opponent.
18. Make your opponents live by their own rules.
19. Tie advocacy group efforts to related events.
20. Have a good time.

Note. From *Public Health Advocacy: Creating Community Change to Improve Health* (pp. 27–35), by D. G. Altman, F. E. Balcazar, S. B. Fawcett, T. M. Seekins, and J. Q. Young, 1994, Palo Alto, CA: Stanford Center for Research in Disease Prevention.

media. Media advocacy strategies focus on earned media and paid placements rather than on public service announcements in which control over the placement and framing of the story is lost. Health educators can achieve news coverage by selecting journalists who are interested in health issues and providing them with accurate information and story ideas. Creating news and piggybacking onto breaking news are also strategies. Elements of newsworthiness include an anniversary, a breakthrough, a celebrity, a controversy, injustice, irony, a local angle, a milestone, a personal angle, or a seasonal angle (Wallach et al., 1993, p. 98). By monitoring the media, health educators can understand which reporters are covering which topics and what the current community concerns are.

In framing for content to give the public health perspective, the individual problem needs to be framed as a social issue, with the primary responsibility shifted away from blaming the individual. For example, the subject should be shifted from teen drinking to the promotion of alcohol. A solution should be presented, including an approach to policy. Story elements to be developed include compelling images, powerful symbols, and social math to show the extent of the problem (e.g., in a year "enough alcohol was consumed by college students to fill 3,500 Olympic-size swimming pools, about 1 on every campus in the United

States," Wallach et al., 1993, p. 108). Also, it is important to use authentic voices of people who are credible because of their experiences but who are deeply involved in the policy aspects of the issue. Using media sound bites of less than 10 seconds to summarize the issue is a skill to be learned (e.g., "You face more danger with the 20 cigarettes that are in your pocket than any six bullets in somebody's gun," Ken McFeeley, quoted in Wallach et al., 1993, p. 112).

Wallach and colleagues also provide practical advice for developing media goals and objectives, pitching the story to journalists, developing media kits, and giving interviews. Their summary rules for working with reporters are that health educators should be honest, should help the press better understand the issues, should comment only on issues that they know about, and should remember that everything they say is on the record (Wallach et al., 1993, p. 141).

POLICY ADVOCACY Now we turn to political science theories to understand more fully how policy agendas are set. Cobb and Elder (1983) have identified two types of policy agendas: a systemic agenda that includes the issues perceived by the political community as meriting consideration and as within the jurisdiction of governmental authority, and the institutional or governmental agenda that is the set of issues that are explicitly up for active consideration by governmental decision makers. Cobb and Elder have identified three models by which an issue comes first to the systemic agenda and then to the institutional agenda: the outside-initiative model, the inside-initiative model, and the mobilization model. Advocacy efforts must be matched to the model by which the issue comes to the agendas and also to whether the goal is to get the issue to the systemic agenda or from the systemic agenda to the institutional agenda.

In the outside-initiative model, public support is needed to bring the issue to the systemic agenda. For public health issues, the methods of grassroots organizing, media advocacy, and professionally driven organizing use the media to show the importance of the issue and its effects on people, the urgency of the problem, and the power and legitimacy of the groups wishing to address the issue. Earlier in this chapter we discussed the strategies and tactics for community organization and advocacy to generate public support.

In the inside-initiative model, the initiative comes from within the government system and moves from there to the institutional agenda without involving the larger public. Here the advocacy work is much more behind the scenes. Health advocates form relationships with legislative staff, persuade them of the importance of the issue, and show how the issue fits with their legislators' agendas. Supplying accurate and timely (according to the legislative staff members' needs) information as the issue moves through the policy process enables the staff to do their jobs to get the issue into play. This process does not require large-scale community mobilization and media, because the issue is likely floating close to the systemic agenda. Here, individual policy entrepreneurs may be as effective as organized community groups. Policy entrepreneurs use the methods we have discussed earlier (e.g., persuasive communication, value discussions, presentation of facts) to get policy-making insiders to place the issue on the systemic and institutional agendas.

In the mobilization model, policy proposals are developed within the government, and then support is sought among the public for policy passage and successful implementation. In this instance, government insiders use the media and community forums to inform and persuade the public of the importance of the issue so that broad-scale support can be mobilized for the policy proposal. The methods are similar to the dual-channel methods (i.e., mass media and interpersonal communication) that were discussed earlier in this chapter.

Issues have a life cycle, and an understanding of the stages and their determinants allows the advocate to move an issue forward more effectively. Cobb and Elder (1983) identified five stages in the cycle: issue awareness, issue recognition, issue resolution, issue realignment, and issue dormancy. In the issue awareness stage, groups and individuals begin to discuss problems and potential issues. For issues to be recognized, a policy maker must decide that the issue should be addressed. Issues are more likely to be recognized if they are defined broadly, have a large social impact, have long-term implications, are not too technical and complex, and are not routine. Interest group characteristics are also important. The group's ideology and values must arouse enough tension concerning the problem for the potential issue to emerge. The more powerful the group is, in terms of size and legitimacy, and the more committed it is to the issue, the more likely it is to influence the policy. Time is important as well. Too rapid an emergence can lead to a crisis in which policy makers are unprepared; some issues require time to "ripen," but too long a period can lead to loss of interest by the public.

At the recognition stage, organizational resources for in-depth analysis and monitoring must be devoted to the issue by the policy maker. Advocates have the opportunity to provide data and policy analysis that can be used by policy makers and their staff members. To reach resolution, a satisfactory policy solution must be adopted. With multiple interest groups, compromise occurs. At this point, delaying tactics by someone in the political system or obstruction by powerful interest groups may move the issue to dormancy. After adoption of the policy, rules and procedures for implementation must be developed and enforced, and funding and personnel allocated. Fine-tuning of the policy and its rules and procedures often occurs during the implementation period. In the dormant stage the issue is out of the public eye unless it re-emerges and enters the cycle again.

In legislative advocacy, as in many other arenas, timing is everything, and opportunity knocks for those advocates who are prepared. Much of the success in placing issues on the systemic and institutional agendas and in achieving policy enactment comes from an understanding of when to act and how to frame the issue. Kingdon's (1995) notion of policy windows, which we discussed in Chapter 4, provides a framework for timing. Kingdon says that policy is placed on the agendas when windows open up between the three streams of politics (including elections, party platforms, and national mood regarding government), problems (all the issues within different policy sectors, including health, housing, economic sectors), and policy solutions (such as school-based clinics and universal health insurance) so that the policy can be put forward. For example, newly elected officials may focus on different problems, for which prepared advocates who have networked with the right gatekeepers can present their solutions. Community advocacy groups can work with each of the streams. For example, they can support candidates for elected office or influence party platforms, build community demand for particular problems to be addressed, and develop and promote well-researched and persuasive policy proposals.

SUMMARY

In this chapter we have presented a selection of intervention methods and some ideas about how to translate them to practical strategies. We make a conscious and conscientious distinction between methods (the change mechanism proposed for an intervention component) and strategies (the ways in which that change mechanism is actually delivered). Three important points need to be made about the distinction between methods and strategies. First, these concepts are often on a continuum rather than in distinct categories; for example, modeling as a method is very closely related to role model stories as a strategy. Second, there are often methods within methods; for example, a role model (a method) may be used to convey attribution retraining (also a method). And finally, at times health educators may be unable to sort out what might be the method and what might be the strategy. These concepts are difficult to unbundle, especially in the higher ecological levels. Nevertheless, unbundling is important, and intervention development at this step should include every effort to recognize which part of the strategy is the method, that is, the part intended to produce the change.

Tasks for Intervention Mapping Step 2:

- Brainstorm methods either by grouping learning and change objectives (guided by determinants) or by grouping methods and strategies together
- Translate methods into practical strategies
- Organize methods and strategies by groups of learning objectives at each ecological level, and check that methods are properly operationalized

REFERENCES

Abraham, C., Sheeran, P., & Johnston, M. (1998). From health beliefs to self-regulation: Theoretical advances in the psychology of action control. *Psychology and Health, 13*(4), 569–591.

Ajzen, I. (1988). *Attitudes, personality, and behavior.* Chicago: Dorsey.

Allegrante, J. P., & Roizen, M. F. (1998). Can net-present value economic theory be used to explain and change health-related behaviors? *Health Education Research, 13*(3), i–iv.

Allen, J., & Bellingham, R. (1994). Building supportive cultural environments. In M. P. O'Donnell & J. S. Harris (Eds.), *Health promotion in the workplace* (2nd ed., pp. 204–216). Albany, NY: Delmar.

Allensworth, D., Lawson, E., Nicholson, L., & Wyche, J. (Eds.). (1997). *Schools and health: Our nation's investment.* Washington, DC: National Academy Press.

Altman, D. G., Balcazar, F. E., Fawcett, S. B., Seekins, T. M., & Young, J. Q. (1994). *Public health advocacy: Creating community change to improve health.* Palo Alto, CA: Stanford Center for Research in Disease Prevention.

Anderson, J. R. (1983). A spreading activation theory of memory. *Journal of Verbal Learning and Verbal Behavior, 22*(3), 261–295.

Axner, M., & Berkowitz, B. (1999, August 18). Developing multisector collaboration. *Community Tool Box,* [On-line], chap. 18, section 11. Available: http://ctb.lsi.ukans.edu

Bandura, A. (1986). *Social foundations of thought and action.* New York: Prentice Hall.

Bandura, A. (1997). *Self-efficacy: The exercise of control.* New York: Freeman.

Bartholomew, L. K., Gold, R. S., Parcel, G. S., Czyzewski, D. I., Sockrider, M. M., Fernandez, M., Shegog, R., & Swank, P. R. (2000). Watch, Discover, Think, and Act: Evaluation of computer-assisted instruction to improve asthma self-management in inner-city children. *Patient Education and Counseling, 39*(2–3), 269–280.

Bartholomew, L. K., Parcel, G. S., Seilheimer, D. K., Czyzewski, D. I., Spinelli, S. H., & Congdon, B. (1993). Development of a health education program to promote the self-management of cystic fibrosis. *Health Education Quarterly, 18*(4), 429–443.

Bartholomew, L. K., Shegog, R., Parcel, G. S., Gold, R. S., Fernandez, M., Czyzewski, D. I., Sockrider, M. M., & Berlin, N. (2000). Watch, Discover, Think, and Act: A model for patient education program development. *Patient Education and Counseling, 39*(2–3), 253–268.

Beyer, J. M., & Trice, H. M. (1978). *Implementing change: Alcoholism programs in work organizations.* New York: Free Press.

Bouman, M., Maas, L., & Kok, G. (1998). Health education in television entertainment—Medisch Centrum West: A Dutch drama serial. *Health Education Research: Theory and Practice, 13,* 503–518.

Bracht, N., & Kingsbury, L., (1990). Community organization principles in health promotion: A five-stage model. In N. Bracht (Ed.), *Health promotion at the community level* (pp. 66–88). Newbury Park, CA: Sage.

Brager, G. A., & Holloway, S. (1978). *Changing human service organizations: Politics and practice.* New York: Free Press.

Brug, J., Glanz, K., Van Assema, P., Kok, G., & van Breukelen, G. J. (1998). The impact of computer-tailored feedback and iterative feedback on fat, fruit, and vegetable intake. *Health Education and Behavior, 25*(4), 517–531.

Brug, J., Van Assema, P., Kok, G., Lenderink, T., & Glanz, K. (1994). Self-rated dietary fat intake: Association with objective assessment of fat, psychosocial factors, and intention to change. *Journal of Nutrition Education, 26*(5), 218–223.

Butterfoss, F. D., Goodman, R. M., & Wandersman, A. (1993). Community coalitions for prevention and health promotion. *Health Education Research, 8*(3), 315–330.

Campbell, M. K., DeVellis, B. M., Strecher, V. J., Ammerman, A. S., DeVellis, R. F., & Sandler, R. S. (1994). Improving dietary behavior: The effectiveness of tailored messages in primary care settings. *American Journal of Public Health, 84*(5), 783–787.

Cobb, R., & Elder, C. (1983). *Participation in American politics: The dynamics of agenda-building.* Baltimore, MD: Johns Hopkins University Press.

Cummings, T. G., & Worley, C. G. (1993). *Organization development and change* (5th ed.). Minneapolis/St. Paul, MN: West.

Daka-Mulwanda, V., Thornburg, K. R., Filbert, L., & Klein, T. (1995). Collaboration of services for children and families: A synthesis of recent research and recommendations. *Family Relations, 44*(2), 219–223.

Derry, S. J. (1984). Effects of an advance organizer on memory for prose. *Journal of Educational Psychology, 76,* 98–107.

Dijker, A. J., Kok, G., & Koomen, W. (1995). Emotional reactions to people with AIDS. *Journal of Applied Social Psychology, 26*(8), 731–748.

Dimeff, L. A., & Marlatt, G. A. (1998). Preventing relapse and maintaining change in addictive behaviors. *Clinical Psychology: Science and Practice, 5*(4), 513–525.

Eagly, A. H., & Chaiken, S. (1993). *The psychology of attitudes.* Fort Worth, TX: Harcourt Brace Jovanovich.

Earp, J. A., Viadro, C. I., Vincus, A. A., Aitpeter, M., Flax, V., Mayne, L., & Eng, E. (1997). Lay health advisors: A strategy for getting the word out about breast cancer. *Health Education and Behavior, 24*(4), 432–451.

El-Basel, N., Ivanoff, A., Schilling, R. F., Borne, D., & Gilbert, L. (1997). Skills building and social support enhancement to reduce HIV risk among women in jail. *Criminal Justice and Behavior, 24,* 205–223.

Eng, E., Parker, E., & Harlan, C. (1997). Lay health advisor intervention strategies: A continuum for natural helping to paraprofessional helping. *Health Education and Behavior, 24*(4), 413–417.

Eng, E., & Smith, J. (1995). Natural helping functions of lay health advisors in breast cancer education. *Breast Cancer Research and Treatment, 35*(1), 23–29.

Evans, R. I., Getz, J., & Raines, B. E. (1991). *Theory-guided models on prevention of AIDS in adolescents.* Paper presented at the Science Weekend of the American Psychological Association Meeting, San Francisco, CA.

Evans, R. I., Rozelle, E. M., Mittelmark, M. B., Hansen, W. B., Bane, A. L., & Havis, J. (1978). Deterring the onset of smoking in children: Knowledge of immediate physiological effects and coping with peer pressure, media pressure and parental modeling. *Journal of Applied Social Psychology, 8*(2), 126–135.

Fisher, R. (1997). Social action community organization: Proliferation, persistence, roots, and prospects. In M. Minkler (Ed.), *Community organizing and community building for health* (pp. 53–67). New Brunswick, NJ: Rutgers University Press.

Fisher, R., & Kling, J. (1991). Popular mobilization in the 1990's: Prospects for the new social movements. *New Politics, 3,* 71–84.

Freire, P. (1973). *Pedagogy of the oppressed.* New York: Seabury Press.

Gadotti, M. (1994). *Reading Paulo Freire: His life and work* (John Milton, Trans.). Albany, NY: State University of New York Press.

Glanz, K., Lewis, F. M., & Rimer, B. K. (Eds.). (1997). *Health behavior and health education: Theory, research, and practice* (2nd ed.). San Francisco, CA: Jossey-Bass.

Glover, J. A., Ronning, R. R., & Bruning, R. H. (1990). *Cognitive psychology for teachers.* New York: Macmillan.

Godin, G., Savard, J., Kok, G., Fortin, C., & Boyer, R. (1996). HIV-seropositive gay men: Understanding adoption of safe sexual practices. *AIDS Education and Prevention, 8*(16), 529–545.

Gollwitzer, P. M. (1993). Goal achievement: The role of intentions. *European Review of Social Psychology, 4*.

Goodman, D. D. (1998). Using the empowerment model to develop sex education for Native Americans. *Journal of Sex Education and Therapy, 23*(2), 135–144.

Goodman, R. M., Steckler, A., & Kegler, M. C. (1997). Mobilizing organizations for health enhancement: Theories of organizational change. In K. Glanz, F. M. Lewis, & B. K. Rimer (Eds.), *Health behavior and health education: Theory, research, and practice* (pp. 287–312). San Francisco, CA: Jossey-Bass.

Gottlieb, N. H., & McLeroy, K. R. (1994). Social health. In M. P. O'Donnell & T. H. Ainsworth (Eds.), *Health promotion in the workplace* (2nd ed., pp. 459–493). New York: Wiley.

Green, L. W., & Kreuter, M. W. (1999). *Health promotion planning: An educational and ecological approach* (3rd ed.). Mountain View, CA: Mayfield.

Habana-Hafner, S., & Reed, H. B. (1989). *Partnerships for community development: Resources for practitioners and trainers.* Amherst, MA: The University of Massachusetts at Amherst, Center for Organizational and Community Development.

Haglund, B. J. A., Finer, D., Tillgren, P., & Pettersson, B. (Eds.). (1996). *Creating supportive environments for health: Stories from the Third International Conference on Health Promotion, Sundsvall, Sweden.* Geneva: World Health Organization.

Hale, J. L., & Dillard, J. P. (1995). Fear appeals in health promotion campaigns: Too much, too little, or just right? In E. Maibach & R. L. Parrott (Eds.), *Designing health messages: Approaches from communication theory and public health practice* (pp. 65–80). Thousand Oaks, CA: Sage.

Hamilton, R., & Ghatala, E. (1994). *Learning and instruction.* New York: McGraw-Hill.

Heaney, C. A., & Israel, B. A. (1997). Social networks and social support. In K. Glanz, F. M. Lewis, & B. K. Rimer (Eds.), *Health behavior and health education: Theory, research, and practice* (2nd ed., pp. 179–205). San Francisco: Jossey-Bass.

Heitzmann, C. A., & Kaplan, R. M. (1988). Assessment of methods for measuring social support. *Health Psychology, 7*(1), 75–109.

Hersey, J. C., Kibanoff, L. S., Lam, D. J., & Taylor, R. L. (1984). Promoting social support: The impact of California's "Friends Can Be Good Medicine" campaign. *Health Education Quarterly, 11*(3), 293–311.

Holtgrave, D. R., Tinsley, B. J., & Kay, L. S. (1995). Encouraging risk reduction: A decision-making approach to message design. In E. Maibach & R. L. Parrott (Eds.), *Designing health messages: Approaches from communication theory and public health practice* (pp. 24–40). Thousand Oaks, CA: Sage.

Hospers, H. J., Kok, G., & Strecher, V. J. (1990). Attributions for previous failures and subsequent outcomes in a weight reduction program. *Health Education Quarterly, 17*(4), 409–415.

Israel, B. A., Checkoway, B., Schulz, A., & Zimmerman, M. (1994). Health education and community empowerment: Conceptualizing and measuring perceptions of individual organizational and community control. *Health Education Quarterly, 21*(2), 149–170.

Johnson, K., Grossman, W., & Cassidy, A. (Eds.). (1996). *Elaborating to improve community health.* San Francisco: Jossey-Bass.

Kegeles, S. M., Hays, R. B., & Coates, T. J. (1996). The Mpowerment Project: A community-level HIV prevention intervention for young gay men. *American Journal of Public Health, 86*(8, Pt. 1), 1129–1136.

Kelly, J. A., St. Lawrence, J. S., Stevenson, L. Y., Houth, A. C., Kuliehman, S. C., Diaz, Y. E., Brasfield, T. L., Koob, J. J., & Morgan, M. G. (1992). Community AIDS/HIV risk reduction: The effects of endorsements by popular people in three cities. *American Journal of Public Health, 82*(11), 1483–1489.

Kingdon, J. W. (1995). *Agendas, alternatives, and public policies* (2nd ed.). Boston: Little, Brown.

Koffka, K. (1933). *Principles of gestalt psychology.* New York: Harcourt Brace Jovanovich.

Kok, G., Den Boer, D. J., De Vries, H., Gerards, F., Hospers, H. J., & Mudde, A. N. (1992). Self-efficacy and attribution theory in health education. In R. Schwartzer (Ed.), *Self-efficacy: Thought control of action* (pp. 245–262). Washington, D.C.: Hemisphere.

Kok, G., Schaalma, H., De Vries, H., Parcel, G., & Paulussen, T. H. (1996). Social psychology and health education. *European Review of Social Psychology, 7*, (pp. 241–282).

Kretzmann, J. P., & McKnight, J. L. (1993). Building communities from the inside out: A path toward finding and mobilizing a community's assets. Chicago, IL: ACTA Publications.

Ladson-Billings, G. (1995). Toward a theory of culturally relevant pedagogy. *American Educational Research Journal, 32*(3), 465–491.

Lerman, C., & Glanz, K. (1997). Stress, coping, and health behavior. In K. Glanz, F. M. Lewis, & B. K. Rimer (Eds.), *Health behavior and health education: Theory, research, and practice* (2nd ed., pp. 113–138). San Francisco: Jossey-Bass.

Lewin, K. (1947). Quasi-stationary social equilibria and the problem of social change. In T. M. Newcomb & E. L. Hartley (Eds.), *Readings in social psychology.* New York: Holt, Rinehart & Winston.

Locke, E. A., & Latham, G. P. (1991). *A theory of goal setting and task performance.* Englewood Cliffs, NJ: Prentice Hall.

Maibach, E. W., & Cotton, D. (1995). Moving people to behavior change: A staged social cognitive approach to message design. In E. Maibach & R. L. Parrott (Eds.), *Designing health messages: Approaches from communication theory and public health practice* (pp. 41–64). Thousand Oaks, CA: Sage.

Maibach, E., & Parrott, R. L. (Eds.). (1995). *Designing health messages: Approaches from communication theory and public health practice.* Thousand Oaks, CA: Sage.

Marlatt, G. A. (1985). Situational determinants of relapse and skill-training interventions. In G. A. Marlatt & J. R. Gordon (Eds.), *Relapse prevention: Maintenance strategies in the treatment of addictive behaviors* (pp. 71–127). New York: Guilford.

Mayer, R. E. (1984). Twenty-five years of research on advance organizers. *Instructional Science, 8,* 133–169.

McAlister, A. (1991). Population behavior change: A theory-based approach. *Journal of Public Health Policy, 12*(3), 345–361.

McCallister, L., & Fischer, C. S. (1978). A procedure for surveying personal networks. *Sociological Methods and Research, 7*(2), 131–148.

McFarlane, J., Fehir, J., & De Madres a Madres (1994). A community primary health care program based on empowerment. *Health Education Quarterly, 21,* 81–94.

McGrath, J. (1995). The gatekeeping process: The right combinations to unlock the gates. In E. Maibach & R. L. Parrott (Eds.), *Designing health messages: Approaches from communication theory and public health practice* (pp. 199–216). Thousand Oaks, CA: Sage.

McGuire, W. J. (1985). Attitudes and attitude change. In M. Lindsay & E. Aronson (Eds.), *The handbook of social psychology* (Vol. 2, pp. 233–346). New York: Random House.

Minkler, M. (1997). Community organizing among the elderly poor in San Francisco's Tenderloin District. In M. Minkler (Ed.), *Community organizing and community building for health* (pp. 230–243). New Brunswick, NJ: Rutgers University Press.

Minkler, M., & Wallerstein, N. (1997). Improving health through community organization and community building: A health education perspective. In M. Minkler (Ed.), *Community organizing and community building for health* (pp. 30–52). New Brunswick, NJ: Rutgers University Press.

Monahan, J. (1995). Thinking positively: Using positive affect when designing health messages. In E. Maibach & R. L. Parrott (Eds.), *Designing health messages: Approaches from communication theory and public health practice* (pp. 81–98). Thousand Oaks, CA: Sage.

Mullen, P. D., Green, L. W., & Persinger, G. S. (1985). Clinical trials of patient education for chronic conditions: A comparative meta-analysis of intervention types. *Preventive Medicine, 14*(6), 753–781.

Mullen, P. D., Mains, D. A., & Velez, R. (1992). A meta-analysis of controlled trials of cardiac patient education. *Patient Education and Counseling, 19*(2), 143–162.

National Health Strategy. (1993). *Pathways to better health* (Research Paper No. 3). Melbourne: Treble Press.

Nutbeam, D., & Harris, E. (1995). Creating supportive environments for health: A case study from Australia in developing national goals and targets for healthy environments. *Health Promotion International, 10*(1), 51–59.

Orum, A. M. (1988). Political sociology. In N. J. Smelser (Ed.), *Handbook of sociology* (pp. 393–423). Newbury Park, CA: Sage.

Parcel, G. S., Simons-Morton, B. G., & Kolbe, L. J. (1988). Health promotion: Integrating organizational change and student learning strategies. *Health Education Quarterly, 15*(4), 435–450.

Pasick, R. J., D'Onofrio, C. N., & Hiatt, R. A. (Eds.). (1996). Promoting cancer screening in ethnically diverse and underserved communities: The Pathways project [Special issue]. *Health Education Quarterly, 23* (Suppl.).

Petty, R. E., & Cacioppo, R. T. (1986). The elaboration likelihood model of persuasion. *Advances in Experimental Social Psychology, 19*. New York: Academic Press.

Petty, R. E., & Wegener, D. T. (1997). Attitude change: Multiple roles for persuasion variables. In D. T. Gilbert, S. T. Fiske, & G. Lindzey (Eds.), *The handbook of social psychology* (4th ed., Vol. 1, pp. 323–390). Boston: McGraw-Hill.

Pilisuk, M., McAllister, J., & Rothman, J. (1997). Social change professionals and grassroots organizing functions and dilemmas. In M. Minkler (Ed.), *Community organizing and community building for health* (pp. 103–119). New Brunswick, NJ: Rutgers University Press.

Porras, J. I., & Robertson, P. J. (1987). Organizational development theory: A typology and evaluation. In R. W. Woodman & W. A. Pasmore (Eds.), *Research in organization change and development* (Vol. 1). Greenwich, CT: JAI.

Prochaska, J. O., DiClemente, C. C., & Norcross, J. C. (1997). In search of how people change: Applications to addictive behaviors. In G. Marlatt & G. R. Van den Bos (Eds.), *Addictive behaviors. Readings on etiology, prevention, and treatment* (pp. 671–696). Washington, DC: American Psychological Association.

Pulley, L., McAlister, A. L., Kay, L. S., & O'Reilly, K. (1996). Prevention campaigns for hard-to-reach populations at risk for HIV infection: Theory and implementation. *Health Education Quarterly, 23*(4), 488–496.

Ramirez, A. G., Villarreal, R., McAlister, A., Gallion, K. J., Suarez, L., & Gomez, P. (1999). Advancing the role of participatory communication in the diffusion of cancer screening among Hispanics. *Journal of Health Communication, 4*, 31–36.

Richard, R., Van der Pligt, J., & De Vries, N. K. (1995). Anticipated affective reaction and the prevention of AIDS. *British Journal of Social Psychology, 34*(Pt. 1), 9–21.

Rogers, E. M. (1995). *Diffusion of innovations* (4th ed.). New York: Free Press.

Rosen, R. H. (1992). *The healthy company.* New York: G. P. Putnam's Sons.

Rothman, J. (1979). Three models of community organization practice, their mixing and phasing. In R. M. Cox, J. L. Erlich, J. Rothman, & J. E. Tropman (Eds.), *Strategies of community organization: A book of readings* (pp. 25–45). Itasca, IL: F. E. Peacock.

Rothman, J. (1987). Three models of community organization practice, their mixing and phasing. In R. M. Cox, J. L. Erlich, J. Rothman, & J. E. Tropman (Eds.), *Strategies of community organization: A book of readings* (4th ed.). Itasca, IL: F. E. Peacock.

Rowling, L. (1996). The adaptability of the health promoting schools concept: A case study from Australia. *Health Education Research: Theory and Practice, 11*(4), 519–526.

Rudd, R. E., & Comings, J. P. (1994). Learner developed materials: An empowering product. *Health Education Quarterly, 21*(3), 313–327.

Ruiter, R., Kok, G., & Abraham, C. (1999). *Fear appeals in health education: Theory and research.* Internal report. Maastricht, The Netherlands: University of Mamastricht, Department of Health Education.

Rumelhart, D. E. (1980). Schemata: The building blocks of cognition. In R. J. Spiro, B. C. Bruce, & W. F. Brewer (Eds.), *Theoretical issues in reading comprehension* (pp. 33–58). Hillsdale, NJ: Erlbaum.

Salovey, P., Rothman, A. J., & Rodin, J. (1997). Health behavior. In D. T. Gilbert, S. T. Fiske, & G. Lindzey (Eds.), *The handbook of social psychology* (4th ed., Vol. 1, pp. 633–683). Boston: McGraw-Hill.

Shaffer, R. (1993). *Beyond the dispensary.* Nairobi, Kenya: Amref.

Shiffman, S. (1984). Cognitive antecedents and sequelae of smoking relapse crises. *Journal of Applied Social Psychology, 14*(3), 296–309.

Simons-Morton, B. G., Greene, W. H., & Gottlieb, N. H. (1995). *Introduction to health education and health promotion* (2nd ed.). Prospect Heights, IL: Waveland Press.

Skinner, C. S., Strecher, V. J., & Hospers, H. (1994). Physicians' recommendations for mammography: Do tailored messages make a difference? *American Journal of Public Health, 84,* (1) 43–49.

Smelser, N. J. (1988). Social structure. In N. J. Smelser (Ed.), *Handbook of sociology* (pp. 103–129). Newbury Park, CA: Sage.

Steckler, A., Allegrante, J. P., Altman, D., Brown, R., Burdine, J. N., Goodman, R. M., & Jorgensen, C. (1995). Health education intervention strategies: Recommendations for future research. *Health Education Quarterly, 22*(3), 307–328.

Strecher, V. J. (1999). Computer-tailored smoking cessation materials: A review and discussion. *Patient Education and Counseling, 36*(2), 107–117.

Strecher, V. J., Kreuter, M., Den Boer, D. J., Kobrin, S., Hospers, H. J., & Skinner, C. S. (1994). The effects of computer-tailored smoking cessation messages in family practice settings. *Journal of Family Practice, 39*(3), 262–270.

Strecher, V. J., & Rosenstock, I. M. (1997). The health belief model. In K. Glanz, F. M. Lewis, & B. K. Rimer (Eds.), *Health behavior and health education: Theory, research, and practice* (2nd ed., pp. 41–59). San Francisco: Jossey-Bass.

Strecher, V. J., Seijts, G. H., Kok, G., Latham, G. P., Glasgow, R., DeVellis, B., Meertens, R. M., & Bulger, D. W. (1995). Goal setting as a strategy for health behavior change. *Health Education Quarterly, 22*(2), 190–200.

Susser, E., Valencia, E., & Torres, J. (1994). Sex, Games, and Videotapes: An HIV-prevention intervention for men who are homeless and mentally ill. *Psychosocial Rehabilitation Journal, 17*(4), 31–40.

Texas Department of Health Coalition Task Force. (1996). *Coalition building: A healthy community is everyone's business.* Austin, TX: Texas Department of Health (1100 West 49th St., Austin, TX 78756).

Van der Pligt, J., Otten, W., Richard, R., & Van der Velde, F. (1993). Perceived risk of AIDS: Unrealistic optimism and self-protective action. In B. J. Pryor & G. D. Reeder (Eds.), *The social psychology of HIV infection* (pp. 39–58). Hillsdale, NJ: Erlbaum.

Wallack, L., Dorfman, L., Jernigan, D., & Themba, M. (1993). *Media advocacy and public health.* Newbury Park, CA: Sage.

Wallerstein, N. B., & Sanchez-Merki, V. (1994). Freirian praxis in health education: Research results from an adolescent prevention program. *Health Education Research: Theory and Practice, 9,* 105–118.

Wallerstein, N. B., Sanchez-Merki, V., & Dow, L. (1997). Freirian praxis in health education and community organizing: A case study of an adolescent prevention program. In M. Minkler (Ed.), *Community organizing and community building for health* (pp. 195–215). New Brunswick, NJ: Rutgers University Press.

Walter, C. H. (1997). Community building practice: A conceptual framework. In M. Minkler (Ed.), *Community organizing and community building for health* (pp. 68–87). New Brunswick, NJ: Rutgers University Press.

Wang, C., & Burris, M. A. (1994). Empowerment through photo novella: Portraits of participation. *Health Education Quarterly, 21*(2), 171–186.

Wang, C. C., Yi, W. K., Tao, Z. W., & Carovano, K. (1998). Photo voice as a participatory health promotion strategy. *Health Promotion International, 13*(1), 75–86.

Weber, M. (1947). *The theory of social and economic organization* (A. M. Henderson & T. Parsons, Trans.). New York: Oxford University Press.

Weiner, B. (1986). *An attributional theory of motivation and emotion.* New York: Springer.

Witte, K. (1995). Fishing for success: Using the persuasive health message framework to generate effective campaign messages. In E. Maibach & R. L. Parrott (Eds.), *Designing health messages: Approaches from communication theory and public health practice* (pp. 145–166). Thousand Oaks, CA: Sage.

CHAPTER 7

Intervention Mapping Step 3: Producing Program Components and Materials

READER OBJECTIVES

- Revisit the intended participants for a health education and promotion program and bring their preferences to program design
- Prepare design documents that will aid different professions in producing materials that meet the needs of the program and adhere to specific guidelines or parameters for particular methods and strategies
- Prepare design documents for programs such as lobbying that require little traditional support material
- Review available program materials for possible match with learning and change objectives, methods, and strategies
- Develop and pretest program materials
- Oversee the production of program materials

The purpose of this chapter is to enable the reader to produce creative materials in support of health education and promotion programs. We speak of materials "in support of" to circumvent the temptation of referring to support materials or products such as newsletters, billboards, and videotapes *as* the program. The program will usually be a multicomponent, complex entity supported by certain products or materials. The goal is that these products are creative, effective pieces of the entire behavior-change and environmental-change puzzle that has been painstakingly planned. A challenge in this step is one of translation—getting the support pieces right so that the methods and strategies are adequately (and sometimes brilliantly) operationalized and the learning and change objectives accomplished.

Planning to this point should enable production of creative products that emerge from the thinking captured in the matrix development and the selection of methods and strategies. In particular, the products should do an excellent job of representing the parameters that pertain to the methods that have been chosen. For example, if a planning team decides to use modeling (method), they must ensure that their participants can identify with the depicted role models (parameter) and that the role-model stories (strategies) have certain characteristics (parameter). The end product of this step should be a plan for a coherent program that remains true to the planning that has been accomplished in Steps 1 and 2.

Another challenge in this step is to ensure that the final program fits with both the populations and the context or contexts in which it will be delivered. This step provides an opportunity to revisit the at-risk groups to ensure that the program materials result in attention, comprehension, and central processing. Only then will there be a chance that the learning and change objectives will be accomplished and behavior and environment affected. Health educators can use this planning moment to check not only the depth of their understanding of the intended participants and contexts but also the status of their linkage system with the people who will adopt and implement the program.

In Chapter 8 we present the development of interventions to influence program adoption and implementation. These interventions are directed to the gatekeepers of organizations who will adopt the new program and to the program deliverers who will implement the new program. In this chapter, we focus on program design and materials development. Although our discussion is centered on the health education program that is directed to the client population, the same creative and technical process needs to be applied to the intervention for program adoption and implementation.

PERSPECTIVES

Using Steps 1 and 2

Often, planning groups will shy away when confronted with the perceived complexity of converting all their planning to a program. Members may tend to revert to overly simplistic thinking, such as "We need a videotape." This dilemma was what the mayor's health educator faced, and one thing that helped was staying focused on the thorough work the team had done on Intervention Mapping Steps 1 and 2. In Step 1 they had developed matrices for the at-risk group—the middle school and high school youth—and matrices for various segments of the environment—parents through churches and neighborhood groups, the city government through the mayor and city council.

In Step 2 the team developed lists of theoretical methods and practical strategies for each matrix. Further, they had adopted the McGuire system of checking all the communications they would develop in Step 3 (McGuire, 1985). With these foundations, they could use Step 3 to ensure good communications that

Chapter 7 Intervention Mapping Step 3

The health educator from the mayor's office thought the last major planning hurdles had been passed. The task group had decided on intervention levels, written performance objectives at all those levels, and then created matrices. They even put the matrices aside for a bit and planned theoretical methods and practical strategies with a lot of energy and creativity. They had found ways to listen to everyone's ideas. What a team! At the end of the year, they had enough energy and goodwill to plan a celebratory picnic to commemorate six months of hard work and productive (and sometimes loud) discussions. That picnic was just before the city hit low gear at winter break and everyone took a breather.

Now it's January 4 and the first meeting of the new year is in full swing. The health educator can't believe what is happening. What is all of this regression to original ideas about what the program should include? Why is the group talking about what the billboards should look like, and what celebrity should narrate the videotape? What billboards? What videotape? The group hadn't decided to have products such as billboards and videotapes as a part of their program, and the health educator thought that some members had learned a thing or two about the characteristics of effective role models, but that was the least of the problems. This meeting was beginning to look like a pitched battle. Before members could become entrenched in these resurfaced old ideas, the health educator had to take action.

incorporated the methods and strategies to accomplish the learning and change objectives. Just as Step 2 has two styles of accomplishing the tasks, Step 3 has at least two styles as well—but none of the new styles means abandoning the previous work. One style is to take each method and strategy, consider it, and develop a program component to deliver it. Another style is to put away all lists, matrices, and other planning papers and allow the group to bring forth all the ideas they have had to this point about what the program should look like. After all, the planning to this point is at its best if it has stimulated many creative thoughts about the nature of the program. If this style is chosen by a work group, then members must check back periodically to their methods, strategies, and learning and change objectives to make sure that their program components are actually delivering what they are supposed to deliver.

Seeking Members of the At-Risk Groups Often and Well

Pilot testing is the process of trying out the program and all its products or support materials with both the intended participants and the implementers *before* final production. Pilot testing is crucially important to determine whether planning to this point has resulted in appealing, understandable messages and whether the program can be implemented. Program materials must be culturally competent as well—not just understandable in a particular culture and not offensive, but making use of particular cultural concepts related to the health, behav-

> The mayor's health educator capitalized on the natural energy of the planning group and encouraged them to "dream" about what their program could look like—without any of their matrices or previous planning materials in front of them. They worked to keep in mind the objectives and the methods they would be trying to deliver. Some of the conversation went like this:
>
> "Well, since we want to reach parents and city government we probably need a coalition of community organizations and agencies. Churches, social service agencies, professional organizations, youth organizations—that sort of thing. The coalition could oversee the program implementation, especially the change directed at the parents and the government approach to the neighborhoods."
>
> "Since I represent the organization of pastors in the areas of the city that have the biggest violence problem, I think that coalition is a good idea. My congregation would like to be very involved, and in speaking with my colleagues, I know they are interested too."
>
> "Yeah, and from our point of view at the schools, we need the support of the school district to reach the age groups of youth we are targeting. I think the youth component should have a school focus. Of course we need a way to reach dropouts as well. The theme could be …"
>
> "Okay, let's get down to basics. What would a school program look like? How would we use our methods of modeling, skill building for problem solving, negotiation, resistance skills, planning and studying, goal setting, self monitoring? Do you think we could use community organization methods in the schools?"
>
> "What about even having the youth from the school program recruit the community agencies for the coalition?"

ior, and community changes inherent in the program and leaving the community with greater capacity than before the program.

Sometimes pilot testing is not done because at the point of production many program planners are experiencing a time crunch. No matter how big the hurry, planners must make time for pilot testing. One of us has had the experience of consulting with an AIDS prevention agency that had an advertising firm develop a series of messages. The agency refused to pilot test and, to make a long story short, produced messages that had the reverse of the intended effect: The messages made people feel that they were safe from AIDS under certain circumstances that were actually irrelevant to risk. The ad campaign might actually have increased risky behavior among the intended audience.

Someone on the planning team may object to pilot testing by pointing out that "we have representatives of the at-risk groups in the planning group." Representatives, however, have probably come to value the program they have developed in a way that colors their objectivity. This step requires going back out into the communities being served and talking to the members often, getting their responses to ideas and to all the various aspects of support materials: graphics, illustration, photography, messages, and delivery.

Going back out into the community at this step has the added advantage of reminding program planners of the characteristics of the setting of their program. What is the school, hospital, community really like? Who are the people who will be involved in implementing the program? Is there any group involved in implementation that has not been involved in development? What additional facts about the setting need to be considered in program design? Step 4, which requires the development of an adoption and implementation plan, really begins at the beginning of program development with consideration of a linkage system (see Chapter 2) and resurfaces here. As program components are conceptualized, the planner needs to consider how they will be implemented and what implementation will require of the implementers. The impact of perceived program characteristics on the gatekeepers—those responsible for adoption decisions—must also be considered (see Chapter 8).

Allowing Creativity to Flourish

Planning should allow creativity to flourish. In this step, program planners liberate all those ideas that have been put on hold during the work of the previous steps. Sometimes they close the books, turn the matrices over, and even close their eyes to dream what a program could look like. The planning group should be cohesive by this point, so it should be okay to come forth with some crazy ideas, to brainstorm some ridiculous themes, and to get carried away with some awful motifs. Out of this creative mess can emerge a great program. The foundation is laid; the design task should be fun. A related point is making use of the real talents of any production contractors the team may have. In this chapter we build on the planning documents developed to this point to create design documents that can guide contractors without hamstringing them.

CREATING A PROGRAM

The first task in Intervention Mapping Step 3 is to translate methods and strategies into program plans that consider implementers and sites. In this section we describe the tasks involved in creating a program. We intend to help the reader understand how to get started as well as understand the types of decisions that must be made in the creation of a program plan. Planners need to come up with program structure, themes, motifs, and vehicles for delivery. They need to consider whether to use computer technology for the program, and they must decide whether to use existing program materials (rather than create their own).

A Summary Program Plan

The product of the first part of this step is a plan that outlines scope and sequence of the program, all program vehicles and materials that must be produced, and the budget and resources not only for the materials, but also for the implementation of the program. The program plan should account for every intended contact of the program participants with some element of the program. Working with the implementation objectives in Step 4 (see Chapter 8), the health educator must specify in as much detail as possible how the people will interact with program components. The health educator looks to specify both the amount of the program that is expected to be delivered and the way the program should "look" at each interface with participants. The format of the summary plan will vary from program to program, but should include at least the program scope and sequence; a description of each population group and program interface with a list of the program materials and staff required for that interaction; and a program budget for materials production and for implementation.

Program Ideas

Gedney and Fultz (1988) address the problem that plagues communicators, that is, how to have a good idea. They suggest: Don't have just one idea, have 100, or even better, 200; use brainstorming to generate ideas that encompass the entire program (We could go to schools and . . .); use brainstorming to address specific methods and strategies (The role-model stories could contain . . .). This step is a good time to throw away all preconceived notions and program restraints. Planners should ask themselves, What would we do if we could do anything that comes to mind? What would be the most powerful things we could do? Brainstorming allows no editorial comments and thereby is a good mechanism to generate, generate, generate. When brainstorming gets stuck, planners can try a paradoxical approach: If we wanted to have the *opposite* effect, what would we do?

The core processes that were presented in Chapter 3 may also be useful here. A literature review can elucidate to some extent the types of strategies and programs others have used. Going back to the theory can generate totally new thoughts about how to apply methods. Finally, going to the potential participants and continuing to fuel the process with their ideas is imperative. Focus groups can be used for this purpose and are particularly suited because stimulus materials in the form of learning and change objectives are available. Questions can be phrased in this way: "If you were trying to figure out how to [*learning or change objective X*], what would you do?" For example, "If you were going to *increase the confidence of teenage girls in negotiating condom use*, what would you do?"

Structure, Themes, and Motifs

Health education and promotion programs have units or modules with an identifiable scope and sequence. However, unlike targets of typical curriculum planning, which are cognitive or academic skills, these program components have more diverse learning and change objectives that cut across domains such as attitudes, beliefs, and skills. Therefore, the modules or units might be, for example, combinations of methods, strategies, and delivery mechanisms aimed at various objectives. A program might comprise one-to-one messages delivered by neighborhood volunteers and mass media messages delivered in public service announcements (PSAs) and billboards, all loosely tied together across time with a theme and various motifs.

For example, Figure 7.1 presents the units, scope, and sequence of a community health education and promotion program in three rural Texas counties designed to increase the probability of acute treatment for stroke (Morgenstern et al., 2000). The program was based on four matrices, one for community residents of the three counties and three for the professional health care community, including emergency medical services, emergency departments, and community physicians. The scope of the program was to change behavior of both community residents and their health care providers in a three-month time period. The sequence required that health care providers change their practice prior to changes in demand for stroke services from the community.

The scope and sequence of the stroke project needed to accommodate the methods and strategies chosen. For the community, these methods and strategies were role models for treating stroke as an emergency, delivered by radio and television PSAs and by billboards and posters; and skill training in recognizing stroke symptoms by one-to-one training, role modeling, and information transfer via brochures and newspapers. Changes in health care provider behavior were supported in three ways: (a) organizational change consultation to assess awareness, increase perceptions of need, and diagnose needed support for change in emergency rooms and emergency medical services. (Most hospitals and emergency medical services needed support for getting revised stroke care guidelines in

---

Intervention Themes: Stroke Is an Emergency. Every Minute Counts. There Is Treatment for Stroke.

Week 1	Weeks 2–4	Weeks 4–6	Weeks 6–12	Weeks 12+
Professional Module 1: Meetings with hospital ERs to plan organizational change	**Professional Module 2:** Orientation meetings with hospital medical staff	**Professional Module 3:** Training meetings for ER and EMS teams	**Professional Module 4:** Review training meetings for ER and EMS teams	**Professional Module 5:** Reinforcement for protocol use using newspaper stories and newsletters
Meetings with local EMS to plan organizational change	Guideline and protocol development meetings with medical staff and quality committees	**Community Module 1:** One-to-one train the trainer meetings at work sites plus brochures and posters	**Community Module 1:** One-to-one train the trainer meetings	**Community Module 2A[1]:** Change out billboards and PSAs
	Guideline and protocol development meetings with EMS directors and medical directors		**Community Module 2:** Placement of billboards and PSAs	**Community Module 3A[1]:** Change out newspaper stories and news releases
			Community Module 3: Newspaper stories and news releases	

[1]These intervention modules have sequences of their own. For example, the newspaper sequence begins with articles about the program, then introduces the new therapy for stroke, teaches how to recognize symptoms, and finally reinforces by providing success stories.

FIGURE 7.1 Scope and Sequence of the T.L.L. Temple Foundation Stroke Project

place, including individualized guideline development and staff training); (b) skill training individualized to provider and setting; and (c) reinforcement. All health care providers also received reinforcement for using new treatment protocols via newsletter and newspaper stories of successes. Of course, all these activities could not happen at once, and many of them depended for their success on prior requisite activities—thus the need for a well-defined program sequence.

A program theme is a general organizing construct for a program, whereas a motif is a recurring subtheme or idea. Both themes and motifs can be based on the health topic, such as the themes for the stroke project (see Figure 7.1). Figure 7.2 shows how one of the stroke themes was portrayed in a community billboard using a community role model.

Themes may be based on the behavioral or community change or learning objective. For example, the Watch, Discover, Think, and Act theme of the asthma computer program became the program title and is based on the self-regulatory processes taught in the program (Shegog et al., 1999). Themes and motifs may be unrelated to the program content. The third grade component of the CATCH program (Perry et al., 1997) used a motif of space creatures that had come to earth to teach earth children about diet and physical activity (Figure 7.3). Themes and motifs may also derive from characteristics of the at-risk groups, cultures, or preferred learning styles. In the Cystic Fibrosis Family Education Program, the theme of the adolescent modules was "Taking Charge" (of one's health and one's life) and was based on an adolescent developmental task (Figure 7.4), whereas the modules for the school-age children emphasized exploration and mastery, a developmental task of children this age (Figure 7.5, p. 238).

The most important factor in choosing themes and motifs for the program is whether the chosen idea will aid attention, awareness, and comprehension on a basic level (Petty & Cacioppo, 1986a; Petty & Wegener, 1997). As a second tier of effectiveness, it is possible that themes can also affect determinants and learning and change objectives directly. For example, in the stroke program materials, the theme of urgency paired with the theme that treatment is available was meant to directly affect certain learning objectives.

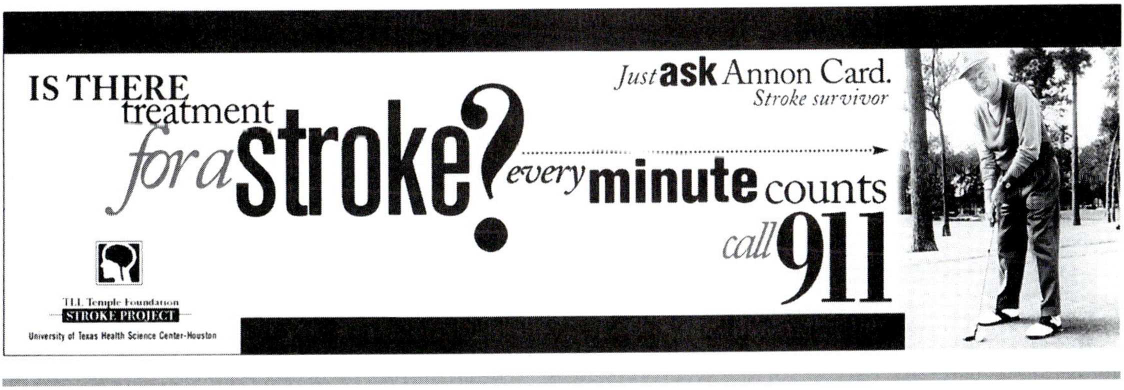

FIGURE 7.2 Billboard for the T.L.L. Temple Foundation Stroke Project

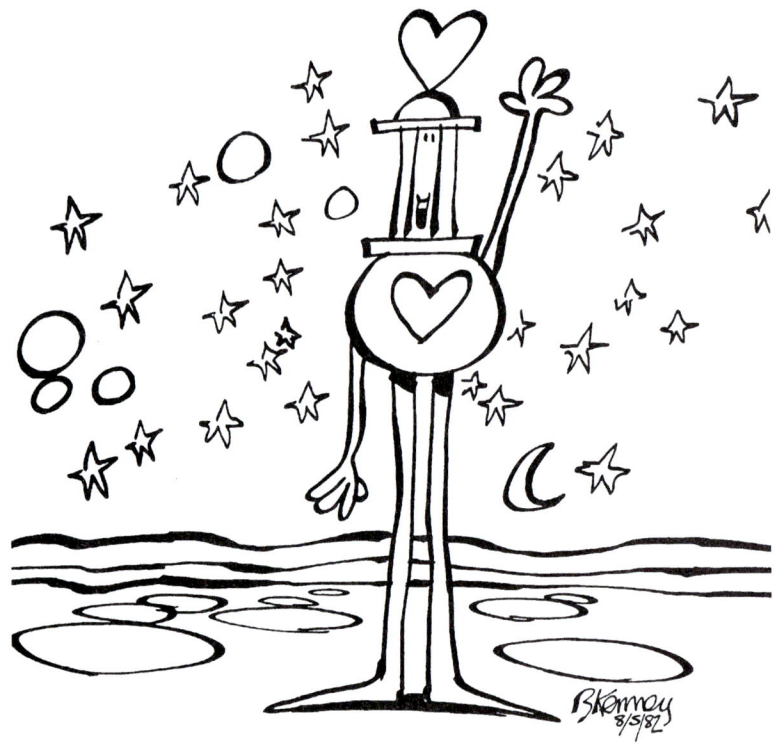

Hi there, Earthlings! I'm Hearty Heart,
With a heart health story I'm about to start.
My planet's called "Strongheart," right next to that star;
When I travel by spaceship, it doesn't seem far.

FIGURE 7.3 Motif Example from CATCH

A good example of the development of a comprehensive program theme designed to appeal to the intended participants is Project PANDA, which is discussed in Chapter 13 (Mullen et al., 1999). When Mullen and her colleagues first characterized a program to help women who had quit smoking during pregnancy not to return to smoking, they thought of the theme "tender loving care for the mother." As they worked on program development and talked to the women, they became even more convinced that a theme that enabled the mother to focus on herself and get ready for the baby would garner the prospective mother's attention, whereas a theme more closely related to cigarette smoking would not.

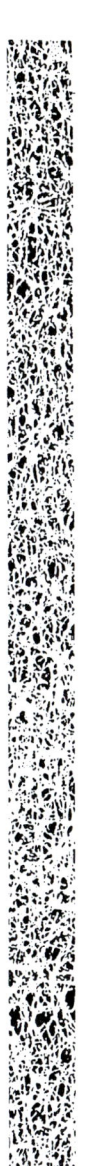

feature story

Finding Your Inner Voice

Finding a personal problem-solving style takes a while. Getting in tune with your own way of solving problems goes hand in hand with gaining more independence.

As Nicole, 23, says, "I was out on my own for a while before I started to listen to my own voice and know what was right and wrong for me. I started to get gut feelings about things: Is this going to work for me? Has it worked in the past?"

Some people like to think over problems for a long time and then try a solution. Others like talking to friends, family, or the medical team before trying out a solution. It all depends on what works for each person.

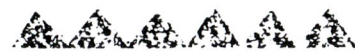

Stopping Problems Before They Happen

No matter what we do, problems happen. But some problems you can almost see coming. What can you do to prevent some of these?

"First of all, you really learn from your mistakes," says Kelly, 16. "I remember going on a trip with my friends. Because nobody wanted to eat as often as I needed to eat, I wasn't getting enough calories. On the next trip with my friends I brought some snacks I could eat between meals. That worked for me."

Thinking through problems ahead of time seems to be a way of avoiding some of them.

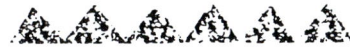

A Step at a Time

Laurel, 22, thinks about problem-solving this way: "I compare it to cleaning the house. If your whole house is a mess and you think, 'I gotta clean this whole place up right away,' you get overwhelmed. So, I divide it up into small tasks. I start by cleaning out a drawer, a closet, or a sink. Then I clean a little bit each day. Pretty soon the whole house is clean. A step at a time."

"I compare problem-solving with cleaning a house. You take it a step at a time."

Creating a Program

FIGURE 7.4 Theme Example from the Cystic Fibrosis Family Education Program (Adolescent)

Channels and Vehicles for Program Methods, Strategies, and Messages

Program design demands decisions not only about themes and motifs, but also about messages and how they will be delivered. A communication channel can be interpersonal or mediated; a vehicle is more specifically how a message is actually

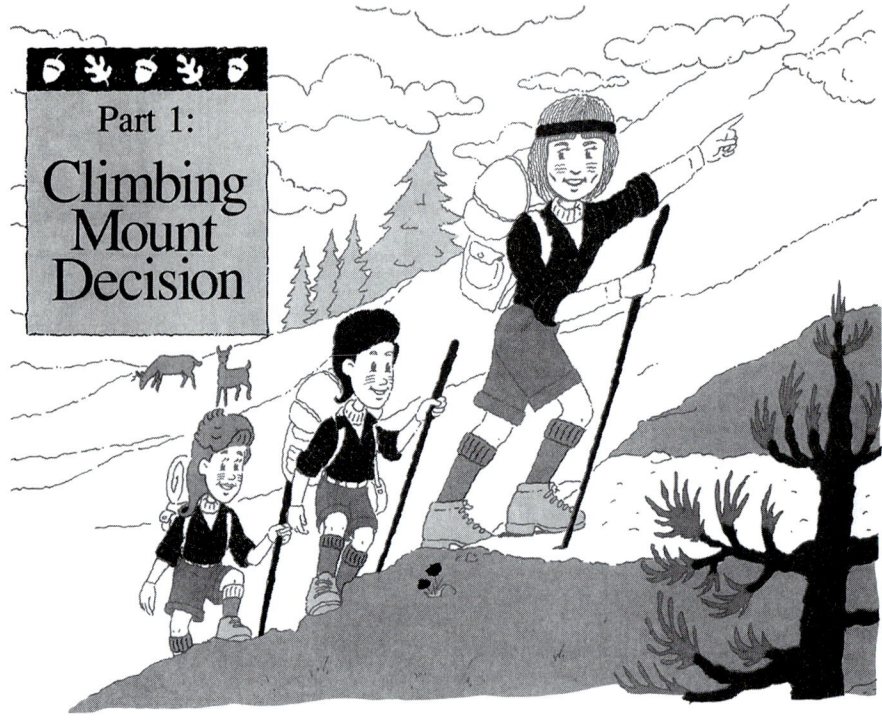

FIGURE 7.5 Motif from the Mastery Theme Cystic Fibrosis Family Education Program (School-Age Children)

packaged and delivered. Various communication vehicles are described in Table 7.1, with examples of the methods and strategies the vehicles often carry. Choosing vehicles is a matter of balancing the needs and preferences of the intended program participants with logistics and budget. With children, for example, planners look to school-based education by using teachers and peer leaders, to health care providers, to magazines, radio, and television targeted to children, and to computer and video games and instruction. Market segmentation techniques can help define the communication vehicles that will reach certain population groups (Lefebvre & Flora, 1988).

One program can use both interpersonal and mediated channels as well as many different vehicles. The *A Su Salud* program used both media (circulating print, radio, and television) and interpersonal communication through community volunteers to promote smoking cessation among Mexican Americans in south Texas (McAlister et al., 1995; Ramirez et al., 1995). Program implementers worked with mass media journalists to produce news and features with information regarding cessation and with stories of real-life people from the population at risk who were in various stages of change regarding the behavior. Trained volunteers then handed out calendars containing the times of the news and talk show broadcasts, tips for quitting, and information of public interest (e.g., the high

Table 7.1
Communication Channels and Vehicles

CHANNELS AND VEHICLES	TYPICAL USES, METHODS, AND STRATEGIES	ADVANTAGES	DISADVANTAGES
Interpersonal: Community volunteers Peer leaders	Skill training Social reinforcing Modeling Tutoring Small group discussion	Is a powerful source of influence and persuasion Is inexpensive Involves community and enhances capacity	Is difficult to train and motivate multipliers
Interpersonal: Teachers	Mastery learning Tutoring Small group discussion Lecture Modeling	Works with experts in teaching techniques Fits organizational context of school	Can be resistant to truly interactive techniques Can be crippled by curriculum time restraints
Interpersonal: Health care providers	Skill training Social reinforcement Modeling Counseling	Is a powerful source of influence and persuasion Works with experts in patient assessment and counseling Caters to a captive audience interested in personal health issues	Is difficult to train and motivate Deals with providers who lack time Can be difficult to integrate counseling techniques if providers are used to a more directive "medical model" Can be perceived as too dissimilar from the patient
Circulating print: Newspapers	Letters to the editor Editorial commentary Role-model stories Information Persuasion Vicarious reinforcement	Is inexpensive Appeals to a wide audience Extends expertise Is detailed Has flexibility Recognizes positive consumer attitudes about vehicle Can be niche based	Depends on literacy Reaches only certain segments Has a short life span Adds to clutter, i.e., many vehicles on the market compete for attention Cannot be used for demonstration Has poor visual quality
Circulating print: Magazines	Letters to the editor and editorial commentary Role-model stories Information Persuasion Vicarious reinforcement	Has good audience segmentation Has high audience receptivity Has credibility and prestige Has long life span Provides good visual quality	Lacks flexibility Lacks control of distribution

(continued)

Table 7.1 Communication Channels and Vehicles *(continued)*

CHANNELS AND VEHICLES	TYPICAL USES, METHODS, AND STRATEGIES	ADVANTAGES	DISADVANTAGES
Circulating print: Newsletters	Letters to the editor and editorial commentary Role-model stories Information Persuasion Vicarious reinforcement	Has good audience segmentation Has high audience receptivity Is a strong possibility for tailoring Offers control of distribution	Requires cultivation of relationships with gate-keepers Requires ability to capitalize on short media attention span for issues Requires high degree of novelty

Display print:
  Billboards
  Posters
	Attention
	Awareness
	Cue to action
		Can be very effective in calling attention to a campaign	Can only effect limited learning and change objectives (e.g., knowledge and awareness)
			Can require significant expense

Display print:
  Brochures
  Flip charts
	Skill training
	Modeling
	Information with extensive detail
	Persuasion
	Vicarious reinforcement
		Can effect a variety of learning and change objectives	Requires plans for distribution because no standard routes exist as they do for circulating print

Radio:
  News items
  Interviews
  PSAs
	Information
	Awareness
	Role-model stories
	Persuasion
		Has good audience segmentation
		Has high audience receptivity
			Requires cultivation of relationships with station gatekeepers
			Requires ability to capitalize on short media attention span for issues
			Has short life span
			Requires high degree of novelty
			Cannot be supported by visuals (role-model stories)

Television:
  News stories
  Talk shows
  Interviews
	Skill training
	Modeling
	Information with extensive detail
	Persuasion
	Vicarious reinforcement
		Has wide distribution
		Offers the possibility for segmentation
			Lacks control over content
			Requires cultivation of relationships with station gatekeepers
			Requires ability to capitalize on short media attention span for issues
			Has short life span
			Requires high degree of novelty
			Competes with broadcast clutter

Table 7.1 (continued)

CHANNELS AND VEHICLES	TYPICAL USES, METHODS, AND STRATEGIES	ADVANTAGES	DISADVANTAGES
Television: Entertainment	Intense role-model stories	Has wide distribution Offers natural segmentation Has norm-changing capabilities	Requires relationship with producers Can be very long
Television: PSAs	To stimulate awareness	Has wide distribution Offers natural segmentation	Loses audience because of channel surfing Must have excellent production quality
Television: Infomercials	Product awareness and persuasion	Can provide large amounts of detail	Loses audience because of channel surfing
Computer-assisted instruction	Skill training Knowledge	Has a very wide and quickly expanding repertoire of vehicles, e.g., CD-ROM, decision support, simulations, games, learner-controlled instruction	Can be costly to develop Requires programming skills, which are in high demand
Videotape: Training Documentary Story	All of the above	Offers control over content	Can be costly Requires plans for distribution

Note. From *Motivating Health Behavior,* by J. P. Elder, E. S. Geller, M. F. Hovell, and J. A. Mayer, 1994, Albany, NY: Delmar; and from *Advertising Principles and Practice* (4th ed.), by W. Wells, J. Burnett, and S. Moriarty, 1998, Upper Saddle River, NJ: Prentice Hall.

school basketball game schedule); encouraged their friends and acquaintances to consider quitting smoking; and reinforced any efforts those friends made.

This approach was also used in the AIDS demonstration projects funded by the CDC (CDC AIDS Community Demonstration Projects Research Group, 1999; Corby, Enguidamos, & Kay, 1996; McAlister et al., 1999; Pulley, McAlister, Kay, & O'Reilly, 1996). In one city, the AIDS project chose runaway youth as the focus, and it targeted condom use and either not shooting up or using clean needles and used micro media in the form of small cards that contained role-model stories (Figure 7.6). Although the role-model stories were true ones obtained by interviews with members of the at-risk groups, the pictures and names were fictitious. In this case, because the chosen at-risk group was small and the behaviors were private, a mass media channel would not be possible or effective.

A major advantage of using role-model stories from the population is that they are culturally appropriate when ascertained properly. The role models speak, think, look, and act like members of the at-risk group because, in fact, they are. By making these early adopters of a healthful behavior more visible to others in the

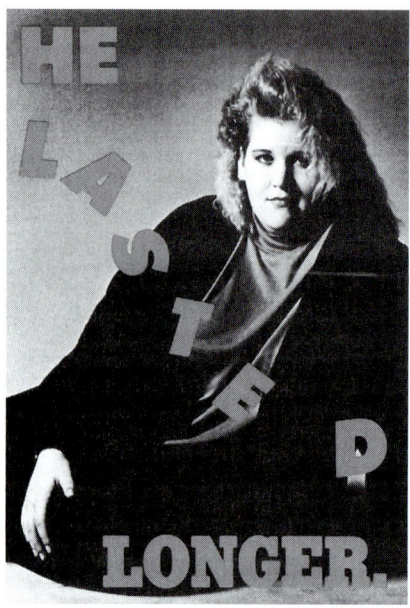
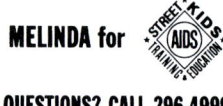

FIGURE 7.6 Role-Model Story for HIV Prevention Project

population, the rate of diffusion of the behaviors in the population is increased (Ramirez et al., 1995).

In addition to community volunteers, interpersonal channels include teachers and health care providers (who also likely use print and video media as well). Teachers may use tutorials (one-on-one instruction), group discussions, and lectures, depending on the context and on the content and objectives of the instruction. Tutorials and small group learning have the advantage over lectures in that learner performance can be elicited and feedback provided with greater individualization.

More abstract and interactive vehicles for change, such as community coalitions, are also parts of most programs. For example, the stroke project described earlier in this chapter included a community committee of people with a stake in stroke treatment, such as health care providers, community groups, and stroke victims. The Walk Texas! program, a community program aimed at getting Texans to exercise, is conducted by local health departments and other community-based organizations. An early task was to identify and connect to partners that would establish local walking groups (Jonas, 1998). Advocacy is a central part of many programs, such as those directed to reducing exposure of youth to tobacco, to increasing support of coordinated school health, and to prevention of various chronic diseases (Altman, 1995a, 1995b). Blueprints for accomplishing these performance objectives are comparable to the program design documents we discuss later in this chapter for the development of media and small group communications. These blueprints include guidelines for selecting coalition members, guidelines for meeting agendas, legislative visit protocols, and sample letters for advocacy. These channels for delivering methods and strategies to accomplish program objectives should be considered as a possible part of every program.

Messages, a part of all health promotion materials, are focused attempts to accomplish a learning or change objective. The following processes can get a health educator started on message development:

- Think about the methods and strategies that have been decided on for a particular set of objectives and that will fit together in a particular vehicle, such as a newspaper story
- Decide what vehicle would be appropriate to deliver the methods and strategies
- Note the learning and change objectives (organized by determinants)
- Draft the specific messages that will be incorporated into the vehicle

For example, Table 7.2 provides an outline of the messages for the stroke project that was introduced earlier in this chapter. For each, the planners thought about what methods and strategies they had decided to use to influence their learning

Table 7.2
Message Development Guide for the T.L.L. Temple Foundation Stroke Project

PROPOSED VEHICLE	LEARNING OBJECTIVES GROUPED BY DETERMINANT	METHODS AND STRATEGIES	MESSAGE CONTENT
Emergency departments and community physicians			
Newspaper article 1	**Social norms:** Recognize that other physicians in the community respond rapidly to symptoms of stroke; believe that other emergency departments are lowering their workup times for stroke	Modeling through role-model stories	I had a stroke patient who got to the hospital on time; the hospital emergency department treated my patient
	Outcome expectations: Expect that stroke patients (especially those presenting with moderate disability) can recover function with acute treatment of stroke	Testimonials	I wasn't sure about this new treatment before, but I am really pleased with the improvement I saw in my patient
	Reinforcement: Prepare and share patient success stories because there may be a lack of feedback to emergency department staff	Vicarious reinforcement	From the patient or family's point of view: I am back (or my family member is back) to full functioning. The doctor saved our quality of life by acting quickly
Community members			
Billboard 1	**Knowledge:** Describe importance of calling 911 for stroke symptoms	Modeling through familiarity of community member	Call 911 Every minute counts Is there treatment for stroke? (Ask Annon Card, stroke victim, who is playing golf)
	Outcome expectations: Expect that getting to the emergency department fast will allow treatment to minimize effects of stroke		

and change objectives. They decided on vehicles to convey those methods and strategies, and partial planning for two of the vehicles is shown in the table. Finally, they composed first drafts of the messages to be contained in the newspaper story and billboard they were planning.

Technology

Computer and telephone technology may help break several important barriers related to individualization and program delivery in health education. The three categories of technology presented here are certainly not exhaustive, but will give the reader an idea about how to consider these program vehicles.

COMPUTER-ASSISTED INTERVENTION The current computer environment in health education is one of great promise. Street and Rimal (1997) define interactive technology as that which includes both user control—the extent to which the user can modify the form and content of the computer environment and can determine what topics and services are selected—and responsiveness. Responsiveness is the extent to which the program takes into account the user's previous activities. A highly responsive program gives feedback and provides opportunities based on the user's input (p. 2). Another aspect of interactive media is that they comprise modular units that are linked together to enable the program to employ an array of databases such as animation, narration, graphics, and services and to enable the user to move from one part to another (Dede & Fontana, 1995). These characteristics are attractive for program development in health education because they provide a powerful medium for delivering methods and strategies that influence a wide range of determinants. Street and Rimal cite the advantages of interactivity as promoting active information processing and satisfaction (Dede & Fontana; Rafaeli, 1988; Schaffer & Hannafin, 1986). These characteristics may contribute to central processing as discussed by Petty and Cacioppo (1986a; 1986b), Chaffe and Roser (1986), and Webber (1990) (see Chapter 4).

Another advantage of interactive multimedia is that a single application can support a wide variety of learner needs (Rimal & Flora, 1997). For example, users who lack sufficient background (including language skills) can supplement text learning with other modalities, such as pictures, and can be presented significant redundancy across modalities. Redundancy is needed because a novice learner is having to construct cognitive schema and then attach new information. On the other hand, users who already have the schema can reduce redundancy and cut to the chase. The computer environment also is an excellent mechanism for balancing novelty (to acquire and maintain attention) and redundancy (to facilitate processing). Rimal and Flora cite Singer and Singer (1979) who compare *Sesame Street* (high novelty) with *Mr. Roger's Neighborhood* (high redundancy). With computer-assisted instruction, both environments are available simultaneously. A further advantage is temporal flexibility. The user can control not only when to get the message, but when and how to manipulate the message. All these types of user control—the ability to control when the program is used and the aspects of novelty and redundancy—can facilitate learning and the development of self-directed learning skills (Lieberman & Linn, 1991).

Despite the potential of computers in health education, Hawkins and colleagues (1997) warn against a "build it and they will come" attitude. They suggest that the program developer build tools, start small, and not be afraid of being captivating. They applied these principles to the Comprehensive Health Enhancement Support System (CHESS), an example of the explicit use of theoretical methods such as problem solving, decision support, self-monitoring, social support, and action planning in a multimedia environment. CHESS also is a good example of developing a carefully limited design and adhering to it across content domains. The program is intended for people who have health crises, and the first problem areas to be developed were breast cancer, HIV, sexual assault, adult children of alcoholics, academic crisis, and stress management (Gustafson, Bosworth, Chewning, & Hawkins, 1987; Gustafson et al., 1993). The program shell consisted of three components: (a) information delivered via an instant library, questions and answers, "ask an expert," and help and support; (b) decision and planning support delivered via decision analysis, action planning, and risk assessment; and (c) social support delivered via personal stories and a discussion group. The HIV component has been evaluated and found to result in better quality of life for the program users as compared to a control group (P. Brennan, Ripich, & Moore, 1991). Quality of life included better cognitive functioning, less degeneration over time in activities of daily living and social activities, more effectively managed medical care visits, and less hospitalization. Other programs, such as one linking caregivers of persons with Alzheimer patients and one providing social support to persons with advanced AIDS (P. Brennan et al.), have also demonstrated the ability to incorporate sound theoretical methods such as social support into computer-assisted health promotion. Furthermore, the programs seem to be used equally across demographic segments, including men and women and both disadvantaged and more advantaged individuals. One study indicated differential use between older and younger, however, with older subjects using the program less often (F. A. Brennan & Fink, 1997).

Other program developers have demonstrated that the computer-assisted instructional environment is a good way to teach self-management skills and to enhance self-efficacy (Brown et al., 1997). Lieberman (1997) describes a series of Health Hero video games that provide simulated self-management environments for diabetes and asthma and that solidify negative attitudes regarding smoking. She notes that children will continue playing games until they can easily complete them. Bartholomew and colleagues had the same experience with the Watch, Discover, Think, and Act program (Bartholomew, Gold, et al., 2000; Bartholomew, Shegog, et al., 2000). Children would often encourage entire families to wait for them in the clinic so that they could "just get one more scene done" in the asthma management program. All these programs have design elements geared toward

Table 7.3

Goals and Related Design Features in Health Hero Video Games

GOALS	DESIGN FEATURES THAT ADDRESS THOSE GOALS
Attention and active processing	
To reduce psychological distance; increase attention to the content; and make the content seem personally relevant to young people	Present content on the popular video game medium in a format young people perceive to be targeted to them
To boost player's self-esteem; increase attention; optimize credibility; and increase the likelihood that young people will emulate the character's behavior	Use attractive, competent role-model characters who have the same health condition as the intended user group and are about 2 to 3 years older
To increase attention, involvement, learning, and retention	Provide cognitive challenges, compelling characters and relationships, experiential learning, user control over the action, and individualized feedback
Motivation	
To make games motivating, engaging, and appealing	Present clear, intriguing, and challenging goals and provide continuous updates on progress toward the goals; provide individualized interaction and feedback
To enhance enjoyment and individualize the learning experience	Allow game players to customize the content according to preference and to match their own health status (e.g., player can select frequency and dose of a diabetic character's daily insulin)
Knowledge	
To teach explicit content	Use direct instruction; include game strategies that require the player to learn information in order to succeed in the game; use very graphic and memorable illustrations such as disgusting tar, plaque, and debris shown in a smoker's body
To teach skills	Present animated demonstrations such as how to use an inhaler for asthma medication; provide opportunities to rehearse skills and solve problems in simulations that show realistic outcomes based on the player's actions

promoting attention and active processing, motivation, knowledge and skills of disease management, self-efficacy, communication, and social support. Watch, Discover, Think, and Act makes use of the computer's capabilities by enabling children to enter their personal asthma characteristics, which the computer then uses to modify the simulations to be more lifelike for the individual child. Table 7.3 is a design document from the Health Heroes series. Chapter 11 describes the Watch, Discover, Think, and Act program.

Table 7.3 *(continued)*

GOALS	DESIGN FEATURES THAT ADDRESS THOSE GOALS
Knowledge *(continued)*	
To ensure that players will retain the information and skills they have learned in the game	Repeat information and animated demonstrations for review when players give a wrong answer; make the game difficult enough that players will repeat game levels dozens of times and therefore will be exposed repeatedly to the same content
To correct mistakes and improve performance	Provide constructive feedback about the player's actions and choices, and offer remediation as needed
To provide background information on demand	Enable easy access to dynamic databases such as a food chart showing the food exchanges in a serving of each food that players may select in the game
To provide a cumulative record of performance in the game; increase the player's understanding; and encourage the use of personal logbooks	Use on-screen, automatically updated logbooks that record, for instance, medications the character has taken and blood glucose or peak flow measurements attained in each game level
Perceived self-efficacy	
To increase player's perceived self-efficacy for prevention and self-care	Create opportunities for players to rehearse new skills and to apply new knowledge in the game until they are successful
To help players feel more confident and willing to discuss their health concerns with peers, parents, and caregivers	Present issues and questions that players must address in the game, thereby allowing them to rehearse the answers while playing alone or to discuss the answers when others are present
To encourage social interaction that can increase peer tutoring, learning, and retention	Offer a two-player option in the game
To provide a springboard for discussion about prevention or self-management	Create an appealing game that young people will want to talk about and will be proud to play

Note. From "Interactive Video Games for Health Promotion: Effects on Knowledge, Self-Efficacy, Social Support, and Health," by D. A. Lieberman, 1977, in R. Street, W. Gold, and T. Manning (Eds.), *Health Promotion and Interactive Technology: Theoretical Applications and Future Directions* (pp. 108–109), Mahwah, NJ: Erlbaum.

COMPUTERIZED TAILORING OF INTERVENTIONS For the past decade, health education researchers have been testing simple computer expert systems that enable the tailoring of communications to match certain characteristics that have been measured in participants (Bental, Cawsey, & Jones, 1999; Strecher, 1999). Although there is need for further research to determine exactly what characteristics are important to tailor on (i.e., what characteristics influence the effectiveness of the intervention), there is enough evidence of effectiveness to continue to work in this area and to import these strategies into common practice with the caveat that the characteristics for tailoring in a particular program must be well justified empirically and theoretically (Brug, Glanz, Van Assema, Kok, & van Breukelen, 1998; Brug, Steenhuis, van Assema, & De Vries, 1998; Dijkstra, De Vries, Roijackers, & van Breukelen, 1998a, 1998b; Kreuter & Strecher, 1996; Rimer et al., 1994; Skinner, Strecher, & Hospers, 1994; Strecher et al., 1994). The literature is somewhat unclear about exactly what aspects of tailored messages have been the effective components, and Table 7.4 provides a summary of the variables that have been used in studies of tailored communications.

Velicer and colleagues (1993) define an expert system as a collection of facts and rules about something and a way of making inferences from the facts and rules. The most common type of expert system in health education is a computer program that generates behavior change messages tailored to specific characteristics of the receiver. In other words, the expert system comprises (a) one or more databases of messages based on theoretical constructs that vary as they apply to different characteristics of individuals and (b) algorithms for matching the messages to the individual. The message channel could, in general, be anything that facilitates delivery of the message. In the expert system by Velicer and colleagues,

Table 7.4
Variables Used in Studies of Tailored Communications

STUDY	CHARACTERISTICS USED IN INTERVENTION
Curry, Wagner, and Grothaus 1991; Curry, McBride, Grothaus, Louie, and Wagner, 1995	Intrinsic motives for quitting, self-efficacy, self-control
Prochaska, DiClemente, Velicer, and Rossi, 1993; Velicer and Prochaska, 1999	Stages and processes of change from the transtheoretical model
Strecher et al., 1994	Smoking behavior, stage of change, perceived benefits, barriers (second study—threat and attributions from previous quitting failures)
Rimer et al., 1994	Stages of changes, quitting needs, and smoking habits
Skinner, Strecher, and Hospers, 1994	Mammography beliefs, stage of change, risk factors and barriers
Brug, Steenhuis, Van Assema, and De Vries, 1996; Brug, Glanz, Van Assema, Kok, and, van Breukelen, 1998	Fat, fruit, and vegetable intake, attitudes, perceived social influences, self-efficacy expectations, and awareness levels
Dijkstra, De Vries, and Roijackers, 1998	Consequences of smoking, benefits of quitting, barriers to quitting, high-risk situations
Bull, Kreuter, and Scharff, 1999	Stage of readiness to change, exercise goal, motives for and perceived barriers to reaching the goal, and preferred type of physical activity

for example, the vehicle is a report, but the message could also be delivered by newsletters, video, or computer-assisted instruction. In the Velicer work, messages were based on the transtheoretical model and included processes of change tailored to the stage of the individual in regard to quitting smoking. Feedback included current smoking status and stage of change, current use of change processes, suggested quitting strategies, and high-risk situations. Feedback was compared against a normative database as well as against the participant's own progress. Another example of delivery is an expert system that is being developed by Abramson and colleagues (2000). This system provides both instructions to physicians who are managing asthma and written tailored feedback in order to support self-management behaviors of children and their parents. All the systems described in the literature are based on similar configurations (Figure 7.7), comprising a theoretical framework and specification of relevant hypothesized determinants of the health behavior; use of the determinant model to create a data collection tool and a series of messages; several databases, including at least a data file and a feedback message file; decision rules and a tailoring program; communications; and delivery vehicles (Dijkstra & De Vries, 1999; Rhodes, Fishbein, & Reis, 1997; Skinner & Kreuter, 1997; Velicer et al., 1993).

TELEPHONE-DELIVERED INTERVENTIONS Soet and Basch (1997) point out that the telephone has been used as an instrument of health care since its debut. They cite a large literature on the use of the telephone as an instrument of health education and promotion, ranging from simple information hotlines, through a

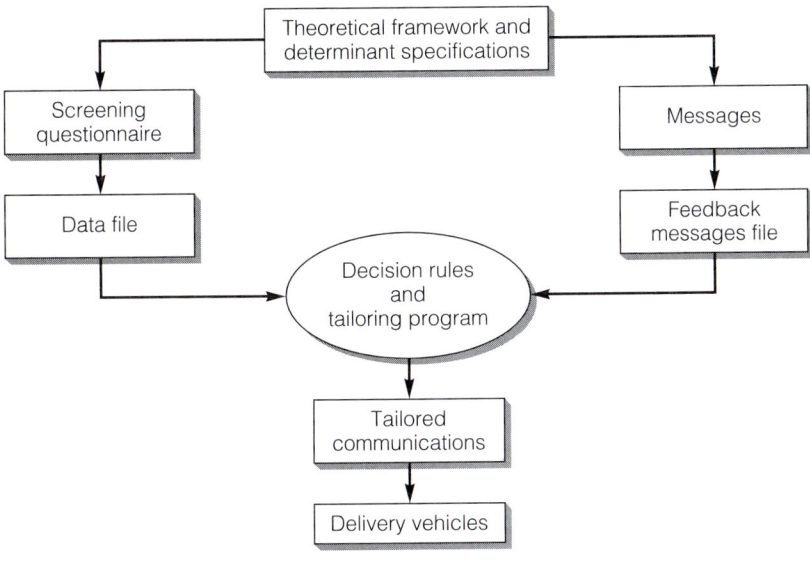

FIGURE 7.7 Developing Tailored Feedback (*Note*. Adapted from "The Impact of a Computer-Tailored Nutrition Intervention," by J. Brug, I. Steenhuis, P. Van Assema, and H. De Vries, 1996, *Preventive Medicine, 25,* pp. 236–242.)

midrange of standardized messages aimed at health behavior, to more complex computerized counseling for behavior change (Ramelson, Friedman, & Ockene, 1999). There are now protocol-supported telephone interventions that support tailoring of messages (Zhu, Balabanis, Rosbrook, Sadler, & Pierce, 1996). The telephone as a delivery mechanism has many advantages. It is interactive, and messages can be not only tailored but also individualized. Visual privacy can make intervention less stressful and more productive for individuals who are reluctant to discuss a particular issue. The telephone also can reach dispersed or homebound populations and can accommodate low literacy and language differences.

There is some risk of loss of meaning in this medium (as there is for print vehicles) because 65% to 95% of social meaning comes from visual cues in face-to-face interaction. However, it is possible that the novelty and different set of expectations for electronic media may liberate the delivery from the burden of interpersonal empathy as long as the messages are developed with appropriate counseling sophistication (Miller & Rollnick, 1991).

Perhaps the most exciting development in telephone delivery is the combination of expert system technology and interactive (digitized voice) telephone counseling. This technology enables a real-time assessment and contingent delivery of messages and feedback regarding attempts to perform a health behavior. Automated systems are being used more and more in managed care situations and other health care settings. For example, Ramelson and colleagues describe the Telephone Linked Communication system that has been used to counsel smoking cessation (Ramelson et al., 1999), improve medication compliance for hypertension (Friedman et al., 1996), help sedentary elderly patients to exercise (Cullinane, Hyppolite, Zastawney, & Friedman, 1994), and promote dietary changes for hypercholesterolemia (Dutton, Posner, Smigelski, & Friedman, 1995). A sample conversation from the smoking intervention is included in Figure 7.8.

Existing Program Materials[1]

Health educators who are considering using existing program materials ask themselves two questions: Do the program materials enable my learning and change objectives and deliver my methods and strategies? and Do the materials fit with my intended audience, that is, are the materials attractive, appealing, and culturally competent? To decide, the health educator reviews materials against matrices and lists of methods and strategies. The match should be almost perfect. Questions to ask include: Are all the messages that are needed to influence learning and change objectives included? Are the required methods executed appropriately? For example, do role-model stories use coping models, and are they derived from a group that matches the community on important characteristics? It is difficult to make all these matches, but sometimes parts of existing programs work well.

Existing materials that match objectives, methods, and strategies can be reviewed for production qualities. If existing materials are based on reading, are

---

[1]Contributed by Karyn Popham, University of Texas–Houston School of Public Health.

they at an appropriate reading level? If the materials are in a language other than English, are they in the appropriate form of that language? Are the layout, design, and typography appropriate for the audience and context? (For instance, items printed on high-gloss paper are difficult to read under the overhead fluorescent lights common to waiting rooms; the elderly appreciate a larger type size than might otherwise be used; many Americans find sans serif type difficult to read in large blocks.) Are the materials culturally sensitive? Do illustrations portray

---

The callers' responses to the questions posed by the system are underlined. The ellipses represent a jump to another part of the conversation.

Figure A: Example of contemplation dialogue

Hello Mr. [name]. I'm glad that you called in today. About how many cigarettes are you now smoking a day?   <u>25</u>

You are smoking more cigarettes than the last time we spoke. I hope you will be able to cut down when we speak next. In the conversation, we will identify reasons that you smoke and reasons why you want to quit. This will help me to give you specific suggestions to help you quit.
. . .

If you haven't smoked for a while, do you get a strong craving or desire to smoke? Press 1 for yes and 2 for no.   <u>1</u>

Write down on your list the words "I smoke to satisfy my craving for a cigarette." Press 1 when you are done.   <u>1</u>

Do you smoke to give yourself a lift or to keep yourself from slowing down? Press 1 for yes and 2 for no.   <u>2</u>

Do you smoke when you are under stress or feeling depressed? Press 1 for yes and 2 for no.   <u>1</u>

Write down on your list the words "I smoke to reduce stress." Press 1 when you are done.   <u>1</u>
. . .

Now I would like to identify reasons why you want to quit. This will help me to give you specific suggestions to help you to quit. Do you want to quit for your health? Press 1 for yes and 2 for no.   <u>2</u>

Dr. [name] recommends that you quit for your health. Passive smoking occurs when you smoke around other people. They inhale your cigarette smoke and the cancer-causing substances in it. Do you want to quit for the health of those close to you? Press 1 for yes and 2 for no.   <u>1</u>

Write down on your list the names of the people who you are thinking about. Press 1 when you are done.   <u>1</u>
. . .

The money that you spend on cigarettes adds up to a lot. Since you started smoking, approximately how many cigarettes on an average day would you say that you have smoked?   <u>30</u>

(continued)

FIGURE 7.8 Computerized Telephone System for Smoking Counseling (*Note.* From "An Automated Telephone-Based Smoking Cessation Education and Counseling System," by H. Z. Ramelson, R. H. Friedman, and J. K. Ockene, 1999, *Patient Education and Counseling, 36*(2), pp. 131–144.)

> Approximately how many years have you been smoking?   25
>
> Do you realize that over the time that you have smoked, you have spent $27,375 on cigarettes. I'll bet that you wish you had that money now. Well, it's not too late to quit smoking and save money now. If you continue to smoke for the next ten years, you will spend another $16,425 on your habit. Do you want to quit to save money? Press 1 for yes and 2 for no.   1
>
> We have finished making our lists. I would like you to put these lists in a place where you will see them every day—like near your telephone or on your fridge. Try to look at them at least once a day. You may think of more reasons why you want to smoke and why you want to quit. Add them to the lists as you think of them.
>
> **Figure B: Example of preparation dialogue**
>
> Did you try to quit [on your quit date]?
> Press 1 for yes and 2 for no.   1
>
> Don't be discouraged. Most smokers need several tries before they quit. Did something unexpected come up that made it hard for you to quit?
> Press 1 for yes and 2 for no.   1
>
> I understand. I hope that you will try again. Are the suggestions that we discussed helping you? Press 1 for yes and 2 for no.   2
>
> We will review the suggestions, and if you want, I will give you some other ones to help you out. After we do this, I will ask you to choose another goal for quitting.
> . . .
>
> You told me that you smoke to satisfy a craving. You wanted to satisfy your craving by taking 10 deep breaths. Did you try this suggestion?
> Press 1 for yes and 2 for no.   1
>
> Did this suggestion help you with your cravings?
> Press 1 for yes and 2 for no.   2
>
> Don't be discouraged. I will give you some other ideas to help you to quit. If you get a strong urge for a smoke, try putting something in your mouth instead of a cigarette. You can carry around with you a carrot, celery, cinnamon sticks, chewing gum, or toothpicks. Do you think you will do this?
> Press 1 for yes and 2 for no.   1
>
> Write down on your list the thing that you will put in your mouth when you get a craving. Examples are carrot, celery, and cinnamon sticks.
> Press 1 when you are done.   1

FIGURE 7.8 Computerized Telephone System for Smoking Counseling *(continued)*

people who look and sound like intended participants? Are the settings familiar to them? Is there anything stereotypical about the materials? (For example, are only mothers portrayed giving certain kinds of care to children? Do the materials display stereotypical power relations, with only males or only females in certain occupations, or with only Whites as physicians while people of color are the patients?) Are inappropriate assumptions made as to the reader's socioeconomic status or environmental resources? Do the materials reflect the quality and production values that the program wishes to embrace? (Glynn & Britton, 1984; Parker, 1988; Strong, 1990; Wells, Burnett, & Moriarty, 1998; White, 1988; R. Williams, 1994.) Doak, Doak, and Root (1995) have a helpful chapter titled

"Assessing Suitability of Materials" that may assist in this evaluation. Finally, these materials must be pretested with the intended participants, just like materials that have been newly developed (U.S. DHHS, 1992).

Before engaging in a thorough evaluation, however, the planner should determine if the materials are available in the needed quantity and time frame. Some agencies may allow reproduction. Some materials may be available in electronic form, for instance, as a PDF file over the Internet. In some cases copyright holders allow materials to be adapted, but any changes must usually be done hand in glove with the copyright owner (Fishman, 1997).

Materials produced by the U.S. government are free for use by U.S. citizens, and more and more such materials are available on the World Wide Web. The National Institutes of Health, for instance, is making a concerted effort to upload its patient education material onto the Web. All copyrights, adaptations, and permissions must be acknowledged on every piece, and it is appropriate to provide courtesy copies to the people who created the original material.

Reading levels are almost always an issue for written materials—actually two issues: What is the reading level, and what should it be? Reading levels indicate a grade level beyond which the message is likely to be difficult to decipher. Ultimately the best course for health educators to follow in determining what the reading level should be is to do the fieldwork necessary to find out the literacy skills of their intended participants (Doak et al., 1995). Health educators who intend to use graphic communication techniques—charts, graphs, tables—must also assess the ability of their audience to use and understand such tools.

The second issue is how to assess the reading level of a document. Many techniques are available; most suffer from the same flaws. In general, evaluations include an assessment of the average number of words in a sentence and the average number of syllables in a word. The former is used as a measure of complexity and the latter as a measure of vocabulary level. There is more to complexity than the length of a sentence, and more to vocabulary level than the number of syllables, but in precomputer days the pioneers developed these methods as workable substitutes. Many word processing and grammar checking programs will now do the math (for instance, Correct Grammar, distributed on CD-ROM by SoftKey Multimedia Inc.), but the programs are still using algorithms set up in the precomputer era. Common protocols include the SMOG formula, the Gunning FOG index, the Fry Readability Graph, the Flesch Reading Ease score, and the Flesch-Kincaid grade level (Flesch, 1949; Fry, 1977). These various protocols will not necessarily give comparable results: a first draft of five paragraphs from this chapter had a Flesch Reading Ease score of 47.7 (grade level required: 13.3, i.e., three months into the first year of college; U.S. adults who understand: 54%). The same five paragraphs had a Flesch-Kincaid grade level of 10.5, and a Gunning Fog index of 13.4 (usually interpreted as a grade level of 13.4). We suggest picking one protocol to use consistently (Trapini & Walmsley, 1981). By using one protocol, the health educator learns over time to write very close to a target grade level and to edit down the grade level of passages.

Many health educators find it simplest to use the protocols included with Word for Windows 95 (and subsequent editions): Tools/Options/Spelling and Grammar/Show Readability Statistics. To fine-tune their assessment, writers can use a graded vocabulary list (e.g., Mogilner, 1992). Such a list gets past the assumption that a longer word is necessarily a harder word ("grandfather" is a first-grade word in the United States, despite its three syllables). Using words at a third-grade level and below ensures capturing an audience with fifth-grade reading skills. Health educators may find such restrictions difficult, but they can inspire genius; it was such an assignment that launched the career of Theodore Geisel as Dr. Seuss.

Several other approaches have been applied to reading levels (Holcomb & Ellis, 1978; Irwin & Davis, 1980; Mosenthal & Kirsch, 1998). A different approach to assessing document complexity is the PMOST/IKIRSCH document readability formula, which looks at both the organizational pattern (simple list, combined list, intersected list, nested list) and density (number of labels and number of items) (Mosenthal & Kirsch). This formula is an attempt to evaluate the readability of charts, graphs, tables, forms, and other nonlinear presentations of written words. In conjunction with the education afforded by Tufte's works (1983, 1990, 1997), it may prove a useful adjunct to standard reading level formulas.

DESIGNING A CULTURALLY COMPETENT PROGRAM

Aiming at Cultural Competence

Another part of operationalizing methods and strategies into a coherent program is to keep an eye on issues of cultural competence. There is no cookbook for ensuring cultural competence in programs. Health educators must explore their personal ethnocentrism, get to know the culture in which they are working, and build reciprocity into programs so that cultural understanding is developmental rather than static.

Often health educators work with groups of people who are members of a cultural group different from themselves. Healthy People 2010 (U.S. DHHS, 1998) highlights the health disparities between racial and ethnic groups, with particular emphasis on eliminating those disparities in infant mortality, cancer screening and management, cardiovascular disease, diabetes, HIV/AIDS, and childhood and adult immunizations. For example, in comparison to Whites, infant mortality rates are 2.5 times higher for African Americans and 1.5 times higher for Native Americans. The prevalence of diabetes in Hispanics is nearly twice that of Whites (U.S. DHHS, 1998). In order to address these priority health issues effectively, health educators must be able to develop culturally appropriate programs. Health educators who wish to look beyond their geographic boundaries and work in international settings must become immersed in the culture in which they are working.

Triandis (1994, p. 13) states that in observing other cultures, we humans see the world through a lens of who we are, rather than seeing the world as it is. Under this condition, it is imperative that health educators learn to see another culture as clearly as possible in order to create programs that are culturally competent. If culture is to society what memories are to an individual (Triandis, p. 15, citing Kluckhohn, 1954, p. 967), then a culturally competent program is one that uses those memories for the empowerment of the individual and the community. A culturally relevant program is one that uses culturally appropriate images and themes to make a program attractive and appealing to a group, thus affecting attention and comprehension. A culturally competent program may go further to stimulate deeper processing of material. A culturally sensitive program can be thought of as the floor of practice—it is simply one that does not stereotype or damage the receiving culture.

Culture can be defined as the implicit and explicit guidelines that individuals inherit as members of a particular society. These guidelines tell people in that culture how to "view the world, how to experience it emotionally, and how to behave in it in relation to other people, to supernatural forces or gods, and to the natural environment" (Helman, 1990, pp. 2–3). The more different that cultures are from one another, the higher the cultural distance is and the less likely it is that people from those different cultures will attach the same meaning to words, gestures, and symbols. Witte and Morrison (1995) have described the specific impact of cultures on health communications including how different cultures explain disease. Ethnomedical systems are personalistic, or naturalistic, or Western scientific. Personalistic systems view supernatural spirits or people as causing disease, and in naturalistic systems, health is described in impersonal terms of equilibrium, for example, hot and cold, active and passive. Western medicine seeks analytical and physiological explanations and cures for disease. Closely related to these explanatory systems are cultural concepts regarding the mind-body connection and the roles of religion and the family. Those concepts, because they mediate how people conceptualize and manage health and illness, are an important context for health education. Pasick (1997), for example, mentions *fatalismo,* a concept of fatalism that can influence health behaviors such as cancer screening: "Why find the cancer if it can't be cured?"

EXPLORING PERSONAL ETHNOCENTRISM Western health educators have a double burden of ethnocentrism. First, they have, like everyone else does, their own personal ethnocentrism. Triandis (1994) describes personal ethnocentrism as a slight superiority in response to stories from other cultures and a boredom at the expectedness of stories from their own culture. This boredom causes them not to seek to understand their own viewpoint or explore their own culture. But in addition to personal ethnocentrism, Western health promotors also have a behavioral and social science ethnocentrism. For example, the theory discussed in this book was generated and tested mostly in the United States and Europe. It may apply only poorly to cultures with significant distance from the generating and testing cultures.

Stereotyping can occur in the incubator of ethnocentrism if individuals begin to ascribe similar attributes to all members of a group. For example, the following statement is at best simplistic and at worst stereotyping: "Members of the Hispanic culture believe in *fatalismo*." Do all members of this hugely diverse group express this belief? How much variation is there among members of the group who do ascribe to this belief? Do members of other cultures ascribe to this belief, and are these beliefs manifested in a way similar to those in Hispanics?

Human beings have much in common as well as much that is different between cultures. In addition, individuals within a culture have many differences from each other. Stereotyping can obscure both of these facts. A superficial effort to draw on elements of another culture in an educational situation may only exacerbate a tendency to stereotype (Rios, McDaniel, & Stowell, 1998). Rios and colleagues recommend a cultural plunge into another culture with concurrent efforts at self-awareness.

Locke (1986, 1992) offers the following set of questions as a guide for a first step at developing cultural self-awareness:

- What is my cultural heritage? What was the culture of my parents and grandparents? With what cultural group do I identify?
- What is the cultural relevance of my name?
- What values, beliefs, opinions, and attitudes do I hold that are consistent with the dominant culture? Which are inconsistent? How did I learn these?
- How did I decide to be a [health] educator? What cultural standards were involved in the process? What do I understand to be the relationship between culture and [health] education?
- What unique abilities, aspirations, expectations, and limitations do I have that might influence my relations with culturally diverse individuals?

Rios and colleagues (1998) argue that the development of an educator progresses from hostility or denial, through awareness, integration, acceptance, respect, and valuing, and finally to commitment to social justice. This growth process requires active motivation to explore personal reactions through writing field notes and journal entries during cross-cultural encounters. In addition, the learning of another language provides an invaluable opportunity for cultural insight.

As a beginning of insight into the culture of the United States and other close cultures, R. M. Williams (1970) has described 15 themes of Anglo-Saxon culture in the United States. Those themes are

- Achievement and success: rags-to-riches stories
- Activity and work: busy people who stress work as a worthy end in itself
- Humanitarian mores: sympathy for the underdog, offering of spontaneous help
- Moral orientation: situations judged in terms of right or wrong

- Efficiency and practicality: getting things done
- Progress: things will get better
- Material comfort: the good life
- Equality
- Freedom
- External conformity: of dress, housing, recreation, manners
- Science and secular rationality
- Nationalism and patriotism
- Democracy
- Individual personality
- Racism and related group superiority

EXPLORING ANOTHER CULTURE Locke (1992) suggests scrutinizing the following 10 cultural elements to begin exploring another culture:

- Degree of acculturation
- Poverty
- History of oppression
- Language and the arts
- Racism and prejudice
- Sociopolitical factors
- Child-rearing practices
- Religious practices
- Family structure
- Values and attitudes

Triandis (1994) presents a different structure for looking at cultures. He describes the cultural syndromes of individualism/collectivism, complexity/simplicity, and tightness/looseness. In an individualist culture such as the United States, the wishes of the individual have a very high priority, whereas in a collectivist culture, the group and its needs are paramount. In a tight culture, there is considerable agreement about norms of correct behavior. Understanding elements of these syndromes may be very helpful for health educators. Characteristics of individualism and collectivism have some specific implications. For example, the role of the group may influence the content of health education messages. If the focus in a culture is doing what the group wants, the message may be directed differently than in a culture in which the emphasis is on the individual. The strong influence of norms and role-relevant goals in collectivist cultures makes for greater interdependence and embeddedness of social behavior. It may be much more difficult for someone of a collectivist culture to participate in a health behavior that is different from the group's.

CULTURE AND COMMUNICATION Like the specific example of *fatalismo* mentioned earlier, many cultural characteristics directly influence both how people communicate and how they understand and respond to communications they receive. For example, communication is very different between collectivist (high-context) cultures and individualist (low-context) cultures (see Table 7.5). In collectivist cultures, communicators are more likely to focus on the perceiver of information (rather than on themselves) and may communicate to please the receiver. In a more individualist culture, the best arguments are presented first in order to gain attention. As Table 7.5 shows, other aspects of communication may differ, including the structure of argument, the use of words, and the standards used to judge credibility. For instance, in high-context cultures the argument is presented climactically, starting with peripheral arguments and ending with the main argument in order not to offend and in order to gauge the response of the listener. Most often, health educators will create messages that match the communication expectations of a cultural group. Occasionally, however, someone may want to consider responding to a message from a different (or from more than one) point of view—for example, a woman may want to consider making a health decision in concert with her family rather than having her family make it for her.

Table 7.5
Communication Preferences by Collectivist and Individualist Attributes of Culture

INDIVIDUALIST	COLLECTIVIST
Important attributes are expert knowledge, credibility, intelligence.	Important characteristics are family, age, gender, status in the group.
Anticlimactic argument style presents best arguments first to get attention.	Climactic argument style builds up from peripheral arguments in order not to offend the perceiver.
Emphasis is on what is said and on specificity and precision in word usage.	Intuition, ambiguity, generality, vagueness, and bland expressions are preferred.
Silence is negative, indicating hostility, rejection, disagreement, weakness, unwillingness, shyness, anxiety, lack of skill.	Emphasis is on the unspoken: too many words spoils their value. Silence is okay.
Inductive argument presents fact, fact, fact, conclusion.	Face-to-face contact is needed because of the importance of paralinguistic communication.
The opinion of the in-group hierarchy is less important.	Deductive argument is used: conclusion, supportive evidence.
	The opinion of the in-group hierarchy is very important.

Interestingly, Triandis (1994, p. 173) points out that message construction can help people respond more or less in a collectivist or individualist fashion.

Health educators must be particularly careful to clearly understand a cultural communication method before using it. Airhihenbuwa (1994) gives the example of the pitfalls of superficial use of oral culture (ear to mouth, versus visual culture of eye to object) storytelling methods. He points out that stories are a reciprocal vehicle that depend on the listeners' interaction with the teller to create the learning. Any adaptation that makes this method a one-way street loses the power of the method. On the other hand, he points out that imposing a method from outside the culture has different pitfalls. For example, if posters are used to convey information in an oral culture, there will be problems with attention, comprehension, and memory because the learner will first have to learn to attend to this novel source of information.

TRANSLATION Translation of health education and promotion materials into another language is usually aimed at symmetry—a translation that is loyal to the meaning of the source language while ensuring equal familiarity and colloquialness in both languages. Another term for this symmetry is decentering (from the source language). Decentering implies a de-emphasis of the developer's language in such a way that the system of symbols supersedes a single culture. At best, decentering eliminates the distinction between source and target language. Decentering requires a multistage translation that allows for paraphrasing the meaning of the source materials and of the translation before deciding on a translated version. The translation is then translated back to the original language, and the versions are compared. The process of translation and back translation are continued until the two versions are acceptable. The goal is a dynamic equivalence in which a cultural symbol in the source language is translated into a cultural symbol in the target language that evokes the same functional response from the reader or listener. For example, Werner and Campbell (1973) relate the problem of finding a Navaho word for measles; a list of symptoms might have evoked a more meaningful response than trying to find one word that does not originally exist in a language. They relate an even more significant problem of meaning when they explain that the literal translation of "meningitis" into Navaho would be "the covering of the brain is getting red."

Translation is at best approximate, and program development is better done using methods and strategies that are built from within the language and culture of the intended participants. When that is not possible, the health educator should use a decentering approach to translation, introduce redundancy into the text, and use a rich context (Werner & Campbell, 1973).

Translation is another good time to work with focus groups to understand the words used to describe certain phenomena. In creating the Spanish version of the Watch, Discover, Think, and Act program, Bartholomew, Shegog, and colleagues (2000) used focus groups to discover the ways people described asthma and related concepts such as "wheezing" and "inhaler." Many of these words related to asthma had no synonyms in Spanish.

RECIPROCITY IN TEACHING AND LEARNING A powerful way to strive for culturally competent health education programs is to be in constant interaction with program participants so that the creation of meaning is both shared and fluid. This interaction does not require that the health educator be of the same ethnic group as the community, and health educators may become complacent if they have a team member who can be the designated cultural match to the community. This unfortunate tokenism does not guarantee any real cultural similarity between the resource group and the community. We are not saying that recruiting ethnic diversity to program development teams is not essential; it is! But it is not enough to ensure culturally competent practice. Culturally competent practice is based on reciprocity in teaching and learning described by Ladson-Billings (1992, 1995). She describes three broad categories of characteristics of culturally competent teachers. In their conceptions of self and others, culturally competent teachers seem to see themselves as members of the community, and they see community members as capable of changing and learning. They believe in the Freirian notion of "teaching as mining," in other words, as facilitating the emergence of existing capabilities and competencies (Freire, 1974, p. 76). They see social relations as fluid within a community of learners, and they encourage program participants to learn collaboratively and be responsible for one another. Finally, they see knowledge as needing to be created jointly between teachers and learners and viewed critically.

If the flow of information is both ways, then health educators have some opportunity to be congruent with the culture of the learner. Wlodkowski and Ginsberg (1995) list a number of methods and strategies that all have the characteristic of the teacher's authentic interest in the experiences of the learner:

- Critical questioning and guided reciprocal peer questioning (Critical questioning requires the skills of analyzing, inferring, synthesizing, applying, evaluating, comparing, contrasting, verifying, substantiating, explaining, and hypothesizing. It promotes central processing of ideas. Questions would be, What do we already know about . . .? What would happen if . . .? What are the strengths and weaknesses of . . .? What would be the effect of . . .? Why is X important? What are the differences between X and Y?)
- Posing a problem (Generative themes grow out of the learners' culture. They use problematic conditions of daily life to frame learning.)
- Decision making
- Authentic research (i.e., in-depth study of something in order to understand, predict, apply, create, or evaluate some phenomenon)
- Invention and artistry
- Simulation

These reciprocal methods make the creation of meaning a mutual task between teacher and learner. Or said another way, with reciprocal methods every participant is both a teacher and a learner. Such methods should be used in every complex health education situation. For example, Majumdar and Roberts (1998) describe a method of AIDS awareness whereby women were organized into like-culture groups with a facilitator from that cultural group. They then planned the way the program would be delivered in their group.

COMMUNICATING PROGRAM DESIGN AND PRODUCING MATERIALS

The next task in Intervention Mapping Step 3 are to develop design documents to guide the process of program creation and to produce the program materials. Sometimes the support materials for health education programs will be developed by members of the planning group. Other times, there will be money in the budget to hire a variety of creative resources. Either way, documents have to be prepared that guide the producers to produce what is intended for the program.

Hiring and Working With Creative Resources

FINDING AND HIRING CREATIVE RESOURCES In an ideal budgetary world, health educators should take the advice of Balderman (1995) who says that if you weren't trained to do something, don't do it. A creative resource should be hired when the health educator does not have the specific skill needed. Commonly used creative resources include graphic design studios, copywriters, instructional designers, video and film writers, and video and film directors. In addition, production resources can include photographers, illustrators, talent (models and actors), location search companies, printers, videographers, and computer programmers.

In order to find the creative or production resources they need, experienced health educators talk to people. Good sources of referrals are printers or other people who have produced work and can introduce a designer, photographer, or illustrator. Often, branching out from the health field can help. Balderman (1995) suggests the following ways to recruit talent to a project:

- Put together a synopsis of the job including approximate budget, length, purpose, concept, and producing agency.
- Send the synopsis with a request for statements of interest. Schedule meetings with the resources who respond. Interviewing this talent is a good way not only to hire for the current job but also to build a file of possible resources for future work.
- Look at the portfolio of work. How does it feel to you? Is there any evidence that this person has conveyed the type of message needed and gotten the desired response? Do you like the work? Does it all look alike? If so, then it is not exactly right. Go elsewhere.

- Ask about the projects that the works represent. Is there a range of budgets? Ask the person to talk about each project. If the type of product you are thinking about is not represented in the portfolio (which is the best of the best), then you probably cannot get it from this vendor.
- Remember that you will not be designing the piece; the creative resource you are hiring will. Health educators should, at no point, have to take over for the creative person. That person should understand the project's intent well enough that he or she brings you something that is even better than what the team imagined. This scenario implies that the person should be not only creative but also willing to thoroughly understand the team's intent. How does this creative person come off? Is he or she purely a salesperson, or does he or she ask *you* questions to understand the nature of your project? Is the person too quick to assume that it is just like other projects he or she has done? Do you get a sniff of arrogance that comes across in statements like "But I'm the TV producer" or "We never do it like that"? If so, proceed cautiously.

A word about second-guessing the creative resources: don't. Health educators should give their creative people the most understandable background possible and then try not to interfere with their creativity. The opportunity to allow a creative resource to create something independently is one of the reasons for all the planning up to this point. The creative people hired for the project will produce their best effort, and fiddling with it will decrease the quality in some way. It is possible that the person hired for a project just cannot deliver acceptable work, and health educators must know when to cut a designer or other creative person loose. If the rough (the preliminary sketch) is not acceptable, the health educator might ask for one more attempt. The project background and the matrices should be gone over again. But after a couple of unsuccessful tries, the health educator should go back to the hiring process.

CONVEYING PROJECT INTENT   The first step in working with a creative resource is conveying initial project parameters. The first design document includes answers to the following questions:

- What are the pieces that will be produced?
- What are the creative and production elements that will be necessary to produce the project, and who will provide them?
- How will each piece be produced? What is the timeline by piece?
- What is the deadline?
- What is the budget?
- What pre-existing pieces or parts can be provided (e.g., videotape, photos, illustrations, logos, copy)?

- Is there a format that needs to be followed? Is there a corporate or agency manual of style?
- Who needs to be acknowledged?
- What and who will be the approval process?

Health educators who are working with creative resources want them to understand the project as well as possible and to wholeheartedly adopt the planning team's intent. They want the creative person to understand what they understand at this point and then to bring his or her talent to producing it. The person's creative additions should bring to life the team's understanding of the problem and its solution, but should never override or misinterpret it. Some creative people are unable to stay within the project parameters. Health educators may encounter the video producer who, no matter what, will try to turn the team's role-model story into her documentary, or the graphic designer who wants the team's newsletter to be his award winner. However, if the health educator has hired well, he or she will not have to deal with such people.

To get started with a creative person, health educators usually invite him or her to a team meeting to talk about the project once the team can give a fairly consistent message. If possible, the health educator takes the creative person to visit with members of the community. Sometimes the creative person can go to focus groups or interviews. The persons encountered at these meetings may end up in the final materials. For example, Figure 7.2 includes Annon Card of Lufkin, an east Texas town where one of us worked on a campaign to increase acute stroke treatment. Mr. Card had suffered a stroke and was a member of the advisory committee as well as a member of a focus group attended by the video producer and copywriter. He ended up in the media campaign.

In an ideal situation, the designer (or writer or producer) can work with the team almost from the beginning of planning, offering ideas as to format and serving as an expert witness on what is (and is not) doable. The next best approach is to bring the designer in when the matrices, strategies, and methods have been hammered out, but before the team has decided on the formats of the support materials. This approach allows the designer to bring his or her creativity to the table as the planning team figures out what precise form the product will take. The earlier the designer can enter the process, the more his or her skills will enrich the process. Designers and other creative consultants need to be compensated for their time in participating in the planning process.

Writing Design Documents

Figures 7.9 and 7.10 are examples of the sequence and type of tasks that are involved in creating two types of products. The figures are drawn to give a sense of the back and forth between the health education and promotion development team and the creative resources that have been contracted to produce the materials, even if the creative people are part of the health education team. These

Chapter 7 Intervention Mapping Step 3

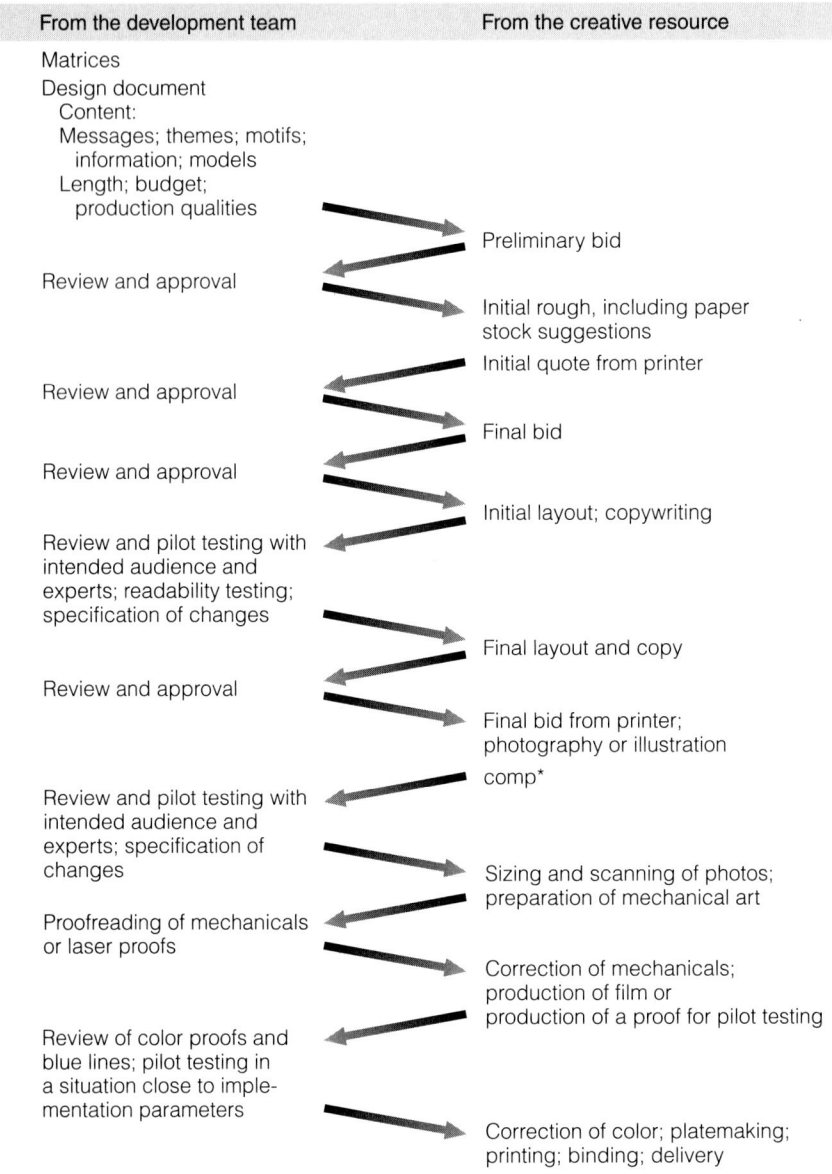

*A comp, or comprehensive, represents the finished product in a more accurate form and detail than does a rough. It shows as closely as possible how the final product will look. Comps are for presentation and pretesting only. They may be required, but will add to the budget.

FIGURE 7.9 Tasks for Producing a Print Piece

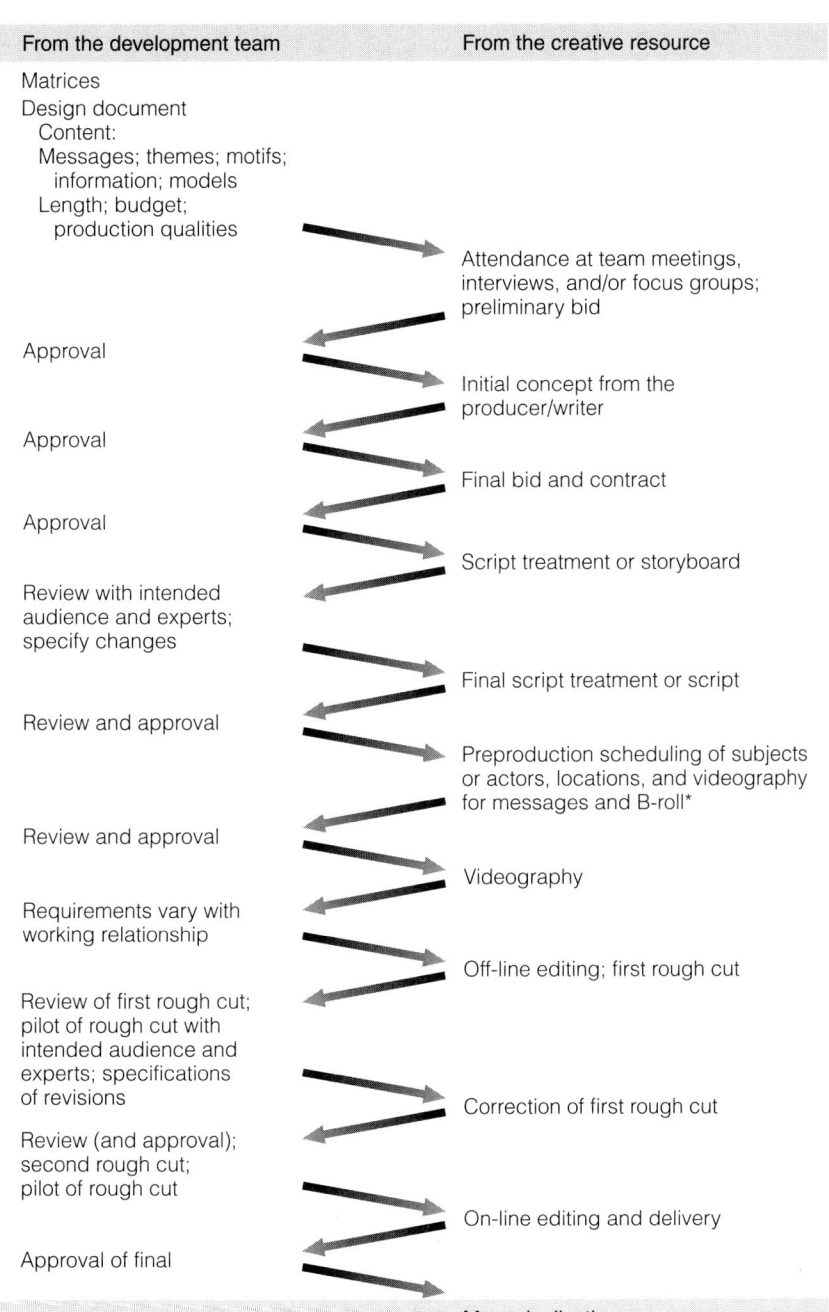

*B-roll is background video to illustrate the point of a voice-over or to make a transition.

FIGURE 7.10 Tasks for Producing a Videotape

figures give an idea of how important the communication of ideas is in this process, and a large part of that communication burden falls on the health educator. He or she must try to communicate in words what someone else will return in various forms of pictures, stories, movement, color, sound, and so forth. It should be noted as well that as the health educator moves down through the figure, inadequate communication or miscommunication becomes more and more costly, so it behooves the health educator to communicate well and in writing at each step.

We have already talked about including the creative people in meetings with the team and the intended audience, but doing so does not alleviate the need for a vehicle to convey the team's intent in detail. We suggest two types of design documents: a series of design documents from the health educator to the creative people and a series of production design documents from the creative people to the health educator. These documents include the matrices, with all the learning and change objectives that are pertinent to a given product highlighted. A second document is a project prospectus that gives the length of the product, a brief description, and the target budget. Tables 7.6 and 7.7 illustrate two of the design documents used for Project PANDA. This project delivered methods through a series of newsletters directed to pregnant women and another series directed to their partners. It also included a videotape for each partner, delivered to their home—the man's prior to the baby's arrival and the woman's just after. The PANDA development team decided to write the first draft of the newsletter copy themselves, so the design document was actually used in-house to convey intent to all the development team members when they had on their copywriter hats (see Table 7.7).

The production design documents that flow from the creative person to the health educator are usually more than written words: They might be written, as in a concept for a videotape, or they might be a combination of words and pictures, as in a storyboard or a rough sketch of a layout. They also might be illustrations or photographs in a layout or rough cut videotape. These documents are all elements of conveying the creative person's image of the final product as it is developed first in the mind of that person and then in some medium. How many of these intermediate production design documents are required will affect the budget.

Creating Design Documents for Abstract Vehicles

At this point, readers who are planning strictly environmental interventions that include only such methods and strategies as policy development, coalition building, and media advocacy are smugly thinking, "All this discussion about design documents doesn't refer to me! I won't be developing traditional materials."

Design documents are also necessary for program components that are not products such as videotapes, PSAs, and the like. Products can be advisory boards, committee meetings, coalitions, or lobbying. Each of these products needs a design document and sometimes more than one. Coalitions, for example, need a design document that specifies how coalition members will be recruited, how meetings

Table 7.6
Project PANDA Design Document for Planning Women's Intervention: Smoking/Time

	29–30 WEEKS	32–34 WEEKS	34–36 WEEKS	IMMEDIATE POSTPARTUM	2 WEEKS POSTPARTUM	4–6 WEEKS POSTPARTUM
Women and smoking	Precontemplator; contemplator; action (model all 3; have them find selves)	Contemplator	Contemplator	Action	Action	Action
Women and ETS control		Contemplator	Action	Action	Action	Action
Outcome	See self as nonsmoker; Attribute success to self; Reassess benefits of not smoking	Be healthier	Acquisition of further skills for not smoking; Preparing for delivery and to return to home as nonsmoker	Relapse prevention: stress reduction; modeling; emotional support	Relapse prevention; specific smoking, cognitive, and behavioral strategies for healthy lifestyle	Relapse prevention; specific strategies for coping with resurfacing of environmental cues
Primary messages	Where are you now?	Personal health/recovery	Aids for creating a nonsmoking environment; cognitive and behavioral strategies for staying off, post-delivery	Having that new baby at home is like nothing before; we've been there; here's what to do for you	Baby and you—a healthier lifestyle; order out of chaos	As you settle in: preparing for return to work or settling into new schedule
Medium	Print	Print	Print	Video	Print	Print

Note. ETS = environmental tobacco smoke.

Table 7.7
Project PANDA Design Document for Planning Women's Intervention #3: Newsletter for 34–36 Weeks

DESCRIPTION	CONTENT	IMPACT
Element 1: Bulletin board Working title: "Let the preparation begin!" Assignment: Sarah	Preparing bags for hospital: hat to bring and what not to bring Preparing house: freeze food; hang no-smoking signs; have some of your favorite things for return from the hospital Seeing home as a place not to smoke; hospital also (don't pack cigs in hospital bag)	Use strategies to enhance environment and control stimuli
Element 2: Feature story Working title: "Using your senses" Assignment: Sarah and Kay	Using senses to experience newborn baby: new baby smell, feel of new skin, etc. Appreciating the role of senses in motherhood; senses that are enhanced after quitting smoking	Focus on benefits of not smoking

Element 3: No-smoking signs (separate from newsletter)
Messages on back of signs
Assignment: Marianna
	For the home and car
	Slogans:
	  "Please don't smoke—tiny lungs at work."
	  Cig with circle and slash
	  "I'm a new mom and I cared enough to quit"
	Effects of passive smoke:
	  "Thanks, Mom, you've saved me from colds and doctor visits"
	  Reasons not to smoke; list from baby's point of view
		Use stimulus control: cues
		Decide not to smoke and to not let others smoke for the baby's sake—protect the baby

Element 4: Tip sheet (detachable) Working title: "Baby's message to relatives and friends" Assignment: Maryann and Angie	Yes, the baby's cute, but mom needs the most attention now Suggestions for helping mom: cooking, grocery shopping, cleaning, laundry	Use tip sheet to structure help after delivery Lessen environmental stress
Element 5: Special feature Working title: "Creating your own smoke-free zone" Assignment: Pat	"Because you know the effects of passive smoke and others may not, you'll need ways to help others not to smoke around your baby" Validate mother's effort to remain smoke-free Provide tips on how to be assertive with others about where they cannot smoke	Recognize that you have the skills to assertively deal with problematic smoking situations Remember passive smoke issues

Table 7.7 *(continued)*

DESCRIPTION	CONTENT	IMPACT
	Phrases to use in certain situations	
	Encourage control over whether smoke that reaches their baby	
	Focus on husband's smoking and how to deal with it	
Element 6: Cartoon Assignment: Sarah	Mom in a tank protecting her baby's "smoke-free zone"	Feel empathy for difficulty of controlling passive smoke
Element 7: Small box Working title: "Baby status report" or "Baby facts" Assignment: Marianna	What's happening with your baby at 34–36 weeks	Stay interested and feel informed

will be run, how minutes or meeting summaries will be constructed and delivered, and much more. A coalition might also need training for membership, and the training session will need a design document. Not only can these documents prevent breakdowns in communication, such as occurred in the mayor's group, but they can also make the processes smooth, productive, and reinforcing to the participants. Figure 7.11 is a coalition design document showing the steps used in recruiting community partners for the Walk Texas! program. Local health departments followed the steps as they tried to establish community walking groups (Jonas, 1998, p. 17). Coalitions must not only recruit members, they must do so in a manner that ensures inclusivity and a broad representation of appropriate stakeholders. Johnson, Grossman, and Cassidy (1996) suggest a three-columned worksheet as a design document. The first column is a listing of appropriate community sectors (e.g., local government, media, parents). The second column is for the name of a recruitment contact within each sector, and the third column is for listing their agreed level of participation. Similar worksheets and other design documents can be deceptively simple but keep the group pointed in the right direction. Another example from Johnson, Grossman, and Cassidy (1996) is the checklist shown in Figure 7.12. It offers a simple but thorough way to assess not only the intentions but the realities of a coalition's inclusivity. Once coalition members are in place, they must create a shared vision for the coalition and its effect on their community. To help community groups develop a shared vision for a drug-free community, for example, Johnson and colleagues (1996, p. 52) suggested such discussion questions as: Five years from now, what will it be like in your community on a Saturday night in the summer? and Five years from now, how will the young people in your community view the future? Such visualization exercises can be empowering to coalition members and energizing to the coalition as a whole.

> Recruiting community partners can be an exciting challenge when you proceed in an organized, well-planned manner. The five steps listed below can help you succeed:
>
> **Step 1:** Determine the characteristics of your ideal partner and list them. Here are some attributes of an ideal community partner.
> - One who reaches the community (i.e., gatekeepers to the audience such as nutrition centers, senior centers, churches)
> - One whose goals and priorities are in line with those of your organization
> - One who is willing to join a partnership
> - One who has credibility (people respect her, she does what she says she will)
> - One with resources (time, money, expertise, facilities, etc.)
> - One who is enthusiastic and willing to work
> - One who is a leader in the community
> - One who can serve as a positive role model
> - One who will champion the cause
>
> **Step 2:** Find potential partners.
> - Satisfied past partners are easy to sell
> - Ask everyone you talk to for more names of potential partners
> - Talk to people who have influence in the community
> - Participate in promotional activities (advertising, booths, etc.)
> - Use lists and directories; don't forget the library
>
> **Step 3:** Do your homework.
> - Gather information about the individual and the organization
>
> **Step 4:** Make an appointment.
> - Schedule a meeting
>
> **Step 5:** Prepare your presentation.
> - Know what you want to accomplish at the meeting
> - Make it clear what's in it for them, but let them express and work through reservations

FIGURE 7.11 Steps for Recruiting Community Partners

A common task of coalition members is advocacy, and examples of advocacy design materials include a guide for interviewing legislators by a three-person team (Figure 7.13). A less elaborate guide can be used for preparing coalition members to make telephone calls to state or national legislators. A typical guide might outline how an advocate should identify him- or herself; "talking points" or brief summaries of relevant data, the conclusion the advocate wishes the legislator to make from this data, a straightforward statement of support (or opposition) to a specific piece of legislation, and an appropriate close (Center for Pediatric Research, 1997). A legislative contact report allows simple but structured record-keeping of such telephone calls and can be used to plan follow-up. A

> The mayor's task force was well on their way to the production of support materials for their multicomponent program. The health educator, while busily looking at portfolios, choosing designers, and trying to understand what the video writer/producer would supply in terms of design documents, received a panicky call from the chair of the group working on the community coalition strategy. She and her cochair were in the neighborhood, so the health educator decided on a spur-of-the-moment face-to-face discussion of whatever was engendering the panic.
>
> "Oh my gosh, we had our first coalition organizational meeting, and it was a free-for-all. I couldn't get hold of the agenda. I know it is supposed to be a participatory agenda. I've read the books. This was participatory all right—participatory by one small group. They took over at the beginning and none of the rest of us could say a thing!"
>
> "Yeah, and one woman felt her ideas were so criticized that she walked out right in the middle of the meeting."
>
> "Several of our most dedicated supporters stopped me afterward and said they didn't know if they could stand to come back."
>
> "And on top of all that, we are not sure whether we all need to start from the beginning together. You know, with all of the groundwork that we have already laid."
>
> The health educator helped the two coalition subgroup chairs plan a strategy. Before their next meeting, the cochairs put together a couple of meeting design documents. One was on how a participatory agenda would be created; the other was a format for meeting summaries that used the meeting that had just occurred. Finally, they put together the coalition overview and task document that would serve as a beginning for group development and task orientation in the coalition.

contact report might, for example, provide room to record the caller's name, who was called, the topic of the discussion, check-boxes for indicating the legislator's overall reaction, space for significant comments or suggestions from the legislator, and the caller's comments or recommendations for follow-up (Public Affairs Committee, Northern Virginia HIV Consortium). Such materials provide how-to information for members and could be used as part of an advocacy training session and, as with legislative contacts, letter and telephone scripts can in themselves serve as micro-media messages.

Working With a Print Designer

Figure 7.9 (page 264) gives an example of the process involved in producing a print piece. Whoever is doing the design and managing the production must have some idea of the content before design starts—for example, a list of the types of stories to appear in each issue or piece and their likely length. This information and many other design elements must be clear to the designer before he or she

Checking for Inclusivity

Now that coalition members are beginning to be in place, you need to assess inclusivity. Place a check mark in the box next to each statement that applies to your group. If you cannot put a check in the box, this may indicate an area for change.

☐ The leadership of our partnership reflects the ethnic and cultural diversity in our community.

☐ We make special efforts to cultivate new leaders, particularly women and people of color.

☐ Our mission, operations, and products reflect diverse cultural and social group contributions.

☐ We fight social oppression within the partnership and in our work with the community.

☐ Members of diverse cultural and social groups are full participants in the group's work.

☐ No speaker from any one group dominates meetings.

☐ The whole community is represented in decision making.

☐ We are sensitive to diverse cultural holidays, customs, and meeting food preferences.

☐ We communicate clearly; people of different cultures share opinions and participate.

☐ We prohibit the use of stereotypes and prejudicial comments.

☐ Ethnic, racial, and sexual slurs or jokes are prohibited.

FIGURE 7.12 Recruiting Coalition Members and Ensuring Inclusivity—Checking for Inclusivity (*Note.* Adapted from Kaye, Gillian and Wolff, Tom. *From the Ground Up! A workbook on Coalition Building and Community Development,* available from AHEC/Community Partners, 24 South Prospect St., Amherst MA 01002)

completes a design. The designer must also be given a clear description of the audience, their special needs, and the contexts in which the material will be used. Material that is to be published in a three-ring binder, for instance, normally calls for a larger size type than does a brochure, because it will be laid on a table to be read. An item that a parent will be consulting while bathing a baby had best be waterproof. All the facts must be clear *before* the design process starts. This second design document includes answers to at least the following questions:

- Who is the audience for this piece? What are they like?
- Where and when will they be using it?
- What is the purpose of the piece? What determinants is it supposed to change? What will the readers or listeners ideally do in response to the piece?
- What are the central messages of the piece?

- What design elements or types of copy will the piece have (e.g., levels of subheads, lists, tables, graphs, charts, illustrations, captions, pull quotes, footnotes or references, interviews, step-by-step instructions)? The more elements there are, the more complicated the design process, though the best result is usually something that does not *look* like a complicated design.
- When and how will the project need updating?
- What are the costs and constraints? The institutional graphics standards? What process will be used to review the piece?
- What aspects of the production process is the team responsible for? Who will produce the camera-ready copy? Will the piece be photocopied or printed?

Next, the designer lists the elements of the design that will be needed to carry the important messages. Will the piece have line illustrations? Photos? Frequent bulleted lists? This list includes all the elements the design will have to accommodate. Should there be places for people to enter personal information? Does the piece serve as a reference tool in which people have to find a particular section quickly?

It is also important to consider how the finished piece will be put together. If a piece is lengthy and requires frequent additions or changes, a three-ring binder is a good choice. If a piece must lay flat, consider wire coil; this plasticized wire comes in a number of colors, does not snag clothing, and allows any page to be flat. Comb binding is inexpensive but not particularly attractive.

Once a designer offers an acceptable design, the content will have to be edited to conform to it. Asking for changes to a completed design is counterproductive: Changing the design will cost more money while decreasing the quality of the result. Also, a good adage to remember is: "You can get it good, you can get it fast, and you can get it cheap, but you can't have all three." Health educators aim for two out of three by talking with suppliers about how long it will take to get the desired quality of product. We also refer the reader to works on basic design principles. Understanding a little about what process designers use can help health educators work *with* rather than against them (Doak et al., 1995; Parker, 1988; White, 1988; Williams, 1994).

Writing and Organizing to Help the Reader

The greatest design in the world can't make up for poor writing or confusing organization. Copywriters should use an active voice. People skim as they read; lists should be understandable without the introductory sentence. For example, in a list of things people should not do, every item should begin with "do not." The writing should be as clear as possible. For example, if the meaning is "do not," copywriters should not use the term "avoid." "Avoid" is often interpreted as "try not to do this, but do it when you have to." The material needs to be presented in the order people need the information. Messages should be matched to the learning and change objectives; everything else should be cut.

The text is broken up, or chunked, through the use of subheads. Descriptive subheads are used within long lists to group items in chunks of 3 to 5 entries each (Doak et al., 1995). Glynn and Britton (1984) suggest a careful hierarchy to support comprehension. They also suggest advance organizers and learning objectives (see Chapter 6) to help the reader integrate text information with relevant personal knowledge. Step-by-step instructions are presented as a numbered list. Checklists can have open boxes in front of each item so that each can literally be checked off. Bullets (solid dots) mark off each item in other kinds of lists; numbered lists are not used for items that can be done in any sequence (Manning, 1981).

The text will be most approachable if it uses one- and two-syllable words and short, simple sentences in active voice. Topic sentences state the main idea at the beginning of a paragraph, and help the reader follow the material. Readers will find it easier to understand a message if sentences are restricted to one idea at a time and if the text includes summaries that are labeled as such. Short slogans help make key points memorable; very important ideas and terms can be highlighted with boldface or italics. Difficult words can be defined by context clues and by appositional phrases and parenthetical statements.

It seems self-evident, but print media shouldn't be used if the intended participants can't read (Torrence & Torrence, 1987). Sometimes technical material is difficult to write below a fifth-grade level without losing meaning and becoming patronizing. Such technical material is perhaps better presented through another medium. Copywriters should avoid the trap of replacing commonly heard words with less commonly heard (but shorter) words; it may lower the computed reading level but will interfere with comprehension. When possible, health educators can prepare the group for the material by determining what the group members need to know *before* they read (e.g., vocabulary) and teaching it and by discussing the point of the material (what readers are supposed to get from it).

Working With Video Writers and Producers

Videotapes can be a good solution to some problems. Many people do not read well enough to learn skills from print materials, for example. The production costs for videotapes are in the master; the individual copies are very inexpensive. The more copies that are needed, therefore, the more cost-effective a medium videotape is. VCRs and televisions are ubiquitous in the United States, and the equipment to make a videotape is also commonplace. Unfortunately, this easy access can lead to the fallacious assumption that making a useful videotape consists of pointing, shooting, and running off copies.

Figure 7.10 (p. 265) presents processes in the production of a videotape. Early in the process, the producer must develop an understanding of what the development team has planned, and optimally the producer has participated in some contacts with the intended audiences. An early step in working with a video producer is the contract. The contract (and therefore, the budget) should include a rough-cut review and approval. A rough cut is usually an off-line edit of the product prior to final on-line editing, which is when all the bells and whistles such as music are added to a tape. In our experience, the rough cut is the moment to perform final pretesting with the development team, the intended participants, and the gatekeepers or program implementers. There must be money in the budget for production of this intermediate stage and for revisions. It helps greatly if the health educator has been at the shoots so that the material included in the rough cut is not a surprise. Other examples of contract considerations are casting approval, credits, and copyright. The program development team (not the video producers) should have the assigned copyright so that video images can be recycled from one medium to another. Any artwork bought for the videotape will also have a contract with it that specifies who owns the material. It is important to

Communicating Program Design and Producing Materials

The interviewing team should consist of three members, each of whom has a specific function. These functions should be thoroughly delineated, and there should be no overlapping of function.

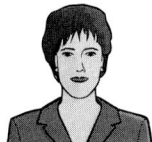

The leader, or team captain:

This person sets the tone of the interview; establishes rapport with the candidate; is a "nice guy" type; must be friendly and courteous and never show any hostility; puts the question—again, objectively—and supplies whatever background information is needed.

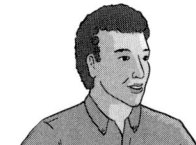

The listener, or reporter:

This person, after saying "How do you do?" doesn't say anything at all; bends all efforts toward being perceptive and toward committing as much of the interview to memory as possible; *does not take notes* (nothing inhibits free discussion more than a pencil and notepad in someone's hands); not only listens to what is said, but also listens for attitudes, for signs of strain (e.g., Every time budget is mentioned, the candidate pulls an earlobe. What could this mean?); tries to spot the candidate's hidden agenda, or why the person is seeking office.

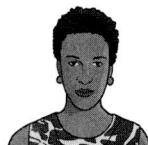

The tracker:

This person has either a big job or a small one, depending on how the conversation goes. The tracker keeps the conversation from meandering fruitlessly. If the interview seems off on a tangent, the tracker can courteously interrupt with phrases such as "you said a moment ago that . . ." "Did you mean . . .?" or "I think Leader meant to ask if . . ." The tracker keeps the interview moving and could signal its change of pace or termination. However, the tracker should not attempt to stifle a discussion that is giving some insights even though it is off track.

Do	Don't
• Be prepared to state your views clearly.	• Don't prolong the interview.
• Have appropriate materials to hand out.	• Don't tip off the "best answer."
• Be on time.	• Don't do all the talking. (Sometimes silence will bring out interesting information.)
• Be friendly, positive, and constructive.	• Don't let the candidate interview you.
• Be specific about your position.	• Don't attempt to exact "rash promises." Obtain reasons for opposition and ask what you can do to help support efforts.
• Be brief! Be brief! Be brief!	

FIGURE 7.13 Organizing the Legislative Interview Team

have legal title and custody of the master tape. Health educators should obtain from the production company copies of all releases—and should make sure that everyone signs a release before setting a foot in front of the camera.

A vital component of videotape production, and a centerpiece of work between a development team and a video producer, is the script or script treatment. A script details the audio and visuals for every scene, whereas a script treatment is for use when stories will be obtained directly from members of the community and edited together. A video script is very different from material that is meant to be read; it is meant to be seen and heard, and people do not talk the way they write. In addition, a video has about 15 seconds to grab the audience's attention, and it has to recapture that attention every 15 seconds after that. To use the video medium to best advantage, it is important that the picture tell the story and that words complete the messages. A video producer should first offer a preliminary script treatment—a scene-by-scene message, a look-and-feel description, or a storyboard with the same information plus visuals. After receiving approval at this stage, the producer can move to final script treatment or script.

Script approval is a formal process and a key point in the creative cycle. Health educators often underestimate the number of people who should approve the video. These same people also should review the script. Reshoots are a budget-buster and in some situations may not even be possible. If the same video is needed in more than one language, the script should be translated as soon as the original is approved. For live-action shots, it can be cost-efficient to shoot all language versions at the same time. For voice-over footage, producers need to allow for the difference in length of the narration and shoot the footage to allow for the longer narration time.

The final script should be compared against the budget, because the more complex the script is or the more difficult it is to shoot, the greater the shooting and editing costs will be. Health educators should consult an experienced videographer before approving the final script. Script approval is also the time for everyone to approve the credits and the copy for the labels and packaging. Although the credits can seem a simple task, if left to the last minute they will invariably have errors, and revising credits can be quite time-consuming for the production house.

Script approval is followed by preproduction. Preproduction includes such tasks as finding locations, actors, and props and scheduling the film crew. Although some preproduction can be done in tandem with script development, there are always items contingent on the final script.

During production, the actual filming will be done neither on film nor on ordinary VHS-quality videotape. If producers were to shoot the original on ordinary videotape, the distributed version would be a copy, and just as with a copy of a photocopy, it would lose some of its clarity and crispness. Currently most productions use half-inch professional videotape (down from three-quarter inch), though the technology is changing rapidly toward digital production.

The first task of postproduction is the creation of a rough cut that can be checked for appropriate execution of methods and strategies and then pretested.

We repeat: Checking the rough cut is a crucial point in program development. For example, in Project PANDA, the videotape for women who had stopped smoking during pregnancy was to be delivered to their homes immediately postpartum, when stress and sleep deprivation are at their height. Even though the program planners had been present during shooting and had seen the raw footage, the rough cut came as a surprise. The development team was looking for *coping models* for the immediate postpartum period, and the video producer (who had not yet had children) had included only the most "together" women. These *mastery models* seemed to have handled the transition to nonsmoking parenthood flawlessly, and they might have caused the self-efficacy of the target women to decrease in comparison. Before pretesting the tape, the development team asked for a second rough cut that would include more models who were moving toward success rather than models who were already there. Following approval of the rough cut, the music soundtrack, graphics, and credits are inserted, and a final master tape is produced.

PRETESTING AND REVISING

The final task in Intervention Mapping Step 3 is to pretest and revise program materials. Atkin and Freimuth (1989) describe two types of formative evaluation research: preproduction and production. Preproduction research discovers characteristics of the intended participants that relate to message, medium, and situation, whereas production testing (pretesting) is a process in which prototypes of program materials are tested for audience reaction.

Preproduction Research

Preproduction research includes (a) identifying the anticipated audience, (b) specifying the health behavior, (c) elaborating the intermediate responses (determinants), (d) ascertaining channel and vehicle use, and (e) conducting a preliminary evaluation of message components. Health educators who have done a careful job of Intervention Mapping to this point have already completed the first three steps of this research. Here we focus on the last two.

Before channels and vehicles for delivery of program components can be chosen, the preferred media use by intended audiences must be ascertained.

- Do they watch television, listen to the radio, and read newspapers and magazines?
- What amount of time do they spend with each medium?
- What content do they attend to (e.g., news, talk shows, PSAs, entertainment)?
- What channels are used to get information about the program topic?

Entertainment programming has become a popular vehicle for health education and promotion. Early in the history of edu-tainment, effort was expended on convincing producers to "do the right thing" about health messages within program content, such as the presence of smokers (Montgomery, 1988, 1990). Now, increasingly, both cartoon and dramatic shows with appropriate health messages are aimed at all age groups in the United States. On a recent episode of *Felicity*, a drama about a college freshman with great appeal to middle schoolers, the title character modeled sexual decision making, including the demonstration of the correct way to use a condom (obtained from the college health service).

In the preproduction research phase, health educators explore interpersonal as well as media channels. Freimuth (1985) also suggests ascertaining credibility of vehicles and sources and the recall of previous messages on a topic. Preproduction testing can include both informal feedback and ratings of sources, messages, themes, persuasive arguments, and stylistic devices. Focus groups are a good mechanism for preproduction testing. Work at this point can be very important in determining program messages. For example, in the development of the Cystic Fibrosis Family Education Program, we held focus groups with children, adolescents, and parents who would be using the program. One issue that stood out was the adolescents' discussion of being different from their peers. The program developers had thought that "worrying about being different" should be dealt with explicitly in the program. However, the adolescents with cystic fibrosis said in no uncertain terms, "We are not different and we will 'trash' anything that addresses this subject." With this and other feedback, it was back to the drawing board for the developers.

Pretesting

Table 7.8 presents various pretesting methods. The first pretesting that health educators conduct is to test initial program concepts, including key phrases and visuals proposed to portray the main ideas. Focus groups and interviews are good for this purpose. A very important reason for this process is to discover the words, phrases, and vernacular used by members of the at-risk group on the topic.

In the next stage of pretesting, the various program components are executed in rough and are tested to determine attention, comprehension, strong and weak points, and personal relevance. At this point, potential objection to sensitive or controversial issues can be gauged. A major dilemma at this stage is how to get materials in final-enough form to be good stimulus material without spending too much extra money. For example, videotapes can be presented in storyboard format, as can PSAs. Radio PSAs can be read aloud, and newsletters can be produced with a word processing format. However, as much of the final product as possible should be included—illustrations, photographs, and graphics for newsletters rather than just the words, for example. It is also important to evaluate individual aspects of materials rather than just the whole. For example, Project PANDA newsletters were reviewed by two panels of consultants, one of

Table 7.8
Pretesting Methods

	CONCEPT TESTING	READABILITY TESTING	EXECUTING THE MESSAGE	IMPACT ON DETERMINANTS	ADOPTION/ IMPLEMENTATION CHARACTERISTICS
Purpose	To develop and test the key phrases and visuals that portray the main ideas; to discover vernacular	To estimate school grade reading level required to read text	To determine whether program material messages are attended to, comprehended, appealing, and culturally relevant	To get a sense of possible impact or to actually measure impact	To see how the materials are perceived in terms of complexity, trialability, observability, and relative advantage by those who will adopt and implement them; to determine problems with implementation
Materials and strategies	Interviews and focus groups	Text and readability program such as FOG or SMOG; computer program	Interviews, focus groups, questionnaires after exposure, theater testing	Interviews, focus groups after exposure; measurement via instruments designed from the determinants columns of the matrices	Interviews and focus groups after review by potential adopters and implementers; observation of trial implementation
How to	Use concept ideas as stimulus materials; ask people how they would convey an idea	Apply the program or formula; apply to each component	Ask people to tell you what they "got" from the product; separate components; assess identification with questions such as "how much were these people like you?" (looked like you, expressed thoughts and feelings you might have, etc.)	(see Chapter 9)	Ask for review by naive potential implementers, not those who have worked on development; make pilot as realistic as possible
Can't be used for	Nothing at this stage is attributable to the executed materials	Determining whether text will be understood by intended readers	Estimating total impact	Only a formative evaluation; without a control group, change is not attributable to the program	Determining actual adoption rate

Familiar Faces, Familiar Routines

About this time, most new mothers feel more like their old selves and are going back to their usual activities. They are no longer getting the special treatment of pregnancy and the first few weeks after giving birth. They are feeling the demands of job and family.

Re-entering life as it was before brings some special challenges. You changed because you gave birth and are now responsible for another, very needy human being. In pregnancy, you were more conscious of your body and how you treated it, you ate more healthful foods, and you stopped smoking.

Although most women would like to stick to these healthy patterns, it's easy to drift back into the old ones. Now is the time to make a conscious decision about what you want for yourself. Don't expect this to be easy, because old habits arise with old routines. For example, your partner and coworkers probably didn't expect you to smoke along with them while you were pregnant. But now they may think there's no reason for you not to.

Women who went through this process tell us that drinking juice or water during coffee breaks with coworkers reduces the temptation to smoke. Another technique is keeping both hands busy with handwork like needlepoint, which interferes with smoking but promotes conversation.

Tell people what you've decided to do, but don't judge them. One mother who returned to work told us, "It's easy to act self-righteous about changing my habits, and get down on others for continuing to smoke or eat unhealthy foods. But I remember how hard and slow the change was for me. It doesn't give me the license to judge someone else for the choices they make. Reminding myself of this helps me think twice before I reach for a cigarette or for another doughnut at the office."

Circle the appropriate number.

This article:

A. was not interesting 1	was moderately interesting 2	was very interesting 3
B. was not easy to understand 1	was moderately easy to understand 2	was very easy to understand 3
C. did not apply to my life 1	moderately applied to my life 2	very much applied to my life 3
D. included information that was not helpful 1	included information that was moderately helpful 2	included information that was very helpful 3

FIGURE 7.14 Article Response Box from Project PANDA Pretest

women and one of partners. Response boxes were included for each newsletter article (see Figure 7.14).

In Intervention Mapping Step 2, decisions were made on theoretical methods and practical strategies. For instance, in the development of the AIDS prevention program (Chapter 10), the developers selected modeling, active learning, and feedback as methods for improving self-efficacy. For the strategies, the developers chose to create an interactive video presentation in which peer models present a scenario on video; the students stop the video and have a group discussion about solutions; the peer models on video present a solution; and the teacher gives the students feedback on their solutions. Although this video presentation is only a part of the program, it requires many decisions and assumptions. For instance, an assumption for the use of peer models is that students will find these models attractive (Bandura, 1986). Pretesting of the program should be an assurance for this assumption, but in practice not all models communicate a positive image. Another assumption for the educational program is that students will pay attention to the program because they have become aware of its personal relevance (McGuire, 1985). Again, pretesting should address this assumption, but it also has to be measured in a process evaluation (Chapter 9).

In addition to the methods of focus groups and in-depth interviews, central location intercept interviewing and theater testing are good for pretesting. In central location intercept, interviewers armed with questionnaires ask for responses from people in high-traffic areas such as malls and grocery stores. In theater testing for television spots, groups of watchers are asked to respond to programs or other television components amid simulated television clutter. For example, spots are aired between two 30-minute television shows. After the first show, spots are interspaced between irrelevant material, and after the next 30-minute show, viewers are tested for recall. Viewers are then shown the messages again and asked about specific characteristics. Day-after recall can also be used to assess what is remembered from various program materials.

Program developers must also conduct gatekeeper reviews and use testing so that the people who will implement and maintain the program review the components; the materials must also be tested in real life or a simulation of real life. This review is to ascertain how the materials are perceived in terms of characteristics that have been shown to influence adoption and implementation. Such testing can also uncover potential problems with implementation plans. (See Chapter 8 for more on adoption and implementation.) For this pretesting, it is important to find potential implementers and gatekeepers who have not been a part of program development.

Making Sense of Pretest Data

At every step of pretesting, there is the likelihood of obtaining conflicting data. Table 7.9 presents one method for organizing data from the participant review. This method does not include the opinions of gatekeepers and implementers, which would be summarized in another table. The point is to use some mechanism to make clear what is being said and how strongly it is being said. The "implications" note reminds the planner to consider what would be left out of the intervention in terms of methods, strategies, and messages if the material was changed on the basis of reviewers' comments. For example, according to Table 7.9, some reviewers did not particularly like the role-model stories. The developer then has to decide whether to leave the stories as they are, to change them, or to

Table 7.9
Making Sense of Pretest Data

MATERIAL NAME: MANAGING HIV IN YOUR CHILD

Component	Category			
	Role modeling	Skill training	Technical content	Other
Module 1: Observing signs and symptoms	Comments: The stories are just a waste of space. (1) The stories are great. I felt exactly like that. (1) In response to specific question about stories: Leave them in. They're okay. Not bad, not good. (8)	Comments: Steps are not broken down enough. (2)	Comments: This is not what I was taught by the nurse. (3)	Comments: It is so nice to have these materials to follow. (6)
	Implications: There would be damage to methods if role modeling were deleted.	Implications: Review to ensure enough detail.	Implications: Ask nurses to review materials again. Plan training.	
Module 2: Treating infections	Comments:	Comments: Steps are not broken down enough. (6) Cards with medications are too easy to lose.	Comments:	Comments:
	Implications:	Implications: How to avoid giving unneeded drug info	Implications:	Implications:
Module 3: Maintaining good nutrition	Comments: Maybe if these mothers can get their children to eat, I can.	Comments: Impractical. (1) Can't do this. (3) My child won't eat these things. (4)	Comments: Yes, this is exactly what the dietitian tells us.	Comments:
	Implications:	Implications: Review again with parents. Add more popular foods.	Implications:	Implications:

Note. Numbers indicate the number of people who made similar comments.

delete them. If the stories are deleted, then the method of role modeling (strategy—role-model stories) is deleted and should be replaced by an equally powerful method or re-executed in a different strategy with different messages. Making appropriate use of pretest data requires working back through messages, strategies, and methods to matrices to ensure that changes in the program materials do not leave holes in the intervention chain of causation.

SUMMARY

Guidance on how to organize programs and produce health education program support materials is a massive topic that requires a text of its own. We have enabled the reader to do what we consider crucial in this step: (a) Revisit the intended participants multiple times in the development of program ideas and the pretesting of materials; (b) struggle to produce culturally competent programs; (c) write excellent design documents to convey planning intent to the production process; and (d) pretest all program components.

Tasks for Intervention Mapping Step 3:
- Operationalize the strategies into plans that consider implementers and sites
- Develop design documents and produce materials
- Pretest programs and materials with target groups and implementers

REFERENCES

Abramson, S., Shegog, R., Bartholomew, L. K., Sockrider, M. M., Czyzewski, D. I., & Mullen, P. D. (2000). *Conceptual basis of an expert system to promote asthma self-management support behavior of asthma health care providers.* Manuscript in preparation.

Airhihenbuwa, C. O. (1994). Health promotion and the discourse on culture: Implications for empowerment. *Health Education Quarterly, 21*(3), 345–353.

Altman, D. G. (1995a). Strategies for community health intervention: Promises, paradoxes, pitfalls. *Psychosomatic Medicine, 57*(3), 226–233.

Altman, D. G. (1995b). Sustaining interventions in community systems: On the relationship between researchers and communities. *Health Psychology, 14*(6), 526–536.

Atkin, C. K., & Freimuth, C. (1989). Formative evaluation research in campaign design. In R. E. Rice & C. K. Atkin (Eds.), *Public communication campaigns* (pp.131–150). Newbury Park, CA: Sage.

Balderman, B. (1995). *Buying creative services.* Lincolnwood, IL: NTC Publishing Group.

Bandura, A. (1986). *Social foundations of thought and action: A social cognitive theory.* New York: Prentice Hall.

Bartholomew, L. K., Gold, R. S., Parcel, G. S., Czyzewski, D. I., Sockrider, M. M., Fernandez, M., Shegog, R., & Swank, P. R. (2000). Watch, Discover, Think, and Act: Evaluation of computer-assisted instruction to improve asthma self-management in inner-city children. *Patient Education and Counseling, 39*(2–3), 269–280.

Bartholomew, L. K., Shegog, R., Parcel, G. S., Gold, R. S., Fernandez, M., Czyzewski, D. I., Sockrider, M. M., & Berlin, N. (2000). Watch, Discover, Think, and Act: A model for patient education program development. *Patient Education and Counseling, 39*(2–3), 253–268.

Bental, D. S., Cawsey, A., & Jones, R. (1999). Patient information systems that tailor to the individual. *Patient Education and Counseling, 36*(2), 171–180.

Brennan, F. A., & Fink, S. V. (1997). Health promotion, social support, and computer networks. In R. Street, W. Gold, & T. Manning (Eds.), *Health promotion and interactive technology: Theoretical applications and future directions* (pp. 157–169). Mahwah, NJ: Erlbaum.

Brennan, P., Ripich, S., & Moore, S. (1991). The use of home-based computers to support persons living with AIDS/ARC. *Journal of Community Health Nursing, 8*(1), 3–14.

Brown, S. J., Lieberman, D. A., Germeny, B. A., Fan, Y. C., Wilson, D. M., & Pasta, D. J. (1997). Education video game for juvenile diabetes self-care: Results of a controlled trial. *Medical Informatics, 22*(1), 77–89.

Brug, J., Glanz, K., Van Assema, P., Kok, G., & Van Breukelen, G. J. (1998). The impact of computer-tailored feedback and iterative feedback on fat, fruit, and vegetable intake. *Health Education and Behavior, 25*(4), 517–531.

Brug, J., Steenhuis, I., Van Assema, P., De Vries, H. (1996). The impact of a computer-tailored nutrition intervention. *Preventive Medicine, 25*(3), 236–242.

Bull, F. C., Kreuter, M. W., & Scharff, D. P. (1999). Effects of tailored, personalized, and general health messages on physical activity. *Patient Education and Counseling, 36*(2), 181–192.

CDC AIDS Community Demonstration Projects Research Group. (1999). Community-level HIV intervention in 5 cities: Final outcome data from the CDC AIDS Community Demonstration Projects. *American Journal of Public Health, 89*(3), 336–345.

Center for Pediatric Research. (1997, April 27–30). Materials for Coalition Training Institute. Eastern Virginia Medical School, Norfolk. VA.

Chaffe, S. H., & Roser, C. (1986). Involvement and the consistency of knowledge, attitudes, and behavior. *Communication Research, 13*(3), 373–399.

Corby, N. H., Enguidamos, S. M., & Kay, L. S. (1996). Development and use of role model stories in a community-level HIV risk reduction intervention. *Public Health Reports, 111*(1, Suppl.), 54–58.

Cullinane, P. M., Hyppolite, K., Zastawney, A. L., & Friedman, R. H. (1994). Telephone linked communication: Activity counseling and tracking for older patients. *Journal of General Internal Medicine, 9*(4, Suppl. 2), 86.

Curry, S. J., McBride, C., Grothaus, L. C., Louie, D., & Wagner, E. H. (1995). A randomized trial of self-help materials, personalized feedback, and telephone counseling with nonvolunteer smokers. *Journal of Consulting and Clinical Psychology, 63*(6), 1005–1014.

Curry, S. J., Wagner, E. H., & Grothaus, L. C. (1991). Evaluation of intrinsic and extrinsic motivation interventions with a self-help smoking cessation program. *Journal of Consulting and Clinical Psychology, 59*(2), 318–324.

Dede, C., & Fontana, L. (1995). Transforming health education via new media. In L. M. Harris (Ed.), *Health and the new media: Technologies transforming personal and public health* (pp. 163–183). Mahwah, NJ: Erlbaum.

Dijkstra, A., & De Vries, H. (1999). The development of computer-generated tailored interventions. *Patient Education and Counseling, 36*(2), 193–203.

Dijkstra, A., De Vries, H., & Roijackers, J. (1998). Long-term effectiveness of computer-generated tailored feedback in smoking cessation. *Health Education Research, 13*(2), 207–214.

Dijkstra, A., De Vries, H., Roijackers, J., & Van Breukelen, G. (1998a). Tailored interventions to communicate stage-matched information to smokers in diffcrent motivational stages. *Journal of Consulting and Clinical Psychology, 66*(3), 549–557.

Dijkstra, A., De Vries, H., Roijackers, J., & Van Breukelen, G. (1998b). Tailoring information to enhance quitting in smokers with low motivation to quit: Three basic efficacy questions. *Health Psychology, 17*(6), 513–519.

Doak, C. C., Doak, L. G., & Root, J. H. (1995). *Teaching patients with low literacy skills* (2nd ed.). Philadelphia: Lippincott, Williams, & Wilkins.

Dutton, J. P., Posner, B. A., Smigelski, C., & Friedman, R. H. (1995). Lowering of total serum cholesterol through the use of DietAid? A telecommunications system for dietary counseling. *Annals of Behavioral Medicine, 17,* s088.

Elder, J. P., Geller, E. S., Hovell, M. F., & Mayer, J. A. (1994). *Motivating health behavior.* Albany, NY: Delmar.

Fishman, S. (1997). *The copyright handbook: How to protect and use written works* (4th ed.). Berkeley, CA: Nolo Press.

Flesch, R. (1949). *The art of readable writing: With the Flesch readability formula.* New York: Harper and Row.

Freimuth, V. S. (1985). Developing the public service advertisement for nonprofit marketing. In R. Belk (Ed.), *Advances in nonprofit marketing* (Vol. 1, pp. 55–95). Greenwich, CT: JAI.

Freire, P. (1974). *Pedagogy of the oppressed.* New York: Seabury.

Friedman, R. H., Kazis, L. E., Jette, A., Smith, M. B., Stollerman, J. E., Torgerson, J., & Carey, K. (1996). A telecommunications system for monitoring and counseling patients with hypertension: Impact on medication adherence and blood pressure control. *American Journal of Hypertension, 9*(4, Pt. 1), 285–292.

Fry, E. (1977). Fry's readability graph: Clarifications, validity, and extension to Level 17. *Journal of Reading, 21*(3), 242–252.

Gedney, K., & Fultz, P. (1988). *The complete guide to creating successful brochures.* Brentwood, NY: Asher-Gallant Press.

Glynn, S. M., & Britton, B. (1984, October). Supporting readers' comprehension through effective text design. *Educational Technology, 24*(10), 40–43.

Gustafson, D. H., Bosworth, K., Chewning, B., & Hawkins, R. P. (1987). Computer-based health promotion: Combining technological advances with problem-solving techniques to effect successful health behavior changes. *Annual Review of Public Health, 8,* 387–415.

Gustafson, D. H., Wise, M., McTavish, F., Taylor, J., Wolberg, W., Stewart, J., Smalley, R., & Bosworth, K. (1993). Development and pilot evaluation of a computer-based support system for women with breast cancer. *Journal of Psychosocial Oncology, 11*(4), 69–93.

Hawkins, R. P., Pingree, S., Gustafson, D. H., Boberg, E. W., Bricker, E., McTavish, F., Wise, M., & Owens, B. (1997). Aiding those facing health crises: The experience of the CHESS Project. In R. Street, W. Gold, & T. Manning (Eds.), *Health promotion and interactive technology: Theoretical applications and future directions* (pp. 79–102). Mahwah, NJ: Erlbaum.

Helman, C. G. (1990). *Culture, health, and illness* (2nd ed.). London: Wright.

Holcomb, C., & Ellis, J. (1978). Measuring the readability of selected patient education materials: The CLOSE procedure. *Health Education, 9*(6), 8.

Irwin, J. W., & Davis, C. A. (1980). Assessing readability, the checklist approach. *Journal of Reading, 24*(2), 124–130.

Johnson, K., Grossman, W., & Cassidy A. (Eds.). (1996). *Collaborating to improve community health workbook and guide.* San Francisco: Jossey-Bass and The Healthcare Forum.

Jonas, J. R. (1998). *WalkTexas! start-up kit.* (Available from Texas Diabetes Program/Council, Texas Department of Health, 1100 West 49th St., Austin, TX 78756 and at http://www.tdh.texas.gov/diabetes/walktx/index.html as of March 2000.)

Kaye, G., & Wolff, T. (Eds.). (1997). *From the ground up! A workbook on coalition building and community development* (Available from AHEC/Community Partners, 24 South

Prospect St., Amherst, MA 01002 and at http://ahecpartners.org/resources/order/index.stm as of March 2000.)

Kluckhohn, C. (1954). Culture and behavior. In G. Lindzey (Ed.), *Handbook of social psychology* (Vol. 2, pp. 921–976). Cambridge, MA: Addison Wesley.

Kreuter, M. W., & Strecher, V. J. (1996). Do tailored behavior change messages enhance the effectiveness of health risk appraisal: Results from a randomized trial. *Health Education Research, 11*(1), 97–105.

Ladson-Billings, G. (1992). Culturally relevant teaching: The key to making multicultural education work. In C. A. Grant (Ed.), *Research and multicultural education: From the margins to the mainstream.* Washington, DC: Falmer Press.

Ladson-Billings, G. (1995). Toward a theory of culturally relevant pedagogy. *American Educational Research Journal, 32*(3), 465–491.

Lefebvre, R. C., & Flora, J. A. (1988). Social marketing and public health intervention. *Health Education Quarterly, 15*(3), 229–315.

Lieberman, D. A. (1997). Interactive video games for health promotion: Effects on knowledge, self-efficacy, social support, and health. In R. Street, W. Gold, & T. Manning (Eds.), *Health promotion and interactive technology: Theoretical applications and future directions* (pp. 103–120). Mahwah, NJ: Erlbaum.

Lieberman, D. A., & Linn, M. (1991). Learning to learn revisited: Computers and the development of self-directed learning skills. *Journal of Research on Computing in Education, 23*(3), 373–394.

Locke, D. C. (1986). Cross-cultural counseling issues. In A. J. Palmo & W. J. Weikel (Eds.), *Foundations of mental health counseling.* Springfield, IL: Charles C. Thomas.

Locke, D. C. (1992). *Increasing multicultural understanding: A comprehensive model* (pp. 119–137). Thousand Oaks, CA: Sage.

Majumdar, B., & Roberts, J. (1998). AIDS awareness among women: The benefit of culturally sensitive educational programs. *Health Care for Women International, 19*(2), 141–153.

Manning, D. (1981). Writing readable health messages. *Public Health Reports, 96*(5), 464–465.

McAlister, A., Fernandez-Esquer, M. E., Ramirez, A. G., Trevino, F., Gallion, K. J., Villarreal, R., Pulley, L. V., Hu, S., Torres, I., & Zhang, Q. (1995). Community level cancer control in a Texas barrio: Part II. Baseline and preliminary outcome findings. *Journal of the National Cancer Institute. Monographs, 18,* 123–126.

McAlister, A., Johnson, W., Guenther-Grey, C., Fishbein, M., Higgins, D., O'Reilly, K., & the AIDS Community Demonstration Projects. (1999). Behavioral journalism for HIV prevention: Newsletter exposure influences risk-related attitudes and behavior in community demonstration studies. Manuscript submitted for publication.

McGuire, W. J. (1985). Attitudes and attitude change. In M. Lindsay & E. Aronson (Eds.), *The handbook of social psychology* (3rd ed., Vol. 2, Special fields and applications, pp. 233–246). New York: Random House.

Miller, W. R., & Rollnick, S. (1991). *Motivational interviewing: Preparing people to change addictive behavior.* New York: Guilford Press.

Mogilner, A. (1992). *Children's writer's word book.* Cincinnati, OH: Writer's Digest Books.

Montgomery, K. (1988). *Target prime-time: Advocacy groups and the struggle over entertainment television.* New York: Oxford University Press.

Montgomery, K. C. (1990). Promoting health through entertainment television. In C. Atkin & L. Wallack (Eds.), *Mass communication and public health: Complexities and conflicts* (pp. 114–128). Newbury Park, CA: Sage.

Morgenstern, L., Wein, T. H., Staub, L., Hickenbottom, S., Groff, J., & Bartholomew, L. K. (2000, February). *Who are the appropriate targets to increase FDA-approved acute stroke therapy?* Paper presented to the 25th American Heart Association International Stroke Conference, New Orleans, LA.

Mosenthal, P. B., & Kirsch, I. S. (1998). A new measure for assessing document complexity: The PMOSE/IKIRSCH document readability formula. *Journal of Adolescent and Adult Literacy, 41*(8), 638–657.

Mullen, P. D., DiClemente, C. C., Carbonari, J. P., Sockrider, M. M., Nicol, L., Richardson, M. Q., & Taylor, W. C. (1999). Project PANDA: Maintenance of prenatal smoking abstinence at 12 months postpartum. Manuscript submitted for publication.

Parker, R. C. (1988). *Looking good in print: A guide to basic design for desktop publishing.* Chapel Hill, NC: Ventana Press.

Pasick, R. J. (1997). Socioeconomic and cultural factors in the development and use of theory. In K. Glanz, F. M. Lewis, & B. K. Rimer (Eds.), *Health behavior and health education: Theory, research, and practice* (2nd ed., pp. 425–440). San Francisco: Jossey-Bass.

Perry, C. L., Sellers, D. E., Johnson, C., Pedersen, S., Bachman, K. J., Parcel, G. S., Stone, E. J., Luepker, R. V., Wu, M., Nader, P. R., & Cook, K. (1997). The Child and Adolescent Trial for Cardiovascular Health (CATCH): Intervention, implementation, and feasibility for elementary schools in the United States. *Health Education and Behavior, 24*(6), 716–735.

Petty, R. E., & Cacioppo, J. T. (1986a). *Communication and persuasion: Central and peripheral routes to attitude change.* New York: Springer-Verlag.

Petty, R. E., & Cacioppo, J. T. (1986b). The elaboration likelihood model of persuasion. *Advances in Experimental Social Psychology, 19,* 124–205.

Petty, R. E., & Wegener, D. T. (1997). Attitude change: Multiple roles for persuasion variables. In D. T. Gilbert, S. T. Fiske, & G. Lindzey (Eds.), *The handbook of social psychology* (4th ed., Vol. 1, pp. 323–390). New York: McGraw-Hill.

Prochaska, J. O., DiClemente, C. C., Velicer, W. F., & Rossi, J. S. (1993). Standardized, individualized, interactive, and personalized self-help programs for smoking cessation. *Health Psychology, 12*(5), 399–405.

Pulley, L. V., McAlister, A. L., Kay, L. S., & O'Reilly, K. (1996). Prevention campaigns for hard-to-reach populations at risk for HIV infection: Theory and implementation. *Health Education Quarterly, 23*(4), 488–496.

Rafaeli, S. (1988). Interactivity: From new media to communication. In R. P. Hawkins, J. M. Wiemann, & S. Pingree (Eds.), *Advancing communication science: Merging mass and interpersonal processes* (pp. 110–134). Newbury Park, CA: Sage.

Ramelson, H. Z., Friedman, R. H., & Ockene, J. K. (1999). An automated telephone-based smoking cessation education and counseling system. *Patient Education and Counseling, 36*(2), 131–144.

Ramirez, A. G., McAlister, A., Gallion, K. J., Ramirez, V., Garza, I. R., Stamm, K., de la Torre, J., & Chalela, P. (1995). Community-level cancer control in a Texas barrio: Part I. Theoretical basis, implementation, and process evaluation. *Journal of the National Cancer Institute. Monographs, 18,* 117–122.

Rhodes, F., Fishbein, M., & Reis, J. (1997). Using behavioral theory in computer-based health promotion and appraisal. *Health Education and Behavior, 24*(1), 20–34.

Rimal, R. N., & Flora, J. A. (1997). Interactive technology attributes in health promotion: Practical and theoretical issues. In R. Street, W. Gold, & T. Manning (Eds.), *Health promotion and interactive technology: Theoretical applications and future directions* (pp. 19–38). Mahwah, NJ: Erlbaum.

Rimer, B. K., Orleans, C. T., Fleisher, L., Cristinzio, S., Resch, N., Telepchak, J., & Keintz, M. K. (1994). Does tailoring matter? The impact of a tailored guide on ratings and short-term smoking-related outcomes for older smokers. *Health Education Research, 9*(1), 69–84.

Rios, R. A., McDaniel, J. E., & Stowell, L. P. (1998). Pursuing the possibilities of passion: The affective domain of multicultural education. In M. Dillworth (Ed.), *Being responsive to cultural differences: How teachers learn* (pp. 160–181). Thousand Oaks, CA: Corwin Press.

Schaffer, L. C., & Hannafin, M. J. (1986). The effects of progressive interactivity on learning from interactive video. *ECTJ, 34,* 89–96.

Shegog, R., Bartholomew, L. K., Gold, R. S., Pierrel, E., Parcel, G. S., Sockrider, M., Czyzewski, D., Fernandez, M., Berlin, N., Combes, R., & Abramson, S. (1999). *Self-management education for pediatric chronic disease: A description of the Watch, Discover, Think, and Act Asthma computer program.* Manuscript submitted for publication.

Singer, J. L., & Singer, D. G. (1979, March). Come back Mister Rogers, come back. *Psychology Today, 12*(10), pp. 56, 59–60.

Skinner, C. S., & Kreuter, M. W. (1997). Using theories in planning interactive computer programs. In R. Street, W. Gold, & T. Manning (Eds.), *Health promotion and interactive technology: Theoretical applications and future directions* (pp. 39–65). Mahwah, NJ: Erlbaum.

Skinner, C. S., Strecher, V. J., & Hospers, H. (1994). Physicians' recommendations for mammography: Do tailored messages make a difference? *American Journal of Public Health, 84*(1), 43–49.

Soet, J. E., & Basch, C. E. (1997). The telephone as a communication medium for health education. *Health Education and Behavior, 24*(6), 759–772.

Strecher, V. J. (1999). Computer-tailored smoking cessation materials: A review and discussion. *Patient Education and Counseling, 36*(2), 107–117.

Strecher, V. J., Kreuter, M., Den Boer, D. J., Kobrin, S., Hospers, H. J., & Skinner, C. S. (1994). The effects of computer-tailored smoking cessation messages in family practice settings. *Journal of Family Practice, 39*(3), 262–270.

Street, R. L., Jr., & Rimal, R. N. (1997). Health promotion and interactive technology: A conceptual foundation. In R. Street, W. Gold, & T. Manning (Eds.), *Health promotion and interactive technology: Theoretical applications and future directions* (pp. 1–18). Mahwah, NJ: Erlbaum.

Strong, L. V. (1990). *The how-to book of advertising: Creating it; preparing it; presenting it* (3rd ed.). New York: Fairchild Publications.

Torrence, D. R., & Torrence, J. A. (1987, August). Training in the face of illiteracy. *Training and Development Journal, 41*(8), 44–48.

Trapini, F., & Walmsley, S. A. (1981). Five readability estimates: Differential effects of simplifying a document. *Journal of Reading, 24*(5), 398–403.

Triandis, H. C. (1994). *Culture and social behavior.* New York: McGraw-Hill.

Tufte, E. R. (1983). *The visual display of quantitative information.* Cheshire, CT: Graphics Press.

Tufte, E. R. (1990). *Envisioning information.* Cheshire, CT: Graphics Press.

Tufte, E. R. (1997). *Visual explanations: Images and quantities, evidence and narrative.* Cheshire, CT: Graphics Press.

U.S. Department of Health and Human Services, Office of Cancer Communications, National Cancer Institute. (1992). *Making health communication programs work: A planner's guide.* (NIH Publication No. 92-1493). Bethesda, MD: U.S. Department of Health and Human Services.

U.S. Department of Health and Human Services. (1998). *Healthy People 2010 objectives: Draft for public comment.* Washington, DC: U.S. Department of Health and Human Services.

Velicer, W. F., & Prochaska, J. O. (1999). An expert system intervention for smoking cessation. *Patient Education and Counseling, 36*(2), 119–129.

Velicer, W. F., Prochaska, J. O., Bellis, J. M., DiClemente, C. C., Rossi, J. S., Fava, J. L., & Steiger, J. H. (1993). An expert system intervention for smoking cessation. *Addictive Behaviors, 18*(3), 269–290.

Webber, G. C. (1990). Patient education: A review of the issues. *Medical Care, 28*(11), 1089–1103.

Wells, W., Burnett, J., & Moriarty, S. (1998). *Advertising principles and practice* (4th ed.). Upper Saddle River, NJ: Prentice Hall.

Werner, O., & Campbell, D. T. (1973). Translation, working through interpreters and the problem of decentering. In R. Naroll & R. Cohen (Eds.), *A handbook of method in cultural anthropology* (pp. 398–422). New York: Columbia University Press.

White, J. V. (1988). *Graphic design for the electronic age: The manual for traditional and desktop publishing.* New York: Watson-Guptill Publications.

Williams, R. (1994). *The non-designer's design book: Design and typographic principles for the visual novice.* Berkeley, CA: Peachpit Press.

Williams, R. M., Jr. (1970). *American society: A sociological interpretation.* New York: Knopf.

Witte, K., & Morrison, K. (1995). Intercultural and cross-cultural health communication: Understanding people and motivating healthy behaviors. In R. L. Wiseman (Ed.), *Intercultural communication theory* (pp. 216–246). Thousand Oaks, CA: Sage.

Wlodkowski, R. J., & Ginsberg, M. B. (1995). *Diversity and motivation: Culturally responsive teaching.* San Francisco: Jossey-Bass.

Zhu, S. H., Balabanis, M., Rosbrook, B., Sadler, G., & Pierce, J. P. (1996). Telephone counseling for smoking cessation: Effects of single-session and multiple-session interventions. *Journal of Consulting and Clinical Psychology, 64*(1), 202–211.

CHAPTER 8

Intervention Mapping Step 4: Planning Program Adoption, Implementation, and Sustainability

READER OBJECTIVES

- Identify potential users of the health promotion program
- Develop a system that links program planners with potential program users
- Specify performance objectives for program adoption, implementation, and sustainability
- Specify determinants of adoption, implementation, and sustainability
- Create program use matrices
- Select methods and strategies to address the determinants
- Design interventions and organize programs to affect learning and change objectives related to program use

Effective health education and promotion programs will have little impact if they are never used or if they are discontinued while still needed to create the desired health impact (Oldenburg, Hardcastle, & Kok, 1997; Parcel, Perry, & Taylor, 1990). In Step 4 of Intervention Mapping the focus is on planning an intervention component to ensure that the program being developed in the previous steps will be put into use and maintained over time as long as it is useful.

The purpose of this chapter is to enable health educators to consider how programs will be initially adopted and implemented and how they will be continued beyond these initial processes. The chapter also guides the use of the Intervention Mapping process in the development of program components that affect the successful use of the program.

PERSPECTIVES

Planning for Program Use Is Essential

The impact of a health education program will be determined not only by the effectiveness of the interventions but also by the quality of program implementation and the proportion of intended participants exposed to the program (Parcel, 1995). In this chapter, we take the perspective that preparing for program use is an essential component of an effective health education or health promotion program. Program failure can often be traced to problems with program adoption and use (Green & Kreuter, 1999). Therefore, program planning must include this step.

The type of objectives needed for program use will depend on how involved the people who will use the program have been in its development. Some health education programs may be totally self-directed and self-selected; however, most programs require someone to deliver the program. Often the person or persons who deliver the program will be different from the program developers; therefore the developers cannot assume that the implementers will know the "what and how" of program implementation. Under these circumstances, especially, planning is needed for interventions to increase the likelihood that the program will be used and continued over time.

Most programs have people who deliver the program and who are actively involved in the program activities. Teachers who present health education programs to students, and nurses who present programs to patients, are examples of program users. In contrast, some programs are delivered without a person implementing intervention activities. However, these mediated programs still need to get to the intended participants through a delivery system. Gatekeepers for delivery systems, even though they are not program users like the teacher and nurse, may still be program adopters because they are necessary to get the program to the end users. For example, the principal in a school may not be the user of a health education curriculum, but his or her support for the program may be critical for adoption. A program manager at a radio station may not be directly involved in conducting a mass media campaign, but his or her support in getting the program on the air is essential.

Planned Interventions Can Make a Difference

We have experience with programs whose implementation was characterized by an echoing lament, "We should have thought about that." Bartholomew and colleagues' computer-assisted instructional program for self-management of asthma was one of these programs. In its first implementation, we relied on research assistants for implementation and underestimated the roles of clinic nurses and physicians. Without having specified in advance what these individuals would need to do to implement the program, and without having delineated determinants (and methods and strategies to change them), we achieved little cooperation from the health care providers (Bartholomew, Gold, et al., 2000).

On the other hand, we have experience with very well conceptualized diffusion interventions that have supported adoption and implementation of programs. For example, Heart Partners was a program to enable schools to adopt and implement programs for prevention of heart disease. The American Heart Association developed a network of school Heart Partners (usually on-site school staff) who acted as program champions to acquire and enable heart health program adoption and implementation. The average number of American Heart Association curriculum kits used in Heart Partner schools was 3.6 as opposed to 1.9 in schools without Heart Partners. The number of Texas schools with Heart Partners increased from 637 the first year of the program to 2,734 the fourth year of the program, and its success in Texas led to the institutionalization of the program nationally (Roberts-Gray, Solomon, Gottlieb, & Kelsey, 1998). Dissemination activities to promote full use of programs as depicted in the Heart Partners program can be planned with Intervention Mapping Steps and core processes.

CONCEPTUAL FRAMEWORK

Terms: Adoption, Implementation, and Sustainability

The work of Rogers (1983, 1995) and others over several decades has laid the groundwork for how to get programs adopted, implemented, and continued over time. Often this process is referred to as diffusion and focuses on program adoption and initial use. However, over the past decade, increasing attention has been given to the processes involved with both program implementation (Monahan & Scheirer, 1988; Roberts-Gray, 1985; Scheirer, 1981, 1990, 1994) and continuation of programs (Goodman, McLeroy, Steckler, & Hoyle, 1993; Goodman & Steckler, 1989; Goodman, Steckler, & Kegler, 1997; Scheirer, Shediac, & Cassady, 1995; Shediac-Rizkallah & Bone, 1998). Diffusion is thought of as moving from awareness of a need or of an innovation, through decisions to adopt the innovation, to initial use and program continuation. Figure 8.1 presents the various stages of program diffusion and use as they are in the literature. There are essentially three stages in program use: (a) adoption, which depends on knowledge of an innovation, awareness of an unmet need, and the decision that a certain innovation may meet the perceived need and will be given a trial (adoption can depend on active dissemination of a program); (b) implementation, that is, the use of the innovation to a fair trial point; and (c) sustainability, that is, the maintenance and institutionalization of a program or its outcomes.

Adoption

DIFFUSION OF INNOVATION An innovation is an idea, practice, or product that is new to the adopter, which may be an individual or an organization. Healthful behavior, for example, physical activity, stopping smoking, and using contraceptives may be innovations for individuals, as may interventions to promote these

	Steckler et al., 1992; Goodman et al.,1997	Shediac-Rizkallah & Bone, 1998	Parcel, 1995; Parcel, Eriksen, et al., 1989; Parcel, Taylor, et al., 1989	Rogers (1983, 1995) Adoption by individuals	Rogers (1983, 1995) Innovation in organizations
Adoption	Awareness Adoption		Dissemination Adoption	Adoption: Knowledge Persuasion Decision	Initiation: Agenda-setting Matching
Implementation	Implementation Maintenance		Implementation	Implementation Confirmation	Implementation: Redefining Clarifying
Sustainability	Institutionalization Renewal	Sustainability: Institutionalization Maintenance of health benefits Capacity building	Maintenance		Routinizing

FIGURE 8.1 Adoption and Implementation Terms

behaviors in organizations. Further, new programs demand change in individuals and organizations. For example, patient self-management programs may change the power relationship between patients and providers (Mullen & Mullen, 1987).

For many years Everett Rogers (1983, 1995) has studied the process of diffusion beginning with a focus on individual adopters of new technology. Rogers's individual model is useful for health education because many program adopters and users are individuals, such as schoolteachers, who can act somewhat independently of their organizations. Rogers describes program adopters as moving through the stages of

- Knowledge of the innovation
- Persuasion or attitude development
- Decision
- Adoption
- Implementation
- Confirmation

Of course, potential adopters can decide not to adopt. This decision can be either an active process or simply a passive failure to become familiar with the innovation and to decide (Rogers, 1995).

Rogers (1995) describes three types of knowledge of an innovation that can be important to a decision to adopt. Awareness knowledge is knowing that the innovation exists. The adopter must also have procedural knowledge, or knowledge about how to use the innovation, and principles knowledge, the underlying mechanism of the innovation or how it works.

Classic diffusion theory has dealt with characteristics of adopters and characteristics of innovations. Adopters adopt at different times following the introduction of the innovation into their social system, and the population can be segmented into innovators, early adopters, early majority, late majority, and laggards based on the point at which they adopt the innovation. Rogers (1995) has described the process of adoption as a normal, bell-shaped distribution, as shown in Figure 8.2, that places early and late majority adopters within one standard deviation on either side of the mean or midpoint of the curve, that places early adopters and laggards two standard deviations away, and that places innovators three standard deviations away. These categories of adopters have been shown to have different characteristics. For example, innovators are venturesome, early adopters are opinion leaders, the early majority are deliberators, the late majority are skeptical, and the laggards are traditional. All individual adopters go through a process of awareness, interest, trial, and adoption of the innovation, but the time required to complete these stages increases across the categories, with innovators having the shortest period between awareness and adoption.

Innovations are often communicated through two different channels, media and interpersonal communication. Initially, media increase awareness of the innovation. As people hear about the innovation and begin to adopt it, they talk with others about their interest and experience. The interpersonal channel, thus, becomes more important as more members of the population adopt the innovation. More potent outreach and incentives are needed for late adopters and laggards, who have not adopted even though the innovation has been communicated through the media and the majority of members of the population have adopted the innovation. Thus, for intervention planning purposes, it is important to know the adopter category (Green, Gottlieb, & Parcel, 1987; Rogers, 1995).

Social cognitive theory provides explanations of the psychological mechanisms by which diffusion occurs (Bandura, 1986). For potential program users to adopt, they must be aware of the innovation, hold positive outcome expectations

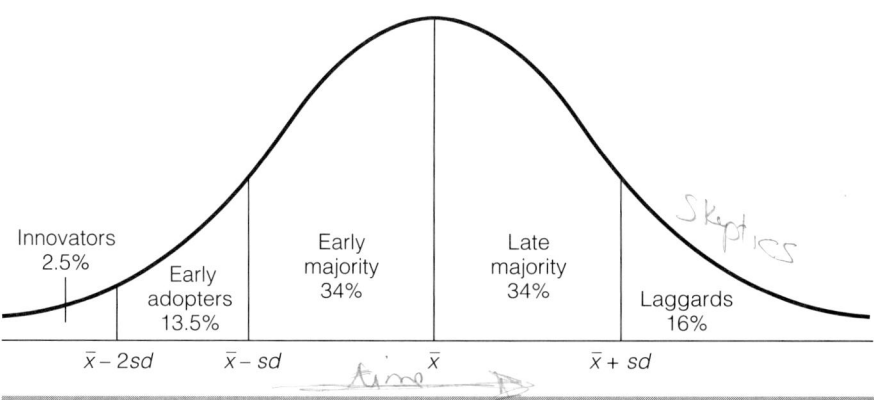

FIGURE 8.2 Bell-Shaped Curve of Adoption (*Note*. From *Diffusion of Innovations* [4th ed., p. 262], by E. M. Rogers, 1995, New York and London: The Free Press.)

and expectancies for it, and have sufficient self-efficacy and behavioral capability for both adoption and implementation. For example, positive outcome expectations by the potential adopters of self-management programs might include beliefs that the program will lead to better self-care and increased health and quality-of-life outcomes among patients and to increased job satisfaction and career enhancement for health care providers. Negative outcome expectations could include beliefs that the program will disrupt patient-provider relationships, lead to inappropriate or detrimental self-care based on faulty self-management decisions, and result in a decline in health status. Expectancies are how much each of the outcomes is valued. Intervention messages would seek to increase positive outcome expectations and values and decrease negative ones. Self-efficacy, or confidence in implementing the innovation, is also important for adoption. However, it increases in importance as a person tries to implement the new program.

Also important in the consideration of interventions to promote diffusion are the characteristics of innovations (Oldenburg et al., 1997; Rogers, 1995). These characteristics are the potential adopters' perceptions of what the program is like. They include relative advantage of the innovation compared to what is being used, compatibility with the intended users' current practice, complexity, observability of the results, impact on social relations, reversibility or ease of discontinuation, communicability, required time, risk and uncertainty, required commitment, and ability to be modified. Each of these characteristics of an innovation must be considered as either a predictor of, or a barrier to, adoption and implementation both in innovation design and in the creation of an intervention to aid diffusion.

DIFFUSION OF INNOVATION IN ORGANIZATIONS In the past ten years, the focus of diffusion research has shifted somewhat from a classical approach of looking at characteristics of individuals and innovations to a focus on organizations. Rogers posits slightly different stages for diffusion of innovations in organizations:

- Agenda setting
- Matching
- Redefining, restructuring
- Clarifying
- Routinizing

This process of organizational change has also been described by Beyer and Trice (1978) and translated to health promotion by Goodman et al. (1997).

Agenda setting is the process of acknowledging organizational problems and issues and prioritizing them for solution. Sometimes organizations are aware of problems and search for solutions, as the term *agenda setting* suggests. Other times, awareness of the existence of a certain innovation may actually stimulate agenda setting and matching, whereby an innovation is selected to match an issue or problem and is tried out by an organization. In the third and fourth stages, the organization modifies the innovation to fit its objectives and structure and formalizes the fit between innovation and organization. Finally, the innovation loses its unique character as it is incorporated into organizational routine.

Other authors have described these stages as dissemination, adoption, implementation, maintenance, and institutionalization (Goodman & Steckler, 1989; Oldenburg et al., 1997; Parcel, Eriksen, et al., 1989; Paulussen, Kok, & Schaalma, 1994; Paulussen, Kok, Schaalma, & Parcel, 1995). Diffusion and program use by organizations is a more complex event than is adoption by individuals, and it often involves key agents who vary with the diffusion process or stage. For example, a team leader may hear about a program at a professional meeting and discuss it with others. The team leaders may then request the curriculum coordinator or superintendent (depending on the size of the district and its personnel structure) to adopt the program. At implementation, the focus turns to the teachers. At maintenance and institutionalization, teachers may continue the program but the program must be included in curriculum plans and budgets, which will likely involve administrative organizational members.

Diffusion within organizations is complex and requires consideration of a variety of organization-level factors. Planners of diffusion interventions must consider the organization's goals, authority structure, roles, rules and regulations, and informal norms and relationships (Rogers, 1983). The different diffusion processes require decision and action from many different organizational roles. The decision to adopt an innovation within an organization can be made by an individual independent of others, collectively by consensus among the members of the organization or a subsystem within it, or by a person or persons with authority for the organization. An intervention to influence an adoption decision must be clearly oriented to how that decision is being made. Implementation success will depend on the degree of ownership felt and support given by those who must carry out the tasks. These attributes may depend in part on how the adoption decision is made.

Certain organizational characteristics have been found to be associated with innovativeness. However, the picture of when these general patterns hold (i.e., for what sorts of innovations, under what conditions) is not simple, and we refer the reader to Rogers (1995) for a summary. With that caveat, we can generalize that organizations most responsive to innovations tend to be large and complex with leaders who are positive toward change. They tend to have decentralized administration, high interconnectedness and informality, and organizational resource availability.

A powerful influence toward the adoption of new programs in organizations can be program champions. Program champions are likely to be sophisticated, analytical individuals with strategic linking locations in organizations. They often have intuitive skills in discovering the program adopters' and users' goals, and they have interpersonal and negotiating skills in order to troubleshoot both adoption and implementation (Goodman & Steckler, 1989). A champion can be a force to facilitate adoption of programs and to prevent discontinuation (Monahan & Scheirer, 1988). Compared to their colleagues, program champions have been described as taking more risks, being more innovative, and initiating more attempts to influence others (Howell & Higgins, 1990). Program champions must be credible to their colleagues, and when an innovation is costly or represents a radical new direction for the organization, the champion must be in a powerful organizational role.

Implementation

In addition to a shift toward studying organizational innovation, a great deal of contemporary thought is focused on what is meant by program implementation, especially what is meant by a well-implemented program (Scheirer, 1981, 1994). Program developers and evaluators are often concerned about two dimensions of implementation—fidelity and completeness (Rossi, Freeman, & Lipsey, 1999; Scheirer, 1981). Fidelity is the degree to which the program is implemented with its methods and strategies intact, whereas completeness indicates the proportion of program activities and components that are actually delivered. For example, in the Cystic Fibrosis Family Education Program, some cystic fibrosis centers taught all the program modules (good completeness) but neglected to perform goal setting with the families (inadequate fidelity) (Bartholomew, Czyzewski, Swank, McCormick, & Parcel, 2000). An important process in developing performance objectives for implementation is to answer these questions: What exactly is the program? and What would constitute a level of fidelity and a level of completeness consistent with program effectiveness?

Program developers must know what constitutes a well-implemented program. On the other hand, a defining characteristic of program implementation is mutual adaptation (Hall & Loucks, 1978). Both the innovation and the organization must adapt to each other's objectives, processes, and structures. Mutual adaptation is so ubiquitous that Rogers (1995) described it as a stage in organizational innovation, calling it reinvention. Quite a bit of reinvention takes place; various studies have found that more than 50% of adopting institutions reinvent the programs they adopt—from small insignificant changes to major revisions. From the perspective of the adopting institution, reinvention is a positive process that fosters program ownership and commitment. In the diffusion of the Cystic Fibrosis Family Education Program, we encouraged cystic fibrosis centers to reinvent the program to fit their ways of practicing (Bartholomew, Czyzewski, et al., 2000). From an intervention perspective, it may be best to anticipate this process and facilitate it within boundaries of program effectiveness. The resulting ownership is important not just for program implementation but for sustainability, which is discussed later in this chapter.

Ottoson and Green (1987) note that the innovation obtains its value only by its interaction with the context. If the program is not shaped to fit the context, it will be of limited value; simultaneously, if the context doesn't change, then the program has not been adopted. Health educators should consider this political process when developing the Intervention Mapping matrix for diffusion. The social interaction among stakeholders who seek to maximize their own goals and interests during adoption and implementation is complex. Organizational decision makers may adopt the program to accomplish the goals of the organization or to reduce pressure from interest groups. Implementers may wish to conduct the program as they would like rather than as the developers designed the program. The decision to retain the program may be in competition with other organizational activities. The program may be a source of career advancement for some, but an undesired added workload for others. In any event, there are multiple competing views of whether to adopt the program, how it will be implemented, and whether it should be retained.

As attention shifts from adoption to the implementation of a health promotion program, the determinants shift to an emphasis on behavioral capability, skills, self-efficacy, and reinforcement. A challenge in planning interventions to promote implementation is to correctly estimate the level of skills and related self-efficacy necessary to implement the program. For example, the Cystic Fibrosis Family Education Program (CF FEP) required many different types of skills for putting this complex program into clinical practice (Table 8.1). Skills were perceived as important determinants of implementation by the clinic coordinators who had to direct its use, and the diffusion intervention emphasized skill building. In comparison, necessary skills were sometimes underestimated in the CF FEP diffusion in spite of careful planning. The planners seriously underestimated the training intensity required to develop skills in communication domains such as mutual goal setting. Skill requirements are also often neglected or taken for granted in community interventions based on activities such as coalitions. Some researchers have suggested that coalition members receive training on how to be part of an effective coalition as a part of the implementation of a coalition-based health promotion program.

Another important determinant of program implementation is reinforcement. Usually, the innovation will eventually be intrinsically reinforcing because the implementers will see its effects. In the CATCH program, the food service workers liked seeing the children choose low-fat foods and were reinforced by the good feelings from their role in creating a healthier environment for the children. However, at the beginning of an implementation, positive reinforcement is delayed and change can be punishing (a hassle, a disruption). Therefore, extrinsic reinforcements may have to be built into a diffusion intervention. Extrinsic reinforcements can sometimes be a process of simply highlighting program outcomes that may be difficult for implementers to see. In a program to improve response to stroke by community and health care providers in east Texas, the diffusion intervention included collecting stories of successful transports and treatments. These stories were then provided as feedback and reinforcement to hospital emergency staff, emergency medical services, and community members through newsletters and community news media. This intervention created a reinforcement contingency where none might have been recognized in a natural sequence of events because stroke patients are rapidly moved after treatment from the emergency department to another part of the hospital.

Table 8.1
Cystic Fibrosis Family Education Program Diffusion Intervention Plan

DIFFUSION STAGE	PERFORMANCE OBJECTIVES	DETERMINANTS ADDRESSED	THEORETICAL METHODS	INTERVENTION STRATEGIES
Adoption—awareness of CF center health care providers	For staff Evaluate patient education needs in their center Know CF FEP exists as a response to need Review program characteristics favorably Learn how to implement the CF FEP	Personal Knowledge Awareness Outcome expectations External Identification of contact person for workshop planning Identification of potential program champion	Persuasion Modeling Cues to participate in training	Pharmaceutical-style product detailing of program to CF centers Contact person recruitment of workshop registrants Distribution of color program guide charts Workshop invitation and confirmation Scientific presentations and exhibit at CF medical meeting

Adoption—decision by CF centers (top down and team buy-in)	For CF centers
	Decide to adopt
	Identify program champion
	For program champion
	Facilitate adoption in CF centers
	Meet with CF center director and team to facilitate decision
		Personal
		Outcome expectations
		Self-efficacy
		Attitudes (positive evaluation of program characteristics)
		Skill set to get center personnel buy-in
		External
		Existence of team
		Team orientation meetings
		Storage and teaching space
		Time and workflow
		Patient to staff ratio
		Decision-making process
		Team leader and program champion
			Persuasion
			Active learning
			Social support
			Dissonance reduction
			Modeling
			Skill building
				Regional workshops
				  Discussion
				  Problem analysis
				  Role playing
				  Social support
				  Presentation
				  Team meeting to plan implementation
				  Problem solving
				  Enactment with guided practice
				Newsletter
				  Role-model stories
				  Resources
				  Information

Implementation with families in CF centers	For team members
	Work with families using the CF FEP with completeness and fidelity
		Personal
		Behavioral capability and self-efficacy for working with families and team
			Modeling
			Skill training
			Reinforcement
			Persuasion
				Regional workshops
				  Role playing
				  Skill building with guided practice
				  Lecture and written guides

(continued)

Table 8.1 Cystic Fibrosis Family Education Program Diffusion Intervention Plan *(continued)*

DIFFUSION STAGE	PERFORMANCE OBJECTIVES	DETERMINANTS ADDRESSED	THEORETICAL METHODS	INTERVENTION STRATEGIES
Implementation with families in CF centers *(continued)*	Design implementation plan Create implementation plan Schedule CF FEP team meetings Orient new or untrained team members to CF FEP Talk about patient care using the CF FEP Document program use to communicate with team members	Outcome expectations External Teaching and storage space Time and workflow Documentation Program champion Implementation team roles Medical staff buy-in		Videotape information and role modeling Guided practice and feedback Regional coordinators Technical and social support Social reinforcement Role modeling Newsletters Role-model stories Resouces Information
Institutionalization	For team members Integrate the CF FEP into center routines Use CF FEP in orientation of new staff Write CF FEP into job descriptions Write CF FEP into care paths or continuous quality improvement plans	Personal Behavioral capability and self-efficacy for program integration into routines Outcome expectations Social reinforcement External CF FEP meetings or routine CF FEP discussions as a part of other meetings Documentation forms	Problem solving Reinforcement Social support	Regional coordinators Technical and social support Social reinforcement Role modeling Newsletters Role-model stories Resources Information

Note. CF = cystic fibrosis; CF FEP = Cystic Fibrosis Family Education Program. From "Maximizing the Impact of the Cystic Fibrosis Family Education Program: Variables Related to Diffusion," by L. K. Bartholomew, D. I. Czyzewski, P. R. Swank, L. McCormick, and G. S. Parcel, 2000, *Journal of Family and Community Health, 22*(4), pp. 1–22.

Sustainability

A final stage of program diffusion has been described as institutionalization, that is, incorporating a program into organizational routines so that it survives beyond the presence of the original program funding, adopters, or program champion (Goodman & Steckler, 1989; Goodman et al., 1997). However, a broader construct, sustainability, can stimulate the health promoter to choose among several possible program continuation goals. Shediac-Rizkallah and Bone (1998) theorize that sustainability includes three possible goals: maintenance of health benefits from a program, institutionalization of a program within an organization's routines, and capacity building in the recipient community. Whereas development of thinking about health promotion programs in the United States has focused on institutionalization (e.g., Goodman & Steckler, 1987, 1989), the international development literature has described sustainability as program continuation that can take diverse forms and transfer the whole program, program parts, or program outcomes to community ownership (Bossert, 1990; Lafond, 1995).

Institutionalization is described by Rogers (1983) as routinization, or the progression of an innovation to an indistinguishable part of the individual or organizational host's practices. However, Goodman and Steckler (1989) pointed out more than a decade ago that health education and promotion interventions can be fragile and expendable innovations unless institutionalization is planned for and nurtured. These authors built on the work of Yin (1979) to define dimensions of institutionalization as extensiveness of the integration of a program into the subsystems of a host organization and intensiveness, or the depth of program integration into each organization subsystem. Degrees of intensiveness are (a) passages—anniversaries of the intervention, such as the number of fiscal year beginnings the intervention has survived; (b) routines—operating structures and functions into which program protocols are embedded; and (c) niche saturation—complete integration into a subsystem's structures and functions.

Once a program has achieved a certain level of health effects, the program continuation goal may be to continue the effects of the program rather than the program itself. Some programs are needed in their original form to continue the effects; Shediac-Rizkallah and Bone (1998) give the example of a measles disease prevention program that was effective in controlling measles outbreaks only while it was functioning. Two years later the rates were at the preprogram level. However, other programs need to change to maintain the effects. In the World Health Organization smallpox eradication efforts, an initial program of mass vaccination was followed by one of surveillance and aggressive follow-up of suspected cases. Both these programs were in service of the same health objective and represent program sustainability. As another example, Lichtenstein, Thompson, Nettekoven, and Corbett (1996) describe efforts to continue tobacco control activities, rather than the actual program, after the COMMIT trial.

Sometimes the best way to sustain a program is to go beyond organizational boundaries. Both intact programs and program components intended to guard health effects may need multiple community agencies to sustain them. Bracht and colleagues (1994) describe how community agency efforts were taken to sustain components of the Minnesota Heart Health Program, a program begun by university-based researchers. Agencies and their networks may need training and technical assistance and developmental support for the expansion of capacity to house new programs. The specific areas of capacity enhancement that may need to be included in diffusion interventions for this type of program continuation are skills, structures, and functions to encourage participation, leadership, group process, conflict resolution, leverage of resources, and network maintenance.

INTERVENTION MAPPING STEP 4: PLANNING FOR PROGRAM USE

Intervention Mapping can be used to promote the diffusion of programs first on a small scale for demonstration and evaluation and subsequently on a wider scale after effectiveness has been demonstrated. Planning for program diffusion involves two aspects. The first is designing the health education program in ways that enhance its potential for being adopted, implemented, and sustained. The second is designing interventions to influence these diffusion stages. To effectively address both aspects of planning, several tasks in Step 4 of Intervention Mapping will need to be integrated into earlier steps. Planners will work with the potential program users and seek to incorporate their concerns during all steps of Intervention Mapping. It is especially critical in Step 3, program design, to know as much as possible about the program users to ensure a good fit. As discussed in Chapter 7, planners need to involve potential program users as part of the planning process, know the context in which the program will be implemented, know how the potential program users typically practice, and pilot test program components with potential users.

A Linkage Approach to Program Diffusion

The first task in Intervention Mapping Step 4 is the development of a linkage system. The importance of developing a linkage system is discussed in Chapter 1 as an essential structure for effective health education program planning. The specific information about developing a linkage system is presented here as the first task in Step 4, but the activities to complete this task should really begin in Step 1 and continue throughout the Intervention Mapping process. The main purpose of a linkage system is to ensure that the program planners have a structure in place to effectively interact with program users. The structure should provide a means to exchange information and ideas between planners and users, to ensure program user access to the planning process, and to facilitate the development of user-friendly programs.

Several authors encourage the development of a linkage system to connect those who are developing the health promotion intervention (the resource system) to those who will use the program (the user system) to encourage collaborative program development ending in effective implementation (Havelock, 1971; Kolbe & Iverson, 1981; Orlandi, 1986; Orlandi, Landers, Weston, & Haley, 1990). The primary function of the linkage system is to create a structure or means for the exchange of knowledge and ideas between the resource system and the user system. The linkage system serves a dual purpose: to enable collaboratively developed user-relevant health education programs and to influence the diffusion process to accomplish program adoption and implementation. The linkage system should be established at the beginning of program planning because it aids the program planners at each stage of the Intervention Mapping process and aids the user system in expressing needs, expectations, and limitations for the health education program.

The resource system is the agency or organization supporting and developing the health education program. The resource system could be a university group, a community group, a governmental office, a hospital department, an educational agency, a service group, or a coalition of groups. The resource system includes the personnel, funding, materials, and services available to support the development of the health education program. The user system includes the individuals or groups who will implement the health education program and might be located in schools, work sites, hospitals, clinics, service agencies, mass media outlets, neighborhoods, or communities. The linkage system comprises representatives of both the resource system and the user system with the addition of any change agents who facilitate collaboration or who may be in positions to influence changes necessary to support the adoption, implementation, and institutionalization of the health education program. Advisory groups, training workshops, and consultation are examples of activities facilitating linkage systems. Schwartz and colleagues (1993) have described a linkage system for translating the findings of research and demonstration programs for cardiovascular disease risk reduction supported by federal public health agencies through the linkage system of state health agencies to communities. Technical assistance, quality assurance, training, funding, and on-site coordination were listed as dissemination activities bringing together the state health agencies and community program implementers.

In Chapter 10, a linkage system is described for the Dutch AIDS prevention program for the schools. To anticipate problems with future adoption and implementation of the program, the program developers formed a linkage board to bridge the gap between the research and development team and the school system. This board was made up of representatives from the research and development team, the school advisory services, the organizations that provide sex and AIDS education to secondary schools, and an association of teachers of biology. The role of the board was to provide feedback on performance and learning objectives of the program and to give advice on implementation issues. The linkage board gave careful consideration to the secondary school context for the program and to the teachers who would use it.

The Heart Partners program created a linkage system of school-based volunteers specifically to mediate between the teachers and the American Heart Association (AHA). The role of the Heart Partner was to promote awareness and use of AHA school-site programs, to conduct training sessions, and to reinforce teachers who conducted the programs. The Heart Partners program also used a linkage system composed of teachers who were knowledgeable about the AHA and its resources, AHA program staff, and university program developers (Roberts-Gray et al., 1998).

Intervention Mapping Step 4: Planning for Program Use

There are a number of ways in which the linkage system can be organized with varying degrees of formality. In its simplest form, potential users of the program can be invited to be members of the program-planning group and participate fully in each step of the Intervention Mapping process. This simple form can be extended by having the user system select members to represent it and by having these representatives report and obtain feedback on the progress of the program development. The size or complexity of the project will influence ways of creating and structuring the linkage system. Another influence will be the goal for sustaining the program. A program that will depend on the hospitality and resources of many agencies should have these community partners present throughout its development in order to foster as much commitment and ownership as possible as well as to foresee implementation barriers and facilitators.

For a very large project, either in scope of the program to be developed or in the number of organizations to be involved in planning and implementation, the linkage system may need to be more formal and a new entity may need to be created to carry out the linkage function. The structure of a linkage system and the makeup of individuals participating in the system will be unique to each program and situation. An important consideration in selecting individuals to participate in the linkage system is to ensure representation of different views and receptivity toward the innovative program. Often, program planners rely entirely on volunteers who are already committed to the implementation of a new program. If individuals who are reluctant or opposed to using the program are not included in the planning process, the program may fail to be adopted and implemented because of divergent views not taken into consideration as part of the planning process. Representation of potential decision makers for adoption and institutionalization, in addition to those who will implement the program, will ensure that the larger organizational perspectives will be considered. The following examples from two health promotion projects illustrate this more formal approach.

The School Asthma Partnership Program (see Chapter 11) is a research and demonstration project to develop and evaluate a multicomponent school-based program to improve the management of childhood asthma. To help develop the interventions and to achieve program adoption and implementation, a linkage system with two components was created. The first was an advisory committee that included the director of school health services, a school nurse, an elementary school principal, the director of risk management, the director of building maintenance and services, and a parent of a child with asthma. The primary role of this group was to engage in planning to develop and carry out interventions to ensure program adoption and implementation. The second component was a small group of selected pilot schools to serve as sources of information on needs, expectations, and limitations of program users and to test components of the intervention. The major role for this group was to ensure that the health promotion program was compatible with program users and was a good fit for the structure and context of the schools. Both of these formal groups functioned as partners in the program-planning process.

The mayor's task force is chugging along with program development. Support materials are being planned, and implementation networks are being considered. The team is really a team now—a model of a cohesive working group. Along the way they have added members with a commitment to inclusiveness. Anyone who wanted to work hard on violence was welcomed. For a while, it seemed that every new meeting generated a new member and every planning success attracted another contingent of community members. The health educator handled this by creating a new member orientation packet with information designed to quickly bring a new member up to date on the planning milestones accomplished and alternate paths considered. So far, so good.

The planning committee members were pleased with their efforts to keep an intact linkage with the community. Members who joined the task force along the way included representatives of churches, community centers, and advocacy groups. However, as the subgroup on implementation began to enumerate the types of people and agencies who might be involved with the program, they were astounded by who was *not* represented around the table. Neighborhood social groups, parent organizations, and (interestingly enough) other arms of the mayor's city government were absent. Where were the police, juvenile justice, child welfare, alternative schools, and city job programs?

The task force went back to the "pavement." The members were assigned to recruitment efforts, and the mayor personally invited colleagues from other city departments to meet and discuss the effort's history with her and the health educator. The mayor encouraged department heads to assign both management and neighborhood specialists to the task force. Fortunately, the group members prided themselves on inclusiveness, and the health educator had been facilitating integration of new individuals all along with the new member orientation packet. The group understood the need to cover old ground and even to engage in program reinvention in order to integrate these new members who were so crucial to the linkage system. Soon the group returned to its groove of progress toward planning the adoption, implementation, and sustainability program objectives.

Intervention Mapping Step 4: Planning for Program Use

The second example is the linkage system from a project designed to promote the diffusion of an effective tobacco prevention program (Brink et al., 1995; Parcel, 1995; Parcel et al., 1995). The project goal of Smart Choices was to influence as many school districts as possible within two educational service regions of the state of Texas to adopt and implement an adolescent smoking prevention program (Parcel, Eriksen, et al., 1989). The linkage system used for this project also had two components. One pilot school served as a model for program adoption and implementation and then shared its experiences with the tobacco prevention program with potential adopting school districts through video and print communications.

The second component of the linkage system comprised the two educational service centers in the regions. Each center employed a health educator with the responsibility of working with schools to help them identify and adopt health education programs. These two health educators served as links between the research group and the school districts in the field. They enabled the planners to have more direct contact with potential adopters and implementers to gain a better understanding of how to design the diffusion interventions. The two also assisted with implementing the diffusion intervention.

Matrices of Proximal Program Objectives

The second task in Intervention Mapping Step 4 is to create matrices that combine objectives and determinants for adoption, implementation, and sustainability.

PERFORMANCE OBJECTIVES The performance objectives for this step are similar to the performance objectives in Step 1 that were specified for health-related behavior except that the behaviors in Step 4 are adoption, implementation, and (depending on goals selected for sustainability) either maintenance, institutionalization, or capacity building for sustaining health effects. The performance objectives make clear what performance will constitute use with acceptable fidelity and completeness.

Adoption is a decision to use an innovation (Rogers, 1995). The adoption of a health education program by an organization or practitioner means that a decision is made by "someone" to use the program. The "someone" could be an individual, such as a practitioner or an administrator, making an independent decision; or it could be a group, such as a committee or governing board, making a collective decision. Program adoption can also be decided sequentially or concurrently at multiple levels of responsibility within an organization. For example, the school board and superintendent may decide to adopt an innovative health promotion program for a district, a principal may make the decision for a school, and a teacher may decide for a classroom. Knowing ahead of time how and who will make the adoption decision will greatly assist the program planners in specifying the performance objectives for adoption.

Program adoption behavior can be specified in this way: The ["someone"] adopts the [innovative program] as indicated by [the evidence or document to indicate adoption]. For example: The *curriculum committee of the Star Independent School District* decides to adopt the *Smart Choices Tobacco Prevention Program* as indicated by *the superintendent signing the program adoption form*. The answer to the following question specifies the performance objectives for adoption: What do the potential program adopters need to do to constitute adoption of the health education program?

The example just given can be used to state the general question more specifically: What does the curriculum committee of the Star Independent School District need to do to perform an adoption of the Smart Choices Tobacco Prevention Program? Answers to this question are possible performance objectives. For example, the curriculum committee will

- review the Smart Choices program materials
- note the program's objectives, methods, and relative advantages
- obtain parent, administrator, and teacher reaction to the program
- obtain information on the experiences of other school districts using the Smart Choices program
- identify barriers for implementation as perceived by potential program users
- seek information and consultation from the linkage system or resource system for addressing barriers and concerns
- gain support for program adoption from teachers (implementers) and key administrators (principals, director of curriculum, superintendent)
- prepare a statement of recommendation for adoption of the Smart Choices program
- complete the adoption form for the Smart Choices program, have it signed by the superintendent, and return it to the resource system for processing

Table 8.1 presents another example of performance objectives for adoption.

Implementation of a health education program can also be stated in behavioral terms. However, to a greater extent than for adoption, implementation is often multiple tasks performed by a variety of individual roles. For the CATCH program, for example, implementation is performed by classroom academic teachers, physical education teachers, food service staff, and administrators (Perry et al., 1997). Parallel to adoption behaviors, implementation behaviors can be stated in this way: The [role of implementer] will [performance of specific implementation task] with fidelity and completeness as indicated by [quality standards for fidelity and completeness]. The question that needs to be answered is: What do the program implementers need to do to perform the implementation of the program with acceptable fidelity and completeness? The planners of Smart Choices asked what teachers and principals need to do to implement the program, and they developed this set of implementation objectives:

- Health teachers will participate in training to prepare for implementing the Smart Choices curriculum.
- Health teachers will schedule and incorporate the Smart Choices curriculum into the lesson plans for all health classes for each semester.
- Health teachers will teach all six lessons in the Smart Choices curriculum using the teaching methods specified in the lesson plans.
- The principal at each middle school will form a policy committee that includes teacher, student, staff, and parent representation to establish policies for tobacco control at the school.

- The policy committee will follow the Smart Choices Tobacco-Free Policy Guidelines to review current tobacco control policies and will revise or form new policies to establish a tobacco-free school.

Before specifying performance objectives for sustaining a program, the planner will decide on a goal—institutionalization, continuation of health effects, capacity building, or some combination. The example we give here is for institutionalization. Institutionalization objectives can be written in response to the question, What do the organizational decision makers need to do to incorporate the program into the routines of the organization for the long term? Here are the performance objectives for institutionalization of the Smart Choices program within a school district:

- District coordinators will include training of new health teachers to implement the Smart Choices curriculum in their yearly plans.
- Book and curriculum warehouse managers will order and maintain inventory of the curriculum.
- Principals will include implementation of the Smart Choices curriculum in teacher job descriptions and evaluations.
- The principal at each middle school will include the Smart Choices program as a line item in the budget.
- The school district curriculum committee will write Smart Choices into the district curriculum guide for middle school science.
- The policy committee will report the results of the program to the parent teacher association on an annual basis.

If the continuation of the program after the initial cycle of funding will be carried on by multiple organizations in the community, the objectives should be written to include those organization decision makers and would represent the category of capacity building within sustainability. For example, at the conclusion of the Stanford Five-City Project, the project group first attempted institutionalization through a nonprofit community health promotion center. When this approach encountered barriers related to continued funding and program development, the focus shifted to capacity building among health educators employed by local organizations with leadership provided by the local health department (Jackson et al., 1994).

DETERMINANTS As with the performance objectives of health-related behaviors, the performance objectives for program use will have a set of determinants, that is, factors that are likely to influence their performance. The determinants may be personal (i.e., located within the individuals responsible for adoption and implementation) or external (i.e., social or structural factors that might serve as barriers or facilitators).

The processes for selecting determinants are the same as the ones recommended for selecting determinants of health-related behavior and environmental conditions. The starting activity is to brainstorm with the planning group (including the linkage system) a list of factors that will facilitate or serve as barriers to accomplishing the performance objectives for each stage. To refine or add to this list, the group should review the literature and the information from potential program users. A review of the literature starts first with studies that report findings of determinants of use of similar programs in similar settings. There is not a large body of literature on program use in health education and health promotion programs, and searching in other fields may be required (Oldenburg, Sallis, French, & Owen, 1999).

Next, the team can review the literature on theories that have been used to explain the diffusion of innovations and the literature from general theories that includes some of the identified determinants. For example, if the preceding review of the literature identified "relative advantage" as a possible determinant of the adoption of an innovation, it would be useful to go to the literature on diffusion theory for which relative advantage is a central construct. A review of diffusion theory may suggest other constructs that might be considered as important determinants of the program adoption and implementation. A review of theory should not be limited to theories of diffusion. For example, in the Smart Choices diffusion project, social cognitive theory (Bandura, 1986) was used to hypothesize determinants of adoption and implementation such as outcome expectations, expectancies, reinforcement for adoption, and behavioral capability and self-efficacy for implementation (Parcel, Eriksen, et al., 1989; Parcel, Taylor, et al., 1989; see Table 8.2).

The application of the theory of planned behavior (TPB; Ajzen, 1991) to the identification of determinants for program adoption and implementation is illustrated in Figure 8.3 and in Chapter 10, which describes a Dutch AIDS prevention program in the schools. Paulussen and colleagues (1994, 1995) hypothesized both endogenous and background variables to influence teacher adoption of an AIDS curriculum. The background variables are thought to influence adoption and implementation through their effects on the TPB variables on the top half of Figure 8.3. Instrumentality refers to the teachers' perceptions of whether the curriculum meets their planning concerns and includes clarity of instructions, anticipated student reactions, time required, and ease of teaching. The authors found that subjective norms, instrumentality, and descriptive norms (perceived colleague behavior) explained a considerable amount of the variability in teachers' adoption of AIDs curricula.

Because program adoption and implementation often involves organizations and community groups making decisions and changing practices to make use of an innovation, the application of organizational change and community development models is critical to identifying the external determinants of program adoption and implementation. The brainstorming and the literature review provide informed but nevertheless hypothesized relationships of determinants to the

Table 8.2
Smart Choices Diffusion Intervention Plan

DIFFUSION STAGE	PERFORMANCE OBJECTIVES	DETERMINANTS ADDRESSED	THEORETICAL METHODS	INTERVENTION STRATEGIES
Dissemination	Teachers and administrators will indicate awareness of the Smart Choices program	Preconditions (knowledge and awareness)	Symbolic modeling Direct modeling	Dissemination videotape Workshop for school personnel
	Teachers and administrators will view the Smart Choices program favorably	Outcome expectations Expectancies	Dual-channel communication	Diffusion network Newsletter
	Teachers and administrators will discuss the Smart Choices program			
Adoption	School districts will adopt the Smart Choices program	Outcome expectations Expectancies Vicarious reinforcement	Symbolic modeling Incentives Contracting	Newsletter Adoption form
Implementation	Teachers will use the Smart Choices program with acceptable completeness, fidelity, and proficiency	Behavioral capability Self-efficacy	Direct modeling Symbolic modeling Guided enactment Self-directed application of acquired skills	Training workshop Training videotape
Maintenance	After one year, teachers will continue to use the Smart Choices program with acceptable completeness, fidelity, and proficiency	Self-efficacy Outcome expectations Expectancies Reinforcement		Recognition Material rewards Special status for school district Feedback on performance

Note. Adapted from "Translating Theory Into Practice: Intervention Strategies for the Diffusion of a Health Promotion Innovation," by G. S. Parcel, W. C. Taylor, S. G. Brink, N. Gottlieb, K. Engquist, N. M. O'Hara, and M. P. Eriksen, 1989, *Journal of Family and Community Health,* 12(3), pp. 1–13.

adoption and implementation objectives. If there is a long list of determinants at this stage, the planner may need to test the hypothesized relationships of determinants in order to select the most important determinants to guide intervention development. If the list of determinants is small, the planner may need to collect data from the potential program users to identify additional determinants. In either case, both qualitative methods and quantitative methods can be used.

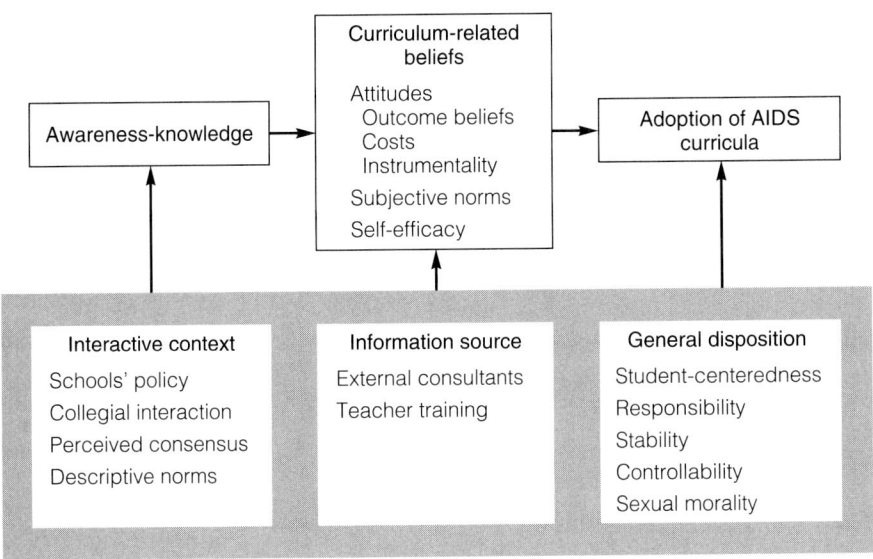

FIGURE 8.3 Model for Explaining Teachers' Adoption of Exemplary AIDS Education Materials (*Note.* From "Diffusion of AIDS Curricula Among Dutch Secondary School Teachers," by T. Paulussen, G. Kok, H. Schaalma, and G. S. Parcel, *Health Education Quarterly, 22*(2), p. 231.)

Qualitative methods, such as focus groups or interviews, can be helpful in generating new ideas for determinants or in checking out some of the findings from the research literature. Quantitative data collection using questionnaires that measure the determinants and interest or intentions to adopt and implement a program can be especially helpful in judging the strength of the association between determinants and potential adoption and implementation. With both types of data collection, planners can obtain some estimate of the presence or absence of the determinant in the user system.

In the Smart Choices diffusion project, for example, the program developers had assumed that teachers and school administrators would need to be convinced that it is important for the schools to conduct programs to prevent student tobacco use. Therefore, modeling and messages were created in the adoption intervention to influence teachers to place a higher value on the schools' conducting tobacco prevention programs. However, the baseline data collected for program evaluation showed that the teachers and administrators already placed high value on tobacco prevention; because this possible determinant was high, it could be reinforced rather than introduced in the intervention (Parcel, Eriksen, et al., 1989; Parcel, Taylor, et al., 1989).

Eventually, the list of determinants must be refined. A long list of determinants is not practical for program development. To assess the list of determinants, planners should begin by rating each determinant in terms of importance (i.e., strength of association with program adoption and implementation) and changeability (i.e., how likely it is that a diffusion intervention influences a change in the determinant). Priority should be given to those determinants that have high importance and high changeability. However, planners may want to retain some determinants with high importance and low changeability because the determinant is likely to be a critical factor in program adoption or implementation. For example, the cost of adopting a health promotion program may be a strong determinant but there may be little that can be done to lower the cost. Because cost may be a major barrier to adoption, it needs to be addressed in the intervention so that the planner can find ways to compensate (i.e., find additional funding sources) or demonstrate that the cost-benefit ratio of the program is worth the investment.

Examples of determinants of program adoption, implementation, and institutionalization are illustrated by the program to diffuse the Cystic Fibrosis Family Education Program (CF FEP; Bartholomew, Czyzewski, et al., 2000). Table 8.1 is an example of a diffusion intervention table that can be prepared instead of a matrix. However, for complex adoption or implementation efforts, we suggest developing matrices before proceeding to develop this type of table. The CF FEP was tested over a period of two years in one cystic fibrosis center using a quasi-experimental evaluation design and was shown to be effective in improving self-management skills and clinical outcomes (Bartholomew et al., 1997). There are more than 100 multidisciplinary cystic fibrosis centers that care for approximately 20,000 cystic fibrosis patients in the United States (*Cystic Fibrosis Foundation patient registry*, 1995). For the CF FEP to have a meaningful impact on helping patients and families self-manage cystic fibrosis, the next phase of program development had to address the adoption, implementation, and institutionalization of the CF FEP in the cystic fibrosis centers throughout the United States. To accomplish the outcomes of program adoption, implementation, and institutionalization, a diffusion intervention was designed to address both personal and external determinants. The personal determinants for adoption of the CF FEP were identified as follows:

- Outcome expectations that the program is effective in helping patients and in helping the health care providers do their jobs better
- Self-efficacy to persuade center personnel to adopt the program
- Positive attitudes toward the program and its characteristics
- Skills to persuade center personnel to adopt the program

The external determinants identified for program adoption included the following:

- Existence of a team to assess and evaluate the relative advantage of the program
- Team orientation meetings to discuss the program and to become more aware of program features
- Space for storage of program materials and for teaching sessions with families

- Time and workflow to schedule program activities
- Patient-staff ratio sufficient to provide staff resources
- Decision-making process for arriving at a decision to adopt the program
- Team leader or program champion to visibly support and encourage adoption of the program

Determinants for implementation of the CF FEP focused on those factors that would be necessary for the health care team to conduct the program, including these personal determinants:

- Behavioral capability and self-efficacy to work with the families and teams that use the program and to engage the families in the learning activities of the program
- Outcome expectations that families will be successful in using the program

External determinants included the following:

- Space for storage and teaching so that there is a place to do the program
- Time and workflow to incorporate the program into patient care routines
- Documentation of patient self-management learning goals, activities, and outcomes to ensure communication across health care providers
- Program champion to keep attention on the program and to promote continued use
- Implementation team roles that are defined and understood; agreement on who will be taking responsibility for different program activities and reinforcing patient and family use of the program
- Medical staff buy-in to ensure that all health care providers, regardless of their involvement in the CF FEP, support the program and reinforce the patients and families for using the skills learned through the program

Determinants for institutionalization of the program also included behavioral capability, self-efficacy, and outcome expectations, but these were related to getting the program into the routines of the organization, for example, writing it into budgets, job descriptions, performance evaluations, and critical pathways and nursing care plans.

MATRICES The adoption and implementation processes for many health promotion programs may be relatively straightforward and may allow the program planners to move from performance objectives and determinants directly to methods and strategies through the use of a table such as the CF FEP or Smart Choices diffusion tables (see Tables 8.1 and 8.2). However, we recommend the creation of matrices that follow the processes used in Step 1, especially for more complex program adoption and implementation situations. Performance objectives and determinants might be quite different for the different stages of program use, so it may be necessary to create separate matrices for program adoption, implementation, and sustainability.

The matrix is created, like the matrices that were developed for planning the intervention, by entering performance objectives on the left side of the matrix and determinants across the top of the matrix. Then the program planner assesses each cell to decide if the determinant is likely to be important to the achievement of the performance objective. Next, the planner writes learning and change objectives for the appropriate cells. The process for writing learning and change objectives is the same for adoption and implementation matrices as for the health education matrices that were described in Chapter 5.

Selection of Methods and Strategies

The third task in Intervention Mapping Step 4 is to select methods and strategies to influence the determinants and accomplish the performance objectives for program adoption, implementation, and sustainability. The same core processes used in other Intervention Mapping steps can be applied here. The program planners start with the list of determinants and brainstorm methods that they think can influence a change. Next, they review the relevant research and practice literature to confirm, refute, or modify the provisional list of methods. The best approach is for planners to start with the literature on the diffusion of health promotion programs and then review diffusion literature related to other innovations that may have some common elements with the adoption and implementation of health promotion programs. Planners also need to explore the literature on theories of change related to specific theoretical constructs on the final list of determinants. For example, self-efficacy may be considered an important determinant of program implementation, but it may not be specifically addressed in the literature on diffusion. However, a review of the theoretical literature on self-efficacy would lead to social cognitive theory, which does have a discussion of methods shown to be effective in changing self-efficacy (Bandura, 1986). Finally, it may be useful and necessary to collect additional data from potential adopters and program users to test out some items on the provisional list of methods to determine acceptability and appropriateness for use in an intervention.

The revised list of methods is then used to design practical strategies to influence program adoption and implementation. As discussed in Chapter 6, the selection of methods and strategies may be a back-and-forth process. In reviewing the adoption and implementation objectives, planners may find that ideas for strategies occur to them before ideas for methods. The strategy can then be assessed in order to link it to a theoretical method. For example, planners of a program are brainstorming methods and strategies to influence families to adopt a program to survey and correct household hazards for childhood injuries. One of the strategies they think would be effective is to communicate through mass media the stories of parents who have been successful in adopting the program and discovering hazards that might have been very harmful to their children. This strategy of role-model stories (Pulley, McAlister, Kay, & O'Reilly, 1996; Ramirez et al., 1995; Suarez, Nichols, Pulley, Brady, & McAlister, 1993) is not a theoretical method, but it can be linked to the method of modeling from social cognitive theory (Bandura, 1986). The planners can then review the theoretical principles that guide the use of modeling in order to influence possible determinants of program adoption such as perceived norms, outcome expectations, and self-efficacy. They can then design interventions that take advantage of what others have learned about the method of modeling and how it can be applied to their idea for using role-model stories as a strategy.

The methods and strategies discussed in Chapter 6 can be applied to interventions to accomplish program adoption, implementation, and institutionalization. Personal determinants such as knowledge of program compatibility and relative advantage, attitudes toward the program, outcome expectations for the program, self-efficacy, and behavioral capability for doing the program activities can be addressed with methods based in social psychology such as persuasive communication, modeling, skills training, incentives, reinforcement, and social comparison (Bandura, 1986; McGuire, 1985; Suls & Wills, 1991). Methods to address external determinants for program adoption, implementation, and institutionalization, such as social support, program advocacy, resources, organizational structures and practices, and policies, can also be found in Chapter 6.

Adoption, Implementation, and Sustainability Plan

The final task in Intervention Mapping Step 4 is to design a plan for an intervention to influence program adoption, implementation, and sustainability outcomes. The plan for getting a program adopted and implemented is as important as the intervention plans discussed in Chapter 7. It should include a scope and sequence of activities, staffing, and budget. Development of the written plan should begin with an intervention matrix or table such as Tables 8.1 and 8.2.

SUMMARY

Without diffusion, the program stays on the shelf—the shelf of the developers if the program is not adopted, or the shelf of the organization if the program is adopted but not implemented. If the program is not sustained, it returns to the shelf after initial implementation. Systematic planning for each stage of diffusion is essential if the program is to optimally affect the population for whom it was designed.

Tasks for Intervention Mapping Step 4:
- Develop a linkage system
- Create matrices of proximal program objectives that combine performance objectives and determinants

- Select methods and strategies and create a diffusion intervention table
- Write an adoption and implementation plan

REFERENCES

Ajzen, I. (1991). The theory of planned behavior. *Organizational Behavior and Human Decision Process, 50,* 179–211.

Bandura, A. (1986). *Social foundations of thought and action: A social cognitive theory.* Englewood Cliffs, NJ: Prentice Hall.

Bartholomew, L. K., Czyzewski, D. I., Parcel, G. S., Swank, P. R., Sockrider, M. M., Mariotto, M., Schidlow, D. V., Fink, R., & Seilheimer, D. K. (1997). Self-management of cystic fibrosis: Short-term outcomes of the Cystic Fibrosis Family Education Program. *Health Education and Behavior, 24*(5), 652–666.

Bartholomew, L. K., Czyzewski, D. I., Swank, P. R., McCormick, L., & Parcel, G. S. (2000). Maximizing the impact of the Cystic Fibrosis Family Education Program: Variables related to diffusion. *Family and Community Health, 22*(4), 1–22.

Bartholomew, L. K., Gold, R. S., Parcel, G. S., Czyzewski, D. I., Sockrider, M. M., Fernandez, M., Shegog, R., & Swank, P. R. (2000). Watch, Discover, Think, and Act: Evaluation of computer-assisted instruction to improve asthma self-management in inner-city children. *Patient Education and Counseling, 39*(2–3), 269–280.

Beyer, J. M., & Trice, H. M. (1978). *Implementing change: Alcoholism policies in work organizations.* New York: Free Press.

Bossert, T. J. (1990). Can they get along without us? Sustainability of donor-supported health projects in Central America and Africa. *Social Science and Medicine, 30*(9), 1015–1023.

Bracht, N., Finnegan, J. R., Rissel, C., Weisbrod, R., Gleason, J., Corbett, J., & Veblen-Mortenson, S. (1994). Community ownership and program continuation following a health demonstration project. *Health Education Research: Theory and Practice, 9*(2), 243–255.

Brink, S. G., Basen-Engquist, K. M., O'Hara-Tompkins, N. M., Parcel, G. S., Gottlieb, N. H., & Lovato, C. Y. (1995). Diffusion of an effective tobacco prevention program: Part 1. Evaluation of the dissemination phase. *Health Education Research: Theory and Practice, 10*(3), 283–295.

Cystic Fibrosis Foundation patient registry: 1995 data report. (1995). Bethesda, MD: Cystic Fibrosis Foundation.

Goodman, R. M., McLeroy, K. R., Steckler, A. B., & Hoyle, R. H. (1993). Development of level of institutionalization scales for health promotion programs. *Health Education Quarterly, 20*(2), 161–178.

Goodman, R. M., & Steckler, A. (1989). A model for the institutionalization of health promotion programs. *Family and Community Health, 11*(4), 63–78.

Goodman, R. M., Steckler, A., & Kegler, M. C. (1997). Mobilizing organizations for health enhancement: Theories of organizational change. In K. Glanz, F. M. Lewis, & B. K. Rimer (Eds.), *Health behavior and health education* (2nd ed., pp. 287–312). San Francisco: Jossey-Bass.

Goodman, R. M., & Steckler, A. B. (1987). The life and death of a health promotion program: An institutionalization case study. *International Quarterly of Community Health Education, 8*(1), 5–21.

Green, L. W., Gottlieb, N. H., & Parcel, G. S. (1987). Diffusion theory extended and applied. In W. B. Ward & F. M. Lewis (Eds.), *Advances in health education and promotion* (Vol. 3, pp. 91–117). Philadelphia: Jessica Kingsley.

Green, L. W., & Kreuter, M. W. (1999). *Health promotion planning: An educational and ecological approach* (3rd ed.). Mountain View, CA: Mayfield.

Hall, G. E., & Loucks, S. F. (1978). *Innovation configurations: Analyzing the adaptations of innovations.* Austin, TX: University of Texas, Research and Development Center for Teacher Education.

Havelock, R. G. (1971). *Planning for innovation through dissemination and utilization of knowledge.* Ann Arbor, MI: University of Michigan, Institute for Social Research, Center for Research on Utilization of Scientific Knowledge.

Howell, J. M., & Higgins, C. A. (1990). Champions of technological innovations. *Administrative Science Quarterly, 35,* 317–341.

Jackson, C., Fortmann, S. P., Flora, J. A., Melton, R. J., Snider, J. P., & Littlefield, D. (1994). The capacity-building approach to intervention maintenance implemented by the Stanford Five-City Project. *Health Education Research: Theory and Practice, 9*(3), 385–396.

Kolbe L.J., & Iverson, D.C. (1981). Implementing comprehensive health education: Educational innovations and social change. *Health Education Quarterly, 8*(1), 57–80.

Lafond, A. K. (1995). Improving the quality of investment in health: Lessons on sustainability. *Health Policy and Planning, 10*(Suppl.), 63–76.

Lichtenstein, E., Thompson, B., Nettekoven, L., & Corbett, K., for the COMMIT Research Group. (1996). Durability of tobacco control activities in 11 North American communities: Life after the community intervention trial for smoking cessation (COMMIT). *Health Education Research: Theory and Practice, 11*(4), 527–534.

McGuire, W. J. (1985). Attitudes and attitude change. In G. Lindzey & E. Aronson (Eds.), *The handbook of social psychology* (3rd ed., Vol. 2, pp. 233–346). New York: Random House.

Monahan, J. L., & Scheirer, M. A. (1988). The role of linking agents in the diffusion of health promotion programs. *Health Education Quarterly, 15*(4), 417–433.

Mullen, P. D., & Mullen, L. R. (1987). Implementing asthma self-management education in medical care settings: Issues and strategies. *Journal of Allergy and Clinical Immunology, 72*(5, Pt. 2), 611–622.

Oldenburg, B., Hardcastle, D. M., & Kok, G. (1997). Diffusion of innovations. In K. Glanz, B. Rimer, & F. Lewis (Eds.), *Health behavior and health education* (2nd ed., pp. 270–286). San Francisco: Jossey-Bass.

Oldenburg, B. F., Sallis, J. F., French, M. L., & Owen, N. (1999). Health promotion research and the diffusion and institutionalization of institutions. *Health Education Research: Theory and Practice, 14*(1), 121–130.

Orlandi, M. A. (1986). The diffusion and adoption of worksite health promotion innovations: An analysis of barriers. *Preventive Medicine, 15*(5), 522–536.

Orlandi, M. A., Landers, C., Weston, R., & Haley, N. (1990). Diffusion of health promotion innovations. In K. Glanz, F. M. Lewis, & B. K. Rimer (Eds.), *Health behavior and health education* (pp. 288–313). San Francisco: Jossey-Bass.

Ottoson, J. M., & Green, L.W. (1987). Reconciling concept and context: Theory of implementation. *Advances in health education and promotion* (Vol. 2, pp. 358–382). Greenwich, CT: JAI Press.

Parcel, G. S. (1995). Diffusion research: The Smart Choices project. *Health Education Research: Theory and Practice, 10*(3), 279–281.

Parcel, G. S., Eriksen, M. P., Lovato, C. Y., Gottlieb, N. H., Brink, S. G., & Green, L. W. (1989). The diffusion of a school-based tobacco-use prevention program: Project description and baseline data. *Journal of Health Education Research, 4*(1), 111–124.

Parcel, G. S., O'Hara-Tompkins, N. M., Harrist, R. B., Basen-Engquist, K. M., McCormick, L. K., Gottlieb, N. H., & Eriksen, M. P. (1995). Diffusion of an effective tobacco prevention program: Part 2. Evaluation of the adoption phase. *Health Education Research: Theory and Practice, 10*(3), 297–307.

Parcel, G. S., Perry, C. L., & Taylor, W. C. (1990). Beyond demonstration: Diffusion of health promotion innovations. In N. Bracht (Ed.), *Health promotion at the community level* (pp. 229–251). Newbury Park, CA: Sage.

Parcel, G. S., Taylor, W. C., Brink, S. G., Gottlieb, N., Engquist, K., O'Hara, N. M., & Eriksen, M. P. (1989). Translating theory into practice: Intervention strategies for the diffusion of a health promotion innovation. *Family and Community Health, 12*(3), 1–13.

Paulussen, T., Kok, G., & Schaalma, H. P. (1994). Antecedents to adoption of classroom-based AIDS education in secondary schools. *Health Education Research: Theory and Practice, 9*(4), 485–496.

Paulussen, T., Kok, G., Schaalma, H., & Parcel, G. S. (1995). Diffusion of AIDS curricula among Dutch secondary school teachers. *Health Education Quarterly, 22*(2), 227–243.

Perry, C. L., Sellers, D. E., Johnson, C., Pedersen, S., Bachman, K. J., Parcel, G. S., Stone, E. J., Luepker, R. V., Wu, M., Nader, P. R., & Cook, K. (1997). The Child and Adolescent Trial for Cardiovascular Health (CATCH): Intervention, implementation, and feasibility for elementary schools in the United States. *Health Education and Behavior, 24*(6), 716–735.

Pulley, L. V., McAlister, A. L., Kay, L. S., & O'Reilly, K. (1996). Prevention campaigns for hard-to-reach populations at risk for HIV infection: Theory and implementation. *Health Education Quarterly, 23*(4), 488–496.

Ramirez, A. G., McAlister, A., Gallion, K. J., Ramirez, V., Garza, I. R., Stamm, K., de la Torre, J., & Chalela, P. (1995). Community-level cancer control in a Texas barrio: Part 1. Theoretical basis, implementation, and process evaluation. *Journal of the National Cancer Institute. Monographs, 18*, 117–122.

Roberts-Gray, C. (1985). Managing the implementation of innovations. *Education and Program Planning, 8*, 261–269.

Roberts-Gray, C., Solomon, T., Gottlieb, N., & Kelsey, E. (1998). Heart Partners: A strategy for promoting effective diffusion of school health promotion programs. *Journal of School Health, 68*(3), 106–110.

Rogers, E. M. (1983). *Diffusion of innovations* (3rd ed.). New York: Free Press.

Rogers, E. M. (1995). *Diffusion of innovations* (4th ed.). New York: Free Press.

Rossi, P. H., Freeman, H. E., & Lipsey, M. W. (1999). *Evaluation: A systematic approach* (6th ed.). Newbury Park, CA: Sage.

Scheirer, M. A. (1981). *Program implementation: The organizational context.* Beverly Hills, CA: Sage.

Scheirer, M. A. (1990). The life cycle of an innovation: Adoption versus discontinuation of the Fluoride Mouth Rinse Program in schools. *Journal of Health and Social Behavior, 31*(2), 203–215.

Scheirer, M. A. (1994). Designing and using process evaluation. In J. S. Wholey, H. P. Hatry, & K. E. Newcomer (Eds.), *Handbook of practical program evaluation* (pp. 40–68). San Francisco: Jossey-Bass.

Scheirer, M. A., Shediac, M. C., & Cassady, C. E. (1995). Measuring the implementation of health promotion programs: The case of the Breast and Cervical Cancer Program in Maryland. *Health Education Research: Theory and Practice, 10*(1), 11–25.

Schwartz, R. S., Smith, C., Speers, M. A., Dusenbury, L. J., Bright, F., Hedlund, S., Wheeler, F., & Schmid, T. (1993). Capacity building and resource needs of state health agencies to implement community-based cardiovascular disease programs. *Journal of Public Health Policy, 14*(4), 480–494.

Shediac-Rizkallah, M. C., & Bone, L. R. (1998). Planning for the sustainability of community-based health programs: Conceptual frameworks and future directions for research, practice, and policy. *Health Education Research: Theory and Practice, 13*(1), 87–108.

Steckler, A., Goodman, R. M., McLeroy, K. R., Davis, S., & Koch, G. (1992). Measuring the diffusion of innovative health promotion programs. *American Journal of Health Promotion, 6*(3), 214–224.

Suarez, L., Nichols, D. C., Pulley, L., Brady, C. A., & McAlister, A. (1993). Local health departments implement a theory-based model to increase breast and cervical cancer screening. *Public Health Reports, 108*(4), 477–482.

Suls, J., & Wills, T. A. (Eds.). (1991). *Social comparison: Contemporary theory and research.* Hillsdale, NJ: Erlbaum.

Yin, R. K. (1979). *Changing urban bureaucracies: How new practices become routinized.* Lexington, MA: D. C. Heath.

CHAPTER 9

Intervention Mapping Step 5: Planning for Evaluation

READER OBJECTIVES
- Describe the purpose of a planned evaluation and how stakeholders will be involved
- Devise an evaluation model based on the products of each step of Intervention Mapping
- Use results from the needs assessment and the matrix of proximal program objectives to formulate effect evaluation indicators and to design measures
- Use assumptions made in Intervention Mapping Steps 2 through 4 to formulate process indicators and to design measures

The product of Intervention Mapping Step 5 is a plan for process and effect evaluation of a health education program based on the products from the previous Intervention Mapping steps. In this chapter, we will *not* go into the details of the general techniques of process and effect evaluation. There is a wealth of literature available for that purpose (Campbell & Stanley, 1966; Cook & Campbell, 1979; Green & Lewis, 1986; Patton, 1997; Rossi, Freeman, & Lipsey, 1999; Wholey, Hatry, & Newcomer, 1994; Windsor, Baranowski, Clark, & Cutter, 1994). The purpose of this chapter is to help planners use the previous steps of Intervention Mapping to facilitate program evaluation. The chapter first addresses the development of a process and effect evaluation model and then describes how Intervention Mapping can be used to formulate process and effect evaluation indicators and measurement instruments.

PERSPECTIVES

Evaluation Terms

The development of an evaluation plan is the final step of Intervention Mapping. However, thinking about the evaluation is a parallel process with program planning and begins with the needs assessment. As a matter of fact, most evaluation texts (see Rossi et al., 1999) include program planning as the first part of evaluation planning. In the process and effect evaluation, planners determine *if* the intervention was or was not successful in meeting program goals and objectives (effect) and *why* the intervention was or was not successful (process). Process evaluation is necessary to understand the results from an evaluation of effect.

Effect evaluation (sometimes referred to as impact or outcome evaluation, or both) describes the differences in outcomes with and without the program. Possible outcomes of interest include quality of life, health indicators, behaviors, environmental conditions, and proximal program objectives (determinants, performance objectives, and learning and change objectives). Effect evaluation involves determining if these factors change as a result of the intervention, which usually means comparing the group that received the program to one that did not. An evaluator does not usually propose to measure all intended program outcomes in an evaluation plan. Proposed measurement will depend on the causal model for the intervention as well as on evaluation resources, stakeholders, and purposes. Effect evaluation can be described as efficacy, meaning a program evaluated under optimal conditions, and effectiveness, meaning a program evaluated under "real-world" circumstances (Flay, 1986; Windsor et al., 1994).

Process evaluation involves several aspects of program design and implementation (Scheirer, 1994). The two categories of process evaluation are program implementation and explanations for the implementation status. Program implementation questions include, Is the program being delivered to the persons for whom it was intended? Is the program being delivered in a form that maintains fidelity to its original design? Further, this aspect of process evaluation includes whether theoretical methods have been appropriately operationalized in the program strategies. Process evaluation also attempts to describe the program, organizational, and implementation factors related to why an intervention is being implemented in a certain way. For example, an intervention can be well designed but not well implemented because the planners misjudged the need in the at-risk group (Glasgow, Lando, Hollis, McRae, & La Chance, 1993). Alternatively, it can be poorly implemented because the implementers lack certain skills or because there is no one to champion the program in an organization (Bartholomew, Czyzewski, Swank, McCormick, & Parcel, 2000). A program can be poorly implemented at a more basic level if the program designers have not adhered to assumptions inherent in the use of the proposed theoretical change methods.

In contrast to effect evaluation, which makes comparisons between groups, process evaluation is concerned with the group that received the intervention. Some process indicators, for example, judgments by the participants about the intervention, can only be found in the intervention group. Researchers may also collect process data in the control group, but mostly to find out if there was any unplanned intervention that may have contaminated the evaluation study.

Planners evaluate the efficiency of programs in terms of their costs and effects. Cost-benefit analysis monetizes both the inputs and the outputs of a program, whereas cost-effectiveness describes only program inputs in terms of money. Cost-effectiveness avoids the controversy involved in computing a monetary value for a health or social effect of a program by describing the program outputs in programmatic units rather than money. For example, a cost-effectiveness evaluation of a health program that seeks to prevent cases of measles would report cost of a case of measles averted rather than determining the monetary value (possibly by determining productivity loss averted). Knowing how program outcomes compare in terms of their cost is very important to deciding whether to expand, continue, or terminate an innovative program. The program plan (see Chapter 7) includes a budget and a description of all other program inputs that should provide a basis for an efficiency analysis. This chapter does not present the methodology for efficiency analyses, and we refer the reader to other references (Green and Kreuter, 1999, chapter 7; Green & Lewis, 1986; Mishan, 1988; Rossi et al., 1999, pp. 365–394; Windsor et al., 1994; Yates, 1996).

Formative and *summative* are terms used to describe the purpose of an evaluation rather than to refer to specific evaluation questions. A formative evaluation is done to obtain information to guide program improvement, whereas the primary purpose of a summative evaluation is to "render a summary judgment" on whether program goals and objectives were met (Rossi et al., 1999, p. 36).

Reasons for an Evaluation

Health education researchers and practitioners may think of evaluation within the context of summative efficacy and effectiveness research or formative pretesting of programs and support materials. However, it is equally important to look at evaluation as essential to program management that enables the most benefit from scarce program resources. The key to accountability and to improving the health promotion program (e.g., fitness program, communication campaign, school-based curriculum) is the framing of performance, learning, and change objectives for both behavioral and environmental outcomes and for program implementation, and then assessing whether or not these objectives are met. Our experience is that successful health promotion practitioners maintain tight monitoring of the implementation and effect of their programs in order to improve them as they are being conducted, to ensure their ongoing quality, and to justify them for continued allocation of resources.

Perhaps the most exciting reason to perform program evaluation is the generation of knowledge. Knowledge about effective programs, good implementation, and useful evaluation methods enriches the field of health education and promotion. A program planner who has used a systematic planning framework, such as Intervention Mapping, should be able to express in the scientific literature the theory of the intervention, its operationalization, and its implementation. If so, a contribution to knowledge will be possible and should depend on the quality of the evaluation, because a poorly conceptualized or described intervention (the downfall of most evaluations) should not be an issue.

An important goal of every evaluation should be that the results are used by someone (Torres, Preskill, & Piontek, 1996). To ensure that evaluation results are used, the evaluator must engage the attention of the evaluation stakeholders. The stakeholders include the program consumers, funders, planners, and implementers. Table 9.1, from Rossi and colleagues (1999, p. 55), describes possible evaluation stakeholders. Getting an evaluation used requires identifying and gaining the participation of stakeholders. Not all types of stakeholders will be relevant for every evaluation, but there are probably always multiple stakeholders. The steps in ensuring stakeholder participation (Reineke, 1991) are:

- Identify stakeholders and involve them early
- Plan structures for involving stakeholders in the ongoing evaluation process
- Help stakeholders plan how to use evaluation data
- Present evaluation results in multiple forms

Some evaluators would argue that the most important stakeholders from an ethical point of view are the intended beneficiaries of a program. These persons stand to be most affected by both formative and summative evaluations. Even

Table 9.1
Evaluation Stakeholders

Policy makers and decision makers	Persons responsible for deciding the fate of a program including funding, start-up, continuation, expansion, and change
Program sponsors and funders	Organizations that initiate and fund a program (may overlap with policy makers and decision makers)
Evaluation sponsors and funders	Organizations that initiate and fund the evaluation (health education program and evaluation sponsors often are the same)
Target groups; beneficiaries	Persons, households, communities, or other units who are intended to receive the intervention and its benefits
Program adopters	Persons in an organization, community, and linkage system who are responsible for deciding to bring the program in, to use it
Program developers	Persons in the resource system and the linkage system who create, choose, or modify the program
Program managers	Personnel responsible for overseeing the intervention
Program staff/ implementers	Personnel responsible for delivering the program components or for supporting those who deliver the program
Program competitors	Organizations or groups who offer competing programs and who compete for available resources
Contextual stakeholders	Organizations, groups, and individuals who form the immediate environment of the program
Health education community	Health education professionals who read the health education literature and learn from the successes and failures of their peers
Evaluation community	Evaluation professionals who read evaluations and learn from their technical contributions

Note. From *Evaluation: A Systematic Approach* (6th ed.), by P. H. Rossi, H. E. Freeman, and M. W. Lipsey, 1999, Newbury Park, CA: Sage.

when their opinions have been sought regarding the program, they often are left out of the evaluation process. Participatory evaluation should include the program's stakeholders, including the at-risk group, and many evaluators are beginning to consider an empowerment approach that includes enhancing the capacity of program stakeholders to perform and use evaluations (Fetterman, Kaftarian, & Wandersman, 1996; Greene, 1988; Mark & Shotland, 1985; Papineau & Kiely, 1996; Torres et al., 1996).

SPECIFYING THE EVALUATION MODEL

The first task in Intervention Mapping Step 5 is the formation of an evaluation model.

Before going into the how of process and effect evaluation, evaluators need to know what to evaluate. Effective evaluators do *not* begin with the generation of effect or impact evaluation questions. They first need to understand the program they are evaluating and what types of program effects can be expected within the time frame of the program implementation and follow-up evaluation. If the evaluators are part of the program development team and if the team has used a systematic framework to plan the program, then understanding the program is a fairly simple descriptive step explained in this section. However, evaluators are sometimes asked to evaluate a program after it has been developed. In this case, the evaluator must backtrack and reconstruct the steps in the planning process. Rossi and Freeman (1993) state, "Clearly, it would be a waste of time, effort, and resources to estimate the impact of a program that lacks measurable goals or that has not been properly implemented" (p. 218). Wholey (1994) suggests an evaluability assessment that includes a description of the program model, assessment of how well defined the model is, and identification of the ability of stakeholders to

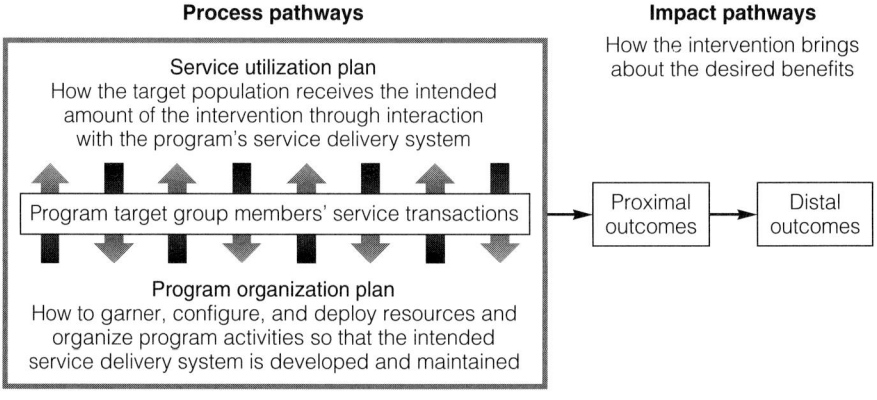

FIGURE 9.1 Overview of Program Pathways (*Note.* From *Evaluation: A Systematic Approach* [6th ed., pp. 99–100], by P. H. Rossi, H. E. Freeman, and M. W. Lipsey, 1999, Newbury Park, CA: Sage.)

use the evaluation results. Evaluators may decide that an evaluation study is unnecessary and useless when the needs assessment, the definition of objectives, the choice of methods, the translation into a program, or the preparation for implementation were not appropriately executed.

Rossi and colleagues (1999) describe the evaluation model as the theory of the program and refer to the logic of the pathways for effecting program outcomes. Other evaluation experts refer to theory of action (Patton, 1997) and causal models (Scheirer, 1994). Program pathways comprise two parts: the impact pathway, how the program is expected to cause change, and the process pathway, how the program is implemented. In addition, the description of the program pathways includes careful specification of the intended participants.

In describing the program pathways, Rossi and colleagues (1999) suggest beginning with the process components and specifically with a description of the intended interactions of the participants with the program. These intended interactions with the delivery system of the program, called the program's utilization plan, are depicted in Figure 9.1. The development of the plan was discussed in Chapter 7. These interactions are the practical program strategies in operation. They are the "acting out" of the methods that the program is intended to deliver to effect change, that is, actualization of the impact pathway. No matter how good the program's utilization plan is, if the interactions with the intended participants do not happen or do not happen according to the parameters necessary to make a method effective, the impact pathway breaks down.

Some program planners will want to begin with a simple causal model of intended program effects. Figure 9.2 is such a model developed from the child restraint device example presented in Chapter 3. (Other models of this type can be found in Rossi et al., 1999, pp. 103–105.)

An evaluation map contains the two program pathways. All the information needed to draw the map should be available from the work done throughout Intervention Mapping. Figure 9.3 presents an evaluation map and a designation of which step in Intervention Mapping contains the relevant information for each part. Following the suggestion of Rossi and colleagues (1999), the planner looks at the evaluation map on the process (left) side first. From Intervention Mapping,

Specifying the Evaluation Model

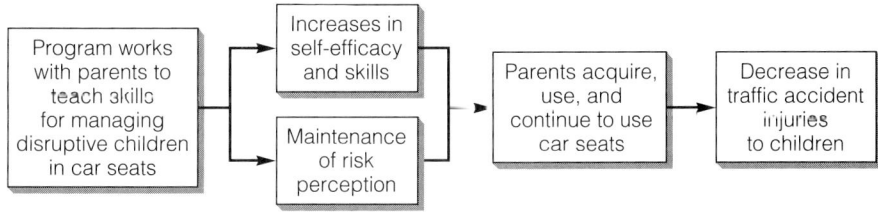

Note: CRD = child restraint device.

FIGURE 9.2 CRD Use Causal Model

> The health educator is hard at work finishing up the program plan to be presented to the city council tomorrow afternoon. As a matter of fact, the floor of the office is serving as a work surface to accommodate matrices and audiovisuals. Just the finishing touches have to be put on the chart that explains the scope and sequence of program activities and the graphic that outlines all the program partners. Then the evaluation plan can be tackled.
>
> The department head drops in just to make sure that everything is in place for tomorrow's meeting. She has no particular concerns until she asks how everything is coming along.
>
> "Oh, just great," the health educator answers. "Sixteen members of the task force will be at the meeting. Here is the agenda for the flow of the presentation. You can see that you are giving the introduction. Then later on, I have you slated to hand out certificates of appreciation."
>
> "Sounds good. Looks like you are just finishing up here."
>
> "Yes, I just have to write the evaluation plan."
>
> "The evaluation plan? What do you mean 'write the evaluation plan'?" the boss asks, just barely under control. "Why did you wait until the last moment?"
>
> The health educator, calm as usual, pulled out the folder for the evaluation part of the presentation. "Look, here's the evaluation map. Of course I didn't wait until the last minute. You know me better than that. The whole process of Intervention Mapping is, in a way, developing the evaluation plan as you go along. See, here are our health and quality-of-life objectives, behavior and environment changes, proximal program objectives, methods and strategies, program and resources. Here are the pages that show how we are going to measure each factor, and here is our plan to monitor the process. I just have to wrap some words around it. The plan has been formulating itself for a long time."

the planner has a description of the intended interactions of the members of the target groups with the program components. The planner should also be able to describe the implementation plan for the program and the program inputs in terms of costs and other resources. Planners should know the theoretical methods they intend to deliver and how those methods were operationalized into deliverable strategies with consideration of the important parameters for the methods.

Next, moving to the right, the planner can specify the proximal program objectives that the methods are supposed to affect. In turn, changes in proximal program objectives (specifically in determinants) are hypothesized to effect change in behavior and environmental causes of the health problem. Proximal program objectives combine hypothesized determinants with desired change, and both should be well specified and documented from Intervention Mapping Step 1. Finally, the needs assessment should have resulted in a set of program objectives pertaining to health and quality of life.

A word of caution: The evaluator who is also the program developer must remember to check out how the program *is* in addition to knowing how it *should be*. Rossi and colleagues (1999) suggest both interview and observation for ascertaining what is actually happening in a program. For example, in the Cystic Fibrosis Family Education Program, the developers considered goal setting to be an important theoretical method on the evaluation map. However, implementers often delivered the program without setting goals with the patients and families (Bartholomew et al., 2000).

Looking at the evaluation map in this way, first the planner needs a correctly implemented intervention (as stated in the adoption and implementation objectives in Chapter 8) in which all the assumptions that were made in the methods and strategies steps are realized (Chapters 6 and 7). Then the planner may expect changes first in the determinants and proximal program objectives (as stated in Chapter 5) and second in behavior and environmental conditions (as stated in the performance objectives in Chapter 5). Finally, changes are expected in health outcomes and quality of life (as stated in the measurable objectives related to the health problem and the quality-of-life indicators in Chapter 2).

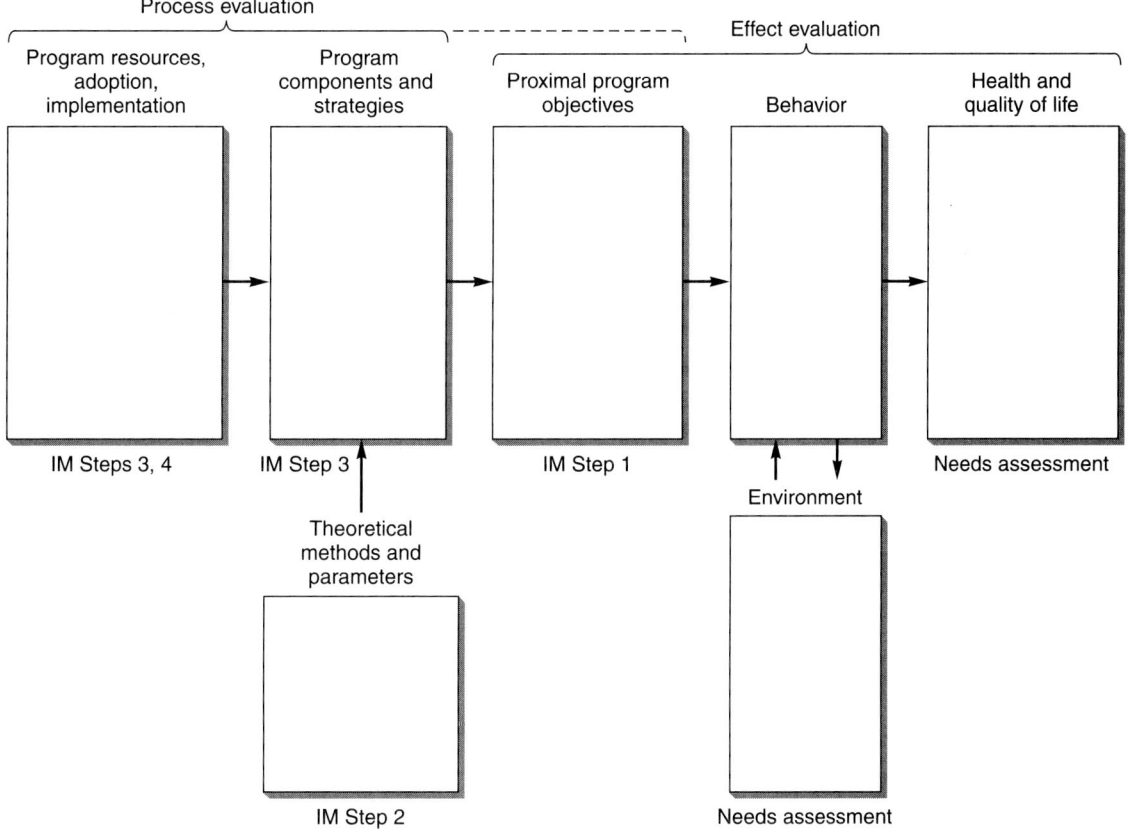

Note: IM = Intervention Mapping.

FIGURE 9.3 Evaluation Map

In the AIDS prevention program for schools, the first evaluation issue was to determine if the program was implemented completely and correctly. After that, the evaluators could explore whether execution of the program met assumptions made in program design, including selection of theoretical methods and practical strategies. If the program was well implemented and the design assumptions were met, the health educators could expect changes in proximal program objectives. In other words, they could expect to observe changes in knowledge, negotiating skills, and self-efficacy as those factors pertain to the performance objectives, and then they could expect changes in behavior, such as buying and using condoms. Finally, the health educators could expect a reduction in HIV infections, in AIDS cases, and in mortality from AIDS, and ultimately they could expect an improvement or maintenance of quality of life. The evaluation model for the school AIDS prevention program is illustrated in Table 9.2 with examples of outcomes or assumptions for each step of Intervention Mapping and the needs assessment.

Evaluating the Program Pathways

Evaluating the integrity of the program pathways is both a first step in determining program evaluability (Wholey, 1994) and the first step in actually evaluating a program. To evaluate program pathways, the planner judges the logic in the causation as well as the evidence and theory used to develop the logic. If Intervention Mapping core processes have been carefully used to access evidence and theory at each step, then the model should be sound. However, when the evaluator determines that the logic is flawed, a possibility is that the evaluation stops at that point and a recommendation is made to correct the program logic. If the intended intervention has little likelihood of creating the desired impact, then resources used to create and execute an evaluation plan to measure the intended impact would be wasted. The evaluator can help program planners and administrators correct the theory of the program, the program intent. Another aspect of evaluating the program pathways is to make sure that the processes being implemented are the ones intended.

Determining an Evaluation Time Frame

The second task of Step 5 is to state the evaluation questions. However, this task cannot be done until the planner thinks about the evaluation time frame. For instance, health and quality-of-life outcomes shown in Table 9.2 could not be evaluated within the time frame of the school HIV prevention project (Schaalma et al., 1996). Because the program was designed to reach students before they began having sexual intercourse, changes in behavior were also outside the initial time frame for program evaluation. The behavior of interest was expected to occur a year or more from the time of the program. Therefore behavior change was not an appropriate short-term evaluation goal even though it certainly belonged in the evaluation model. The actual short-term impacts expected by

Table 9.2
Evaluation Map for a School AIDS Prevention Program

INFORMATION SOURCE	PROCESS EVALUATION	EFFECT EVALUATION
Needs assessment and Intervention Mapping	Program is delivered to target population	Program has differential effect on treatment over comparision groups

Intervention Mapping: Step 4, program implementation
Observation and interviews of program being delivered
Questionnaires for implementers and recipients
	Assumptions:
	  Schools adopt the program
	  Teachers conduct all four lessons as designed
	  Students read the magazine
	  Students do homework assignments
	  Teachers and students like the program
		NA

Intervention Mapping: Steps 2–3, methods-strategies, and program
Review of program support materials
Observation of program delivery
	Assumptions:
	  Modeling is operationalized well:
	    Students attend to, remember, and identify with role models in print and video
	    Role models show appropriate responses
	  Skill training is operationalized well:
	    Students can make counter-arguments against risk
	    Students practice refusal skills, applying a condom
		NA

Intervention Mapping: Step 1, proximal program objectives	Assumptions:
	  Chosen determinants are the correct ones
	  All important behavioral domains are covered
		Proximal program objectives related to:
		  Knowledge
		  Skills
		  Self-efficacy

Needs assessment: behavior and environment	Assumptions: Behavior and environmental change are specified correctly	Condom use objectives Condom availability
Health[a]	NA	HIV infections AIDS cases Mortality
Quality of life[a]	NA	Quality of life related to worry about AIDS Quality of life related to AIDS

Note. NA = not applicable.
[a] Not included in the final evaluation model because of time frame.

designers of the program were changes in knowledge, self-efficacy, and skills. The program developers expected the program to have a longer-term impact that would be observable when the students reached an age at which they were beginning to have intercourse (within a year or two).

Having a clear understanding of the time frame for being able to create certain program effects is important to making sure that the expectations for measuring program effects in an evaluation are realistic. Some program funders, planners, and other stakeholders are satisfied with positive outcomes in the process evaluation, such as participation of the at-risk group; others will not be satisfied before there is a relevant reduction in the health problem and improvement in quality of life (Fishbein, 1996). Our position is that the evaluation should be realistic and take into account the complexity in influencing a health problem. First, intervention effects require time to develop. For example, even if a planner could, theoretically, expect one transition in the stages of change (Prochaska & DiClemente, 1984) to happen in one year, it might take longer to influence an effect in behavior. Second, health education is often directed at people's future behavior at a time when a risk behavior has not yet emerged. In this case, the desired changes may become observable only years after the intervention. An example of this situation is the promotion of condom use in adolescents who have not yet become sexually active. Third, all variables in the chain of effect have multiple causes, and the planner has tried to focus on the most plausible and relevant. However, the more relevant a cause, the more difficult it often is to change. For instance, knowledge is quite easy to improve, but often insufficient, whereas self-efficacy is often very important but quite difficult to improve. Finally, the intervention itself needs time, especially when the intervention is targeted for long-term change, such as empowerment and community development.

The question about the reality of evaluation goals is not an easy one. On the one hand, the planner wants to show effects that have meaning in relation to the health problem. On the other hand, the planner may not reasonably expect certain changes in health outcomes or risk factors shortly after an intervention. An essential part of the evaluation plan is to decide in advance on the level of effects that can be expected within a given time frame. In the example of the AIDS prevention program for schools, the final evaluation goals after two years are for behavior change, in this case consistent condom use, and changes in determinants, that is, knowledge, self-efficacy, and skills. Schaalma and colleagues (1996) did not include any health or quality-of-life outcomes in the evaluation plan because they did not expect health changes in that respect from the program within the given time frame.

When health changes are not expected or measured in the evaluation plan, the planner must have strong evidence and logical arguments to justify any assumption of causation that is beyond the scope of the evaluation. For instance, the planner must document the relation between skills improvement now and the use of condoms and a reduction in HIV infections later. The need for epidemiological or experimental evidence and arguments could include (a) the relation between behavior or environment change and change in the health problem, (b) the relation between change in determinants and change in behavior or environment, and (c) the relation between methods and change in determinants. That last type of evidence is often difficult to document, but may be based on earlier intervention studies. For instance, there is now evidence that tobacco prevention programs that influence adolescents' perceptions of norms, self-efficacy, and refusal skills will lead to a reduction in the onset of smoking (U.S. Department of Health and Human Services, 1994).

FOCUSING THE EVALUATION AND FRAMING THE QUESTIONS

The second task in Intervention Mapping Step 5 is to state process and effect questions. The evaluation map lays out the sequence and logic of program effect and process, and all questions refer back to the map. However, program evaluation questions will not be formulated for every part of the model. Several issues must be addressed before the evaluator formulates questions for the evaluation to answer. These issues include definition of a realistic time frame for anticipated effects, a statement of the purpose of the evaluation, that is, how and by whom evaluation results will be used, and a determination of available resources.

Measuring and attributing outcomes to a program, without insight into what program was actually delivered and how it was delivered, is a "black box" evaluation (Patton, 1997). A black box evaluation contributes little to any field because the evaluator does not know why a program was successful (or not). If a program was not successful, the cause could be in the program's impact pathways (i.e., the program's theoretical methods and practical strategies cannot cause the intended effects). Or it can be a problem with the process pathways. Patton offers one extreme example in which the effect of a parenting program was measured before and after the program against a group that did not receive the program, and the results were presented to policy makers who canned the program because of its ineffectiveness. Several years later the evaluators found that the program had never been implemented at all because of political sensitivities. This situation is an outstanding example of a black box evaluation.

Process Evaluation

The process evaluation will carefully check all the decisions and assumptions that the program developers have made within the Intervention Mapping process in Steps 2, 3, and 4. That information is essential for the interpretation of the outcomes of the effect evaluation. If the program fails to show an intervention effect, the process evaluation data can help determine why the program failed. A better understanding of why the program does not work can improve decision making about program modifications. It is very important to the field of health education and promotion that planners critically analyze programs that are not effective to learn from these programs and share the learning with other program planners.

Process evaluation has a place in both formative and summative evaluations and a place in both one-time evaluations and ongoing program monitoring. Process questions generally focus on two points: the amount of the program that is going to the intended participants, and the fidelity of the program that is being delivered. Process evaluation can also include exploration of why programs are being delivered the way they are (i.e., with or without sufficient quantity and fidelity). Because the focus of Intervention Mapping is on program development, health educators are also very concerned in process evaluation with determining if, and to what degree, the decisions they have made about program methods and strategies were appropriate. Further, they want to ensure that the necessary parameters have been met as the methods and strategies are translated into a program.

FIDELITY AND REACH The first task in asking process questions is to fully describe the program that should be delivered. What is each program component? What are the program support materials? What is entailed in complete and acceptable delivery of the program? How should the program methods be translated in order to ensure that they produce change? For example, a program might include four meetings with individual families whose children with diabetes were experiencing frequent high blood sugar. A description of the program would include the specifications that the meetings would follow a defined schedule of a meeting every two weeks for two months. Each of the meetings would follow a format in which a self-management problem is delineated and problem-solving steps are used to address the problem.

Process evaluation questions related to the program reach would include: What proportion of the intended groups are participating in the program? Are any families who are not members of the intended groups participating in the program? How much of the program are intended participants receiving? Are the people receiving the program representative of the intended populations (Glasgow, Vogt, & Boles, 1999)?

Process evaluation questions related to fidelity could include questions related to both the program utilization plan and the program organization plan. Questions related to the program organization include: Are the type of staff delivering the program those specified in the plan? Do the staff have available program materials? Is time scheduled for the program? Questions related to utilization include: Is the protocol followed in program delivery? How often is the protocol, or parts of the protocol, omitted? Which parts are omitted?

Inherent in any process evaluation are performance standards, the minimum level of performance described by experts in a special area (Windsor et al., 1994). In the diabetes example just discussed, the program manager could express performance standards or acceptable levels of adherence to both the visit schedules and the protocol elements within the visits. Windsor and colleagues suggest the creation of an implementation index that combines the reach of the program with the performance standard.

Table 9.3 presents a calculation of implementation indices from the hypothetical diabetes program. In the program, 200 children were screened by medical

Table 9.3
Process Evaluation of Hypothetical Diabetes Counseling Program

Procedures: INITIAL IMPLEMENTATION	Eligible (A)	Exposed (B)	Percent reached (B/A) = C	Performance standard for reach (D)	Implementation reach index C/D = E	Average percent of protocol followed[a] C[f]	Performance standard for fidelity D[f]	Implementation fidelity index C[f]/D[f] = E[f]
Screening for poor control	200	200	100	80	1.20	NA	NA	NA
Enrollment contact	75	75	100	100	1.00	63	80	0.79
Counseling session 1	75	70	93	95	0.98	72	80	0.90
Counseling session 2	75	67	89	90	0.99	80	80	1.00
Counseling session 3	75	60	80	85	0.94	62	80	0.78
Counseling session 4	75	59	79	80	0.99	64	80	0.80
Counseling session 5	75	58	77	75	1.03	70	80	0.88
Counseling session 6	75	55	73	70	1.04	62	80	0.78

Procedures: PROGRAM MAINTENANCE	Eligible (A)	Exposed (B)	Percent reached (B/A) = C	Performance standard for Reach (D)	Implementation reach maintenance C/D = E	Average percent of protocol followed[a] C[f]	Performance standard for fidelity D[f]	Implementation fidelity index maintenance C[f]/D[f] = E[f]
Screening for poor control	125	125	100	100	1.20	NA	NA	NA
Enrollment contact	25	25	100	100	1.00	72	80	0.90
Counseling session 1	25	18	72	95	0.76	72	80	0.90
Counseling session 2	25	16	64	90	0.71	80	80	1.00
Counseling session 3	25	15	60	85	0.71	79	80	0.90
Counseling session 4	25	14	56	85	0.66	70	80	0.88
Counseling session 5	25	14	56	85	0.66	70	80	0.88
Counseling session 6	25	14	56	85	0.66	71	80	0.89

Note. Adapted from *Evaluation of Health Promotion, Health Education, and Disease Prevention Programs* (2nd ed.), by R. A. Windsor, T. Baranowski, N. Clark, and G. Cutter, 1994, Mountain View, CA: Mayfield.

[a] Average percent across all family sessions in the initial implementation.

record review to judge who met the criteria of frequent poor blood glucose control, and 75 children were selected for the program. Their parents were notified of the new program and encouraged to enroll. Those who enrolled were invited to counseling sessions every two weeks for two months. The performance standards were that 80 percent of those invited enrolled, and that the proportion completing each session showed no more that a 5% loss from the session before. The implementation index for program reach was calculated by dividing the proportion reached by the performance standard. In addition, the manager set the standard that 80% of the program's intended characteristics should be met in each counseling session. Table 9.4 shows the observation sheet for implementation characteristics that the manager used to judge the implementation. The implementation index for fidelity was calculated by dividing the proportion of implementation guidelines adhered to by the performance standard.

Further, the manager, concerned that the program be maintained over time, extended the process evaluation table to include a second implementation (the bottom half of Table 9.3). In the first implementation during the maintenance period of this program, not as many children were eligible because most of the children who fit the criteria had participated in the first go-round. However, there were some newly eligible children and also some children whose parents had dropped out of the program in the first go-round. As can be seen in Table 9.3, the group was somewhat more difficult to involve, and reach was not as good. On the other hand, the manager had tightened the training requirements for the staff who implemented the protocol, and the fidelity index improved. The performance standard column of Table 9.3 is the average across all families of the proportion of implementation criteria met in each session. Table 9.4 indicates clearly

Table 9.4
Implementation Checklist for Counseling Sessions

	PRESENT	ABSENT
1. Asks how the family has been since last session or from intake	☐	☐
2. Establishes or reviews goal statement	☐	☐
3. Reviews progress on each step of the problem-solving framework or, if first session, teaches framework	☐	☐
4. Reviews data collected or presents forms for self monitoring	☐	☐
5. Reinforces approximations to the problem-solving steps	☐	☐
6. Shows video sequence with role-model story	☐	☐
7. Has family practice appraisal	☐	☐
8. Has family practice alternative generation	☐	☐
9. Has family practice alternative evaluation	☐	☐
10. Elicits family's thoughts and feeling about the process	☐	☐

that the checklist was devised from both Step 2 and Step 3 of Intervention Mapping because it represents both implementation guidelines and attention to the detail of how the health educator meant methods such as role modeling to be operationalized.

In the AIDS prevention program evaluation, Paulussen, Kok, Schaalma, and Parcel (1995) asked teachers about program adoption and use (Table 9.2). For instance, they asked about familiarity with the program and whether the teachers used the program in the last year. Fidelity was assessed with the question, "How did you use the program?" and the following answer choices: "took some ideas," "took many ideas," "as guiding principle," "followed most of the instructions," "followed the instructions completely." The teachers were also asked, "Have you used other materials along with the program materials?"

REASONS FOR FIDELITY AND REACH In the next part of the process evaluation, the evaluator will want explanatory data for the extent and fidelity of implementation. What barriers were there for implementation? For example, in the Cystic Fibrosis Family Education Program study of program diffusion and implementation, the evaluators found that the program was implemented with only moderate fidelity. A major reason for the lowered fidelity was the lack of skills of program implementers to engage in the goal-setting process (Bartholomew et al., 2000). In the AIDS program evaluation (Schaalma et al., 1996; Schaalma, Kok, Poelman, & Reinders, 1994), teachers were also asked questions that could explain implementation failure, such as: "Is AIDS prevention a structural part of your curriculum?" (answer choices were "yes" or "no"); "The program is sufficiently flexible to be used in classes with substantially different subgroups (ethnicity, sexual experience)" (answer choices were "agree" or "disagree"). Schaalma and colleagues actually interviewed teachers a second time, based on their responses on the questionnaire, to better understand implementation barriers.

METHODS AND STRATEGIES Questions related to the decisions made in program planning—questions about program methods and strategies and their operationalization—have been addressed to some extent in the pretesting and formative evaluation of the program (see Chapter 7). The only difference is that now the planner can test the intervention in its final form and its final setting instead of in a provisional form and in a simulated setting. Again, evaluators do not deal with *effects* here, but with judgments, such as satisfaction, positive emotional reaction to the materials, an understanding of the message, whether the program was of help, or conversations with peers about the program. Data from the intermediate program users may complement the picture.

Effect Evaluation

Questions related to effect come off the right side of the evaluation map. These questions are concerned with the program's impact on proximal program objectives and determinants, on changes in behavioral and environmental causes of the health problem, and finally, on health and quality-of-life outcomes. Program goals and objectives written about desired changes in these factors form the basis for evaluation questions: How much was the health or quality-of-life problem changed in the designated time frame? What changes in behavior and environmental conditions were achieved? What changes did the program create in the hypothesized determinants of the behavior or of the environmental condition?

In the AIDS evaluation example (Table 9.2), the following effect evaluation questions were derived from the column on the right:

- Questions covering determinants: Did the teens who received the program increase their knowledge of condom use as compared to teens who did not receive the program? Did teens who received the program increase their skills and self-efficacy as compared to teens who did not receive the program?
- Questions concerning behavior change, in this case condom use: Did teens who had sexual intercourse use condoms more often as compared to the control group of teens? For teens who had not begun to have intercourse at the time of the program, the question could cover intention to use condoms at first intercourse, or the time frame could be extended.
- Environment: Was condom availability enhanced by the program?
- Health outcomes: In this particular program, the epidemiological evidence that links condom use to reductions in HIV and other STD infection is adequate.

The investigators were justified in not including outcome questions related to these health factors. However, in other programs health effect questions would be important. For example, a doctoral student hypothesizes that better coping during pregnancy will influence perinatal outcomes. The evidence concerning these linkages is equivocal, and the student will want to ask evaluation questions concerning determinants, behavior (i.e., coping), and health outcomes.

DEVELOPING INDICATORS AND MEASURES

The third task in Intervention Mapping Step 3 is to develop or select indicators and measures using the Intervention Mapping matrices. A planner usually sets program goals that are stated in terms of health status, functional status, and behavior and environmental change. These goals may specify an amount of change and a time frame, but they usually do not specify an indicator of the change. The first task in determining an indicator is to define the construct being measured. For example, a program goal may be to increase the functional status of elementary school children with asthma by 25% in two years. Now the problem is, what is an indicator of functional status in children that can be measured in a program evaluation? The construct of functional status can be defined as the ability to conduct normal activities of daily living unlimited by disease. Children are usually not limited by disease if they can attend school, can have achievement congruent with aptitude, and can engage in playtime and physical activity with other children. So, indicators of functional status in children with asthma could be school days attended, grades, achievement, participation in physical education, and time spent playing after school.

A measure is a device for quantifying or categorizing an indicator. A measure usually entails applying numbers to indicators. For example, an evaluator interested in grades achieved could measure this construct in many different ways. A measure could be a year-end achievement test, an average of numerical grades achieved in all subjects, an average of numerical grades achieved in math and language arts (core subjects), and so forth. Likewise, the indicators of functional status can be measured in numerous ways. Using the asthma program goal from the previous paragraph, the indicator of participation in physical education could include number of days in attendance, number of days with doctor- or parent-excused absence, time spent in moderate to vigorous movement, and so forth.

This section presents some guidelines for defining constructs from Intervention Mapping and for developing the measures of the constructs. However, advice on measurement theory and on the ways similar constructs have been measured by other evaluators must come from the measurement literature (DeVellis, 1991) and from the literature on a specific construct.

Reliability and Validity

Validity in measurement basically means that the evaluators are measuring what they think they are measuring. Rossi and colleagues (1999) describe four types of measurement validity: (a) consistency with the past work using the construct, (b) consistency with alternative measures of the construct that have been used effectively by other evaluators, (c) internal consistency, or substantial correlation between various items used to measure a construct, and (d) consequential predictability, or the ability to predict certain related attributes or behaviors. Intervention Mapping very carefully specifies the constructs that will eventually be measured; therefore, it is a good basis for these types of validity in measurement because it helps the planner achieve clarity in behavioral, environmental, and determinant definition. Intervention Mapping Step 3 also provides the basis for clarity about what the program is, and Step 4 covers how it is to be implemented—constructs that will be important in process evaluation.

Reliability, on the other hand, is stability in measurement. If evaluators measure the same construct at two points in time, or if two different observers record the same event, will they get the same answer? Reliability concepts include consideration of sources of error. For example, a child may understand questions about symptoms or self-efficacy or any other construct differently at two points in time based on the complexity of the question, distraction in the environment, or help received. Reliability can also be diminished through procedural problems, such as asking the question in different ways or transcribing data inaccurately.

Intervention Mapping contributes much less to the consideration of reliability of measurement than to validity questions, and again we refer the reader to the evaluation and measurement literature.

Selecting Versus Creating Measures

Often researchers receive requests to use measures from their program evaluations from health educators who are looking for "valid and reliable" measures with which to evaluate their interventions. These requests always bring forth the question of how close a match is the instrument under consideration to the purpose of the program they are trying to evaluate. Certainly, considerable effort goes into the development and pilot testing of measures, but even a highly reliable measure will do an evaluator no good if it is not valid for the intended measurement purpose. For example, if an evaluation team wants to assess whether a program has met its goal of increasing asthma knowledge among school-age children, it must decide whether to use an existing measure or to create one.

The team looks at a recently published (hypothetical) report of a measure of asthma knowledge for children. It has good reported internal consistency and test-retest reliability. It also was found to be sensitive to pretest and post-test program change. Should the team use it? Well, that depends. What does it measure? What were the items on the measurement blueprint from which the items for the measure were sampled? What domains of asthma knowledge do they represent? How well do the domains and items match the knowledge that was taught in the program the team is assigned to evaluate? Table 9.5 represents the domains of asthma knowledge in which the evaluators were interested compared to the domains of the published article. There is not a good match; therefore, there is no chance that the validity of the published measure is adequate for the new purpose. This point about validity to the purpose will become even more clear as we describe measurement development from Intervention Mapping in the next section.

Effect Measures

In the planning for the effect evaluation, evaluators will have stated questions related to program impact on quality-of-life and health problems from the measurable goals defined in the needs assessment. They also will have stated questions related to change in behavior and environmental conditions that are thought to have an impact on quality-of-life and health problems, and they will have identified questions related to the hypothetical determinants that must be changed in order to have an impact on behavior and environment. The evaluators' next task is to develop indicators and measures that will enable them to generate answers to each of the questions.

DETERMINANTS   Learning and change objectives are the most specific objectives for program development *and* for the effect evaluation. Using the same principle as for intervention development, the evaluator organizes the learning and

Table 9.5
Comparison of Domains of Asthma Knowledge

PUBLISHED MEASURE DOMAINS	DOMAINS UNDERLYING THE PROGRAM TO BE EVALUATED
Anatomy of the respiratory system	Monitoring asthma symptoms
Physiology of asthma	Figuring out personal triggers
Causes of asthma exacerbations	Using an asthma action plan
Rescue and control medicines for asthma	Managing an episode
	Staying in control

change objectives by determinant to create a blueprint for each measure related to evaluation questions concerning change in determinants. So, for example, if there is an evaluation question about change in knowledge, then the learning objectives for knowledge (the knowledge column in a matrix) can be used as a blueprint for the measurement of knowledge. Looking at the columns of a matrix as blueprints for measuring a construct in the specific way it was used for program development is a good way to begin developing construct validity for the specific evaluation purpose. Thus, the indicators for program evaluation are the determinants specified in Step 1, and the learning and change objectives linked to each of the determinants serve as the basis for items in a scale to measure the determinants. The program evaluator then constructs scales for each of the determinants following the measurement methodologies typically applied to the specific type of determinant. For example, if learning objectives for adolescents in an STD prevention program included self-efficacy for performance objectives related to condom acquisition, use, negotiation, disposal, refusal, and so on, then the blueprint includes self-efficacy learning objectives for all these behaviors. However, the evaluator must go to the literature on self-efficacy to determine how the construct is typically measured and use this literature as a guide for the actual instrument development (Basen-Engquist et al., 1999; Forsyth & Carey, 1998; Maibach & Murphy, 1995; Maurer & Pierce, 1998).

The sunscreen protection matrices presented in Chapter 5 can be used as an example. To devise measures of determinants of sunscreen behavior, the evaluator can look down the columns on the matrix for learning objectives related to determinants such as knowledge ("Identify all places where sunscreen can be purchased"; "Explain how to interpret the sun protection factor on the label"), norms ("Perceive that family, friends, other parents, preschool teachers, and YMCA think that it is important to purchase sunscreen for child"), and cues ("Place sunscreen packets, bottles in visible storage area by door"; "Place mark on sunscreen dispenser to remind parents to purchase more sunscreen when that mark is reached"). For every learning or change objective in a column, the evaluator may formulate one or more questions. To measure some of the learning objectives just stated, for instance, the evaluator may ask people what they think they know: "I know where I can purchase sunscreen," with answer categories from "strongly agree" to "strongly disagree." The evaluator may also ask more directly, "Where can you purchase sunscreen?" and provide people with a list of alternatives or ask it as an open-ended question. To measure other learning objectives, the evaluator may ask people's perception of other parents' behavior and of other parents' expectations, for instance, "Most other parents I know purchase sunscreen for their child" and "Most other parents I know expect me to purchase sunscreen for my child" (answer choices are "agree" or "disagree").

BEHAVIOR AND ENVIRONMENTAL CONDITIONS Most health problems have a combination of behavioral and environmental causes. Sometimes it is easy to choose a behavioral evaluation objective, for instance, the consistent use of a child restraint device to prevent serious damage to the child in case of an accident. Often the decision is more complex, for example, a healthy diet to prevent cardiovascular diseases and cancer. A behavior evaluation objective could be a reduction of fat intake by consumers; an environmental condition evaluation objective could be a reduction of the percentage of fat in some popular foods (by the industry). The best indicator for behavior is the list of performance objectives for behavior changes in Intervention Mapping Step 1, task 2, and the best indicator for environmental conditions is the list of performance objectives for environmental changes, also in Intervention Mapping Step 1, task 2.

For some behaviors, the measurement issues and methods are complex and will require the program planner to become knowledgeable about the scientific basis for their measurement. For example, behaviors such as smoking (Prokhorov, Murray, & Whitbeck, 1993), nutrition (McPherson, Hoelscher, Alexander, Scanlon, & Serdula, in press; Thompson & Byers, 1994), and physical activity (Mâsse et al., 1998; Pereira et al., 1997; Sidney et al., 1991) have established and tested standardized instruments or methods for measurement. For each of these behaviors there is extensive scientific literature on measurement. The program evaluators will need to review this literature and decide if existing measurement tools match well with the stated performance objectives. If several options are available, then the decision will be to choose the one that best fits the performance objectives and program participants. If there is not a good fit with the performance objectives, then the evaluators may find it necessary to develop new questions or instruments to measure the behaviors. The design of reliable and valid instruments to measure the evaluation objectives is beyond the scope of this chapter; however, there are several texts that can be used to help guide program evaluators (DeVellis, 1991; Mahoney, Thombs, & Howe, 1995; National Cancer Institute, 1989; Osterlind, 1989; Tryon, 1985; Windsor et al., 1994).

A similar approach can be applied to environmental outcomes. For example, if the change objective is to substitute low-fat milk for regular milk (in this case by the school food service staff), the planner would focus part of the intervention on the lunch program. The effect evaluation would measure whether, as a result of the intervention, low-fat milk has been substituted for regular milk.

From the list of performance objectives, measurement items can be selected based on importance of the objective, pilot testing of the measure, and feasibility.

The evaluator should make sure that items are selected to represent all domains of objectives and that domains are not underrepresented after the planners have tested the measure and deleted poorly performing items.

Based on Project SPF's needs assessment of sun exposure in young children, a number of behaviors for parents and teachers (the child's interpersonal environment) were identified to reduce sun exposure for the child (there were no expected short-term effects in terms of health and quality of life; McCormick, Carvajal, Tripp, Parcel, & Gritz, 1999; see Chapter 5, Table 5.2). The following behaviors were chosen for parents and teachers in the children's interpersonal environment:

- Apply sunscreen (SPF 15 or higher) to child at least 30 minutes before child goes outside.
- Reapply sunscreen to child every 1.5 to 2 hours after the child has been swimming or sweating profusely.
- Dress child in protective clothing such as caps, hats, or shirts.
- Direct child to play in the shade.
- Eliminate avoidable sun exposure.

Questions to measure these behaviors could include actual behavior or intentions, for instance, "I (plan to) apply sunscreen (SFP 15 or higher) to my child at least 30 minutes before going outside" with answer categories of "always," "frequently," "sometimes," "rarely," and "never," and "I (plan to) reapply sunscreen to my child every 1.5 to 2 hours after the child has been swimming or sweating profusely," with the same answer categories. These five behaviors related to sun exposure can be described in more detail that identifies performance objectives. For example, the performance objectives for the first behavior, "Apply sunscreen (SPF 15 or higher) to child at least 30 minutes before child goes outside" are:

- purchase or obtain sunscreen (SPF 15 or higher)
- spread sunscreen evenly
- cover all exposed areas from head to toe

So, to measure the behaviors (or intentions) in more detail, questions about these performance objectives could include, "I (plan to) purchase or obtain sunscreen (SPF 15 or higher)" with answer categories of "always," "frequently," "sometimes," "rarely," and "never," and "I (plan to) spread sunscreen evenly over my child," with the same answer categories.

These questions are examples of a self-report approach to measuring behavior. Observation of behavior is usually a more valid measurement technique, but it is also usually more resource intensive. When self-report forms are used, they should, when feasible, be validated against observation. In the sunscreen example, parents may think that they apply the sunscreen correctly, while in fact they do not; or parents may answer the questions in a socially desirable way so that they make a good impression on the researchers, while in fact their actual behavior is different from what they report. Observing the actual behavior—for example, of the parents in the sunscreen program—may be a necessary additional measure of behavior.

HEALTH AND QUALITY OF LIFE The primary source for deciding what to measure to determine if the health promotion program had an effect on health is the needs assessment (Chapter 2). In the needs assessment the program planners identified the health conditions that contributed to quality-of-life outcomes and were caused by behavior and environmental conditions. The needs assessment led to the statement of measurable goals for health and quality-of-life outcomes. Choosing measurable evaluation indicators that are related to the health problem, as was done in the needs assessment, can be simple or difficult. In an example of fireworks injuries on New Year's Eve, a reasonable health outcome indicator is injuries caused by fireworks. In an example of patient education for chronic diseases, a health outcome indicator could be a reduction in emergency visits to the hospital, which also can be accomplished in a fairly short time frame (Mesters, van Nunen, Crebolder, & Meertens, 1995). However, in cancer prevention, a health outcome indicator is more difficult to establish. A reduction in cancer morbidity and mortality could only be described over an extended time period (10 to 25 years or more). Therefore, the best short-term indicators for cancer morbidity and mortality are probably to be found in behavior changes, such as smoking and diet, and not in health outcomes.

Sometimes planners can identify indicators for the health problem that are measurable at an earlier stage. AIDS diagnoses, for example, follow the infection after about 10 years, but a measurable short-term indicator would be a reduction of cases of HIV infection after a limited number of years, depending on the intervention. An alternative would be to use STD cases as an indicator. For cardiovascular diseases, indicators could be serum cholesterol levels, blood pressure, and overweight. However, the consensus on these indicators is not always strong. Moreover, many health education programs are directed at younger people, anticipating effects on future behavior, which means that the health outcome evaluation goals are all long-term goals.

Once the indicators are selected, the evaluator develops a protocol for measurement. For example, a typical protocol for the measurement of lung function would include the daily calibration of the spirometer, the performance of three measures, and the use of the best score.

The selection of indicators for the measurement of quality of life is also based on the needs assessment. In the needs assessment, specific outcomes were identified that are considered to be the consequences of the health problem or the behavioral factors and environmental conditions (see Chapter 2; Green & Kreuter, 1999). The indicators may be stated at the individual level, such as days lost from work, happiness, self-esteem, and alienation, or at a societal level, such as crime, crowding, discrimination, and unemployment. Thus measurement can be made by collecting data from the population to evaluate the outcomes of the program for individuals as well as by collecting data from organizations or governmental agencies that track potential social indicators of quality of life. The field of quality-of-life measurement is developing at a fast pace, concurrent with the incorporation of this type of measurement into many clinical trials. In public health, quality of life is increasingly being considered as an important outcome for health promotion and disease prevention programs (Glasgow et al., 1999; Hennessy, Moriarty, Zack, Scherr, & Brackbill, 1994). Recently, extensive efforts have been directed at the development of measures of quality of life that are especially relevant to and sensitive to health-related factors. The Centers for Disease Control and Prevention have developed indices for health-related quality of life (HRQOL) based on a series of survey questions that are used in the Behavioral Risk Factor Surveillance System (Centers for Disease Control and Prevention, 1994; Hennessy et al., 1994; Hough, 1999). The advantage of using a standard measure of quality of life, such as the HRQOL measure, is that results from one study or program evaluation can be compared with data from the Behavioral Risk Factor Surveillance System or to findings from other studies. Such a comparison allows the program evaluators to know how quality-of-life indices for their population compare to other populations and allows evaluators to determine if quality of life improves as a result of the program. The disadvantage of a standardized measure of quality of life is that it may not be specific to the health problem being addressed by the program and therefore not sensitive to change even if the health outcomes do improve.

The measurement of quality of life has important time-related factors that need to be considered when developing a program evaluation model. The time needed to detect an improvement in quality-of-life outcomes, as in health outcomes, may be long after the actual conduct of the health promotion program, especially for broad societal measures that may require decades of intervention to make a difference. Some of the individual-level indicators, such as happiness or days lost from work, may be more sensitive and therefore measurable within the time frame for evaluating the health promotion program. The point is to select those measures of quality of life that are sensitive to change within the time period allocated to evaluate the effectiveness of the program.

DESIGNING AND PLANNING THE EVALUATION

The fourth task in Intervention Mapping Step 5 is to develop the design for an evaluation study and to write the evaluation plan.

Qualitative Methods for Process Evaluation

Up to this point, we have focused on quantitative methods and measures for intervention evaluation. The objectives produced in Intervention Mapping allow for clear specification of process indicators and indicators of impact and outcome. However, as seen in Chapter 2, qualitative methods using words rather than numbers can add richness and depth to explanations of processes occurring in local contexts (Miles & Huberman, 1994).

Qualitative research paradigms range from an inductive method (Lincoln & Guba, 1985; Strauss & Corbin, 1990) that uses grounded theory in which theoretical propositions emerge from the empirical research, to a deductive approach (Miles & Huberman, 1994; Yin, 1994) that uses conceptual models of the objective world. Qualitative methods include the case study, focus groups, interviews, observations, document review, and open-ended surveys.

Like the data obtained using quantitative measures, the data obtained using qualitative methods must bear scrutiny in terms of reliability and validity. Qualitative study designs must enable the accumulation of valid and reliable observations. Reliability has been defined as the extent to which the same observational procedure in the same context yields the same answer however and whenever it is carried out (Kirk & Miller, 1986); other approaches to reliability emphasize dependability or auditability, meaning that other researchers can follow the decision trail of the original investigator (Lincoln & Guba, 1985). Validity is viewed as the truth value or credibility of the findings. Credibility is increased through prolonged engagement, through the investment of sufficient time to understand the phenomenon being studied, through persistent observation to understand what aspects of the situation are most relevant, and through triangulation of sources, methods, investigators, and theories. Other techniques include peer debriefing and member checks (Lincoln & Guba). Construct validity can also be viewed as the relationship between the conceptual model being studied and the evidence collected in the field (Yin, 1994). A study of a human experience is credible when people who have had the experience can recognize the description as their own or, if they have not had the experience, can recognize it even though they have only read the study (Sandelowski, 1986). Internal validity, which relates to causal relationships, is closely related to truth value and credibility. Yin suggests the techniques of pattern matching and explanation building to enhance internal validity.

Gottlieb, Lovato, Weinstein, Green, and Eriksen (1992) used focus groups, structured interviews, and written comments of surveys to identify factors associated with the implementation of a restrictive work-site smoking policy. They used a conceptual model in which the smoking policy concept and organizational context produced an implementation process, including communication, administrative procedures, and management support, that resulted in intended and unintended outcomes. A quantitative survey assessed exposure of communication regarding policy, beliefs, policy-related behaviors, and tobacco use among employees. The triangulation of these methods enabled the investigators to gain a clearer understanding of the policy implementation and impact.

The Purpose of Designs for Effect Evaluation

The purposes of designs for process evaluations and for effect evaluations are different. In an effect evaluation the purpose of a design is to enable the evaluator to answer two questions: How do indicators of desired program effects compare before and after the program? and Can changes noted be attributed to the intervention being evaluated? The first question requires a design in which the evaluators measure program outcomes before the program is implemented (usually referred to as baseline or pretest measures) as well as after the program has been conducted (follow-up or post-test measures). Sometimes, multiple follow-up measures are made to monitor how long it takes for change to take place or how long change is sustained once it does occur.

However, change in the outcome measures over time may result from influences other than the health promotion program being evaluated—thus the second question and the need for designs that include a comparison group. For example, if a smoking cessation program is implemented and evaluated during the same time period in which there is a national trend in reduced rates of smoking, the possibility exists that the observed evaluation outcomes are the results of secular trends rather than the interventions in the program. Therefore, the evaluator also needs to know if there is a difference between people participating in the program and those not participating. This added feature leads to a design containing pre- and post-program measures in exposed and nonexposed groups. An important methodological principle in program effect evaluation is ensuring comparability between treatment and control groups on all factors that may influence the outcomes of interest. This principle is most easily adhered to by using an experimental design with random assignment of participants to the intervention group and a control group. However, it can also be accomplished with a number of quasi-experimental designs in which the treatment group is compared to itself at more than two time points or is compared to another group that is not defined by random assignment (Campbell & Stanley, 1966; Cook & Campbell, 1979).

In health education practice, the random assignment of individuals is sometimes impossible. For instance, students from secondary schools cannot randomly be assigned to a school program or a control program, because the program is schoolwide or at least classwide. In that case, it is possible to randomly assign *units* to the program condition or the control condition. When randomization of individuals or units (i.e., schools, clinics, work sites, communities) is not possible, a variety of quasi-experimental designs allow the evaluator to compare two or more groups that are as similar as possible. Evaluators have to expect that the groups are not completely equivalent, meaning not completely comparable on a number of relevant characteristics, and evaluators cannot even assume that they know all the relevant characteristics. Statistically, evaluators can control for most of these differences, but only when the differences are measured before the program starts (Cook & Campbell, 1979; see Schaalma et al., 1996, for an example). The reader is encouraged to refer to texts on program evaluation (Cook & Campbell, 1979; Rossi et al., 1999; Windsor et al., 1994) for more specific guidance on selecting a design for program evaluation.

Whether evaluators use a random assignment or a quasi-experimental design, they sometimes want to find out if their intervention is more successful than the standard program or practice. In this situation, the control condition is not a condition without a program but a condition with the usual program. The evaluators are estimating program effects for the new program compared to usual care or practice. This group is usually called a comparison group rather than a control group. Randomized experimental design using these two groups provides the strongest basis for straightforward answers to the question, "Did the program have an effect?" However, an experimental design for program evaluation is not always possible and not always the preferred design for all program evaluations.

The Evaluation Plan

An evaluation plan includes the evaluation questions, design, indicators and measures, and timing of the measures. The plan should also include how the resulting data will be analyzed and presented to the stakeholders. Finally, the plan should outline the resources required to conduct the evaluation. Table 9.6 provides an outline for the evaluation plan and includes examples from the school AIDS prevention program that was presented in the discussion of evaluation maps earlier in this chapter (Schaalma et al., 1996; Schaalma et al., 1994). Just like the intervention plan (Chapter 7), the evaluation plan should contain details about how the evaluation will be carried out—what data will be collected, who will collect it, what resources will be needed, and how the data will be analyzed and reported.

For example, the plan in Table 9.6 suggests that a survey instrument will be developed that includes scales to measure the personal determinants of knowledge and self-efficacy and questions to measure the performance of using a condom. The survey will be administered to subjects in an intervention group and a control group at baseline before the intervention and at follow-ups 6 months and one year after the intervention. An observation instrument will be developed and used to measure an increase of condom machines in locations where adolescents have access and to measure the placement of posters that serve as cues for using condoms. Finally, health department reports on STD cases in adolescents will be used as a proxy measure of HIV infections at 3, 4, and 5 years following implementation of the intervention. The plan also includes the decisions not to measure quality of life, because the time period would not allow for AIDS prevention to have an impact, and not to measure skills, because it would be difficult to develop a reliable and valid measure of skills that could be applied to a large number of people.

SUMMARY

Program evaluation is an essential component for the practice of health education. Health education practitioners have a responsibility to the program participants, supervisors, general public, and funding agencies to collect and provide information that will enable all interested parties to judge the effectiveness of a health promotion program. Program planners need this information not only to

Table 9.6
Evaluation Plan Summary for a School AIDS Prevention Program

PROCESS EVALUATION PLAN

Evaluation questions, variables, and proposed design	Measures	Sources	Data collection timing and resources	Data analysis	Reporting
Adoption					
Awareness	Survey	Teachers	Prior to program	Frequencies on surveys and record review	To the linkage system
Agreement to conduct program	Record review	Project records	Project research assistant		
Participation in teacher training	Observation	Teacher training		Summary memos on observations	
Implementation					
Lessons completed	Teacher records	Teachers	During program	Frequencies	To the development team
Activities executed	Observation	Research staff	Project research assistant		In the scientific literature
Time per lesson	Surveys	Students			To the schools
Scheduling of lessons	Interviews				To the funder
Use of video					
Intervention assumptions					
User evaluation—teachers	Surveys	Teachers	One week following program	Frequencies	To the research team
User evaluation—target population	Interviews	Students	Project research assistant	Comment summaries	To the scientific literature
Participant exposure					To the schools
Method and strategy assumptions		Changes in determinants			To the funder
					To the participants

(continued)

Table 9.6 Evaluation Plan Summary for a School AIDS Prevention Program *(continued)*

EFFECT EVALUATION PLAN

Outcomes/indicators	Measures	Sources	Data collection timing and resources	Data analysis	Reporting
Quality of life					
Quality of life	Not measured				
Health					
HIV infection	Not measured				
AIDS cases	Health department registry of STD infections	Health department surveillance	Baseline, yrs 3, 4, 5	Change in pre and post incidence rates compared between groups	To research team, schools, funders, scientific literature
STD cases					
Behavior					
Condom use	Survey questions	Intervention and control groups	Basline, 6 mo, and 1 yr follow-up	Pre and post change scores compared between groups	To research team, schools, funders, scientific literature
Environmental condition					
Availability of condoms (condom machines)	Observations	Businesses	Baseline, 1 yr follow-up		
Determinants					
Knowledge	Knowledge scale	Intervention and control groups	Baseline, 6 mo and 1 yr follow-up	Pre and post change scores compared between groups	To research team, schools, funders, scientific literature
Skills	Not measured				
Self-efficacy	Self-efficacy scale				
Cues	Observation				

assess program effectiveness but also to determine why programs are or are not effective in order to improve and further develop future health promotion programs. The purpose of Intervention Mapping Step 5 is to develop a plan for evaluating the health promotion program. In this chapter we did not attempt to cover all the relevant information or to address the skills necessary for conducting program evaluation. There is an extensive body of literature on program evaluation in general and a well-developed literature on program evaluation in health education and promotion. We encourage readers of this text to refer to the textbooks and papers referenced in this chapter for more detailed coverage of methods and procedures for program evaluation. For students, we encourage enrollment in courses that explicitly address program evaluation and applied research methodology.

Step 5 of Intervention Mapping is structured to assist the program planner in making effective use of the outcomes and products of the needs assessment and the previous Intervention Mapping steps to guide the planning for evaluation of the program. The same analysis and decision making used to plan the program can also inform specific aspects of program evaluation. Using the Intervention Map as a tool for both program development and program planning helps to ensure a congruence between these two important aspects of health education practice.

Tasks for Intervention Mapping Step 5:

- Develop an evaluation map from Intervention Mapping
- State process and effect questions (consider the time frame)
- Develop or select indicators and measures using the Intervention Mapping matrices
- Specify evaluation designs and write the evaluation plan

REFERENCES

Bartholomew, L. K., Czyzewski, D. I., Swank, P. R., McCormick, L., & Parcel, G. S. (2000). Maximizing the impact of the Cystic Fibrosis Family Education Program: Factors related to program diffusion. *Journal of Family and Community Health, 22*(4), 1–22.

Basen-Engquist, K., Mâsse, L. C., Coyle, K., Kirby, D. Parcel, G. S., Banspach, S., & Nodora, J. (1999). Validity of scales measuring the psychosocial determinants of HIV/STD-related risk behavior in adolescents. *Health Education Research: Theory and Practice, 14*(1), 25–38.

Campbell, D. T., & Stanley, J. C. (1966). *Experimental and quasi-experimental designs for research.* Chicago: Rand McNally.

Centers for Disease Control and Prevention. (1994). Quality of life as a new public health measure—Behavioral Risk Factor Surveillance System, 1993. *Morbidity and Mortality Weekly Report, 43*(20), 375–380.

Cook, T. D., & Campbell, D. T. (1979). *Quasi-experimentation: Design and analysis issues for field settings.* Boston: Houghton Mifflin.

DeVellis, R. F. (1991). *Scale development: Theory and applications.* Newbury Park, CA: Sage.

Fetterman, D. M., Kaftarian, S. J., & Wandersman, A. (Eds.). (1996). *Empowerment evaluation: Knowledge and tools for self-assessment and accountability.* Thousand Oaks, CA: Sage.

Fishbein, M. (1996). Great expectations, or do we ask too much from community-level interventions? [Editorial]. *American Journal of Public Health, 86*(8), 1075–1076.

Flay, B. R. (1986). Efficacy and effectiveness trials and other phases of research in the development of health promotion programs. *Preventive Medicine, 15*(5), 451–474.

Forsyth, A. D., & Carey, M. P. (1998). Measuring self-efficacy in the context of HIV risk reduction: Research challenges and recommendations. *Health Psychology, 17*(6), 559–568.

Glasgow, R. E., Lando, H., Hollis, J., McRae, S. G., & La Chance, P. A. (1993). A stop-smoking telephone help line that nobody called. *American Journal of Public Health, 83*(2), 252–253.

Glasgow, R. E., Vogt, T. M., & Boles, S. M. (1999). Evaluating the public health impact of health promotion interventions: The RE-AIM framework. *American Journal of Public Health, 89*(9), 1322–1327.

Gottlieb, N. H., Lovato, C. Y., Weinstein, R., Green, L. W., & Eriksen, M. P. (1992). The implementation of a restrictive worksite smoking policy in a large decentralized organization. *Health Education Quarterly, 19*(1), 77–100.

Green, L. W., & Kreuter, M. W. (1999). *Health promotion planning: An educational and ecological approach* (3rd ed.). Mountain View, CA: Mayfield.

Green, L. W., & Lewis, F. M. (1986). *Measurement and evaluation in health education and health promotion.* Palo Alto, CA: Mayfield.

Greene, J. C. (1988). Stakeholder participation and utilization in program evaluation. *Evaluation Review, 15*(4), 471–481.

Hennessy, C. H., Moriarty, D. G., Zack, M. M., Scherr, P. A., & Brackbill, R. (1994). Measuring health-related quality of life for public health surveillance. *Public Health Reports, 109*(5), 665–672.

Hough, J. F. (1999, February). *"Healthy Days" measures and data: New tools for population surveillance and research. Disability surveillance using the BRFSS disability module.* Paper presented at the Ninth Prevention Research Centers Conference, Altanta, GA.

Kirk, J., & Miller, M. L. (1986). *Reliability and validity in qualitative research.* Newbury Park, CA: Sage.

Lincoln, Y. S., & Guba, E. G. (1985). *Naturalistic inquiry.* Newbury Park, CA: Sage.

Mahoney, C. A., Thombs, D. L., & Howe, C. Z. (1995). The art and science of scale development in health education research. *Health Education Research, 10*(1), 1–10.

Maibach, E., & Murphy, D.A. (1995). Self-efficacy in health promotion research and practice: Conceptualization and measurement. *Health Education Research, 10*(1), 37–50.

Mark, M. M., & Shotland, R. L. (1985). Stakeholder-based evaluations and value judgements. *Evaluation Review, 9*(5), 605–626.

Mâsse, L. C., Ainsworth, B. E., Tortolero, S., Levin, S., Fulton, J. E., Henderson, K. A., & Mayo, K. (1998). Measuring physical activity in midlife, older, and minority women: Issues from an expert panel. *Journal of Women's Health, 7*(1), 57–67.

Maurer, T. J., & Pierce, H. R. (1998). A comparison of Likert scale and traditional measures of self-efficacy. *Journal of Applied Psychology, 83*(2), 324–329.

McCormick, L. K., Carvajal, S., Tripp, M., Parcel, G., & Gritz, E. (1999). *Validation of an instrument to assess determinants of parents' sun protection behavior toward their children.* Manuscript submitted for publication.

McPherson, R. S., Hoelscher, D. M., Alexander, M., Scanlon, K. S., & Serdula, M. K. (in press). Dietary assessment methods among school-aged children: Validity and reliability. *Preventive Medicine.*

Mesters, I., van Nunen, M., Crebolder, H., & Meertens, R. (1995). Education of parents about paediatric asthma: Effects of a protocol on medical consumption. *Patient Education and Counseling, 25*(2), 131–136.

Miles, M.B., & Huberman, A.M. (1994). *Qualitative data analysis* (2nd ed.). Newbury Park, CA: Sage.

Mishan, E. J. (1988). *Cost-benefit analysis* (4th ed.). London: Allen & Unwin.

National Cancer Institute. (1989). *Making health communications work: A planner's guide* (NIH Publication No. 89-1493). Bethesda, MD: National Institutes of Health.

Osterlind, S. J. (1989). *Test item bias.* Beverly Hills, CA: Sage.

Papineau, D., & Kiely, M. C. (1996). Peer evaluation of an organization involved in community economic development. *Canadian Journal of Community Mental Health, 15*(1), 83–96.

Patton, M. Q. (1997). *Utilization-focused evaluation: The new century text* (3rd ed.). Thousand Oaks, CA: Sage.

Paulussen, T., Kok, G., Schaalma, H., & Parcel, G. S. (1995). Diffusion of AIDS curricula among Dutch secondary school teachers. *Health Education Quarterly, 22*(2), 227–243.

Pereira, M. A., FitzGerald, S. J., Gregg, E. W., Joswiak, M. L., Ryan, W. J., Suminski, R. R., Utter, A. C., & Zmuda, J. M. (1997). A collection of physical activity questionnaires for health-related research. *Medicine and Science in Sports and Exercise, 29*(6, Suppl.), s1–s205.

Prochaska, J. O., & DiClemente, C. C. (1984). *The transtheoretical approach: Crossing traditional boundaries of therapy.* Homewood, IL: Dow Jones–Irwin.

Prokhorov, A. V., Murray, D. M., & Whitbeck, J. (1993). Three approaches to adolescent smoking detection: A comparison of "expert" assessment, anonymous self-report, and comeasurement. *Addictive Behaviors, 18*(4), 407–414.

Reineke, R. A. (1991). Stakeholder involvement in evaluation: Suggestions for practice. *Evaluation Practice, 12,* 39–44.

Rossi, P. H., & Freeman, H. E. (1993). *Evaluation: A systematic approach* (5th ed.). Newbury Park, CA: Sage.

Rossi, P. H., Freeman, H. E., & Lipsey, M. W. (1999). *Evaluation: A systematic approach* (6th ed.). Newbury Park, CA: Sage.

Sandelowski, M. (1986). The problem of rigor in qualitative research. *Advances in Nursing Science, 3*(3), 27–37.

Schaalma, H. P., Kok, G., Bosker, R., Parcel, G. S., Peters, L., Poelman, J., & Reinders, J. (1996). Planned development and evaluation of AIDS/STD education for secondary school students in the Netherlands: Short-term effects. *Health Education Quarterly, 23*(4), 469–487.

Schaalma, H., Kok, G., Poelman, J., & Reinders, J. (1994). The development of AIDS education for Dutch secondary schools: A systematic approach based on research, theories and co-operation. In D. R. Rutter (Ed.), *Social psychology and health: European perspectives* (pp. 175–194). Aldershot, UK: Avebury.

Scheirer, M. A. (1994). Designing and using process evaluation. In J. S. Wholey, H. P. Hatry, & K. E. Newcomer (Eds.), *Handbook of practical program evaluation* (pp. 40–68). San Francisco: Jossey-Bass.

Sidney, S., Jacobs, D. R., Jr., Haskell, W. L., Armstrong, M. A., Dimicco, A., Oberman, A., Savage, P. J., Slattery, M. L., Sternfeld, B., & Van Horn, L. (1991). Comparison of two methods of assessing physical activity in the Coronary Artery Risk Development in Young Adults (CARDIA) study. *American Journal of Epidemiology, 133*(12), 1231–1245.

Strauss, A., & Corbin, J. (1990). *Basics of qualitative research: Grounded theory procedure and techniques.* Newbury Park, CA: Sage.

Thompson, F. E., & Byers, T. (1994). Dietary assessment resource manual. *Journal of Nutrition, 124*(11, Suppl.), 2245s–2317s.

Torres, R. T., Preskill, H. S., & Piontek, M. E. (1996). *Evaluation strategies for communicating and reporting: Enhancing learning in organizations.* Thousand Oaks, CA: Sage.

Tryon, W. W. (1985). *Activity measurement in psychology and medicine* (Springer Series on Behavior Therapy and Behavioral Medicine No. 15). New York: Plenum Press.

U.S. Department of Health and Human Services, 1994. *Preventing tobacco use among young people: A report of the Surgeon General.* Washington, DC: U.S. Government Printing Office.

Wholey, J. S. (1994). Assessing the feasibility and likely usefulness of evaluation. In J. S. Wholey, H. P. Hatry, & K. E. Newcomer (Eds.), *Handbook of practical program evaluation* (pp. 15–39). San Francisco: Jossey-Bass.

Wholey, J. S., Hatry, H. P., & Newcomer, K. E. (Eds.). (1994). *Handbook of practical program evaluation.* San Francisco: Jossey-Bass.

Windsor, R. A., Baranowski, T., Clark, N., & Cutter, G. (1994). *Evaluation of health promotion, health education, and disease prevention programs* (2nd ed.). Mountain View, CA: Mayfield.

Yates, B. T. (1996). *Analyzing costs, procedures, processes, and outcomes in human services.* Thousand Oaks, CA: Sage.

Yin, R. K. (1994). *Applied social research methods series: Vol 5. Case study research: Design and methods* (2nd ed.). Newbury Park, CA: Sage.

CHAPTER 10

A School AIDS Prevention Program in the Netherlands

Herman Schaalma and Gerjo Kok

READER OBJECTIVES

- Conceptualize how to perform a study of determinants for program planning
- Use theory to guide the selection of determinants and methods
- Translate methods into practical strategies

HIV infection and AIDS in the Netherlands are mainly limited to men having sex with other men. In 1994, when this program was developed, in the Netherlands 337 people were diagnosed with AIDS; 63.7% were men having sex with other men (NCAB, 1995). However, there seems to be a small increase in the AIDS prevalence among the heterosexual population. In 1994, 17.5% of the diagnosed AIDS cases were attributed to heterosexual contact; 12.4% to intravenous drug use.

Despite the low prevalence of AIDS cases among young people, there are several reasons to address AIDS prevention programs to this population. A significant spread of HIV among the heterosexual population cannot be ruled out. Young adults diagnosed with AIDS may have contracted HIV as teenagers because of the long incubation period of HIV (by November 1994 in the Netherlands, 22.3% [527] of the people diagnosed having AIDS were young adults ages 20 to 29). A considerable proportion of the general population, including young people, still does not practice HIV preventive behaviors (Brugman, Goedhart, Vogels, & Van Zessen, 1995; Vogels & van der Vliet, 1990), and because of the

---

This project was supported by funds from the Dutch Ministry of Welfare, Health, and Cultural Affairs (grant #90020) and the Dutch AIDS Fund.

growing epidemic of HIV infection, young people today face increased risk of exposure. In addition, health education programs seem to be most effective when the population has not yet formed risky behavior patterns and habits (Basch, 1989). Finally, it is relatively easy to expose a large proportion of young people to AIDS prevention activities through the school system; whereas it is rather difficult to reach them after they have finished their secondary school career.

This chapter presents the development of an AIDS prevention program in Dutch secondary schools. At the time we began this project, one of us (Kok) also was developing Intervention Mapping. We were following Intervention Mapping steps without necessarily naming them so, and this chapter represents, in part, a post hoc analysis of the program development in Intervention Mapping terms.

PERSPECTIVES IN THIS CASE

Health educators and promoters are often in the position of developing programs with the barest suspicion of the determinants of behavior or environment relevant to the health problem. The emphasis in this chapter is the use of a careful study of determinants in program development. Even though health educators are not always able to perform an extensive determinants study, attention to developing a strong (hypothetical) list of facilitators and barriers to behavior is always necessary.

NEEDS ASSESSMENT

Behavioral and Environmental Risk Factors

For Dutch young people the behavioral risk factors related to HIV infection are having vaginal or anal sex without using a condom, performing oral sex so that sperm, vaginal fluid, or menstrual blood enters the mouth, injecting drugs with shared hypodermic needles, and receiving a tattoo with infected needles. Of these behaviors, unprotected heterosexual intercourse, primarily vaginal intercourse, is the most prevalent mode of HIV transmission (Brugman et al., 1995; Vogels & van der Vliet, 1990).

In 1986 the Alan Guttmacher Institute presented the results of an international comparative study on teenage pregnancy (Jones, 1986; Jones, Forrest, Henshaw, Silverman, & Torres, 1988). The Netherlands was reported to have the lowest rate of unwanted pregnancies among teenagers of all industrialized countries. According to the researchers of the Guttmacher Institute, this low rate of unwanted pregnancies was attributed to a relatively effective use of contraceptives, especially birth control pills. The Institute report further attributed the contraceptive use to a pragmatic and liberal attitude toward sexuality and sex education, the high quality of information and education on sex and contraception at secondary schools and in the mass media, and the wide availability of con-

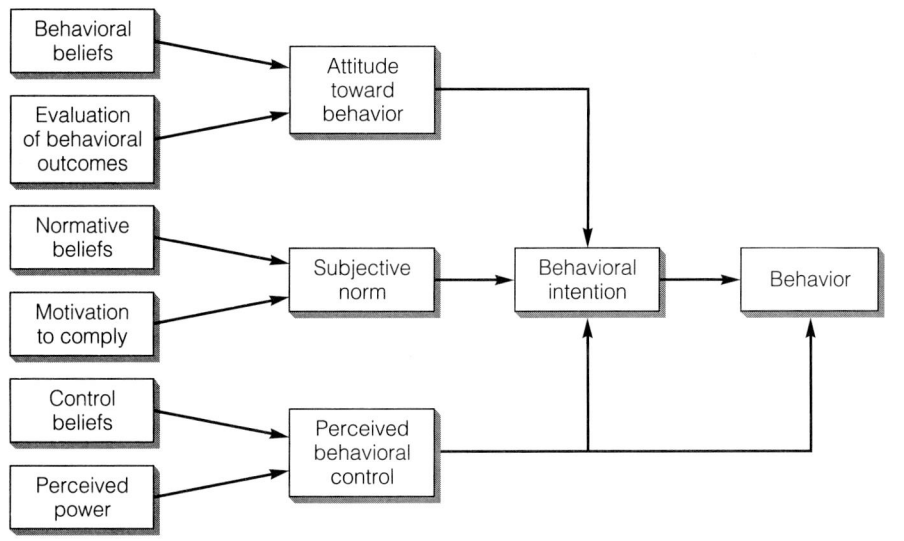

FIGURE 10.1 Theory of Planned Behavior (*Note.* From "The Theory of Reasoned Action and the Theory of Planned Behavior," by D. E. Montaño, D. Kasprzyk, and S. H. Taplin, 1997, in K. Glanz, F. M. Lewis, and B. K. Rimer, Eds., *Health Behavior and Health Education: Theory, Research, and Practice* [2nd ed., p. 92], San Francisco: Jossey-Bass.)

fidential and low-cost contraceptive services. In line with this liberal climate regarding sex education, the large majority of schools provide education on AIDS prevention (Paulussen, Kok, Schaalma, & Parcel, 1995), and condoms can be purchased in every drugstore and in almost every supermarket. Neither school policy favoring AIDS education nor condom availability seem to be major environmental risk factors for HIV infection among young people, but both may be positively related to young people's safer sex behavior.

Determinants of Safe Sex

When we began program development, there were very few studies of the determinants of safe sex behaviors among Dutch youth (Schaalma, Kok, Braeken, Schopman, & Deven, 1991). Therefore, we needed to explore these determinants before undertaking intervention development. We hypothesized major determinants of behavior based on the theory of planned behavior (Ajzen, 1991; see Figure 10.1). These determinants were attitudes toward safe sex, beliefs concerning the consequences of practicing safe sex, beliefs about social influences regarding practicing safe sex, perceptions of the sexual behavior of others, and beliefs about self-efficacy with regard to practicing safe sex (Bandura, 1986; Fishbein & Ajzen, 1975).

We used both qualitative and quantitative methods (see Chapter 2 and Figure 10.2). First, we conducted a review of the literature using the topic or issues

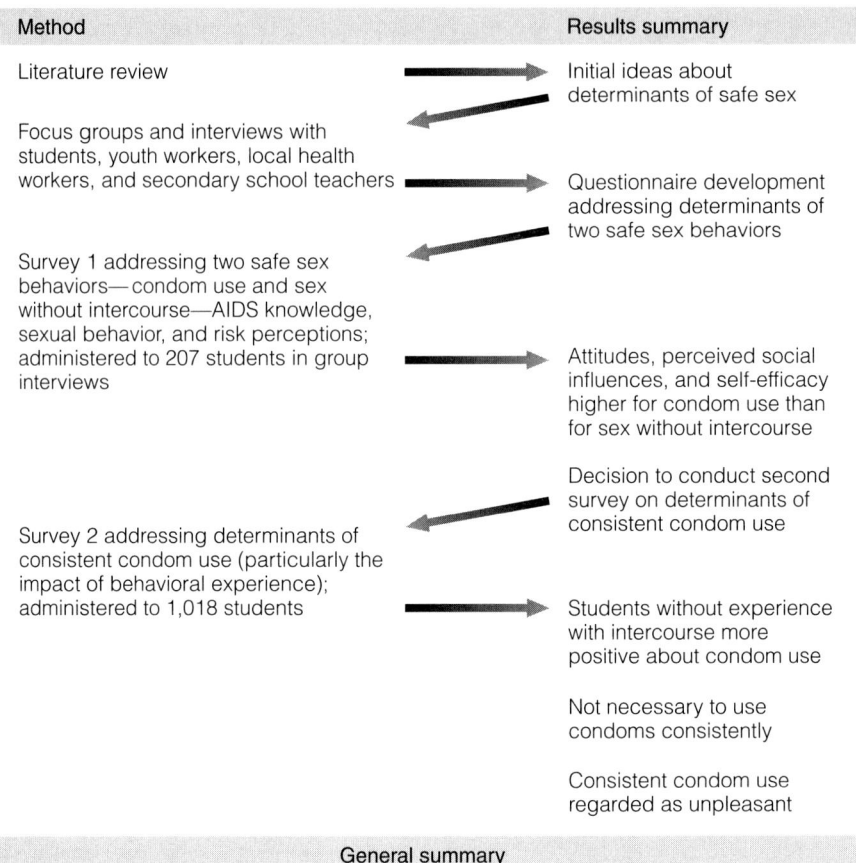

FIGURE 10.2 An Iterative Approach to Determinant Study Methods

approach (Chapter 3) about young people's contraceptive and HIV preventive sexual behavior to get initial ideas about the determinants of safe sex. To highlight and broaden these ideas, we used focus group interviews with students and interviews with youth workers, local health educators, and secondary school teachers. Table 10.1 provides an outline of focus group and interview questions. Subse-

Table 10.1
Examples of Focus Group and Interview Questions

Do you think young people should practice safe(r) sex when having sexual intercourse? Do you think that the prevention of HIV and other STDs is relevant for people your age? Why? Why not?

Do you think that infection with HIV or another STD is relevant for you personally? Why? Why not?

What are, in your view, the most important advantages of condom use when having sexual intercourse? Why?

What are, in your view, the most important disadvantages of condom use when having sexual intercourse? Why?

Do you think that your peers, classmates do practice safe sex to prevent HIV and other STDs? Have you ever discussed safe sex with your friends? If so, can you elaborate on that?

What is, in your view, the opinion of your parents/brothers/sisters with regard to safe sex and young people? Have you ever discussed safe sex with your family? If so, can you elaborate on that?

Have you ever had sexual intercourse? Did you practice safe sex? Why? Why not?

Suppose you decide to practice safe sex in the future, when or in what situations may this be a difficult thing to do? Do you expect any difficulties with bringing safe sex into practice? Which? When? Why?

quently, we administered two surveys to the youth: The first addressed the determinants of condom use and sex without intercourse, AIDS knowledge, sexual behavior, and risk perceptions. The second addressed condom use.

Table 10.2 provides an outline of the first survey questionnaire. The questionnaire was pretested by means of group interviews with students to assess comprehensibility, length, and language. We then administered it to 207 students (mean age 15.8 years). This survey revealed that attitudes, perceived social influences, and self-efficacy expectations concerning condom use were more positive than attitudes, social influences, and self-efficacy expectations concerning sex without intercourse. Consequently, students' intention to use condoms was significantly higher than their intention to have sex without having intercourse. This finding implies that AIDS education should emphasize condom use to prevent HIV because this behavioral option seems to be the most realistic for young people. We therefore decided to focus a second survey on the use of condoms to prevent HIV infection.

The second survey emphasized the impact of behavioral experience on the determinants of consistent condom use (Schaalma, Kok, & Peters, 1993). Experience of intercourse may affect beliefs about condom use, perceived social norms, and self-efficacy (Bandura, 1990; Fishbein & Ajzen, 1975). Information about the impact of behavioral experience on the determinants of condom use is sparse, even though it may be particularly relevant for AIDS education. A questionnaire was administered to 1,018 students (mean age 15.1 years).

Table 10.2
Outline of Determinants Survey Questionnaire

VARIABLES	QUESTIONNAIRE ITEMS
Demographics	What school do you attend?
	What grade level?
	What is your age?
	What is your religious background?
Knowledge (yes/no/don't know)	You can tell from a person's looks whether or not he or she is infected with AIDS.
	You can contract AIDS by sharing toilets or bathrooms with an AIDS patient.
Risk (very little/a big chance; 5-point scale)	Suppose you have unprotected sexual intercourse with a one-night stand.
	What are, in your view, the odds of contracting AIDS?
Attitude (agree/disagree; 7-point scale)	The use of condoms reduces the pleasure of lovemaking.
	If you want to use condoms because of AIDS, you distrust your sex partner.
Social influence (they do/they do not; 7-point scale)	Do you think your parents want you to use condoms consistently to prevent HIV infection?
	Do you think your best friends use condoms consistently to prevent HIV infection?
Self-efficacy (yes/no; 7-point scale)	Do you think you have the guts to buy condoms in a drugstore?
	Do you think you are able to use condoms when you are drunk?
	Suppose you are on holiday with a nice boy/girl. One night you both want to have sex. You took condoms along and planned to use them.
	Do you think you are able to bring up the subject of condom use?
	Do you think you are able to resist pressure to have sex without a condom?
Behavioral intention (yes/no; 7-point scale)	Suppose you want to have sex with a girl whom you have been dating for a couple of months. She is using oral contraceptives.
	Do you plan to use a condom?
Sexual behavior	Have you ever had sexual intercourse?
	If so, what was your age when you had intercourse for the first time?
	Did you use a condom?
	How many times have you had sexual intercourse? With how many people?
	The times you had sexual intercourse, did you use condoms? Why? Why not?

The results confirmed the suggestion that, apart from attitudes, perceived social influences and self-efficacy expectations were important determinants of intentions to use condoms, and the results provided detailed information about beliefs and expectations that differentiated students with positive intentions from those with negative intentions.

On average, Dutch students seemed to be quite well informed about AIDS and HIV prevention. However, misunderstandings existed with regard to the distinction between having AIDS and being HIV positive, the incubation period of HIV, and HIV transmission. Although students were generally well aware of the risk of HIV transmission, they did not consider it to be their problem, especially not when having a relationship they regarded as being steady. They did not seem to endorse the fact that their relationships are usually short (about 3 months) and that being monogamous within these relationships is not an effective method of HIV prevention.

Students without experience with intercourse generally had positive attitudes toward consistent condom use, but there was a marked decline in the popularity of condom use after students had begun having sexual intercourse. Although students with experience regarded using condoms consistently as a sensible thing to do, they did not consider it necessary to use condoms consistently, especially when having intercourse with a relatively well-known partner. Moreover, they were likely to regard consistent condom use as being unpleasant, creating an annoying interruption, reducing sensitivity, and decreasing pleasure.

Most students endorsed the health-related advantages of condom use. These advantages, however, did not differentiate students who used condoms and those who did not. Beliefs about the disadvantages of condom use in general (e.g., reduced pleasure), disadvantages of condom use because of AIDS (e.g., distrust), and beliefs about the necessity of condom use in specific situations (e.g., when having intercourse with a regular date) did differentiate students with low intentions to use condoms from their counterparts with high intentions.

Although perceived social influences with regard to using condoms consistently were moderately positive, young people did not perceive condom use as current practice among their peers. Generally, students had the idea that their parents, peers, and friends might favor safe sex, although a lot of them had no idea of what others think or do with regard to AIDS prevention. The positive social influence of parents was striking and conflicting with the general assumption that young people tend to become more independent of adults and to conform to their peer group. Perceived social influences of young people without experience with intercourse were more positive than those of their counterparts with experience of intercourse.

Although most students without sexual experience were quite optimistic about practicing safer sex, a considerable proportion of students with sexual experience had trouble resisting social pressures to practice unsafe sex. Generally, students' self-confidence in their ability to negotiate condom use was strongly related to their intentions to use condoms. A considerable proportion of the students expected problems with purchasing condoms, carrying them regularly, maintaining consistent use, and negotiating their use. Students without sexual experience, especially girls, were the most likely to expect difficulties with purchasing and regularly carrying condoms, whereas students with experience of intercourse were the most likely to expect difficulties in maintaining consistent use within a steady relationship.

When age and educational levels were considered, the study showed that young teenagers in vocational schools especially and, to a lesser degree, students in schools for lower general secondary education were potentially at risk for infection with HIV or other STDs (Schaalma et al., 1993). Among these teenagers we found the lowest levels of AIDS knowledge and a relatively high prevalence of sexual intercourse without condom use, or even without using oral contraceptives. These findings are similar to those of other studies (Brugman et al., 1995; Vogels & van der Vliet, 1990).

INTERVENTION MAPPING STEP 1: CREATING MATRICES OF PROXIMAL PROGRAM OBJECTIVES

Selection of a Population

On the basis of data-based and practical considerations we decided to direct a new AIDS education program to students in the lower grades of schools for lower secondary education. The large majority, about 80%, of these students do not have experience with sexual intercourse. However, these young teenagers in schools for lower secondary education and vocational schools are potentially at the highest risk for HIV infection (Schaalma et al., 1993; Vogels & van der Vliet, 1990). These students start their sexual career at a younger age than students in other schools do, and the prevalence of unprotected sexual intercourse is fairly high. Their level of AIDS knowledge is fairly low, and their attitudes toward condom use to prevent HIV infection are somewhat negative. From a practical point of view, it was desirable to develop a prevention program for these students because most Dutch programs had been developed for young people in the higher grades of secondary schools.

When demographic variables are considered, this population of teenagers can be characterized as having, on average, a low socioeconomic status and a variety of religious affiliations (nonreligious, Protestant, Catholic, and Islamic). They are from various ethnic backgrounds, especially in the big cities (native Dutch, Turkish, Moroccan, Surinamese, Antillean).

We considered whether or not to differentiate the intended audience on the following variables: experience with sexual intercourse, age, ethnicity, and gender. The question regarding differentiation is whether either the determinants or the performance objectives differ by group. If they do, then if the effects are large, different matrices must be developed for the group; if the effect is small, it can be handled within a matrix (see Chapter 5).

We already had seen from the needs assessment that it might be useful to differentiate between young people with and without experience with sexual intercourse, because these two groups differ to a large extent on the psychosocial determinants related to practicing safe sex (Schaalma et al., 1993). Experience with sexual intercourse was related to more negative attitudes and perceived social influences toward using condoms consistently. In addition, young people without experience with sexual intercourse primarily anticipated difficulties with buying condoms and initiating a conversation about condom use, whereas experienced students primarily anticipated difficulties with using condoms consistently within a steady relationship. Because sexual experience is to some extent related to age and grade level, it might have been possible to develop different programs for students in the lower and higher grades. However, from a practical point of view, it would be more costly to create two programs, and possibly it would have impeded widespread diffusion of the program. The population was differentiated on the variable of sexual experiences, and differences were considered within the matrices and during program development, so that different messages could be included for the two groups. The age variable was handled by focusing on young teens.

Differentiation also could have been gender-based. Although behaviors of boys and girls with regard to AIDS prevention were not very different, the needs assessment did demonstrate significant gender differences with regard to buying condoms and taking responsibility for condom use. Again, even though from a practical point of view gender-specific education may not be a feasible option for classroom practice, the differences were taken into consideration during matrix and program development.

Although the role of parents in AIDS education is not very clear, it may be worthwhile to include them in a prevention program. However, involving parents and increasing parent-child communication about sexual topics may be very difficult to accomplish (Kirby et al., 1994). Moreover, Dutch schools are not familiar with the inclusion of educational activities that go beyond the classroom, and a community-based education approach may impede widespread implementation because it is very time-consuming and in need of intensive organization.

Another possibility would be differentiation based on religious affiliation or ethnicity. Although the needs assessment did not reveal significant differences between the beliefs and behaviors of nonreligious, Catholic, and Protestant students, it demonstrated differences between students with a Dutch background and those with a Muslim background. We did not want different programs based on ethnicity to interfere with the nationwide character of the program. Moreover, Muslim girls strongly stated that they did not like the idea that they would be treated as a special group. Therefore, again we considered these differences within the matrices and during program development to ensure appropriate role models and messages.

Health Behaviors and Environmental Conditions

Because the needs assessment clearly indicated that condom use is the most realistic option for young people to prevent HIV infection, we decided to focus the program primarily on condom use. After the program, students should use condoms when having sexual intercourse, and they should continue condom use during—at least—their teenage years. Because the population has a mixed religious affiliation, the program should not only address condom use, but also nonpenetrative sex and abstinence. This decision was primarily based on implementation considerations: The inclusion of various safe sex options would facilitate widespread diffusion of the program among religious schools.

Regarding environmental conditions, condom use might be increased by a school policy favoring AIDS education and by an easy availability of condoms in schools. Because condoms are relatively easy to access in the community, we decided to address condom availability as an external determinant and to focus on students' self-confidence and skills regarding purchasing condoms instead of condom availability in schools. Interviews with teachers revealed that there would be strong opposition by school management to making condoms available in their schools. School policy on AIDS education had improved in the last several years: For national schools AIDS education had become compulsory, and this education had to go beyond a mere transfer of information.

Performance Objectives, Determinants, and Matrices

In order to effectively use condoms, students should be able to do the following:

- Make an adequate decision about future condom use to prevent HIV infection
- Buy condoms
- Carry condoms regularly
- Communicate about condom use with potential sex partners within the context of both one-night stands and regular dates
- Use condoms correctly and consistently
- Maintain condom use in their teenage years
- Use condoms in relationships that are perceived as steady

Our needs assessment and other studies showed that risk perceptions, attitudes, social influences, and self-efficacy expectations are relevant determinants of young people's intentions to use condoms to prevent HIV infection, as well as determinants of actual condom use. Research also showed that young people's attitudes toward condoms, condom use, and communicating about condom use are moderately positive, and that they perceive norms that are slightly favoring safe sex. However, many young people do not seem to regard AIDS and HIV prevention as something that affects them personally. Although they generally regard using condoms as a sensible thing to do, many associate condoms primarily with casual sex. Research also revealed that many young people, especially girls, expect difficulties with buying condoms and with carrying them regularly. Furthermore, a lot of young people seem to expect difficulties with communicating condom use, because this is an embarrassing thing to do and seems to indicate a lack of trust in the partner, especially for steady relationships.

Although research showed that levels of AIDS knowledge do not differentiate students who practice safe sex and those who do not, basic knowledge is a prerequisite for risk perceptions and other determinants. Therefore, AIDS education should influence knowledge about AIDS and HIV prevention, and it should establish that young people do regard HIV prevention as personally relevant. Subsequently, it should develop and reinforce attitudes and social norms favoring safe sex, and it should enhance students' self-efficacy beliefs with regard to the various behaviors that are related to safe sex.

Most of the research information is about determinants of the individual decision making or planning with regard to condom use to prevent HIV infection. There is little information about the antecedents of the specific behaviors related to safe sex that we formulated as performance objectives: buying condoms, carrying them regularly, communicating condom use, condom use, and maintenance. Our needs assessment provided some information about attitudes toward communicating condom use (e.g., is embarrassing, implies lack of trust, and is difficult to counter the "reduction of pleasure" notion) and condom use (e.g., annoying). It did provide specific self-efficacy information about buying condoms, taking them along, communicating and negotiating condom use, and maintaining condom use. Self-efficacy expectations of students without experience with sexual intercourse were quite low with regard to interrupting sex to put on a condom and with regard to the use of condoms when drunk or when having sexual intercourse with a sex partner for the first time. Furthermore the needs assessment showed that these students had low self-efficacy expectations with regard to buying condoms in drugstores or from vending machines, although they generally thought that they could manage to get a condom if they would like to. Self-efficacy expectations with regard to carrying condoms regularly (e.g., when having a date or a party) were generally low. Although young people were generally optimistic about their communication skills, a lot of them expected difficulties with resisting social pressure to practice unsafe sex (especially boys) and with maintaining safe sex within a steady relationship. In summary, the AIDS education program should address the following determinants of students' condom use:

- AIDS knowledge and risk perceptions
- Attitudes, especially attitudes regarding the consistent use of condoms for the purpose of HIV prevention
- Perceived social influences, again especially influences regarding the consistent use of condoms for the purpose of HIV prevention
- Self-efficacy beliefs regarding students' ability to buy condoms, take them along regularly, negotiate their use, and use them adequately

Table 10.3
Final Determinant Delineation Regarding Behavior Performance Objectives

DETERMINANTS	IMPORTANCE	CHANGEABLE	EVIDENCE
Knowledge	+	+++	Basic knowledge about AIDS and HIV prevention is a precondition for a positive attitude toward safe sex behavior
Risk perceptions	+	+	Students should at least endorse the fact that HIV prevention is also their concern, also when having sex with relatively well-known sex partners (serial monogamy)
Attitudes	+++	+	Positive attitudes are a major antecedent of condom use, communicating condom use, and maintaining condom use; buying condoms is seen as a male responsibility
Social influences	++	+	Attitudes and intentions toward condom use are related to perceived social norms; it takes two to tango
Self-efficacy	+++	++	Among students without sexual experience, intentions to use condoms are strongly determined by self-efficacy regarding buying condoms, carrying them, and using them
			Among students who have sexual experience, condom use is strongly related to self-efficacy regarding use, communication, and maintenance

See Table 10.3 for a final determinant delineation.

The last task in this step in Intervention Mapping is the translation of performance objectives and determinants into the most immediate focus for program impact—learning and change objectives. One matrix was developed for this program (Table 10.4).

INTERVENTION MAPPING STEP 2: SELECTING THEORY-BASED INTERVENTION METHODS AND PRACTICAL STRATEGIES

The next step in Intervention Mapping is to link the desired learning outcomes and change objectives to theoretical methods. We selected theoretical methods based on a review of theories about changing behavior in general and changing behavior by means of education in particular (general approach to theory se-

Table 10.4
Proximal Program Objectives

PERFORMANCE OBJECTIVES	KNOWLEDGE	RISK	ATTITUDE	PERCEIVED SOCIAL NORMS	SELF-EFFICACY	AVAILABILITY
Plan condom use	Explain the difference between HIV-positive and AIDS (i.e., HIV incubation) Describe other STDs, e.g., which are the most serious; how to catch, prevent, recognize, cure Discuss basic facts about contracting and preventing HIV infection, e.g., how it is contracted, what works for prevention, how it affects the immune system	Recognize that HIV/STD infection is related to behavior, not to risk group; know who can contract HIV or another STD Describe accurate perceptions of the prevalence and incidence of AIDS and other STDs (what are the odds?) Recognize the possibility of landing in situations in which contracting HIV/STD can't be ruled out	Perceive that condom use has advantages that are not related to health (e.g., no feelings of regret, lower chance of early ejaculation, no postcoital discharge of sperm) Have a strong perception of the health-related advantages of condom use and other safe sex options Recognize that the advantages of safe sex outweigh the disadvantages Anticipate disadvantages of condom use	Describe peers who plan to use condoms		
Buy condoms	Describe where to buy condoms				Express confidence in buying condoms and coping with embarrassment	Describe where to buy condoms
Carry condoms regularly				Describe peers as carrying condoms	Express confidence in carrying condoms regularly Describe a plan of where to carry them	

(continued)

Table 10.4 Proximal Program Objectives *(continued)*

PERFORMANCE OBJECTIVES	KNOWLEDGE	RISK	ATTITUDE	PERCEIVED SOCIAL NORMS	SELF-EFFICACY	AVAILABILITY
Communicate about condom use				Discuss accurate perceptions of what young people think, fear, and do with regard to AIDS/STD prevention Describe the process of social influence and conformity Adduce arguments countering proposals to have unsafe sex	Demonstrate negotiation of condom use or other safe sex options with potential sex partners (bringing up the subject; resisting proposal to have unsafe sex)	
Correctly and consistently use condoms	Describe how to put on, take off, and dispose of a condom				Demonstrate/describe adequate condom use	
Maintain condom use			Describe a plan to cope with the disadvantages of condom use		Express confidence in regard to practicing safe sex in difficult situations	
Use condoms with regular partners		Describe personal sexual behavior; can be characterized as serial monogamous (rather than monogamous)			Express confidence in being able to negotiate condom use with regular partner	

lection; see Chapter 3). In addition, we reviewed school-based programs on sex education and health education that had been shown to be effective (issue-related approach to theory selection; see Chapter 3).

This review suggested that an AIDS prevention program based on social cognitive theory and social influence theory can be effective (Flay, 1985; Gilchrist & Schinke, 1983; Kirby et al., 1994). This approach posits that the likelihood of an action such as using condoms is affected by (a) an understanding of what must be done to avoid infection with HIV or another STD (knowledge), (b) a belief in the anticipated benefits of risk-reducing sexual behavior (outcome expectations, beliefs about advantages and disadvantages), (c) perceived and actual social influences, and (d) the belief that risk-reducing sexual behaviors can effectively be practiced (self-efficacy). This theory is consistent with the behavioral determinants we have focused on in this program and is useful because it also posits change methods. These are the basic social cognitive methods of social modeling/peer modeling, skills training, and guided practice applying information and skills in difficult situations.

In addition to this general theoretical approach, more specific theories suggested a variety of intervention methods (concept-related theory selection; see Chapter 3). For example, theoretical insights on risk perception and "unrealistic optimism" suggested various methods to communicate risk and to attract young people's attention to the program (Hendrickx, 1991; van der Pligt, 1994; Weinstein, 1989). Theories of attitude change suggested methods for the presentation of information (Petty & Cacioppo, 1986). Theories of fear-arousing communication suggested methods to motivate young people for action (Janz & Becker, 1984; Leventhal, 1984; Rogers, 1983). Theories about social comparison (Suls & Wills, 1991) and conformity (Turner, 1991) suggested methods to deal with social influences. These methods are discussed in detail later in this chapter.

The next task in Intervention Mapping includes the translation of theoretical methods into practical strategies, such as classroom exercises and educational materials. An essential feature in this step is that theoretical methods are operationalized into effective communication variables (McGuire, 1985, 1986). Although there is extensive information on teaching methods and activities that are frequently used in school-based primary prevention projects (Sussman, 1991), little is known about the effectiveness and practicability of specific teaching strategies. Program developers can overcome the information gap (a) by developing their programs in collaboration with teachers, educational experts, and students; (b) by diagnosing teachers' wishes, needs and abilities; and (c) by carefully pretesting strategies and materials (Kok & Green, 1990).

In general, students' attention may be enhanced by a positive message and by attractive and appealing information sources and materials. Messages should be geared to students' levels of sexual experience, and the program should use appealing media formats such as popular TV programs and teen magazines. To enhance attraction and comprehension, the program should match students' language and their priorities and values, taking into account differences between genders, ethnic groups, and educational levels (Bunton, Murphy, & Bennett,

Intervention Mapping Step 2: Selecting Theory-Based Intervention Methods and Practical Strategies

1991). Strategies to enhance comprehension are clear organization of information, repetition, and explicit conclusions (Burgoon, 1989). Print materials added to video and class activities may also enhance comprehension, and peers may be a useful source for translating expert knowledge into comprehensible information. Furthermore, teaching strategies based on active learning and participation, such as inquiry teaching and classroom discussion, can enhance elaboration of the message and, consequently, comprehension (Petty & Cacioppo, 1986). Table 10.5 summarizes our choices of methods and strategies.

Risk Perception Change

Considering the communication aspects of the process of behavior change, a major problem that had to be dealt with was students' perceptions of invulnerability. Although adolescents are generally very eager to receive education about AIDS and AIDS prevention, most students seem to regard themselves as personally invulnerable (Abrams, Abraham, Spears, & Marks, 1990).

Theories of risk perception suggest that these perceptions of invulnerability may be due to unrealistic optimism (Weinstein, 1989). Students may consider themselves as being invulnerable because of an underestimation of what others do to protect themselves and because of a stereotypical image of high-risk groups. With regard to the first, the needs assessment showed that a considerable proportion of students had no knowledge of the protective behavior of their peers. With regard to the latter, the needs assessment showed that students' AIDS risk perceptions were strongly related to their ideas about monogamy and promiscuous sex. In their view, HIV prevention is especially relevant for people having many one-night stands, and people who have sex only within steady relationships may be not at risk. To deal with risk perceptions and unrealistic optimism, we provided information about the protective behavior of similar others (peers) and about the risks of certain behaviors (such as serial monogamy), so that the adolescents could come to feel that they are not protected by not being in certain risk groups.

Studies on risk perception and decision making suggested that people not only base their risk judgments on frequency-based risk information (probability statistics), but also on "information that may aid the construction of an image of the ways in which a particular outcome may occur" (Hendrickx, 1991, p. 28). Various studies have revealed that the cognitive availability of an explanation for an event (e.g., catching a disease) increases the assessment of the likelihood of that event, and that events that are rated as easy to imagine are judged as more likely to occur than events that are rated as difficult to imagine (Carroll, 1978; Hendrickx; Sherman, Cialdini, Schwartzman, & Reynolds, 1985). According to Tversky and Kahneman (1983, p. 307), "a scenario that includes a cause and an outcome could appear more probable than the outcome on its own." Experiments on risk judgments and decision making concerning personally controllable, small-scale risks revealed that frequency information was dominated by available scenario information (Hendrickx). These studies on risk perception guided us to provide the

Table 10.5
Methods and Strategies

METHOD	THEORY (PARAMETERS)	PRACTICAL STRATEGIES
For risk perception		
Secnario-based risk information	Risk perception; unrealistic optimism (use controllable, small-scale risks)	Role-model stories in textbooks; videotaped role modeling
Fear appeals	Fear-arousing communication (present effective coping strategies)	Inquiry teaching; role-model stories in textooks; videotaped role modeling
Frame in terms of "losses"	Judgment under uncertainty	Role-model stories in textbooks; videotaped role modeling
For attitude change		
Active processing of information	Elaboration likelihood (provide high motivation, sufficient cognitive ability)	Inquiry teaching; group discussion; questionnaire; quiz; interviews
Short-term consequences; two-sided messages; argument ordering; logic; number of arguments; moderate message discrepancy	Persuasive communication; social judgment theory (promote high involvement)	Information in print materials; role-model stories in textbooks; videotaped role modeling
Linking beliefs with enduring values	Congruity theory	Role-model stories in textbooks; videotaped role modeling
Eliciting potential affective responses	Theories of economic decision making	Role-model stories in textbooks; videotaped role modeling; group discussion
Mere exposure	Learning theory	Print material; classroom demonstration; video demonstration
Associating attitude object with other positive stimuli	Learning theory	Erotic instruction in print material; erotic innuendo in videotape
For dealing with social influences		
Information about others' attitudes and behavior	Social comparison theory; group polarization (ensure favorable initial group position)	Role-model stories in textbooks; videotaped role modeling; group discussion
Enhancement of refusal skills	Social inoculation theory	Counterarguments in print material; group discussion; role-model stories in textbooks; videotaped role modeling; video-guided role playing
For skills and self-efficacy		
Enactive learning	Social cognitive theory	Video-guided role playing; small-group discussion
Social modeling, peer modeling	Social cognitive theory (use attractive, positive role modeling and feedback about positive outcomes)	Role-model stories in textbooks; videotaped role modeling

adolescents with scenarios that include a cause and an outcome to make certain contingencies seem more likely.

We used fear-arousing messages that adolescents are personally vulnerable to AIDS and to the losses that would occur with HIV infection. However, we also provided coping methods for reducing the threat and taught the skills for applying the coping methods. Theories of fear-arousing communication suggest that fear appeals may enhance acceptance of health recommendations, but that high levels of fear may elicit persuasive-inhibiting responses such as defensive avoidance (Eagly & Chaiken, 1993; Leventhal, 1984; Rogers, 1983). Reactions to fear appeals and fear-reducing recommendations are mainly dependent on people's outcome expectations regarding the recommendations (what will happen if I follow the recommendations) and their self-efficacy expectations (how confident am I that I can follow the recommendations). Studies on judgment under uncertainty suggest that communication describing the losses that may result from not complying with the recommendations may be most effective in encouraging risk-reducing behavior (Meyerowitz & Chaiken, 1987; Tversky & Kahneman, 1983).

To arouse moderate levels of fear, we personalized the risk information by using the strategies of inquiry teaching, peer-led teaching, role-model stories in print, and videotaped role modeling. We used strategies to enhance elaboration of the information, including classroom and small group discussion and exercises in which students have to apply the information that is provided, such as completing a quiz or questionnaire, developing an information brochure, and interviewing classmates. Inquiry teaching is preferable to the didactic approach because it reduces resistance to the message and encourages discussion and consensus among group members, which in turn promotes more central processing (see, for example, Flay et al., 1988). We used various sources to provide information. Teachers or experts may be most useful for providing factual information, but peer models or peer educators seem to be most useful for providing scenario-based information. Peer modeling can be included in videotape or in print material by means of role-model stories.

Attitude Change

We chose persuasion, exposure to condoms associated with positive stimuli, stimulation of anticipatory regret, and the promotion of elaborative processing of persuasive arguments that are not too discrepant from the students' current beliefs to change students' attitudes. Theories of attitude formation and attitude change (for an overview, see Eagly & Chaiken, 1993) suggest that attitudes may change because of new persuasive arguments, preferably regarding short-term consequences of the behaviors involved (McGuire, 1985), and because of the enhancement of the salience of information already possessed, for instance, by linking beliefs with enduring personal values (Rokeach, 1980). Reception of information, and its persuasiveness, may be enhanced by motivating students to engage in elaborative or systematic processing of the information (Chaiken,

Liberman, & Eagly, 1989; Petty & Cacioppo, 1986). This implies that the AIDS prevention program should not be based on a one-sided transfer of information, but that students should be motivated to actively elaborate the information that is presented. Framing arguments as rhetorical questions, repetition of arguments, and active learning techniques may enhance message-relevant thinking.

Theories of attitude change do not provide clear suggestions for other factors that may affect the persuasiveness of a message, such as the organizational structure of the message, the ordering of arguments, logic, the number of arguments, and the explicitness of conclusions (Burgoon, 1989). However, a two-sided message acknowledging the advantages and disadvantages of condom use may be most valid and as such most preferable because most students will have been, or soon will be, exposed to arguments opposing the use of condoms.

Social judgment theory (Sherif & Hovland, 1961) suggests that people's existing attitudes distort their perception of the positions advocated in communicators' messages. The theory posits an inverted U-shaped relation between message discrepancy and attitude change: Moderate message discrepancy may cause the highest attitude change; extreme levels of discrepancy might even result in boomerang change. This premise implies that the discrepancy between AIDS preventive recommendations and students' current attitudes should not be too large.

Theories of economic decision making (Bell, 1982; Loomes & Sugden, 1982) suggest that choices between behavioral options are determined by the anticipated regret associated with each of these options. Attitudes may change when the potential affective responses to the behavioral options are aroused. We used this principle by enhancing the link between unsafe sex and negative affective reactions, such as regret and worry, as well as the link between safe sex and positive affective reactions, such as relief.

Classical learning theories suggest that attitudes toward condoms may be modified by means of mere exposure (Zajonc, 1968) and by associating condom use with other positive stimuli (Zimbardo & Leippe, 1991). The first premise implies that students should be exposed to condoms frequently. The latter can be accomplished by means of erotic instructions (Tanner & Pollack, 1988). Therefore, we exposed students to condoms and paired the exposure with scenes of positive relationships and pleasant sexual behavior.

Change in Perceptions of Social Influences

Methods to influence the way students deal with social influence are information on group norms and skill training for refusal skills. Social comparison theory assumes that people tend to conform to the attitudes and behavior of similar others, partly because those others provide information about social reality and partly because conformity may be socially rewarding (Suls & Wills, 1991). Young people, however, do not usually communicate about sexuality and AIDS prevention, and most of them have only vague ideas about what their peers think and do. We cleared up perceptions of group norms regarding safe sex by providing information about the way peers respond to sexuality and AIDS prevention and by enhancing communication among young people about sexuality and AIDS prevention.

Research on group polarization has shown that group discussions may strengthen the initial position of the group members because of an exchange of arguments favoring the prediscussion position and because of a comparison of views (Isenberg, 1986). This finding implies that group discussion may lead to a risky shift when the average prediscussion position of the group favors unsafe sex. We helped teachers to be alert for shifts to discussion favoring unsafe sex. Teachers were trained to give up group discussions when the majority of their students strongly favor unsafe sex. Teachers learned that they also might break with an undesired shift by supporting arguments and views favoring safe sex and by presenting support from other reference groups.

A useful method for dealing with social pressure to practice unsafe sex is the enhancement of students' refusal skills. Skills training based on psychological inoculation (McGuire, 1964) and social inoculation (Evans, Getz, & Raines, 1991, 1992) may improve students' ability to cope with their peers' influence toward unsafe sex. The concept of social inoculation (Evans et al., 1992) suggests a method to increase young people's resistance to social influences to practice unsafe sex by "inoculating" them with both knowledge and a repertoire of social skills to help them resist such pressures. Evans, Smith, and Raines (1984) suggest different coping mechanisms for different levels of perceived peer pressure: (a) low-level peer pressure: simple refusal ("Just say no"); (b) moderate-level peer pressure: persistent refusal, delay of decision, and making excuses; and (c) high-level peer pressure: avoidance and counterpressure.

Strategies for social influence methods in our program included classroom and small group discussion, paper-and-pencil exercises, and role-model stories in print and on videotape. The interchange of attitudes and values among peers was dealt with by means of classroom and small group discussion. We included exercises in which values and attitudes were anonymously communicated, such as exercises in which students respond on paper to statements about safe sex, and use these exercises as the basis of subsequent group discussion. Strategies used to accomplish social modeling were role-model stories in print material and role models on videotape. Psychological inoculation was accomplished by the provision of counterarguments by teachers, experts, or peers presented by means of print material, videotape, and small group or classroom discussion. Role-playing techniques provided students with opportunities to practice counterarguments. Videotapes that showed peer models negotiating safe sex in troublesome situations offered models of negotiating skills. Various subskills, for example, purchasing condoms, were enacted in easy situations followed by group discussion or feedback provided by teachers.

Self-Efficacy Enhancement

Methods for self-efficacy enhancement include skills training, mastery experiences, and modeling—all with feedback and reinforcement. To increase their self-belief regarding condom use and related skills, students need encouragement and successful experiences with the purchase of condoms, taking them along on a date, negotiating their use, and using them adequately (Basen-Engquist & Parcel, 1992; Schaalma et al., 1993). Bandura (1986) suggests a teaching process in which four phases can be distinguished: (a) breaking up complex behavior into subskills that are more easy to handle; (b) modeling to facilitate comprehension of the behavior; (c) guided enactment of the behavior in easy situations, followed by feedback; (d) guided enactment of the behavior in more difficult situations, followed by feedback. Social modeling and peer modeling seem to be effective methods to enhance skills (Gilchrist & Schinke, 1983). Adequate feedback and reinforcement may be essential elements in the acquisition of skills.

In the class situation, we limited skills training regarding safe sex to behaviors that are *related* to the actual sexual behavior, such as decision making, communication, and resisting social pressures. To compensate for this limitation, we included materials that explicitly demonstrated condom use and how to handle lifelike high-risk situations.

INTERVENTION MAPPING STEP 3: CREATING A COHERENT PROGRAM

Program Plan

Dutch secondary schools can be categorized by religious affiliation and by educational level. Although most of the AIDS education programs that have been developed for different school types are similar with respect to goals and methods, possible differences in norms and values should be taken into account. We encountered these differences when the organization of Protestant schools refused to distribute an AIDS program because of what it saw as a one-sided emphasis on condom use. We therefore decided to embed AIDS prevention into the broader context of relationship formation and to pay attention to prevailing norms and values regarding sexuality and related matters.

The analysis of the school system further revealed the following issues:

- Schools generally have limited instruction time for AIDS education (about four classroom periods; 4 to 6 hours).
- Most teachers are not familiar with role-playing techniques and they are reluctant to implement role playing.
- Teachers are not willing to invest a lot of time in program preparation or teacher training for an AIDS program.
- The predominant teaching strategies are the didactic approach and the use of textbooks and videotape.
- Most teachers perceive problems with initiating classroom discussions about sexuality.

- Teachers perceive that students in the lower grades of schools for lower secondary education are not able to concentrate on one topic for a long time.
- Students in the lower grades of schools for lower secondary education may have difficulty putting their attitudes and opinions in writing.

Program Scope, Sequence, and Delivery

On the basis of the review of potentially useful strategies and the practical limitations of the school system, we decided to design an AIDS/STD program that consisted of four one-class-period lessons that are embedded in a comprehensive program on sexuality (Schaalma, Kok, Poelman, & Reinders, 1994). The sexuality program covers topics such as falling in love, the first intercourse, and homosexuality. The four lessons of the AIDS/STD program are presented in Table 10.6.

The AIDS/STD program consists of the following support materials: (a) a teacher manual providing background information and fully worked-out lessons in terms of objectives, materials, and methods; (b) a student magazine, similar to popular teen magazines, that presents information about facts, attitudes, and values regarding sexual behavior and AIDS/STD prevention; and (c) a videotape showing the process of social influence and conformity, introducing positive role models, and demonstrating dialogues concerning safer sex in lifelike troublesome situations. Both the magazine and the video deal with young people's beliefs and values concerning safe sex, reasons for having risk-taking sex, barriers to the practice of safe sex, communication about safe sex, and standing up to direct and indirect pressures to practice risk-taking sex. Besides facts about AIDS and other STDs, the magazine provides information about attitudes and values regarding sexual activity and AIDS/STD prevention by means of peer role-model stories about values, attitudes, expectations, problems, and experiences.

In order to introduce skills training in the classroom, we developed a dramatized two-part videotape. The first part presents a group of young people making a television program for a local broadcasting company. The video shows them interviewing peers about safe sex and discussing these interviews during the production of their program. The video also presents a girl demonstrating condom use on the fingers of her boyfriend, and a computer animation of condom use. The second part of the video presents four scenes concerning standing up to social pressures regarding sex. First, a realistic high-risk situation is introduced, for example, a boy pressing his girlfriend to have intercourse. Halfway through the dialogue the teacher stops the tape, and students complete the dialogue in subgroups guided by specific questions. After these discussions the video is resumed and presents a positive outcome to the situation. The dialogues, viewing exercises, and teacher instructions for the discussions are based on a framework for resistance to increasing peer pressure based on social inoculation (Evans et al., 1991, 1992) and are intended to help students build their resistance to social pres-

Table 10.6
Program Scope and Sequence

LESSON NO. AND GOAL	STRATEGIES
Lesson 1: Increase knowledge and change risk perceptions	Inquiry teaching
	Classroom discussion
	Exercises to apply the information that is provided (e.g., making an information brochure, completing a quiz, interviewing peers)
	Lectures by teachers and information in print from experts
Lesson 2: Change attitudes about condom use and safer sex in general	Classroom discussion on the basis of a homework assignment addressing facts about AIDS/STD prevention
	Role-model stories in print material covering attitudes about safe sex and problems with practicing safe sex
	Classroom discussion on the basis of statements about practicing safe sex (students respond to statements orally or in writing)
	Pencil-and-paper subgroup discussion
Lesson 3: Enhance values, social influences, and communication skills regarding the prevention of AIDS and STDs	Homework assignment that requires students to respond to situations addressing social pressures ("What would you do when …")
	Classroom discussion subsequent to homework
	Teacher-delivered information about the process of social influence (didactic approach or inquiry teaching)
	Peer models discussing safe sex and telling about their attitudes, values, and experiences by means of dramatized videotape and subsequent classroom discussion about videotape modeling
Lesson 4: Enhance students' self-efficacy regarding negotiating and condom use skills	Homework assignment on buying condoms
	Subsequent classroom discussion about buying experiences
	Demonstration and practice of condom use on fingers
	Video-animation of adequate condom use
	Interactive videotape showing peer models negotiating real-life troublesome situations and subsequent classroom discussion

sure against safe sex: (a) say what you want, (b) think about the arguments, (c) stick to your opinion, (d) present alternatives, (e) give counterpressure, and if that does not work, (f) walk away (avoidance).

Pretesting and Production

An essential element in program development is pretesting, because it allows the reactions of experts and members of the population to be gauged at an early stage in a program's life. We tested the intervention materials for attractiveness, comprehensibility, relevance, credibility, acceptability, undesired side effects, and workability with the adolescents. We also tested the feasibility of the program with teachers and educational experts. Interviews addressed the suitability of teaching methods and examined expectations about how long preparation and instruction would take. Some of our originally proposed strategies, such as role plays, were deemed to be too radical a departure from usual teaching. Consequently, we revised the program and slightly narrowed the variety of strategies.

The student magazine was first pretested on 147 students, who completed a questionnaire that addressed the layout of the pages and the attractiveness of the illustrations. Generally, the magazine was evaluated positively: 79% of the students liked it; 54% liked the illustrations; 69% found it well organized; and 88% liked the balance between text and illustrations. In a second pretest, the comprehensibility and persuasiveness of the magazine were tested on 119 students using a pretest and post-test control group design. Respondents completed a questionnaire that assessed students' level of AIDS knowledge, and they evaluated the magazine's quality, clearness, usefulness, newsworthiness, and closeness to real life. Both pretests led us to make content and style changes to the magazine.

A synopsis of the video was pretested by means of two group interviews with students. Respondents evaluated the ideas that the video contained and provided suggestions for translating the synopsis into a scenario. A model scenario was pretested among 44 students, using content response coding (U.S. DHHS, 1984), and the off-line montage was previewed by 83 students, who assessed it for attractiveness, credibility, and closeness to real life. Again, pretesting led to changes. A student panel was also frequently consulted during the later development of the program.

Several people contributed to the actual production of the program. A research and development team, including researchers and school health educators, produced the teacher manual. The student magazine was developed in cooperation with a professional text writer, graphic designers, and an illustrator. The videotape was developed in cooperation with a professional scenario writer and a film producer. To guarantee the linkage between materials and theoretical methods and strategies, the research and development team closely supervised all activities.

INTERVENTION MAPPING STEP 4: SPECIFYING ADOPTION AND IMPLEMENTATION PLANS

Linkage Board

To anticipate problems with adoption and implementation of the program, we formed a linkage board to bridge the gap between the development team and the school system (Orlandi, Landers, Weston, & Haley, 1990). This board was made up of representatives from the development team, the school advisory services, the organizations that provide sex and AIDS education to secondary schools, and an association of teachers of biology. A member of the development team acted as change agent. The role of the board was to provide feedback on performance and learning objectives of the program and to give advice on implementation issues.

Performance Objectives, Determinants, and Learning Objectives

The next tasks in developing an adoption and implementation plan begin with a decision about performance objectives based on a description of what would occur if the program is well adopted and implemented. Once performance objectives are determined, developers can hypothesize determinants of the performance and create a matrix of learning objectives by combining the performance objectives with the determinants. In order to do these tasks, we explored the determinants of teachers' intentions to teach AIDS education.

In the Netherlands the autonomy of schools and teachers is the prevailing norm within the educational system. No external authority can interfere in the details of the curriculum in schools. Dutch teachers are not mandated to provide AIDS education, but they are able to make individual or small-team decisions to adopt and implement AIDS education programs. Teachers of biology, social studies, religious education, or health education are the usual providers of education on sex and AIDS, on a voluntary basis. Therefore, teachers should be the ones to adopt and implement a program such as ours. The performance objectives for teachers were the following: (a) become aware of the availability of the new program, (b) adopt the new program, and (c) teach the new program according to guidelines provided by the development team.

A questionnaire survey among a sample of 956 Dutch secondary school teachers provided insight into the determinants of their intentions to provide classroom AIDS education (Paulussen, Kok, & Schaalma, 1994). This study, based on a theoretical model similar to the theory of planned behavior (Ajzen, 1991), addressed determinants of awareness and adoption of four nationally disseminated AIDS programs. It revealed that teachers' knowledge about AIDS programs was largely dependent on diffusion networks within schools. Both the perceived behavior of colleagues and the frequency of interaction with colleagues played an important role in acquiring information about AIDS prevention programs. Adoption of AIDS education in general was associated with perceived subjective norms, self-efficacy beliefs, perceptions of responsibility, sexual morality, and formal school policy toward AIDS education. Neither teachers' general intentions to provide AIDS education nor their intentions to adopt a specific program were associated with beliefs about learning outcomes. This finding suggests that teachers are more motivated by immediate concerns such as ease of program implementation and student response than by expected health or other beneficial outcomes.

A cross-sectional survey of Dutch secondary school teachers revealed that most of the teachers who were aware of national AIDS curricula (60%) had received information about the curricula by written communication (publishers' overviews, direct mail); 16% had received information by personal communication with external experts. A considerable proportion of teachers named colleagues as an information source; 63% of them knew about a colleague using one of the curricula, and 34% had discussed the materials with a colleague. Teachers' awareness was most strongly related to descriptive norms and frequency of collegial interaction (Paulussen et al., 1995).

One out of two teachers had initially implemented one of the AIDS curricula. A teacher's decision to use one of the curricula was associated with subjective norms and perceived instrumentality. A teacher's decision to use a particular curriculum was most strongly related to curriculum-specific beliefs about instrumentality, social norms, and financial costs. The limited impact of teachers' perceptions of the feasibility and importance of student learning outcomes is in line with other research of teacher planning behavior showing that teacher planning is guided by program content and activities, and not by program objectives. Teacher planning appears to be directed by their estimated ability to maximize students' participation and enjoyment (Borko, Livingston, & Shavelson, 1981; Clark & Peterson, 1986; Shavelson & Stern, 1981).

Based on our review of teachers' intentions to provide AIDS education, we hypothesized that targeting the following determinants would be important to facilitate program adoption and implementation:

- Knowledge of the program characteristics including a strong perception of the advantage of the innovation program
- A perception that the program is easy to implement
- A perception that the youth would like it
- Knowledge of how to get the program
- Skills to easily implement the program
- Confidence in the ability to implement the program

Implementation Support

The adoption and implementation plan for postevaluation diffusion included written materials to make teachers aware of the program and its characteristics. The reach of written materials was enhanced by addressing information to individual teachers and to their subject departments as suggested by Stokking and Leenders (1992) and by stimulating teacher collaboration. We used brochures with role models who demonstrated short-term benefits, effective use, and positive student participation and learning. In order to facilitate program implementation, we linked it to a national teacher training program that was specific to the performance objectives and to a large degree based on social learning techniques.

It must be noted that these efforts were not made for the research evaluation implementation but only for the national postevaluation diffusion of the program, which is not covered in this chapter.

INTERVENTION MAPPING STEP 5: GENERATING AN EVALUATION PLAN

Examples from the evaluation of this program are included in Chapter 9.

Evaluation Model and Questions

We were able to evaluate potential program effects in a quasi-experimental field experiment that included 51 secondary schools (Schaalma et al., 1996). Because our program was intended to reduce sexual risk behavior among young adolescents and because prevalence of sexual risk behavior among these young people is quite low, the emphasis of the program was on changing cognitions and skills. Therefore evaluation questions related to program effects on behavior, health, and quality-of-life indicators were beyond the scope of our demonstration project.

In addition to expected program effects, we were interested in students' and teachers' evaluation of the program. Does the program match students' reality? Do students like working with the program? Do they perceive the program as personally valuable? Does the program match teaching practice? Do teachers like working with the program? Do they perceive the program as an improvement of their classes on sexuality and AIDS/HIV prevention? Furthermore, we were interested in the way the various strategies were actually implemented by teachers.

Effect Evaluation Design and Results

The potential program effects were evaluated using a pretest and post-test control group design (Schaalma et al., 1996). Participating schools were matched in pairs on the basis of school type, participating grade levels (9 and 10), religious affiliation, degree of urbanization, number of participating students, boy-girl ratio, proportion of ethnic minorities, and the qualifications of participating teachers. Within these pairs, schools were randomly assigned to the experimental or the control condition. Experimental schools provided education about AIDS, STDs, and prevention by using the experimental program; control schools provided education about AIDS, STDs, and prevention as they had in the past.

Fifty-four schools from a stratified random sample of 415 schools for lower secondary education agreed to participate in the study (13%). Nineteen schools were Catholic schools, 12 were Protestant schools, 21 were nonreligious schools, and two schools had a mixed religious affiliation. Three schools were excluded from the analyses because they failed to provide either baseline data or follow-up data. In sum, 77 teachers participated in the study; 39 were male, 38 female. Most were teachers of biology (23%), health education (38%), or social studies (19%).

Students were requested to complete a questionnaire in their classroom about one month before the education on AIDS, STDs, and prevention was provided (baseline assessment). They had to complete a comparable second questionnaire 4 to 8 weeks after the education had been given (follow-up assessment). The teachers supervised completion of the questionnaires. The questionnaire was to a large extent based on a model of behavioral determinants distinguishing attitude, social influence, and self-efficacy beliefs (Schaalma et al., 1993).

The baseline questionnaire was completed by 3,142 students; the follow-up questionnaire by 2,786 students. The final participating study sample consisted of 51 schools and all students whose baseline and follow-up questionnaire could be correctly matched (N = 2,430; 77% of baseline sample). Matching criteria were (a) school, (b) class, (c) date of birth, (d) initials of mother's name, and (e) profession of father. Unavailability for follow-up was primarily due to absenteeism, transfer to other schools, or missing data on matching variables.

Multilevel regression analyses of students' baseline and follow-up questionnaires revealed that our program had a significant favorable impact on students' AIDS/STD knowledge, on their beliefs and intentions regarding consistent use of condoms, and on their sexual risk-taking behavior. The AIDS/STD program produced its most pronounced effects within the area of knowledge and attitudes. The changes in perceived social influences, self-efficacy beliefs, intentions, and sexual risk-taking were smaller but still significant. Figure 10.3 presents the effect sizes from the evaluation study.

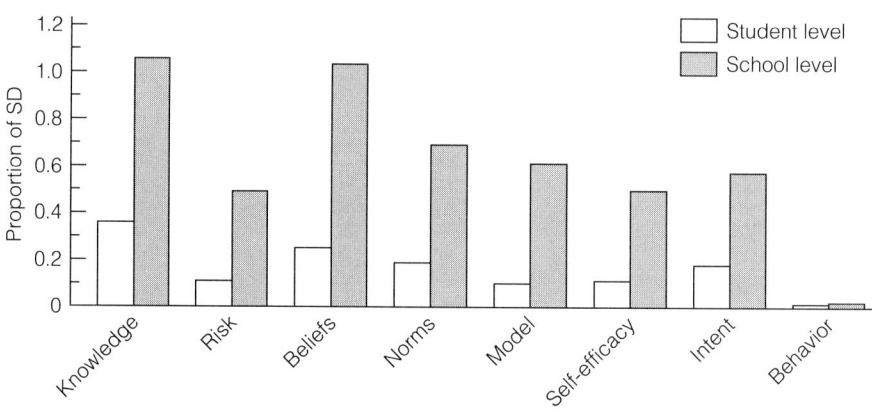

FIGURE 10.3 Effect Sizes (*Note.* Effect sizes are computed as the difference between experimental and control student change scores divided by the pooled SD for these students. Effect sizes at school level are computed as the difference between experimental and control schools' average change scores divided by the pooled SD for these schools.)
SD = standard deviation.

Process Evaluation

In addition to the effect evaluation, the program was subject to a process evaluation. A survey among 1,481 students showed that we managed quite well to match the program to students' perception of their environment. About 75% of the students evaluated the program as informative, good, and clear. Only 10% of them evaluated the program as difficult and unpleasant, and about 25% judged it boring. The student magazine, especially, was positively evaluated: 69% of the students evaluated the magazine as attractive, 43% as beautiful, 82% as informative, 76% as good, 83% as clear-cut, 8% as difficult, and 21% as boring. The video was also positively evaluated, although to a lesser degree: 58% evaluated the video as attractive, 59% as informative, 58% as good, 63% as clear, 19% as lifelike, and 30% as boring.

A survey among 38 teachers revealed that we also managed quite well to match the program to teachers' wishes, needs, and opportunities. Most teachers liked the lessons as suggested by the program (82%), most of them had the impression that their students had liked the lessons (84%), and most of them perceived the program as an improvement of their classes on the prevention of AIDS and STDs (76%). Most teachers evaluated the program as well-organized (92%), realistic (90%), comprehensive (84%), applicable in heterogeneous groups of students (68%), and superior to other programs (61%). However, most teachers also evaluated the length of the program as too long (74%). Opinions about the time required for class organization and preparation were mixed. Despite this positive evaluation of the program, teachers' perceptions of the impact of the program on their students' sexual behavior were only moderately positive.

In addition to this survey, three other methods were used for process evaluation: Classroom observations were conducted using a matrix-sampling procedure; twenty-three teachers who completed the AIDS/STD program were individually interviewed; and implementation of the program was monitored by means of structured teacher self-reports. Teachers recorded the number of lessons, the activities they had executed, teaching time per lesson and per activity, and the course of the lessons and activities. These self-reports revealed that 97% of the teachers had implemented the lesson on AIDS/STD knowledge and risk perception (average instruction time, or ait, was 76 minutes); 96% implemented the lesson on attitudes toward safe sex and condom use (ait 65 minutes); 96% implemented the lesson on values, social influences, and communication skills (ait 65 minutes); and 90% implemented the lesson on assertiveness and refusal skills (ait 60 minutes). These self-reports also revealed positive reactions to the course of the lessons and most of the basic program activities. Notably, only a few teachers implemented the homework assignments that addressed buying condoms (25%) and interviewing shopkeepers who sell condoms (13%).

On the basis of the results of these evaluation activities, the program was further matched to classroom practice. Some of the exercises that had not been used by any of the teachers were excluded; other exercises were adjusted in

Intervention Mapping Step 5: Generating an Evaluation Plan

accordance to teachers' comments and suggestions. Because the video turned out to be too long, it was re-edited. In addition, video-viewing exercises were somewhat simplified.

SUMMARY

The results of the program evaluation showed that a well-planned development process may improve the quality of AIDS/STD prevention practice. The effects of the program, developed according to the guidelines of the model of planned health education, were significantly more favorable than the effects of current AIDS/STD education, on a psychosocial level as well as on a behavioral level. In comparison with previous AIDS/STD education, our program produced a significantly larger increase in students' knowledge about AIDS and STDs; greater changes in their attitudes, perceived social influences, self-efficacy, and intentions regarding consistent condom use because of AIDS and STDs; and a more favorable behavioral change regarding the prevention of AIDS and STDs.

But program development is just a start. To contribute to the prevention of a further spread of HIV and other STDs, the program has to be implemented on a large scale. Research has revealed that a widespread diffusion of innovative school-based HIV/STD prevention programs requires strategies that go beyond current mass media promotion activities (Paulussen et al., 1994, 1995). Funding agencies, however, are slow to recognize the importance of widespread diffusion. Despite little financial support, we were able to develop a brochure based on persuasive communication and social modeling, and Dutch secondary schools finally adopted our program.

This chapter may inadvertently suggest that Intervention Mapping just goes through the protocol in one direction. However, this chapter's more or less straight-line presentation is only for the sake of clarity. In practice, Intervention Mapping goes back and forth again and again, and sometimes it even goes two steps forward and three steps back. The protocol leads to a reconsideration of decisions that were made time and again, and one strength of Intervention Mapping is that it keeps the development process well-organized despite its iterative nature.

REFERENCES

Abrams, D., Abraham, C., Spears, R., & Marks, D. (1990). AIDS invulnerability: Relationships, sexual behavior, and attitudes among 16- to 19-year-olds. In P. Aggleton, P. Davies, & G. Hart (Eds.), *AIDS: Individual, cultural, and policy dimensions* (pp. 35–51). London, UK: Falmer Press.

Ajzen, I. (1991). The theory of planned behavior. *Organizational Behavior and Human Decision Processes, 50,* 179–211.

Bandura, A. (1986). *Social foundations of thought and action: A social cognitive theory.* Englewood Cliffs, NJ: Prentice Hall.

Bandura, A. (1990). Perceived self-efficacy in the exercise of control over AIDS infection. *Evaluation and Program Planning, 13,* 9–17.

Basch, C. E. (1989). Preventing AIDS through education: Concepts, strategies, and research priorities. *Journal of School Health, 59*(7), 296–300.

Basen-Engquist, K., & Parcel, G. S. (1992). Attitudes, norms, and self-efficacy: A model of adolescents' HIV-related sexual risk behavior. *Health Education Quarterly, 19*(2), 263–277.

Bell, D. E. (1982). Regret in decision making under uncertainty. *Operations Research, 21,* 961–981.

Borko, H., Livingston, C., & Shavelson, R. J. (1981). Teachers' thinking about instruction. *Remedial and Special Education, 11,* 40–49.

Brugman, E., Goedhart, H., Vogels, T., & Van Zessen, G. (1995). *Jeugd en sex* [Youth and sex]. Utrecht, The Netherlands: SWP.

Bunton, R., Murphy, S., & Bennett, P. (1991). Theories of behavioral change and their use in health promotion: Some neglected areas. *Health Education Research, 6*(2), 153–162.

Burgoon, M. (1989). Messages and persuasive effects: Review of issues in message-effects research in the social influence literature. In J. J. Bradac (Ed.), *Message effects in communication science* (pp. 129–164). Newbury Park, CA: Sage.

Carroll, J. S. (1978). The effects of imagining an event on expectations for the event: An interpretation in terms of the availability heuristic. *Journal of Experimental Social Psychology, 14*(1), 88–96.

Chaiken, S., Liberman, A., & Eagly, A. H. (1989). Heuristic and systematic processing within and beyond the persuasion context. In J. S. Uleman & J. A. Bargh (Eds.), *Unintended thought* (pp. 212–252). New York: Guilford Press.

Clark, C. M., & Peterson, P. L. (1986). Teachers' thought processes. In M. C. Wittrock (Ed.), *Third handbook of research on teaching* (pp. 255–296). New York: Macmillan.

Eagly, A. H., & Chaiken, S. (1993). *The psychology of attitudes.* Orlando, FL: Harcourt Brace Jovanovich.

Evans, R. I., Getz, J. G., & Raines, B. S. (1991, August 16–20). *Theory guided models on prevention of AIDS in adolescents.* Paper presented at the Science Weekend at the American Psychological Association meeting, San Francisco, CA.

Evans, R. I., Getz, J. G., & Raines, B. S. (1992, March 25–28). *Applying social inoculation concepts to prevention of HIV/AIDS in adolescents: Just say no is obviously not enough.* Paper presented at the Society of Behavioral Medicine, New York.

Evans, R. I., Smith, C. K., & Raines, B. S. (1984). Deterring cigarette smoking in adolescents: A psychosocial-behavioral analysis of an intervention strategy. In A. Baum, J. Singer, & S. Taylor (Eds.), *Social psychological aspects of health* (pp. 301–318). Hillsdale, NJ: Erlbaum.

Fishbein, M., & Ajzen, I. (1975). *Belief, attitude, intention, and behavior: An introduction to theory and research.* Reading, MA: Addison Wesley.

Flay, B. R. (1985). Psychosocial approaches to smoking prevention: A review of findings. *Health Psychology, 4*(5), 449–488.

Flay, B. R., Brannon, B. R., Johnson, C. A., Hansen, W. B., Ulene, A. L., Whitney-Saltiel, D. A., Gleason, L. R., Sussman, S., Gavin, M., Glowacz, K. M., Sobol, D. F., & Spiegel, D. C. (1988). The television, school, and family smoking prevention and cessation project: 1. Theoretical basis and program development. *Preventive Medicine, 17*(5), 585–607.

Gilchrist, L. D., & Schinke, S. P. (1983). Coping with contraception: Cognitive and behavioral methods with adolescents. *Cognitive Therapy and Research, 7*(5), 379–388.

Hendrickx, L. (1991). *How versus how often.* Groningen, The Netherlands: Van Denderen.

Isenberg, D. J. (1986). Group polarization: A critical review and meta analysis. *Journal of Personality and Social Psychology, 50,* 1141–1151.

Janz, N. K., & Becker, M. H. (1984). The Health Belief Model: A decade later. *Health Education Quarterly, 11*(1), 1–47.

Jones, E. F., for the Alan Guttmacher Institute. (1986). *Teenage pregnancy in industrialized countries.* New Haven, CT: Yale University Press.

Jones, E. F., Forrest, J. D., Henshaw, S. K., Silverman, J., & Torres, A. (1988). Unintended pregnancy, contraceptive practice, and family planning service in developed countries. *Family Planning Perspectives, 20*(2), 53–67.

Kirby, D., Short, L., Collins, J., Rugg, D., Kolbe, L., Howard, M., Miller, B., Sonenstein, F., & Zabin, L. S. (1994). School-based programs to reduce sexual risk behaviors: A review of effectiveness. *Public Health Reports, 109*(3), 339–360.

Kok, G. J., & Green, L. W. (1990). Research to support health promotion in practice: A plea for increased cooperation. *Health Promotion International, 5,* 303–308.

Leventhal, H. (1984). A perceptual-motor theory of emotion. In L. Berkowitz (Ed.), *Advances in experimental social psychology: Vol. 17. Theorizing in Social Psychology: Special Topics* (pp. 117–182). New York: Academic Press.

Loomes, G., & Sugden, R. (1982). Regret theory: An alternative theory of rational choice under uncertainty. *Economic Journal, 92,* 805–825.

McGuire, W. J. (1964). Inducing resistance to persuasion: Some contemporary approaches. In L. Berkowitz (Ed.), *Advances in experimental social psychology* (Vol. 1, pp. 191–229). New York: Academic Press.

McGuire, W. J. (1985). Attitudes and attitude change. In G. Lindzey & E. Aronson (Eds.), *The handbook of social psychology* (Vol. 2, pp. 233–346). New York: Random House.

McGuire, W. J. (1986). The myth of massive media impact: Savagings and salvagings. In G. Comstock (Ed.), *Public communication and behavior* (Vol. 1, pp. 175–234). Orlando, FL: Academic Press.

Meyerowitz, B. E., & Chaiken, S. (1987). The effect of message framing on breast self-examination attitudes, intentions, and behavior. *Journal of Personality and Social Psychology, 52*(3), 500–510.

Montaño, D. E., Kasprzyk, D., & Taplin, S. H. (1997). The theory of reasoned action and the theory of planned behavior. In K. Glanz, F. M. Lewis, & B. K. Rimer (Eds.), *Health behavior and health education: Theory, research, and practice* (2nd ed., pp. 85–112). San Francisco: Jossey-Bass.

NCAB (Nationale Commissie AIDS Bestrijding). (1995). *Epidemiogie in Nederland* [Epidemiology the Netherlands]. *AIDS Bestrijding, 20,* 12–13.

Orlandi, M. A., Landers, C., Weston, R., & Haley, N. (1990). Diffusion of health promotion innovations. In K. Glanz, F. M. Lewis, & B. Rimer (Eds.), *Health behavior and health education: Theory, research, and practice* (pp. 288–313). San Francisco: Jossey-Bass.

Paulussen, Th. G. W., Kok, G. J., & Schaalma, H. P. (1994). Antecedents to adoption of classroom-based AIDS education in secondary schools. *Health Education Research, 9*(4), 485–496.

Paulussen Th. G. W., Kok, G. J., Schaalma, H. P., & Parcel, G. S. (1995). Diffusion of AIDS curricula among Dutch secondary school teachers. *Health Education Quarterly, 22*(2), 227–243.

Petty, R. E., & Cacioppo, J. T. (1986). The elaboration likelihood model of persuasion. In L. Berkowitz (Ed.), *Advances in experimental social psychology* (Vol. 19, pp. 123–205). New York: Academic Press.

Rogers, R.W. (1983). Cognitive and physiological processes in fear appeals and attitude change: A revised theory of protection motivation. In J. T. Cacioppo & R. E. Petty (Eds.), *Social psychophysiology: A sourcebook* (pp. 153–176). New York: Guilford.

Rokeach, M. (1980). Some unresolved issues in theories of beliefs, attitudes, and values. In H. E. Howe, Jr. & M. M. Page (Eds.), *Nebraska Symposium on Motivation, 1979* (Vol. 27, pp. 261–304). Lincoln: University of Nebraska Press.

Schaalma, H. P., Kok, G. J., Bosker, R., Parcel, G., Peters, L., Poelman, J., & Reinders, J. (1996). Planned development and evaluation of AIDS/STD education for secondary school students in the Netherlands: Short-term effects. *Health Education Quarterly, 23*(4), 469–487.

Schaalma, H. P., Kok, G. J., Braeken, D., Schopman, M., & Deven, F. (1991). Sex and AIDS education for adolescents. *Tijdschrift voor Seksuologie* [Journal of Sexology], *15*, 140–149.

Schaalma, H. P., Kok, G. J., & Peters, L. (1993). Determinants of consistent condom use by adolescents: The impact of experience with sexual intercourse. *Health Education Research, 8*(2), 255–269.

Schaalma, H. P., Kok, G., Poelman, J., & Reinders, J. (1994). The development of AIDS education for Dutch secondary schools: A systematic approach based on research, theories, and co-operation. In D. R. Rutter & L. Quine (Eds.), *Social psychology and health: European perspectives* (pp. 175–194). Aldershot, UK: Avebury Publishers.

Shavelson, R. J., & Stern, P. (1981). Research on teachers' pedagogical thoughts, judgments, decisions, and behavior. *Review of Educational Research, 51*(4), 455–498.

Sherif, M., & Hovland, C. I. (1961). *Social judgment: Assimilation and contrast effects in communication and attitude change.* New Haven, CT: Yale University Press.

Sherman, S. J., Cialdini, R. B., Schwartzman, D. F., & Reynolds, K. D. (1985). Imagining can heighten or lower the perceived likelihood of contracting a disease: The mediating effect of ease of imagery. *Personality and Social Psychology Bulletin, 11*(1), 118–127.

Stokking, K. M., & Leenders, F. J. (1992). *Heeft de verspreiding van informatie zin?* [Does the spread of information make sense?] Utrecht, The Netherlands: ISOR.

Suls, J., & Wills, T. A. (1991). *Social comparison: Contemporary theory and research.* Hillsdale, NJ: Erlbaum.

Sussman, S. (1991). Curriculum development in school-based prevention research. *Health Education Research, 6,* 339–351.

Tanner, W. M., & Pollack, R. H. (1988). The effect of condom use and erotic instructions on attitudes toward condoms. *Journal of Sex Research, 25*(4), 537–541.

Turner, J. C. (1991). *Social influence.* Milton Keynes, UK: Open University Press.

Tversky, A., & Kahneman, D. (1983). Extensional versus intuitive reasoning: The conjunction fallacy in probability judgment. *Psychological Review, 90*(4), 293–315.

U.S. Department of Health and Human Services. (1984). *Pretesting in health communications: Methods, examples, and resources for improving health messages and materials.* Bethesda, MD: National Cancer Institute.

van der Pligt, J. (1994). Risk appraisal and health behavior. In D. R. Rutter & L. Quine (Eds.), *Social psychology and health: European perspectives* (pp. 131–152). Aldershot, UK: Avebury Publishers.

Vogels, T., & van der Vliet, R. (1990). *Jeugd en sex* [Youth and sex]. The Hague, The Netherlands: SDU.

Weinstein, N. D. (1989). Effects of personal experience on self-protective behavior. *Psychological Bulletin, 105*(1), 31–50.

Zajonc, R. B. (1968). Attitudinal effects of mere exposure. *Journal of Personality and Social Psychology, 9*(2, Pt. 2), pp. 1–27.

Zimbardo, P. G., & Leippe, M. R. (1991). *The psychology of attitude change and social influence.* Philadelphia, PA : Temple University Press.

CHAPTER

11

Partners in School Asthma Management Program

Chris Markham, Shellie Tyrrell, Ross Shegog, Maria Fernandez, and L. Kay Bartholomew

READER OBJECTIVES

- Specify behavioral factors and environmental conditions related to chronic disease
- Develop matrices for environmental conditions
- Use theory to specify behavioral performance objectives
- Consider computer technology as a program vehicle

Asthma is the most common chronic medical condition that affects children in the United States. Childhood asthma morbidity and mortality have increased substantially in the past twenty years (Weiss, Gergen, & Wagener, 1993), and the estimated annual prevalence of asthma among children in the United States is 1% to 11% (Crain et al., 1994; Gergen & Weiss, 1990; Weiss, Gergen, & Wagener). Asthma morbidity, mortality, and hospitalization rates are disproportionately high among minority, inner-city populations (Gergen & Weiss; Centers for Disease Control and Prevention [CDC], 1996), and inner-city children are less likely to have good continuity of primary care. Asthma is the leading cause of school absenteeism, and children with asthma are twice as likely to experience grade failure compared to well children (Public Health Service, 1991, pp. 317, 449). This picture is a frustrating one because asthma is a manageable disease.

This work was supported by the National Heart, Lung, and Blood Institute, National Institutes of Health, Contract No. NO1-HR-56079.

The keys to good asthma management among children are reliable diagnosis, consistent physician management with appropriate prescription of asthma medications, and good self-care by children and their families. Because children spend more than one-third of their day at school, a supportive school environment is also crucial for asthma management. The school site provides an ideal setting to identify children with asthma problems, to educate children and families about asthma care, and to provide a linkage system between the child, family, and physician to promote good care.

In this chapter, we describe how the Intervention Mapping process was used to develop and implement the Partners in School Asthma Management program, a school-based, multicomponent program for inner-city children with asthma. The program was a demonstration project to develop and test a feasible model for elementary schools nationwide. The project goals were to identify children with asthma and to develop partnerships with families and physicians to provide appropriate asthma care. This chapter shows how each step of the Intervention Mapping process was used to conceptualize and develop the program elements and to strategize program adoption, implementation, and evaluation.

PERSPECTIVES IN THIS CASE

Partners in School Asthma Management is a unique program in that it emphasizes the management of asthma-related environmental factors in addition to the behaviors of children, parents, and physicians involved in managing asthma. This program addresses change at the individual level (child), interpersonal level (family, physician, school nurse, and other school personnel), and organizational level (school environment, school district policies and practices). The resulting program has four components: case finding, asthma self-management education for the child and family, linkage system for physician care, and school environmental intervention.

The program represents innovations in asthma management because it utilizes interactive computer technology to individualize self-management education. This computer-assisted technology (CD-ROM) allowed us to teach children using their unique asthma symptoms, triggers, and treatment characteristics. Further, this program uses self-regulatory theory to specify performance objectives and to enable the explicit teaching of self-regulatory processes.

NEEDS ASSESSMENT

The asthma needs assessment was done according to the PRECEDE model and began with a documentation of the scope and seriousness of the rising number of asthma cases and the impact on health and quality-of-life of certain populations (Green & Kreuter, 1999). From the perspectives of self-management or secondary prevention, we also asked, What behaviors and environmental factors are related to better management of asthma and better health and quality-of-life outcomes? The needs assessment model for asthma was presented in Chapter 2.

Asthma-Related Health and Quality-of-Life Issues

Asthma morbidity and mortality rates are rising. The National Heart, Lung, and Blood Institute (NHLBI) expert panel's report (NHLBI, 1991) reported an increase in the prevalence of asthma among people less than 20 years of age. The rate rose from approximately 35 per 1,000 persons in 1980 to a rate of approximately 50 per 1,000 in 1987. A report from the Centers for Disease Control and Prevention (CDC) established that the asthma death rate among children 5 to 14 years of age almost doubled between 1980 and 1993, from 1.7 deaths per million to 3.2 (CDC, 1996).

A study by Crain and colleagues (1994) reported an asthma prevalence (8.6%) among inner-city children in the Bronx, New York, twice the typical estimated rate for all U.S. children. Many studies have implicated urban residency, minority status, and lower socioeconomic status as risk factors for increased prevalence of asthma (Crain et al.; Wood, Hidalgo, Prihoda, & Kromer, 1993). Poor and minority populations, particularly African Americans, living in urban areas have experienced a disproportionately high prevalence of asthma and an increase in morbidity and mortality compared to whites (CDC, 1996; Crain et al.; Cunningham, Dockery, & Speizer, 1996; Gergen & Weiss, 1990; Weitzman, Gortmaker, & Sobol, 1990) Depending on age, African Americans are 3 to 5 times more likely than Caucasians to die from asthma (NHLBI, 1991). Race was found to be a significant predictor of the diagnosis of asthma in a study by Cunningham and colleagues (1996) in which, after adjustment for other demographic and environmental factors, being African American was a significant predictor of active diagnosed asthma among 1,416 African American and Caucasian children aged 9 to 11. The study by Crain and colleagues also showed that the cumulative prevalence of asthma was significantly higher among Hispanics and children from the lowest-income families from the Bronx, New York. The study by Wood and colleagues found that children with lower socioeconomic status exhibited an excess of severe asthma as well as a greater amount of functional morbidity, such as school absenteeism.

Of chronic childhood diseases, asthma is the leading cause of school absenteeism and poor academic performance (Pope, Patterson, & Burge, 1993; Taylor & Newacheck, 1992). It has been estimated that children with asthma average 7.6 school days absent, compared with 2.5 days for children without asthma (Fowler, Davenport, & Garg, 1992). Asthma is also responsible for more than 500,000 emergency room visits each year (Weiss, Gergen, & Hodson, 1992). Asthma hospitalization rates for 1979 were 1.73 per 1,000 among infants to 17-year-olds, and by 1987 that rate had increased to 2.57 per 1,000 (Gergen & Weiss, 1990). Data from the 1988 National Health Interview Survey on Child Health also showed that poor children have diminished accessibility to appropriate health services and higher rates of asthma morbidity, as measured by hospitalization and bed days (Halfon & Newacheck, 1993).

Environment

The risk factors for asthma are multifactorial, comprising genetic susceptibility, early history of pulmonary problems, poor medical management, and environmental factors such as indoor and outdoor aeroallergen and irritant exposure (NHLBI, 1991; Sherman, Tosteson, Tager, Speizer, & Weiss, 1990; Weitzman et al., 1990).

Sensitivity to specific allergens is quite common among persons with asthma, and estimates are that as many as 80% of children with asthma have some allergic hypersensitivity to aeroallergens (Burrows, Martinez, Halonen, Barbec, & Cline, 1989; Gergen & Turkeltaub, 1992; Platts-Mills, 1994; Pollart, Chapman, Fiocoo, Rose, & Platts-Mills, 1989). Because children spend most of their time indoors, the home and school environments are important sources of allergen exposure for children with asthma. Asthma has been significantly associated with reactivity to house dust mites, mold, cockroaches, cat dander, and pollens (Gergen & Turkeltaub; Ingram et al., 1995; Kang, Johnson, & Veres-Throner, 1993; Platts-Mills; Platts-Mills & Pollart Squillace, 1997; Rosenstreich et al., 1997). For example, in inner-city residents of Chicago, both indoor and outdoor aeroallergen sensitivity was observed in 75% of children less than 15 years of age with asthma, and sensitivity to cockroach allergen was observed in 59% of children less than 15 years (Kang et al.). A study of inner-city houses in Atlanta found significant levels of either mite or cockroach allergen in 86% of homes (Call, Smith, Morris, Chapman, & Platts-Mills, 1992). These types of studies are only now being conducted in schools, but the same conditions are thought to exist (University of Texas Health Science Center–Houston, 1996).

Environmental tobacco smoke has been consistently reported to cause increased lower respiratory infections and increased risk for asthma and asthma exacerbations in children (Emerson et al., 1994; Murray & Morrison, 1989; Overpeck & Moss, 1991; Samet, Cain, & Leaderer, 1991). A study by Cuijpers, Swaen, Wesseling, Stumans, and Wouters (1995) found passive smoking (during a child's entire life) to be significantly correlated with impairments to all spirometry parameters tested. Smoking in the child's environment should be eliminated, as it has been shown to be an irritant to airways (Hovell et al., 1994). The National Cooperative Inner-City Asthma Study showed that exposure to environmental tobacco smoke is common among inner-city children with asthma: 59% reported at least one smoker in the home. Additionally, at the study's baseline testing, 48% of children had a cotinine/creatine ratio above 30 ng/mg, a level of significant exposure to tobacco smoke in the last 24 hours (Kattan et al., 1997).

Irritants include strong odors such as outside air pollution, paint fumes, chalk, perfume, scented talcum powder, hair sprays, and pesticides (Pope et al., 1993; Swanson & Thompson, 1994). Pesticides must be used with caution in the indoor environment because unsuspected surface contamination of pesticides may occur via air transport through venting ducts, which can become repeated point sources of contamination (U.S. Environmental Protection Agency [EPA], 1995). A steady supply of uncontaminated outside air is recommended by many indoor air studies to keep allergens and irritants to a minimum and carbon dioxide levels to less than 1,000 parts per million (Ruhl, Chang, Halpern, & Gershwin, 1993; U.S. EPA, 1991). The air ventilation recommendations from the 1989 ASHRAE Standard 62 for classrooms is 15 cubic feet per minute (American Society of Heating, Refrigeration, and Air-Conditioning Engineers, 1989).

To confirm suspected asthma-related environmental conditions in local schools, we conducted environmental surveys in 60 elementary schools and dust sampling and allergen assays in a subsample of 20 schools. Especially high levels of dust mite allergen and mold were found in many schools, and moderate levels of cockroach allergen were found in some schools. The presence of environmental irritants was also a problem in many schools. Factors that seemed to underlie these conditions included high humidity, poor ventilation, dirty HVAC systems, and water and carpet damage (Tortolero et al., 2000; Tyrrell et al., 2000).

Eliminating exposure to allergens and irritants has been identified as an important factor in managing asthma in children. Recommendations for control of indoor allergens such as dust mites, cockroaches, and mold include regular vacuum cleaning, washing bedding and stuffed animals weekly and at a high temperature, removing carpet, and reducing humidity. Extensive cleaning and dust-proofing have been shown to reduce asthma symptoms and medication requirements (Bahir et al., 1997; Murray, 1988; Peroni, Vallone, Antolini, & Warner, 1994; Sarsfield, Gowland, Toy, & Normal, 1974). However, simple hygiene measures are usually ineffective, and although it has been shown that rigorous measures can reduce allergen levels and symptoms, most of these measures are difficult for families and schools to accomplish. There has been little research on allergens and irritants in inner-city elementary schools or on recommendations for the reduction of these contaminants in the school environment (Dungy, Kozak, Gallup, & Galant, 1986; Neuberger et al., 1991; Norback, Torgen, & Edling, 1990). No studies are available on school environmental intervention to reduce asthma morbidity. Investigations and recommendations for one elementary school in Kansas City were reported in 1991; however, this investigation focused on sick-building syndrome and did not look at allergens in the school environment, nor were all the irritants investigated specific to asthma (Neuberger et al.).

Asthma Management

The cornerstone of good medical management of asthma is appropriate pharmacological therapy to control the airway inflammation that underlies asthma episodes (Global Initiative for Asthma, 1995; NHLBI, 1991). For acute exacerbation, bronchodilators act quickly to relieve constriction and the accompanying cough, chest tightness, and wheezing. However, bronchodilators are not recommended as the only treatment for persistent moderate to severe asthma (NHLBI, 1991). Recent studies strongly suggest that anti-inflammatory agents, particularly inhaled corticosteroids, are the most effective medications in controlling persistent asthma (Britton, Earnshaw, & Palmer, 1992; Djukanovic et al., 1992; Global Initiative for Asthma, 1995; Juniper et al., 1990; Salmeron et al., 1989). In spite of the fact that asthma treatment guidelines from the National Institutes of Health have been publicized and widely disseminated to primary care physicians and specialists in 1991 and 1997, there are still misconceptions among physicians about optimal pharmacological therapy, and as a result, anti-inflammatory agents may be underutilized (Finkelstein et al., 1995; NHLBI, 1991). In particular, Latino and African American children aged 1 to 6 years are less likely than non-Hispanic whites to have used either beta agonists or steroids prior to hospitalization for asthma or to be prescribed a nebulizer on discharge (Finkelstein et al.). Inner-city minority children are not very likely to be treated with anti-inflammatory medications; the reported rates vary from 11% to 17% of children with moderate to severe asthma (Homer et al., 1996; Huss et al., 1994; Lieu et al., 1997). Furthermore, even though written action plans with medication schedules and criteria have been shown to be associated with lower hospitalizations and emergency department visits, they are seldom provided to patients and families (Wasilewski et al., 1996; Dawson, Van Asperen, Higgins, Sharpe, & Davis, 1995).

Many urban minority children with asthma may be unable to obtain appropriate diagnosis or treatment for asthma (Crain et al., 1994). For example, in a survey of Baltimore public school children, 52% of first graders and 45% of sixth graders with asthma had received care in emergency rooms rather than from a consistent primary health care provider (Mak, Johnston, Abbey, & Talamo, 1982). Among African Americans, 44% used the emergency room as the primary source of care compared with 24% of whites, and those using emergency rooms also reported a greater number of school days missed (Mak et al.). Wood and colleagues (1993) indicated that Mexican American parents were more likely to use emergency department services as the primary source of care than were non-Hispanics.

Even though school nurses are in a position to assist the child and family with adherence to asthma medications and to serve as a liaison with primary health care personnel to obtain appropriate care for asthma, their role is largely overlooked by families and physicians. Case-finding data from the Partners in School Asthma Management program showed that 62% of students identified as having asthma or having symptoms of asthma were unknown to the school nurse (Bartholomew et al., 1999). This finding means that a large number of students who develop asthma symptoms during the school day are unable to receive timely treatment to reduce or prevent more serious exacerbations.

Child and family behavior should play a crucial role in asthma management. However, the foregoing discussion should make it clear that without environmental support, families cannot do their part to manage asthma. In general, families need support to recognize asthma symptoms and to take steps to prevent the onset or escalation of symptoms. These steps include following prescription guidelines for use of routine control (preventive) medications and relief medications for symptoms or episodes; avoiding and controlling indoor and outdoor irritants and allergens; and maintaining a medical care relationship for the primary care of asthma. These behaviors require time and commitment from the child and family. For example, to manage indoor irritants, parents must protect their children from environmental tobacco smoke, and older children must do their part to avoid it. Because children at different ages have different capacities to manage their own daily treatment regimens, another important asthma management behavior is the transfer of specific responsibilities from parent to child as the child matures.

Needs Assessment Summary

Based on the increasing prevalence of asthma in inner-city children of color and on the burden of the disease in this group, we focused our intervention on these children. We abstracted from the health and quality-of-life factors the following program objectives: reduced hospitalizations, emergency room visits, and daytime and nighttime symptoms; and increased school attendance and performance. The needs assessment made it clear that the greatest impact on health and quality of life would occur from changes in the child's environment, including the medical care environment. These environmental changes are necessary in order for the parent and child to be able to do their parts to manage asthma. Therefore in this project we focused on children and their immediate context—parents, physicians, and schools—to bring about behavioral and environmental change.

INTERVENTION MAPPING STEP 1: MATRICES OF PROXIMAL PROGRAM OBJECTIVES

In the needs assessment we identified environmental conditions that needed changing, such as inadequate medical care and the presence of asthma triggers in the child's physical surroundings at home and school. We also identified the role of parents and children in asthma self-management. For comprehensive program development, we had two sets of planning matrices: the at-risk group (i.e., the child and the parents), and the child's interpersonal and organizational environment (i.e., medical care and school). Because elementary school children are dependent to some extent on their parents to manage asthma, parents were considered together with the children in the at-risk group, and because of their role in medical care, parents were considered to be part of the interpersonal environment as well. To accommodate this complexity, we first discuss the behavior, performance objectives, determinants, and matrices for the child; then we discuss the environmental change, performance objectives, and matrices at the interpersonal levels (medical care change) and organizational levels (school environment change).

BEHAVIOR AND PERFORMANCE OBJECTIVES In the needs assessment, we identified such asthma-specific behaviors as identifying triggers and taking medication, but as we began to develop the intervention we elaborated our conceptualization of behaviors using self-regulation theory. We developed two categories of behaviors: asthma-specific behaviors such as taking preventive medication, removing environmental triggers, and taking medication to deal with an episode or exacerbation; and the broader self-regulatory processes of monitoring behavior and symptoms, comparing with a standard, identifying a problem, and trying and evaluating a solution (Clark & Starr-Schneidkraut, 1994; Creer, 1990; Kotses, Stout, McConnaughy, Winder, & Creer, 1996; Thoresen & Kirmil-Gray, 1983). When we combined these asthma-specific and self-regulatory behaviors, we had a more comprehensive picture of what was required for effective asthma self-management as well as a self-regulatory framework to guide the children's application of asthma-specific behaviors.

We then designed a conceptual framework that would integrate both types of processes, reduce redundancy, and expose any gaps in the delineation of behaviors. Figure 11.1 is an asthma decision tree that combines both types of asthma self-management behaviors. The self-regulatory behaviors of goal setting, monitoring, problem identification, solution identification, action, and evaluation are represented to the left of the framework. These behaviors are the processes by which asthma-specific behaviors such as taking medicine, monitoring peak flow, or avoiding triggers take place. For example, monitoring asthma involves the child watching his or her overall condition. The asthma decision tree in Figure 11.1 shows that the child uses asthma-specific skills, such as peak flow measurement, to monitor for symptoms. The child also monitors the environment for triggers and monitors his or her behavior with respect to taking medications as prescribed and keeping medical appointments.

Using this comprehensive picture of what is involved in asthma management, we combined asthma-specific behaviors with self-regulatory processes in order to create performance objectives. In order to narrow the scope of the target behaviors, we collapsed self-regulation to three steps (monitoring and problem identification, solution development, and action) and prioritized the categories of behavior as symptom resolution, asthma control, and trigger avoidance. Table 11.1 presents the first level of performance objectives, and the following example shows the level of detail in the performance objectives:

1.a. Monitor objectively using a peak flow meter

1.a.1. Set a schedule for peak flow monitoring

1.a.2. Obtain a peak flow meter

1.a.3. Put the mouthpiece between the lips and blow hard until all the air possible is released

1.a.4. Repeat three times

1.a.5. Record the highest number

Intervention Mapping Step 1: Matrices of Proximal Program Objectives

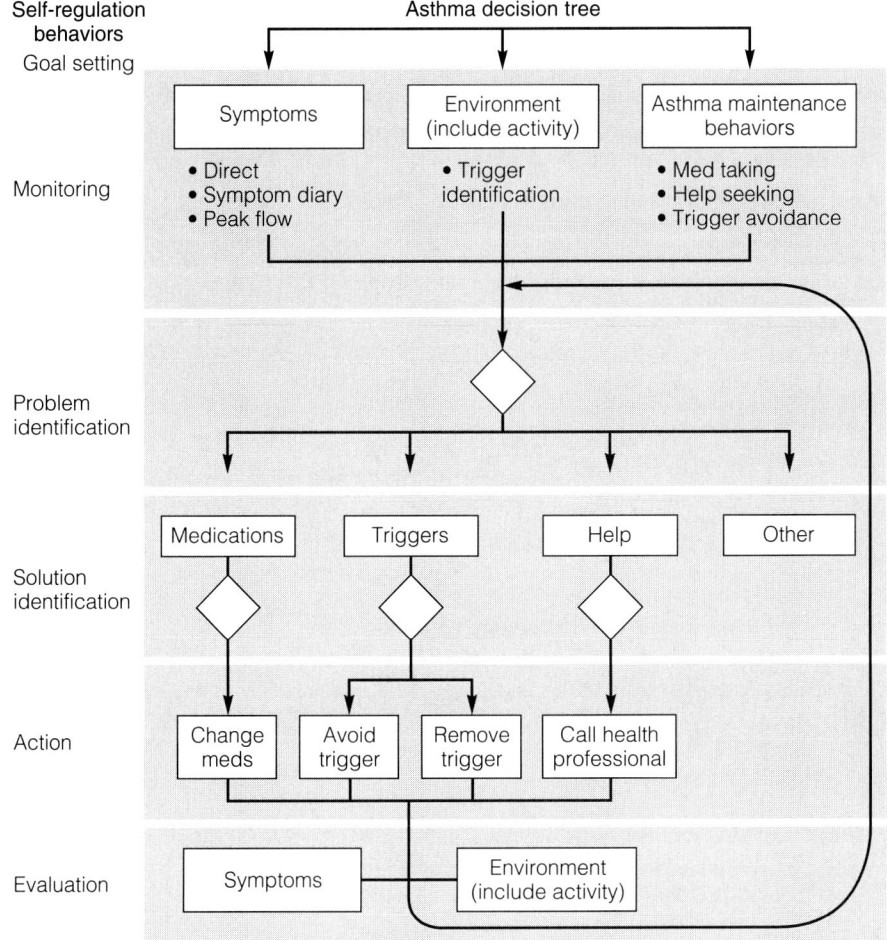

FIGURE 11.1 Asthma Self-Management Behavioral Framework (*Note.* From "Watch, Discover, Think, and Act: A Model for Patient Education Program Development," by L. K. Bartholomew, R. Shegog, G. S. Parcel, M. Fernandez, R. S. Gold, D. I. Czyzewski, M. M. Sockrider, and N. Berlin, 2000, *Patient Education and Counseling, 39*(2–3), 253–268.)

DETERMINANTS OF CHILD AND PARENT MANAGEMENT BEHAVIOR Our next step was to discover important and changeable factors associated with asthma management by the child and family. These factors are knowledge, self-efficacy, outcome expectations, perceptions of seriousness and chronicity, patient/provider interaction including teaching and reinforcement of self-management skills, cultural orientation to illness and health care, and income and socioeconomic status (Clark, 1989; Clark et al., 1988; Evans et al., 1987; Kotses, Lewis, & Creer, 1990; Manson, 1988; McNabb, Wilson-Pessano, & Jacobs, 1986; Wissow, Gittelsohn, Szklo, Starfield, & Mussman, 1988). We added attributions to our list of determinants from the needs assessment because of their demonstrated interaction with self-management for other chronic illnesses and health problems

Table 11.1
Performance Objectives for Child and Parent

Monitor symptoms of asthma and compare to personal standard

Monitor symptoms and compare to personal standard using objective measures (i.e., peak flow meter)

Monitor for personal environmental triggers

Monitor self-management efforts and compare to personal standard

Identify when a problem exists (with any of the above)

Implement solutions:
    Keep regular appointments with health care providers
    Refer to asthma action plan
    Maintain chronic medication as prescribed
    Maintain "normal" exercise level
    Make medication adjustments including administration of rescue medication (based on symptoms, environment, or both) as prescribed
    Avoid or remove asthma triggers
    Call health care professional in acute situation
    Communicate with family members and with health care providers

Evaluate actions and return to monitoring

(Hospers, Kok, & Strecher, 1990; Kuttner, Delamater, & Santiago, 1990; Weiner, 1985). We wanted the child's attributions of success to be internal and attributable to effort—"Working with my parents, doctor, and school nurse, I can control my own asthma. I don't need grown-ups to do it for me."

At this step, we also had to decide whether to differentiate the population on one or more descriptive variables. The decision was based on whether performance objectives or their determinants would vary for subgroups of the at-risk population. Based on the needs assessment, we wanted the asthma partnership program to reach both African American and Hispanic American inner-city youth, and therefore we needed to decide whether there was evidence that the determinants or desired behaviors were different in these two ethnic groups. Must we influence different sets of determinants? Or, do we simply need to vary the strategies to be culturally acceptable? In other words, at this point in the planning process, do we have an ethnocentric intervention or a multiethnic one? Based on our needs assessment, we had no evidence that behaviors or determinants were different for the two groups of children; therefore we did not differentiate. We did need to address ethnic differences in program design, including graphics and messages, to ensure that the program would be acceptable and appealing.

Another consideration in determining how to differentiate the population was the wide age range—school-age children, 6 to 11 years. This age group includes a wide range of cognitive, social, and emotional development. However, because all these children manage asthma as a team with parents, we decided that the performance objectives were not so different that they could not be handled with different versions of the same program rather than with different matrices and potentially different programs. See Step 3 for a description of the two versions (one for grades 1 through 3 and one for grades 4 and 5).

PROXIMAL PROGRAM OBJECTIVES   The next task was to create the matrix of proximal program objectives for the behavioral conditions. Conceptually, the matrix represents the learning and change necessary to influence the child's asthma self-management behavior. To form the matrix we entered the performance objectives on the left side of the table and the determinants across the top. Table 11.2 shows both personal determinants (those within the child) and external determinants (those in the child's environment that are related to the specific performance objectives). We assessed each cell of the matrix to judge whether the determinant was likely to influence the performance objective, and we wrote proximal program objectives in the appropriate cells—learning objectives for personal determinants and change objectives for external determinants. For example, in the cell in Table 11.2 where the performance objective "monitor for symptoms of asthma" is paired with the personal determinant "self-efficacy," we asked the question, What do the participants in the program need to learn related to self-efficacy to be able to use a peak flow meter? Answers to this question include the learner's experience of enhanced self-efficacy that he or she can do the actions necessary to observe symptoms.

Matrices at the Interpersonal and Organizational Levels

AGENTS AND PERFORMANCE OBJECTIVES   The goals for environmental change were identified from the needs assessment and included changes in medical care (interpersonal level) and changes in the school environment (organizational level). We worked with a school district advisory committee to understand what environmental changes were feasible.

Needed changes in medical care focused on appropriate diagnosis of asthma and asthma severity using the National Asthma Education and Prevention Program (NAEPP) guidelines; prescription of both rescue and control medications when necessary; use of an asthma action plan; and increased communication between the patient, family, school nurse, and physician based on the plan (NHLBI, 1991). Three agents were needed to perform these changes: the school nurse, the parent, and the physician. Performance objectives related to medical care changes are presented in Table 11.3.

The following changes were required in the physical environment of the school: eliminating the allergens of mold, dust mites, cockroaches, and rodents; eliminating pollutants such as strong odors and their sources; eliminating contaminants that enter the building via the air handling systems or originate in the systems; and increasing the circulation of fresh air in the building. Organizational-level environmental change agents or decision makers (school personnel) were then differentiated to include principals, plant operators, and teachers. The environmental conditions of concern in the schools are the same for all school

Table 11.2
Matrix for Children with Asthma (Sample Cells)

	PERSONAL DETERMINANTS					EXTERNAL DETERMINANTS	
PERFORMANCE OBJECTIVES	Perceived susceptibility and seriousness	Behavioral capability	Skills and self-efficacy	Outcome expectations	Attributions	Physician and parent behavior	Reinforcement
Monitor for symptoms of asthma	Describes asthma as a serious disease that does not go away Describes own asthma as involving inflammation of the lungs—can't be seen but is always there	Identifies possible personal symptoms of asthma Identifies early symptoms and late symptoms	Demonstrates comparing current respiratory status to baseline Expresses confidence in recognizing symptoms	Expects that by monitoring symptoms, asthma control can be better Expects that action can be taken to prevent asthma episodes if symptoms are monitored	Attributes ability to monitor for asthma symptoms to self ("Children can tell when they have symptoms.") Attributes failure to monitor to temporary state or unstable causes ("I can get back to monitoring.")	Remind child to use peak flow monitoring Assist younger children with direct observation and peak flow	Parent, physician, and intervention reinforce for monitoring symptoms of asthma
Monitor objectively using a peak flow meter	Thinks asthma episodes can be serious	Identifies personal peak flow numbers that are congruent with asthma	Demonstrates using a peak flow meter	Expects that peak flow will allow early detection of decline and episode prevention	Attributes ability to use peak flow to self	Parent and physician look at and discuss peak flow numbers	Parent and physician look at and discuss peak flow numbers
Set a schedule for peak flow monitoring	Thinks asthma is serious enough to monitor regularly and to catch decline in lung function early	Describes schedule for peak flow monitoring Plans when to measure peak flow in daily schedule	Expresses confidence that peak flow monitoring can fit into current schedule	Expects that monitoring peak flow on a certain schedule will result in the ability to predict and prevent asthma episodes	Attributes ability to measure peak flow on a schedule to self Attributes difficulties in keeping to a schedule to unstable causes		Parent congratulates child for keeping to schedule

Table 11.2
(continued)

PERFORMANCE OBJECTIVES	PERSONAL DETERMINANTS					EXTERNAL DETERMINANTS		
	Perceived susceptibility and seriousness	Behavioral capability	Skills and self-efficacy	Outcome expectations	Attributions	Physician and parent behavior	Reinforcement
Obtain a peak flow meter	Thinks asthma is serious enough to monitor and to catch decline in function early	Describes the uses of a peak flow meter	Expresses confidence to negotiate with physician for peak flow meter				
Perform correct peak flow technique		Describes the steps of using a peak flow meter	Demonstrates correct technique Expresses confidence in ability to obtain and use a correct number			Physician teaches peak flow technique Parent teaches use of peak flow meter	Parent and physician reinforce correct technique
Take control (anti-inflammatory) medication	Sees the inflammatory process as serious, as needing to be controlled	Describes purpose of control meds Identifies asthma meds (types) States when to use each asthma med	Demonstrates correct procedure for use of inhaler Expresses confidence that inhaler can be used correctly	Expects control meds to reduce episodes Expects few side effects Expects to be able to decrease control meds with doctor	Sees asthma as something that can be controlled by own efforts Sees lack of asthma control due to inadequate meds	Physician prescribes control (anti-inflammatory) meds Parent gives child control meds	

(continued)

Table 11.2
Matrix for Children with Asthma (Sample Cells) *(continued)*

PERFORMANCE OBJECTIVES	PERSONAL DETERMINANTS					EXTERNAL DETERMINANTS	
	Perceived susceptibility and seriousness	Behavioral capability	Skills and self-efficacy	Outcome expectations	Attributions	Physician and parent behavior	Reinforcement
Take control medication according to asthma action plan	Recognizes that control meds should be taken according to plan, not symptoms			Expects meds to work better if taken as prescribed	Expects to be able to follow action plan. Attributes failure to temporary state	Physician gives action plan with control med section	
Continue control medications when symptoms are not present	Recognizes that control meds should be taken according to plan, not symptoms	Recognizes that control meds are to manage inflammation that cannot be seen or felt				Physician is clear on action plan about when to take meds	Physician, parent, and intervention reinforce taking meds

Table 11.3
Performance Objectives for Medical-Care Change

PARENT	PHYSICIAN	SCHOOL NURSE
Obtain asthma action plan and have completed by doctor	Use NAEPP Assessment and Modified Severity guidelines to diagnose identified students	Ensure that child completes a doctor visit
Get prescriptions filled	Prescribe long-term control medicines and quick relief medicines according to severity	Ensure that child has a functional asthma action plan and proper medications at school
Take completed action plan, inhaler, spacer, and peak flow meter (if needed) to school nurse	Identify concerns the patient and family may have about being diagnosed with asthma, and educate them regarding this new diagnosis	Review action plan with child and parents
Work with child, doctor, school nurse, teachers, and other school personnel to identify, avoid, and remove child's triggers		Assist child to use inhaler and spacer or nebulizer correctly
		Assist child to use peak flow meter correctly
Give all medications as ordered	Agree on treatment goals with patient and family	Administer routine medications
Help child use peak flow meter and help determine child's personal best	Explain how to discover triggers and how to avoid them	Respond to asthma episodes and administer relief medications as needed
Clean inhalers, spacers, and nebulizers properly	Explain to patient how to watch for early warning signs and asthma symptoms	Manage school environment to remove triggers and help child avoid triggers
Record details of asthma episodes to share with doctor	Follow up with patient on performance of asthma action plan	Review performance of action plan with child, parent, and physician
Keep all follow-up doctor appointments		
Talk with school nurse and physician about asthma problems as they arise		

personnel identified at the organizational level; however, performance objectives differ because of the aspects each is able to control. Table 11.4 takes one environmental change and compares performance objectives for plant operators, principals, and teachers.

DETERMINANTS AND MATRICES Using social cognitive theory, we specified internal determinants as behavioral capability, skills, self-efficacy, and outcome expectations. Behavioral capability is the procedural knowledge for the various performance objectives, for example, for the physician to set a goal or for the plant operator to identify and remove sources of allergens and irritants. Self-efficacy is the confidence that the agents experience for each task, and outcome expectations are what the agents expect to occur as a result of their performance. Self-efficacy is expected to be related to the initiation of the performance objectives and persistence in making the changes (Bandura, 1986). An external determinant is something outside the individual, such as reinforcement (Bandura). The actions in environmental cleanup should be a source of negative reinforcement (i.e., removing an aversive stimulus, in this case, sources of respiratory irritants and illness). For example, a teacher removes potted plants with mold in them from

Table 11.4
Plant Operator, Principal, and Teacher Environmental-Change Performance Objectives (Partial)

PLANT OPERATOR	PRINCIPAL	TEACHER
Plant operator prevents air contaminants from entering the school building	**Principal ensures that air contaminants are prevented from entering the building**	**Teacher monitors building for signs that air contaminants are entering building (i.e., children who have asthma symptoms and obvious contaminants)**
Appraise air-handling units for nearby contaminants	Relocate holding area for buses, loading dock, etc., if near outdoor air intake or windows	Report children with asthma symptoms to school nurse and note time of day and potential exposures
Clear outdoor air intakes of nearby pollutant sources and debris	Ensure that plant operator and personnel are keeping air intakes clear of nearby pollutant sources (such as mold) and debris	Report odors to principal
Check filter for clogs or gaps		Routinely check HVAC in classroom
Replace filters every 3 months—including hard-to-reach units		Notice and report outside sources of contaminants to the principal
Install local exhaust and seal off returns in area of activities that emit odors	Work with district to schedule and change filters in all HVAC units every three months	
Schedule activities that emit odors during unoccupied times	Work with district and contractors during activities that emit odors to ensure that local exhaust is temporarily installed, returns are sealed off in area, and work is done during unoccupied times	
Relocate dumpsters or incinerators 50 feet from any air intake		
Secure openings on exterior of building for rodent or bird entry (especially along roofline and crawl space)	Work with plant operator to relocate dumpsters or incinerators that are near air supplies or windows (should be 50 feet from any air intake)	
Schedule painting, reroofing, and pest control to unoccupied times	Ensure that openings on exterior of building for rodent or bird entry are secured (especially along roofline and crawl space)	
Close outdoor air damper for reroofing	Schedule painting, reroofing, maintenance, and pest control to unoccupied times	
Maintain drain traps to prevent odorous dry traps by pouring water down floor drains once per week; run water in sinks and flush unused toilets once per week	Ensure that outdoor air damper is closed during reroofing	
Evaluate if above action items are completed consistently	Ensure drain trap maintenance	
	Evaluate if above action items are completed consistently and compliment plant operator for completed items	
	Add items to plant operator job description and evaluation	

underneath the classroom air-intake, thereby decreasing the spread of mold spore and, consequently, her allergy symptoms and those of the children. Sometimes there is a significant time lag between the removal of the contaminant and improvement in health. Therefore, to be reinforcing, the contingencies may need to be pointed out to the environmental agents. Other reinforcements include those from the social environment, such as approval expressed by the principal for the plant operator's efforts. Other external determinants at the organizational level include the availability of nonscented products, such as cleaners, and equipment that helps eliminate contaminants, such as vacuum cleaners with HEPA filters. The school district advisory committee meetings, along with other interviews, were crucial in identifying availability of appropriate products. For example, we found that a plant operator must have nonscented germicides available for order through the school district warehouse if he or she is to be able to discontinue using bleach (a strong-scented cleaner) inside the school building. External determinants for physician practice included office policy and barriers, particularly length of visits for asthma.

At the interpersonal level, these determinants were crossed with performance objectives in matrices for physicians, school nurses, and parents. Table 11.5 shows an example from a physician's matrix. At the organizational level, determinants were crossed with performance objectives for plant operators, school principals, and schoolteachers. Table 11.6 shows an example from a plant operator matrix.

INTERVENTION MAPPING STEP 2: THEORETICAL METHODS AND PRACTICAL STRATEGIES

The second step in Intervention Mapping is to delineate theoretical methods and match them with practical strategies, making sure that methods to impact each learning and change objective are specified. Tables 11.7, 11.8, and 11.9 present selected methods and strategies that were identified for the program objectives at the individual, interpersonal, and organizational levels.

INTERVENTION MAPPING STEP 3: PROGRAM DESIGN

Review of Asthma Management Programs

Before beginning to work on this new program, we reviewed the literature on health education and promotion interventions for asthma. Educational programs to enhance self-management of childhood asthma have had some impact on the following variables: anxiety about asthma, children's responsibility for asthma management, school attendance, school performance, acute episodes of reactive airways, and medical costs (Clark et al., 1986a, 1986b; Clark, Feldman, Evans, Wasilewski, & Leveson, 1984; Creer et al., 1988; Fireman, Friday, Gira, Vieshaler, & Michaels, 1981; Hindi-Alexander, 1984; Lewis, Rachelefsky, Lewis, de la Sota, & Kaplan, 1984; McNabb et al., 1986; Parcel & Nader, 1977; Parcel, Nader, & Tiernan, 1980; Wilson-Pessano et al., 1987). The development process for these and other programs has contributed greatly to the understanding of asthma management. However, the volume of program objectives and related lessons may deter

Table 11.5

Matrix at the Interpersonal Level: Physician (Sample Cells)

PERFORMANCE OBJECTIVES	PERSONAL DETERMINANTS			EXTERNAL DETERMINANTS	
	Behavioral capability	Skills and self-efficacy	Outcome expectations	Barriers	Office policy
Agree on treatment goals with patient and family Determine family goals for asthma management (ask what patient would like to do but can't because of asthma)	Describes how including patient's input in goal setting leads to greater compliance	Expresses confidence and demonstrates ability to determine appropriate treatment goals from patient information	Believes that creating patient treatment goals leads to better control of asthma	Allow enough time per scheduled exam to educate patients on optimal expectations and to set treatment goals with them Have interpreter readily available	Have printed materials available that explain general treatment goals that patients and families should strive for and expect to achieve
Explain to family the physician's goals for managing asthma Explain that child should sleep through the night, should have no or few emergency room visits or days absent from school, and should feel well and have near-normal lung function	Lists reasons to treat persistent asthma as a chronic illness	Expresses confidence in being able to persuade parents and child that good function is possible when asthma is well treated	Expects that good treatment will produce the outcomes described	Allow time in schedule to review goals at each visit	
Note the family's goals in the child's action plan	Shows familiarity with action plan Describes characteristics of a good goal	Expresses confidence in being able to use plan at each visit	Believes that using plan will enable child and parents to better manage asthma	Allow time to complete action plan	Have action plan in child's chart ahead of asthma visit and have plans accessible in every exam room

Table 11.6
Matrix at the Organizational Level: Plant Operator (Sample Cells)

PERFORMANCE OBJECTIVES	PERSONAL DETERMINANTS			EXTERNAL DETERMINANTS	
	Behavioral capability	Self-efficacy and skills	Outcome expectations	Reinforcement	Policy and availability of materials and equipment
Prevent air contaminants from entering school building	Describes how to appraise air-handling rooms and exhaust fans Describes 10 procedures to prevent air contaminants from entering the school building Describes type of filters to use Describes how to change filters	Expresses confidence in ability to investigate air-handling systems Demonstrates filter change	Believes that protecting children and staff from airborne contaminants will improve their health Expects that the principal will appreciate efforts to improve air quality	Principal praises plant operator for efforts to improve air quality Efforts to improve air quality are responded to positively on district level	Custodial crew policy to reflect the need for compliance with proper air ventilation standards All HVAC system parts to be available for immediate replacement when necessary
Remove existing air contaminants from the building	Describes how to appraise air-handling units and rooms Describes 10 items to check for contaminants Describes how to remove mold and other contaminants from the building	Expresses confidence in and demonstrates ability to investigate air-handling systems and rooms for air contaminants	Believes it important to have clean, well-running ventilation systems for clean air and therefore good health	Principal checks systems and praises plant operator for good conditions	District responds rapidly with requests for parts and help with cleaning

Note. HVAC = heating, ventilation, and air conditioning

Table 11.7
Brainstorming Methods and Strategies for Child and Parent Matrix

METHODS FROM THEORY	EXAMPLES OF PRACTICAL STRATEGIES
Goal setting	Asthma action plan
Modeling	Character in computer game who is learning to manage asthma
	Coach in computer game who has managed asthma
Skill training	Computer game simulation teaches self-regulatory skills and asthma-specific skills
	Video clips in game for psychomotor skills
Self-monitoring	Asthma action plan
	Monitoring of asthma status of character in the game
Persuasive communication	Coach in computer game encourages player
Cues to action	Asthma action plan
Reinforcement	Computer game provides symptom feedback, score, and certificates of congratulation
	Computer game provides feedback on child's game progress so that physicians can socially reinforce child
Attribution training	Coach is an older child who successfully manages asthma
	Child is encouraged throughout game to manage asthma
	Characters in game model the management of their own asthma and are reinforced with symptom reduction

health care providers or school personnel from using them to teach children and parents. Also, the programs do not deal directly with change in the child's school environment. Furthermore, most approaches to asthma self-management are not easily individualized; they require that all children learn the same skills, regardless of individual characteristics or asthma management needs. Little is known about which intervention components contribute to behavior change and thereby to the noted outcomes (Creer, Kotses, & Wigal, 1992). Some programs are group oriented; others make little or no use of information about the child's asthma precipitants, prescribed treatment, or orientation to self-management of asthma. Furthermore, there has been minimal success in implementing these programs within schools or medical care practices. Based on this review, we knew that we wanted a program with the following characteristics:

- Can be individualized and tailored to use the child's own data and meet the specific needs of a child and family
- Is designed to help a child progress to more advanced asthma management
- Is able to be implemented in a variety of settings

Table 11.8
Brainstorming Methods and Strategies for the Interpersonal-Level Matrices

METHODS FROM THEORY	EXAMPLES OF PRACTICAL STRATEGIES		
	Parents	Physicians	School nurses
Goal setting	Asthma action plan	Asthma action plan	Asthma action plan
Persuasive communication	Narrator in video encourages parent to take child to doctor Project staff and school nurse encourage parent to take child to doctor	Narrator in video encourages physician to use asthma action plan to increase patient's compliance with self-management	Project staff encourage nurse to implement program to decrease students' symptoms and absenteeism
Modeling	Role models in video show parent and child discussing asthma action plan with doctor Role models in video show parent and child reviewing action plan at home and placing it in a prominent position	Role model in video shows physician examining child for asthma and using NAEPP guidelines to diagnose severity Role model in video shows physician discussing asthma action plan with families	At in-service training, respiratory therapists model correct techniques for using inhalers, spacers, and peak flow meters At in-service training, project staff model school nurse's interaction with child on computer game
Cues to action	Child brings home action plan and video from school Project staff or school nurse calls parent about action plan	Action plan and video mailed directly to physician Action plan placed in child's medical chart	Project staff deliver log sheets to record interactions with students
Self-monitoring	Asthma action plan		Nurse records interaction with students on log sheets
Skill training	Video models step-by-step use of the action plan	Video provides detailed information on how to use NAEPP guidelines to diagnose asthma and asthma severity Video provides detailed instructions on how to complete asthma action plan	At in-service training, school nurse practices correct techniques for using inhalers, spacers, and peak flow meters At in-service training, school nurse role-plays discussing action plan with parents and physician
Reinforcement	Project staff and school nurse provide feedback on child's asthma management at school	Parent and school nurse provide feedback to physician on child's asthma management	Project staff and school district personnel recognize nurse's efforts

Note. NAEPP = National Asthma Education and Prevention Program.

Table 11.9
Brainstorming Methods and Strategies for the Organizational-Level Matrices

METHODS FROM THEORY	EXAMPLES OF PRACTICAL STRATEGIES		
	Principals	Plant operators (P.O.s)	Teachers
Goal setting	Environmental action committee agreement	Environmental action committee agreement	Environmental action committee agreement
Skill training	At environmental action committee meetings, project staff instruct members on ways to identify and remove irritants and allergens from the school building and grounds Project staff provide feedback on actions taken	At P.O. training, proper cleaning techniques and prevention techniques are demonstrated by speakers and project staff Project staff provide feedback on actions taken	At teacher in-service, project staff present steps to identify and remove irritants and allergens in the classroom Project staff provide feedback on actions taken
Consciousness raising	At principal and superintendent meeting, data are presented concerning levels of irritants and allergens found in schools Individualized environmental "school report card" gives information on irritants and allergens in general and informs of specific problems identified in school building and grounds At environmental action committee meetings, members including principal brainstorm solutions to identified problems and identify additional problematic conditions	At P.O. training, project staff provide educational materials on irritants and allergens P.O.s participate in brainstorming sessions to identify problems and solutions under the control of custodial staff Individualized environmental "school report card" gives information on irritants and allergens in general and informs of specific problems identified in school building and grounds At environmental action committee meetings, members including the P.O. brainstorm solutions to identified problems and identify additional problematic conditions	At teacher in-service, project staff provide educational materials and information on irritants and allergens in the classroom Teachers participate in brainstorming sessions to generate solutions Individualized environmental "school report card" gives information on irritants and allergens in general and informs of specific problems identified in school building and grounds At environmental action committee meetings, members including teachers brainstorm solutions to identified problems and identify additional problematic conditions
Modeling	At environmental action committee meetings, project staff present testimonials from other elementary schools encountering problematic conditions and discuss the solutions they developed	At P.O. training, former plant operator gives testimonial of problems he encountered in the schools and solutions he used to reduce irritants and allergens	Teacher in-service includes testimonials of teachers who have encountered and remedied problematic conditions

(continued)

Table 11.9
(continued)

METHODS FROM THEORY	EXAMPLES OF PRACTICAL STRATEGIES		
	Principals	Plant operators (P.O.s)	Teachers
Modeling *(continued)*		Pest control worker for district gives testimonials on pest control strategies	
		Demonstrations of proper cleaning techniques are provided	
Facilitation	Project staff work with district on policy change	Project staff facilitate purchase orders and maintenance requests at the district level	
Persuasive communication	Project staff encourage principal to ensure follow-through on items from environmental action committee agreement	Project staff encourage P.O.s to follow through on needed purchase orders identified from environmental action committee agreement	Project staff encourage teachers to remove irritants and allergens from classroom
			Teachers are reminded of the risks to staff and student health if not done consistently

- Includes a tie to the child's medical care
- Includes a direct environmental change component

Program Components and Support Materials

After reviewing the strategies and proximal program objectives, we determined that there should be three primary program components: child self-management; a linkage system with physician care; and a school environment intervention. Because we knew that the program was to be implemented in an inner-city school setting, we also had to consider the constraints and limitations that this setting placed on program design. Inner-city schools usually lack resources of space, personnel, and discretionary funds; therefore, the program had to fit into the school setting with minimum interruption to regular school activities, minimum burden for school personnel, and minimum cost to the school administration.

CHILD SELF-MANAGEMENT TRAINING COMPONENT   The principal delivery mechanism for the child self-management component was an interactive computer-assisted program (computer game) that was tailored to characteristics of the individual children. For the child self-management component, we used a program that would stimulate children's interest and allow them to identify with role models from their own ethnic group—African American or Hispanic. We expected reading skills of some of the children to be below grade level. Furthermore, some of the children spoke only Spanish, according to estimated enrollment in English as a second language classes in the school district. In order to accommodate ethnic differences, children could choose attractive Hispanic or African American, male or female, character role models who were about 12 years of age, and coach role models who were about 16 years of age. School nurses could help the child choose whether to play the game in English or Spanish.

The theme of the program—Watch, Discover, Think, and Act—is based on the self-regulatory sequence and is depicted as icons in the program. The icons guide the children to watch (monitor), discover (identify problems and causes), think (decide on solutions), and act (act to solve the problem). Figure 11.2 is a screen from the computer game. These themes are repeated in feedback to the child and in the asthma action plan. The scope and sequence of the computer program is four computer-simulated venues in which children must manipulate their characters to manage asthma—home, community, school, and the fantasy castle (Shegog et al., 1999). The school nurse enters information about the child's own triggers, symptoms, and medications. As the game progresses through the scenes and venues, the learner manages asthma by avoiding or eliminating triggers, taking control and relief medications, visiting the doctor, and making appointments for well visits to the doctor.

The major motif of the computer program is the mission to the castle of Dr. Foulair. In addition to managing their asthma, children collect items required on their mission to liberate an air-cleaning machine from the menacing castle of the inventor-turned-bad guy. Once in the castle, the learner must continue to manage asthma in the face of very unusual obstacles and asthma triggers. Fantasy and adventure-game playing in education have been reported to motivate learners (Parker & Lepper, 1992).

We were interested in using computer-assisted instruction for this program in order to tailor the intervention to each child's asthma symptoms and triggers. Even with this delivery method in mind, however, we had to determine theoretical methods that could produce change in the determinants we had specified in the matrix. Methods used in the computer self-management program were modeling, skill training, goal setting, self-monitoring, persuasive communication, reinforcement, cues to action, and attribution training (see Table 11.7).

Symbolic modeling was chosen as a principal method to elicit change in the child's knowledge and skills, self-efficacy, outcome expectations, and attributions (Bandura, 1986). The models—the child's chosen character and coach in the computer program—were used to teach skills and to reinforce the child's asthma management, thereby enhancing self-efficacy and outcome expectations. The models also illustrated that asthma management behavior is internal, controllable, and unstable in terms of attribution for failure (Weiner, 1985). Children are reminded by the role models that personal effort plays the major role in the management of asthma, that self-management begins with them, and that asthma is

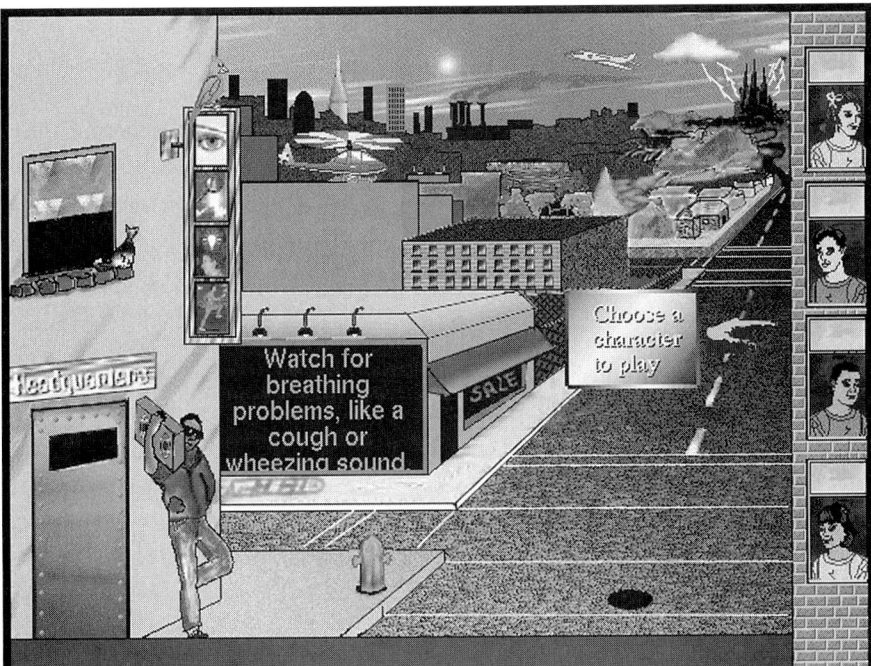

THE OPENING SCREEN

The opening screen is a city street scene. The activities in this scene include:

- **Clicking on various objects that animate when clicked (e.g., helicopter, airplane, castle).** This is an exploratory activity, intended to peak the child's interest in the program.
- **Clicking on the billboard to hear the asthma rap.** Clicking on the billboard will play the *Asthma Rap*. Clicking elsewhere on the screen will stop it.
- **Selecting a character.** The child selects a character by clicking on one of the four characters.
    - ☐ Hispanic/Latina female
    - ☐ Hispanic/Latino male
    - ☐ African American female
    - ☐ African American male
- **Clicking on the door to begin the mission.** A "psst" prompts the child to click on the door.

FIGURE 11.2 Watch, Discover, Think, and Act

something they can control. Further, when self-management failure occurs, it is controllable and unstable; it can be avoided in the future.

Reinforcement occurs throughout the program by vicarious reinforcement of the program role models, by simulated symptom reduction for the character in the game, and by accumulated points. The program also generates a report of the child's progress to stimulate reinforcement by parents and health care providers. The asthma action plan is also designed to elicit social reinforcement for the child's self-management behavior until the desired behavior becomes an internally reinforced part of the daily routine. Goal setting as a part of the asthma action plan is a means to improve the behavioral change effort, persistence, and concentration (Locke & Latham, 1990; Strecher et al., 1995).

PHYSICIAN LINKAGE COMPONENT The principal delivery mechanism for the physician linkage component is the asthma action plan, which was developed at a low reading level in English and Spanish. Once completed by the child's physician, the action plan provides written, individualized guidelines for the child's asthma care. Action plans were sent home to the parent with an accompanying video, which modeled taking the plan to the physician and reviewing it with the school nurse. A short video was mailed to children's homes to persuade parents of the importance of having the child's physician complete an action plan. The video included modeling of parents making a physician appointment, discussing the action plan with the physician, and reviewing the plan at home with the child. The video also provided modeling for interaction between the parent and school nurse discussing the action plan and medication use at school. Persuasive communication and reinforcement strategies were used by project staff and the school nurses to encourage parents to work with the physician on the action plan.

If the child was under physician care, an action plan was also mailed to the physician's office accompanied by the physician training video. The physician was instructed to place the action plan in the child's medical records chart for completion at the next office visit. The school nurse was also able to fax an action plan to the child's physician and request that the information be completed.

Video was also used as a mechanism for delivering program components that were designed to change physician behavior. The video modeled physicians using NAEPP guidelines to judge asthma severity and to objectively monitor asthma symptoms. The video also emphasized the use of a written asthma action plan to increase adherence for self-management.

School nurses play a central role in the intervention to link children to medical care; therefore project staff provided nurses with modeling and guided practice related to use of medication and peak flow meters, communication with parents and physicians to evaluate effectiveness of action plans, and effective communication with students to increase self-management skills. Cues to action, such as medication logs and computer player logs, were provided to prompt the school nurse to implement program activities.

Because many families participating in the study lacked a primary care provider or medical health insurance, the school nurse and project staff also assisted families to identify free or low cost medical services and to apply for Medicaid or other assistance. Families were contacted by telephone and by meetings at school to encourage participation. Once completed action plans were obtained from the physician, the school nurse retained a copy of each plan at the school and periodically reviewed it with the child, family, and physician to determine its effectiveness in reducing asthma exacerbations.

SCHOOL ENVIRONMENTAL CHANGE   Included in the environmental change intervention were the following:

- School-level environmental action committees
- Feedback of environmental survey data on a school "report card"
- Trainings for plant operators and teachers
- District-level policy change
- Facilitation of purchasing and maintenance at the district level

Raising the awareness of school personnel toward the potential harm of allergens and irritants to asthmatics was paramount. To accomplish this awareness, school committees were established and comprised the principal, plant operator, school nurse, and a teacher. Individualized school conditions were reported to the committees on environmental report cards that summarized the findings of allergens, irritants, and carbon dioxide levels found during the environmental survey. The cards had four columns: Three columns contained general information on irritants and allergens, actual school findings, and low-cost action recommendations; and one column was for item completion documentation. This report card was laminated in banner size, and action committees were encouraged to display it in the school as a document to monitor improvement and show commitment (Figure 11.3).

The committees set goals and established an environmental action committee agreement. To enable school personnel to obtain the skills and self-efficacy to implement the agreement, we trained plant operators in the steps for identification of allergens and irritants and removal techniques. At training sessions for plant operators and teachers, role models from each group provided testimonials about their problems and solutions. Project staff provided checklists for inspecting air-handling systems; checklists for identifying and removing mold, moisture, leaks, and spills; clipboards; and face masks. At action committee meetings, project staff encouraged school policy to be changed when needed to reflect action recommendations, such as enforcing a no-food rule in classrooms to reduce cockroaches and other pests.

The project staff helped schools overcome barriers by working on policy at the district level (such as developing suppliers of environmentally friendly items) and helped speed purchase orders and requests for maintenance through the district procedures.

Teachers at each school were provided an in-service workshop in which they were updated on environmental conditions, informed of children enrolled in the study in their class, and trained to identify and remove triggers of asthmatic children. Materials provided to teachers included asthma trigger information, checklists to inspect air-handling systems, checklists to identify and remove allergens and irritants in the classrooms, and a classroom product recommendation list.

Should you improve moisture and mold conditions? | Identify and complete action tasks

AIR FACTS	SCHOOL FINDINGS	ACTION RECOMMENDATIONS	NEEDS TO BE COMPLETED?
◆ Many people have allergic reactions to mold. ◆ Mold can hide from sight but not usually from smell, since mold spores give off a strong moldy, musty smell. ◆ Where there is moisture there is usually mold. Mold and mildew can grow almost anywhere that offers a food source and a small amount of moisture, whether from leaks, spills, or condensation.	% of classrooms surveyed with: ◆ mold smell................83.3% ◆ visible mold..................0% (usually on ceiling or floor tiles, around HVAC systems, or in/around cabinets) ◆ mold in the HVAC........50% ◆ visible water damage.....................20% Other areas in your school where mold smell detected: Standing water next to the school building? ❏yes ❏no Evidence of moisture found in the exterior walls of the building? ❏yes ❏no Mold or mildew on the exterior of the building? ❏yes ❏no	◆ Use the enclosed *Checklist to Detect Mold and Signs of Moisture, Leaks, or Spills* to identify problems ◆ Use proper cleaning practices on floors—using standard of no mold is acceptable. ◆ Fix leaks immediately (call district contact person: _____ ph#: _____ if needed for extra fast service.) ◆ Remediate wet materials or dry rapidly ◆ Wash outside or inside mold from buildings with a bleach/borax solution—including T-buildings ◆ Fill in drainage ditches with dirt or landscaping—do not allow standing water around buildings—including T-buildings ◆ Use anti-mold paints—do not paint over mold	❏yes ❏no BY_____DONE❏ ❏yes ❏no BY_____DONE❏ ❏yes ❏no BY_____DONE❏ ❏yes ❏no BY_____DONE❏ ❏yes ❏no BY_____DONE❏ ❏yes ❏no BY_____DONE❏ ❏yes ❏no BY_____DONE❏

FIGURE 11.3 Environmental Report Card

Program materials were reviewed by project staff and district personnel and were previewed by three elementary school principals.

Program Scope and Sequence

Each of the program components had a scope and sequence, but they also were coordinated into an overall program scope and sequence. The intervention was implemented at 30 elementary schools over 24 months. The sequence of program activities is depicted in Table 11.10.

Pretesting

The computer game Watch, Discover, Think, and Act was tested by children with asthma 6 to 12 years of age prior to final production and implementation. Determination was made as to whether children could understand the program directions and information and whether they could follow the watch, discover, think, and act self-regulatory process. Estimates were made as to how well the child made decisions and how engaged the child was in the process.

Table 11.10
Program Scope and Sequence

	QUARTER 1	QUARTER 2	QUARTER 3	QUARTER 4	QUARTERS 5–8
School environmental change	Surveys of schools Meeting between superintendent and principals	District advisory committee	Environmental report card School environmental committee District advisory committee	Training of plant operators, teachers, and principals Repeat meetings of school environmental committee	Continuation of school environmental committees and district advisory committee meetings Facilitation of purchasing and facilities services at the district level
Self-management training		Survey of asthma symptoms School nurse training on computer	Computer game playing Action plan sent home with video Phone calls to parents	Computer game playing Phone calls to parents of symptomatic children	Continuation of computer game playing and phone calls to parents of symptomatic children
Physician linkage		Action plan and video to physicians Action plan mailed to home Nurse training on action plans	Letter to physicians	Letter and repeat action plan mailing	

Materials such as the asthma action plan were reviewed by members of the school district advisory committee, participating school nurses, and physicians on the research team. Spanish-language focus groups were held before translation to explore commonly used words to describe asthma, and back translation of Spanish language materials was conducted.

INTERVENTION MAPPING STEP 4: ADOPTION AND IMPLEMENTATION

Linkage System

The fourth step in Intervention Mapping involves developing a plan to ensure program adoption and implementation by identifying adopters and implementers, defining potential barriers, developing a linkage system, and preparing an implementation plan. Because Partners in School Asthma Management was to be implemented in an elementary school setting, the first part of creating a linkage system was to include school district personnel on the program development team so that their perspectives of asthma management and the realities of working in schools were represented. The school district advisory committee played an important role in conceptualizing program development and implementation and assisted in the identification of additional school district personnel who would be instrumental for program adoption. The school district advisory committee consisted of directors and personnel from the departments of health and medical services, risk management, environmental affairs, construction management, and health education and curriculum development as well as a school nurse, elementary school principal, and parent advocate. The advisory committee provided insight into the culture and practice of the school district community.

Program Adopters and Implementers

To identify program adopters and implementers, we conducted a series of meetings, first with the school district area superintendents and then with elementary school principals in each of the school district areas. Often principals expressed interest in the program but indicated that they would leave the decision to their school nurses. From these meetings and later meetings with nurses, we hypothesized that adoption and implementation would be influenced by the following factors:

- Ease and low cost of implementation
- Outcome expectations such as perceived student benefits and better health for staff
- Lack of increased burden for school personnel
- No fear of negative publicity from the environmental intervention
- The feeling of doing something good for children with asthma

The school nurse was the key adopter as well as implementer of the program, and we addressed our recruitment efforts to the nurses with the messages that the program would be easy to implement, they would get help with the computer, the environment could benefit, and children and staff would possibly be healthier. In addition, in order to reduce the burden placed on the school nurse to implement the computerized self-management component, project staff trained school parent volunteers to assist children in playing the game. Each participating school was provided with a computer with CD-ROM capability, specifically for program implementation, to reduce administrative costs, and to alleviate competition for limited computer resources. To minimize disruption of the child's academic activities, it was recommended that students play the game during ancillary periods or during their regular computer class period.

INTERVENTION MAPPING STEP 5: MONITORING AND EVALUATION HIGHLIGHTS

The fifth step in Intervention Mapping involves the development of a plan for monitoring and evaluation that makes use of the previously developed Intervention Map. Our evaluation model is included in Figure 11.4.

The Partners in School Asthma Management program described in this chapter is currently under evaluation. However, outcome data are available from a related study that evaluated the impact of the computerized child self-management program in a similar inner-city population (Bartholomew, Gold, et al., 2000). This study was conducted in four inner-city asthma clinical sites with a slightly older range of children (mean age 10.9 years; range from ages 7 to 17). Results showed that children in the intervention group, who worked with

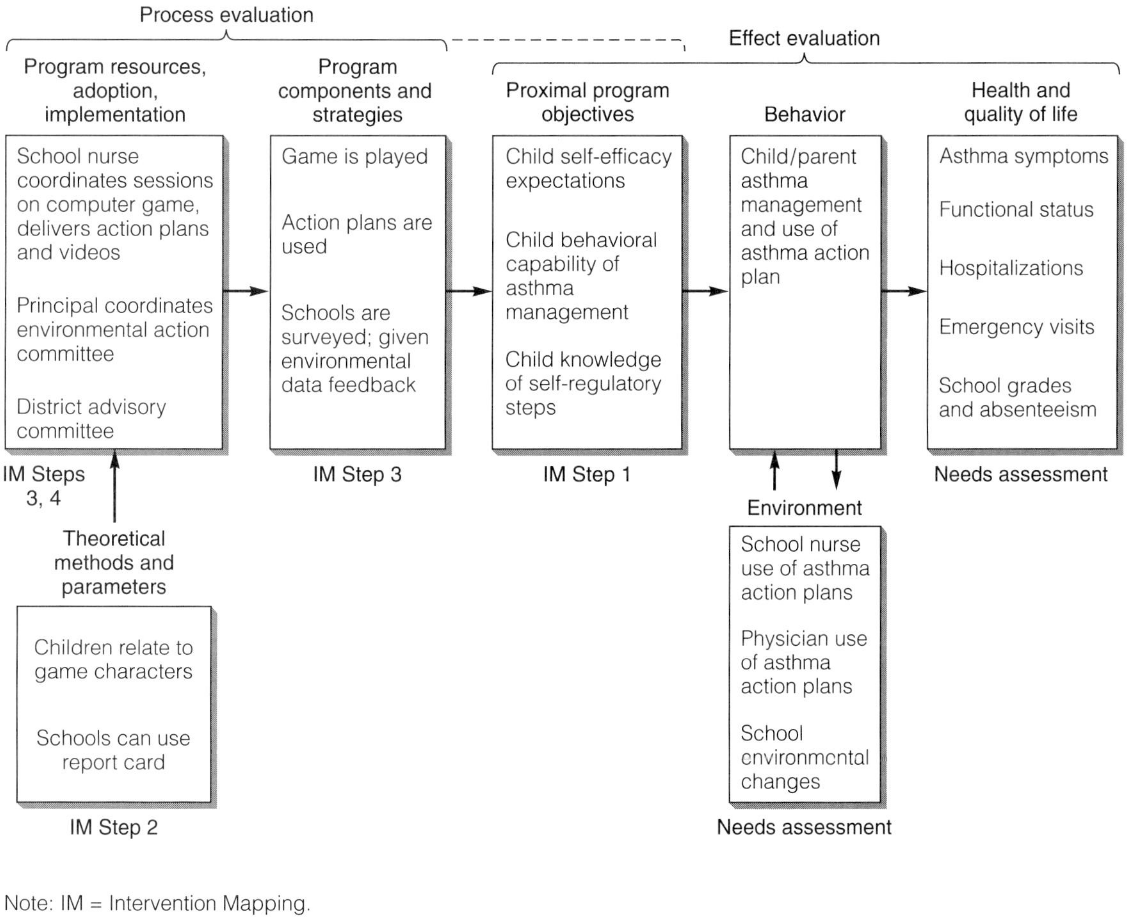

Note: IM = Intervention Mapping.

FIGURE 11.4 Evaluation Map

the computerized program, improved over a comparison group in their self-management of asthma and in their asthma outcomes.

The clinical sites study provided other indicators of planning success, including the observation that children liked to use the computer program and seemed to encourage their parents to bring them to the clinic, thereby improving their appointment-keeping rates. The assumptions that seemed to be appropriate included the use of self-regulatory and social cognitive theory to specify behavior and to create change methods. Further, the translation of the methods into strategies seemed to be successful. For example, the development of both simulations and fantasy components of the program taught skills and ensured the children's attention and interest. The children were generally true to our expectation that they would appreciate and choose role models of their own gender and ethnicity, and this choice may have contributed to their ability to identify with the characters (Bartholomew, Gold, et al., 2000).

SUMMARY

This chapter shows how the Intervention Mapping process was used to develop and implement a school-based asthma management program that addresses the environment and behavior of an at-risk population. Successive steps of the Intervention Mapping process were used to conceptualize program elements, to strategize program adoption, and to direct program implementation and evaluation. This process provides a model that can be used for other childhood chronic disease management programs, such as diabetes. Such an integrated process facilitates the development of creative programs that are deliverable and that have a higher likelihood of producing the desired health behavior outcomes.

REFERENCES

American Society of Heating, Refrigerating, and Air-Conditioning Engineers. (1989). *Standard 62-1989. Ventilation for acceptable indoor air quality.* Atlanta, GA: Author.

Bahir, A., Goldberg, A., Mekori, Y. A., Confino-Cohen, R., Morag, H., Rosen, Y., Monakir, D., Rigler, S., Cohen, A. H., Horev, Z., Noviski, N., & Mandelberg, A. (1997). Continuous avoidance measures with or without acaricide in dust mite–allergic asthmatic children. *Annals of Allergy, Asthma, and Immunology, 78*(5), 506–512.

Bandura, A. (1986). *Social foundations of thought and action: A social cognitive theory.* Englewood Cliffs, NJ: Prentice Hall.

Bartholomew, L. K., Gold, R. S., Parcel, G. S., Czyzewski, D. I., Sockrider, M. M., Fernandez, M., Shegog, R., & Swank, P. R. (2000). Watch, Discover, Think, and Act: Evaluation of computer-assisted instruction to improve asthma self-management in inner-city children. *Patient Education and Counseling, 39*(2–3), 269–280.

Bartholomew, L. K., Shegog, R., Parcel, G. S., Fernandez, M., Gold, R. S., Czyzewski, D. I., Sockrider, M. M., & Berlin, N. (2000). Watch, Discover, Think, and Act: A model for patient education program development. *Patient Education and Counseling, 39*(2–3), 253–268.

Bartholomew, L. K., Tortolero, S., Sockrider, M. M., Markham, C., Abramson, S., Fernandez, M., & Parcel, G. S. (1999, April). Screening children for asthma: Results from 60 elementary schools. Paper presented at the annual meeting of the American Thoracic Society, San Diego, CA.

Britton, M. G., Earnshaw, J. S., & Palmer, J. B. (1992). A 12-month comparison of salmeterol with salbutamol in asthmatic patients. *European Respiratory Journal, 5,* 1062–1067.

Burrows, B., Martinez, F. D., Halonen, M., Barbec, R. A., & Cline, M. G. (1989). Association of asthma and serum IgE levels and skin test reactivity to allergens. *New England Journal of Medicine, 320*(5), 271–277.

Call, R. S., Smith, T. F., Morris, E., Chapman, M. D., & Platts-Mills, T. A. (1992). Risk factors for asthma in inner-city children. *Journal of Pediatrics, 121*(6), 862–866.

Centers for Disease Control and Prevention. (1996). Asthma mortality and hospitalization among children and young adults—United States, 1980–1993. *Morbidity and Mortality Weekly Report, 45*(17), 350–353.

Clark, N. M. (1989). Asthma self-management education: Research and implications for clinical practice. *Chest, 95*(5), 1110–1113.

Clark, N. M., Feldman, C. H., Evans, D., Duzey, O., Levison, M. J., Wasilewski, Y., Kaplan, D., Rips, J., & Mellins, R. B. (1986a). Managing better: Children, parents, and asthma. *Patient Education and Counseling, 8*(1), 27–38.

Clark, N. M., Feldman, C. H., Evans, D., Levison, M. J., Wasilewski, Y., & Mellins, R. B. (1986b). The impact of health education on frequency and cost of health care use by low-income children with asthma. *Journal of Allergy and Clinical Immunology, 78*(1, Pt. 1), 108–115.

Clark, N. M., Feldman, C. H., Evans, D., Wasilewski, Y., & Leveson, M. J. (1984). Changes in children's school performance as a result of education for family management of asthma. *Journal of School Health, 54*(4), 143–145.

Clark, N. M., Rosenstock, I. M., Hassan, H., Evans, D., Wasilewski, Y., Feldman, C., & Mellins, R. B. (1988). The effect of health beliefs and feelings of self-efficacy on self-management behavior of children with chronic disease. *Patient Education and Counseling, 11*(2), 131–139.

Clark, N. M., & Starr-Schneidkraut, N. J. (1994). Management of asthma by patients and families. *American Journal of Respiratory and Critical Care Medicine, 194*(2, Pt. 2), s54–s66.

Crain, E. F., Weiss, K. B., Bijur, P. E., Hersh, M., Westbrook, L., & Stein, R. E. (1994). An estimate of the prevalence of asthma and wheezing among inner-city children. *Pediatrics, 94*(3), 356–362.

Creer, T. L. (1990). Strategies for judgment and decision making in the management of childhood asthma. *Pediatric Allergy and Immunology, 4*(4), 253–264.

Creer, T. L., Backial, M., Burns, K. L., Leung, P., Marion, R. J., Miklich, D. R., Morrill, C., Taplin, P. S., & Ullman, S. (1988). Living with asthma: I. Genesis and development of a self-management program for childhood asthma. *Journal of Asthma, 25*(6), 335–362.

Creer, T. L., Kotses, H., & Wigal, J. K. (1992). A second-generation model of asthma self-management. *Pediatric Allergy and Immunology, 6*(3), 143–165.

Cuijpers, C., Swaen, G., Wesseling, G., Stumans, F., & Wouters, E. F. (1995). Adverse effects of the indoor environment on respiratory health in primary school children. *Environmental Research, 68*(1), 11–23.

Cunningham, J., Dockery, D., & Speizer, F. (1996). Race, asthma, and persistent wheeze in Philadelphia schoolchildren. *American Journal of Public Health, 86*(10), 1406–1409.

Dawson, K. P., Van Asperen, P., Higgins, C., Sharpe, C., & Davis, A. (1995). An evaluation of the action plans of children with asthma. *Journal of Pediatrics and Child Health, 31*(1), 21–23.

Djukanovic, R., Wilson, J. W., Britten, K. M., Wilson, S. J., Walls, A. F., Roche, W. R., Howarth, P. H., & Holgate, S. T. (1992). Effect of an inhaled corticosteroid on airway inflammation and symptoms in asthma. *American Review of Respiratory Disease, 145*(3), 669–674.

Dungy, C. I., Kozak, P. P., Gallup, J., & Galant, S. P. (1986). Aeroallergen exposure in the elementary school setting. *Annals of Allergy, 56*(3), 218–221.

Emerson, J. A., Wahlgren, D., Hovell, M. F., Meltzer, S. B., Zakarian, J. M., & Hofstetter, C. R. (1994). Parent smoking and asthmatic children's exposure patterns: A behavioral epidemiology study. *Addictive Behaviors, 19*(6), 677–689.

Evans, D., Clark, N. M., Feldman, C. H., Rips, J., Kaplan, D., Levison, M. J., Wasilewski, Y., Levin, B., & Mellins, R. B. (1987). A school health education program for children with asthma aged 8–11 years. *Health Education Quarterly, 14*(3), 267–279.

Finkelstein, J. A., Brown, R. W., Schneider, L. C., Weiss, S. T., Quintana, J. M., Goldmann, D. A., & Homer, C. J. (1995). Quality of care for preschool children with asthma: The role of social factors and practice setting. *Pediatrics, 95*(3), 389–394.

Fireman, P., Friday, G. A., Gira, C., Vierthaler, W. A., & Michaels, L. (1981). Teaching self-management skills to asthmatic children and their parents in an ambulatory care setting. *Pediatrics, 68*(3), 341–348.

Fowler, M. G., Davenport, M. G., & Garg, R. (1992). School functioning of U.S. children with asthma. *Pediatrics, 90*(6), 939–944.

Gergen, P. J., & Turkeltaub, P. C. (1992). The association of individual allergen reactivity with respiratory disease in a national sample: Data from the second National Health and Nutrition Examination Survey, 1976 to 1980 (NHANES II). *Journal of Allergy and Clinical Immunology, 90*(4, Pt. 1), 579–588.

Gergen, P. J., & Weiss, K. B. (1990). Changing patterns in hospitalizations among children: 1979–1987. *JAMA, 264*(13), 1688–1692.

Global Initiative for Asthma. (1995). *Global strategy for asthma management and prevention* (NHLBI/WHO Workshop Report; Publication No. 95-3659). Available: http://www.ginasthma.com/xwork.html

Green, L. W., & Kreuter, M. W. (1999). *Health promotion planning: An educational and ecological approach* (3rd ed.). Mountain View, CA: Mayfield.

Halfon, N. & Newacheck, P. (1993). Childhood asthma and poverty: Differential impacts and utilization of health services. *Pediatrics, 91*(1), 56–61.

Hindi-Alexander, M. C. (1984). Evaluation of a family asthma program. *Allergy and Clinical Immunology, 74*(4), 505–510.

Homer, C. J., Szilagyi, P., Rodewald, L., Bloom, S. R., Greenspan, P., Yazdgerdi, S., Leventhal, J. M., Finkelstein, D., & Perrin, J. (1996). Does quality of care affect rates of hospitalization for childhood asthma? *Pediatrics, 98*(1), 18–23.

Hospers, H. J., Kok, G., & Strecher, V. J. (1990). Attributions for previous failures and subsequent outcomes in a weight reduction program. *Health Education Quarterly, 17*(4), 409–415.

Hovell, M. F., Meltzer, S. B., Zakarian, J. M., Wahlgren, D. R., Emerson, J. A., Hofstetter, C. R., Leaderer, B. P., Meltzer, E. O., Zeiger, R. S., & O'Connor, R. D. (1994). Reduction of environmental tobacco smoke exposure among asthmatic children: A controlled trial. *Chest, 106*(2), 440–446. (Published erratum in *Chest, 1995, 107*(5), 1480.

Huss, K., Rand, C. S., Butz, A. M., Eggleston, P. A., Murigande, C., Thompson, L., Schneider, S., Weeks, K., & Malveaux, F. J. (1994). Home environmental risk factors in urban minority asthmatic children. *Annals of Allergy, 72*(2), 173–177.

Ingram, J. M., Sporik, R., Rose, G., Honsinger, R., Chapman, M. D., & Platts-Mills, T. A. (1995). Quantitative assessment of exposure to dog (Can f 1) and cat (Fel d 1) allergens: Relation to sensitization and asthma among children living in Los Alamos, New Mexico. *Journal of Allergy and Clinical Immunology, 96*(4), 449–456.

Juniper, E. F., Kline, P. A., Vanzieleghem, M. A., Ramsdale, E. H., O'Byrne, P. M., & Hargreave, F. E. (1990). Effect of long-term treatment with an inhaled corticosteroid (budesonide) on airway hyperresponsiveness and clinical asthma in nonsteroid-dependent asthmatics. *American Review of Respiratory Disease, 142*(4), 832–836.

Kang, B. C., Johnson, J., & Veres-Thorner, C. (1993). Atopic profile of inner-city asthma with a comparative analysis on the cockroach-sensitive and ragweed-sensitive subgroups. *Journal of Allergy and Clinical Immunology, 92*(6), 802–811.

Kattan, M., Mitchell, H., Eggleston, P., Gergen, P., Crain, E., Redline, S., Weiss, K., Evans, R., 3rd, Kaslow, R., Nercsmar, C., Leickly, F., Malveaux, F., & Wedner, H. J. (1997). Characteristics of inner-city children with asthma: The National Cooperative Inner-City Asthma Study. *Pediatric Pulmonology, 24*(4), 253–262.

Kotses, H., Lewis, P., & Creer, T. L. (1990). Environmental control of asthma self-management. *Journal of Asthma, 27*(6), 375–384.

Kotses, H., Stout, C., McConnaughy, K., Winder, J. A., & Creer, T. L. (1996). Evaluation of individualized asthma self-management programs. *Journal of Asthma, 33*(2), 113–118.

Kuttner, M. J., Delamater, A. M., & Santiago, J. V. (1990). Learned helplessness in diabetic youths. *Journal of Pediatric Psychology, 15*(5), 595–604.

Lewis, C. E., Rachelefsky, G., Lewis, M. A., de la Sota, A., & Kaplan, M. (1984). A randomized trial of A.C.T. (Asthma Care Training) for kids. *Pediatrics, 74*(4), 478–486.

Lieu, T. A., Quesenberry, C. P., Capra, M. A., Sorel, M. E., Martin, K. E., & Mendoza, G. R. (1997). Outpatient management practices associated with reduced risk of pediatric asthma hospitalization and emergency department visits. *Pediatrics, 100*(3), 334–341.

Locke, E. A., & Latham, G. P. (1990). *A theory of goal setting and task performance.* Englewood Cliffs, NJ: Prentice Hall.

Mak, H., Johnston, P., Abbey, H., & Talamo, R. C. (1982). Prevalence of asthma and health utilization of asthmatic children in an inner city. *Journal of Allergy and Clinical Immunology, 70*(5), 367–372.

Manson, A. (1988). Language concordance as a determinant of patient compliance and emergency room use in patients with asthma. *Medical Care, 26*(12), 1119–1128.

McNabb, W. L., Wilson-Pessano, S. R., & Jacobs, A. M. (1986). Critical self-management competencies for children with asthma. *Journal of Pediatric Psychology, 11*(1), 103–117.

Murray, A. B. (1988). Dust mite avoidance in the treatment of asthma. *Annals of Allergy, 60*(1), 84.

Murray, A. B., & Morrison, B. J. (1989). Passive smoking by asthmatics: Its greater effect on boys than girls and older than younger children. *Pediatrics, 84*(3), 451–459.

National Heart, Lung, and Blood Institute. (1991). *Expert panel report: Executive summary. Guidelines for the diagnosis and management of asthma* (Publication No. 91-3042A). Bethesda, MD: National Institutes of Health.

Neuberger, J. S., Newkirk, D. D., Cotter, J., Thorpe, A., Wood, C., & Irwin, J. C. (1991). Diminished air quality and health problems in a Kansas City, Kansas, elementary school. *Journal of School Health, 61*(10), 439–442.

Norback, D., Torgen, M., & Edling, C. (1990). Volatile organic compounds, respirable dust, and personal factors related to prevalence and incidence of sick building syndrome in primary schools. *British Journal of Industrial Medicine, 47*(11), 733–741.

Overpeck, M. D., & Moss, J. A. (1991). *Children's exposure to environmental cigarette smoke before and after birth: Advance data from Vital and Health Statistics #202.* (DHHS Publication No. 91-1250). Hyattsville, MD: National Center for Health Statistics.

Parcel, G. S., & Nader, P. R. (1977). Evaluation of a pilot school health education program for asthmatic children. *Journal of School Health, 47*(8), 453–456.

Parcel, G. S., Nader, P. R., & Tiernan, K. (1980). A health education program for children with asthma. *Journal of Developmental and Behavioral Pediatrics, 1*(13), 128–132.

Parker, L. E., & Lepper, M. R. (1992). Effects of fantasy contexts on children's learning and motivation: Making learning more fun. *Journal of Personality and Social Psychology, 62*(4), 625–633.

Peroni, D. G., Boner, A. L., Vallone, G., Antolini, I., & Warner, J. O. (1994). Effective allergen avoidance at high altitude reduces allergen-induced bronchial hyperresponsiveness. *American Journal of Respiratory and Critical Care Medicine, 149*(6), 1442–1446.

Platts-Mills, T. A. (1994). How environment affects patients with allergic disease: Indoor allergens and asthma. *Annals of Allergy, 72*(4), 381–384.

Platts-Mills, T. A., & Pollart Squillace, S. (1997). Allergen sensitization and perennial asthma. *International Archives of Allergy and Immunology, 113*(1–3), 83–86.

Pollart, S. M., Chapman, M. D., Fiocoo, G. P., Rose, G., & Platts-Mills, T. A. (1989). Epidemiology of acute asthma: IgE antibodies to common inhalant allergens as a risk factor for emergency room visits. *Journal of Allergy and Clinical Immunology, 83*(5), 875–882.

Pope, A., Patterson, R., & Burge, H. (Eds.), and Committee on the Health Effects of Indoor Allergens, Division of Health Promotion and Disease Prevention, Institute of Medicine. (1993). *Indoor allergens: Assessing and controlling adverse health effects.* Washington, DC: National Academy Press.

Public Health Service. (1991). *Healthy People 2000: National health promotion and disease prevention objectives* (Full report with commentary; DHHS Publication No. PHS 91-502212). Washington, DC: U.S. Department of Health and Human Services.

Rosenstreich, D. L., Eggleston, P., Kattan, M., Baker, D., Slavin, R. G., Gergen, P., Mitchell, H., McNiff-Mortimer, K., Lynn, H., Ownby, D., & Malveaux, F. (1997). The role of cockroach allergy and exposure to cockroach allergen in causing morbidity among inner-city children with asthma. *New England Journal of Medicine, 336*(19), 1356–1363.

Ruhl, R., Chang, C., Halpern, G., & Gershwin, M. E. (1993). The sick building syndrome: II. Assessment and regulation of indoor air quality. *Journal of Asthma, 30*(4), 297–308.

Salmeron, S., Guerin, J. C., Godard, P., Renon, D., Henry-Amar, M., Duroux, P., & Taytard, A. (1989). High doses of inhaled corticosteroids in unstable chronic asthma: A multicenter, double-blind, placebo-controlled study. *American Review of Respiratory Disease, 140*(1), 167–171.

Samet, J., Cain, W., & Leaderer, B. (1991). Environmental tobacco smoke. In J. Samet & J. Spengler (Eds.), *Indoor air pollution: A health perspective* (pp. 131–169). Baltimore: Johns Hopkins University Press.

Sarsfield, J. K., Gowland, G., Toy, R., & Normal, A. L. (1974). Mite-sensitive asthma of childhood: Trial of avoidance measures. *Archives of Disease in Childhood, 49*(9), 716–721.

Shegog, R., Bartholomew, L. K., Gold, R. S., Pierrel, E., Parcel, G. S., Sockrider, M., Czyzewski, D., Fernandez, M., Berlin, N., Combes, R., & Abramson, S. (1999). *Self-management education for pediatric chronic disease: A description of the Watch, Discover, Think, and Act asthma computer program.* Manuscript submitted for publication.

Sherman, C. B., Tosteson, T. D., Tager, I. B., Speizer, F. E., & Weiss, S. T. (1990). Early childhood predictors of asthma. *American Journal of Epidemiology, 132*(1), 83–95.

Strecher, V. J., Seijts, G. H., Kok, G. J., Latham, G. P., Glasgow, R., DeVellis, B., Meertens, R. M., & Bulger, D. W. (1995). Goal setting as a strategy for health behavior change. *Health Education Quarterly, 22*(2), 190–200.

Swanson, M., & Thompson, P. (1994). Managing asthma triggers in school. *Pediatric Nursing, 20*(2), 181–184.

Taylor, W. R., & Newacheck, P. W. (1992). Impact of asthma on health. *Pediatrics, 90*(5), 657–662.

Thoresen, C. E., & Kirmil-Gray, K. (1983). Self-management psychology and the treatment of childhood asthma. *Journal of Allergy and Clinical Immunology, 72*(5), 596–610.

Tortolero, S. R., Bartholomew, L. K., Abramson, S., Sockrider, M. M., Whitehead, L., & Markham, C. (2000). *Environmental characteristics of urban elementary schools: A focus on asthma.* Manuscript submitted for publication.

Tyrrell, S., Bartholomew, L. K., Tortolero, S., Markham, C., Abramson, S., Whitehead, L., & Sockrider, M. M. (2000). *A program to improve the asthma-related environment of urban elementary schools: An application of the Intervention Mapping framework.* Manuscript submitted for publication.

U.S. Environmental Protection Agency, Indoor Air Division. (1991). *Building air quality: A guide for building owners and facility managers.* Washington, DC: U.S. Government Printing Office.

U.S. Environmental Protection Agency. (1995). *Indoor air quality tools for schools: Action kit.* (EPA Publication No. 402-K-95-001). Cleveland, OH: National Service Center for Environmental Publications.

University of Texas Health Science Center–Houston. (1996, March 31). *Interventions to improve asthma management and prevention at school* (First Technical Progress Report, Contract No. NO1-HR-56079; submitted to the National Heart, Lung, and Blood Institute, National Institutes of Health).

Wasilewski, Y., Clark, N. M., Evans, D., Levison, M. J., Levin, B., & Mellins, R. B. (1996). Factors associated with emergency department visits by children with asthma: Implications for health education. *American Journal of Public Health, 86*(10), 1410–1415.

Weiner, B. (1985). An attributional theory of achievement motivation and emotion. *Psychological Review, 92*(4), 548–573.

Weiss, K. B., Gergen, P. J., & Hodgson, T. (1992). An economic evaluation of asthma in the United States. *New England Journal of Medicine, 326*(13), 862–866.

Weiss, K. B., Gergen, P. J., & Wagener, D. K. (1993). Breathing better or wheezing worse? The changing epidemiology of asthma morbidity and mortality. *Annual Review of Public Health, 14,* 491–531.

Weitzman, M., Gortmaker, S., & Sobol, A. (1990). Racial, social, and environmental risks for childhood asthma. *American Journal of Diseases of Children, 144*(11), 1189–1194.

Wilson-Pessano, S. R., Scamagas, P., Arsham, G. M., Chardon, L., Coss, S., German, D. F., & Hughes, G. W. (1987). An evaluation of approaches to asthma self-management education for adults: The AIR Kaiser-Permanente study. *Health Education Quarterly, 14*(3), 333–343.

Wissow, S., Gittelsohn, A. M., Szklo, M., Starfield, B., & Mussman, M. (1988). Poverty, race, and hospitalization for childhood asthma. *American Journal of Public Health, 78*(7), 777–782.

Wood, P. R., Hidalgo, H. A., Prihoda, T. J., & Kromer, M. E. (1993). Hispanic children with asthma: Morbidity. *Pediatrics, 91*(1), 62–69.

CHAPTER 12

Project Northland: Alcohol Use Prevention With Older Adolescents

Sara Veblen-Mortenson, Randi Bernstein Lachter, Guy S. Parcel, and Cheryl Perry

READER OBJECTIVES

- Identify environmental conditions that contribute to adolescent alcohol use
- Describe personal and external determinants that influence these environmental conditions
- Give examples of learning and change objectives as proximal targets for a health promotion program that focuses on community change
- Consider methods and strategies for environmental change to reduce adolescent alcohol use

Alcohol is the drug of choice for American adolescents. Despite being illegal for essentially all high school students, 52% of 8th graders, 70% of 10th graders, and 81% of 12th graders report having used alcohol in their lifetime. Furthermore, 23%, 39%, and 52% of 8th, 10th, and 12th graders in the United States report having used alcohol in the past 30 days (Johnston, O'Malley, & Bachman, 1999). The widespread use of alcohol is a significant public health problem in this country, accounting for a substantial portion of the total morbidity and mortality during adolescence (Dryfoos, 1990; "Trends in Drug and Alcohol Use," 1993; Perry, Williams, et al., 1993; Wagenaar & Perry, 1994).

Public health approaches involve community-wide interventions that may include both demand and supply reduction strategies (Perry, Williams, et al.,

---

Project Northland was funded by the National Institute on Alcohol Abuse and Alcoholism (RO1-AA08596).

1993), reflecting the multiple factors that contribute to adolescent drinking. Project Northland–Phase II (1996–1998), a community-based research project to reduce older adolescents' alcohol use, used a multicomponent approach to address this problem and incorporated both individual and environmental change to achieve the project's goals. The program consisted of five intervention components: (a) school-based curriculum; (b) parent education; (c) media; (d) direct action community organizing; and (e) youth development.

This chapter describes, using an Intervention Mapping approach, two of the five intervention components utilized in Phase II of Project Northland: direct action community organizing, and youth development involving high school students in youth action teams. These two components were chosen because they most directly targeted environmental changes to reduce drinking among older teens. These program components were implemented to limit youth's ability to obtain alcohol in the Project Northland communities and to involve them in the environmental change process. The general planning approach we used for Project Northland and other youth health promotion programs is described in a text on health promotion program planning for children and youth (Perry, 1999). Many of the planning processes described by Perry are similar to steps and tasks included in Intervention Mapping; therefore, the description of Project Northland can serve as an example of how Intervention Mapping can be applied to a retrospective description of health promotion programs. Even if Intervention Mapping is not used as the planning framework for a health promotion program, it is possible to analyze the program and reconstruct the products for Intervention Mapping to assist the program planners in describing and communicating to others specific aspects of the program.

PERSPECTIVES IN THIS CASE

This case study focuses on community change. The framework of the research, the hypotheses and theoretical model, the intervention, and the evaluation strategies were established prior to doing an analysis of the program using the steps and tasks of Intervention Mapping (Komro et al., in press). As part of the program development, the researchers worked with the participating communities to develop environmental prevention strategies to change youth alcohol use behavior. Effective efforts to reduce youth drinking and associated health and social problems must focus on change at multiple levels: family, social groups, community, and society. Attempting to change drinking behavior without direct attention to the socioenvironmental conditions supporting alcohol use are of limited utility; at best, short-term changes in small segments of the population are achieved (Wagenaar & Perry, 1994).

It is clear from more than a decade of public health research that the best way to achieve and sustain prevention is to focus on both individuals and their environments (Gardner, Green, & Marcus, 1994), and that demand and supply factors must be targeted simultaneously. The complement of individual and environmental changes, accompanied by widespread community acceptance and support of these prevention initiatives, may be the key to effective and long-lasting prevention efforts. Unfortunately, multilevel interventions that include both individual behavior change (demand) and environmental change (supply) strategies are not common in alcohol prevention programs (National Institute on Alcohol Abuse and Alcoholism [NIAAA], 1994).

NEEDS ASSESSMENT

Health Problems and Quality of Life

The health problems associated with adolescent alcohol use contribute to a substantial portion of the total morbidity and mortality during adolescence. Motor vehicle crashes are the leading cause of death for adolescents with one-third to one-half involving alcohol (National Highway Traffic Safety Administration, 1990). Many of the other causes of death and long-term disability during adolescence (e.g., suicides, homicides, assaults, drowning, and recreational injuries) involve alcohol in notable proportion (Adger, 1991; Brent, Perper, & Allman, 1987; "Trends in Drug and Alcohol Use," 1993), although exact quantification of the health burden of underage alcohol consumption is difficult. Adolescent alcohol use is also associated with violence, delinquency, family problems, and risky sexual behavior resulting in sexually transmitted diseases, including HIV/AIDS, and in teenage pregnancies (Semlitz & Gold, 1986). Equally important is the impact of alcohol use on cognitive and psychosocial development.

Project Northland communities were located in northeastern Minnesota and were chosen because they are in counties that have the highest alcohol-related morbidity and mortality rates in the state (Caces, Stinson, & Elliott, 1991). By the cohort's 10th-grade year, two years after the end of Phase I of Project Northland (6th–8th-grade years), the project's positive outcomes had attenuated. At the end of the cohort's 10th-grade year, 40.3% of all the students who were nondrinkers at the start of Project Northland reported having used alcohol in the past week.

The need to address alcohol use beginning in adolescence also stems from the increased problems associated with early use. A 1998 National Institute on Alcohol Abuse and Alcoholism study found that the younger someone starts drinking, the greater is the chance that teen will develop a clinically defined alcohol disorder. Those students who began drinking before age 15 were four times more likely to develop alcohol dependence than were those who began drinking at age 21. In addition, the risk of alcohol abuse was more than doubled for those who started drinking before age 15 versus age 21 (Grant & Dawson, 1997). Early onset of alcohol use is a crucial risk factor for progression to more serious forms of drug use, a finding that has been replicated across different populations, historical periods, and cultural groups (Kandel & Yamaguchi, 1993). Alcohol use negatively impacts a community's quality of life by contributing to the previously mentioned health and social problems. Reducing adolescent alcohol use could improve the health and well-being of teenagers, their families, schools, and the community.

Behavioral and Environmental Conditions

For adolescents, the primary behavioral condition related to the health problems previously discussed is any level of alcohol use. Adolescent alcohol use is a public health problem in that all teens are at potential risk when using alcohol, not just those who have traditionally been labeled as "high risk." The nature of adolescent drinking makes it a risky behavior. Teenage drinking is a social and normative behavior and is widely accepted by teens and adults despite its being illegal. Blatant disregard for the 21-year-old drinking age is widely accepted in most communities, sending an inconsistent, potentially harmful message to those who are under 21.

The idea that teenagers can drink safely has been consistently disproved. Teenagers have the highest rates of hazardous or risky drinking of all age groups. Results from a 1996 national survey found that during a 2-week period, 14% of 8th graders, 24% of 10th graders, and 32% of 12th graders consumed five or more drinks in a row (Johnston et al., 1999). This type of heavy, risky drinking represents 53% of all drinking (Greenfield, 1996). Beer is the beverage of choice for American teens and is affordable, is easily accessible, and can be distributed in large quantities through keg parties (Kusserow, 1991). Adults need to be informed about the prevalence and nature of teenage drinking and the potential risks involved. Consistent messages need to be communicated in the school, family, and community settings in order to address this normative behavior.

Environmental conditions are defined as those factors within the environment that support or encourage alcohol use. Organizational and community policies, practices, and norms contribute to adolescent alcohol use by sending inconsistent messages to teenagers about the acceptability of alcohol use; serving as role models for alcohol use; focusing recreational activities on adults (e.g., community festivals, adult-centered establishments); making it easy for teens to purchase, obtain, or use alcohol from social sources (i.e., access); and inconsistently enforcing policies and laws regarding underage alcohol use (Wagenaar & Perry, 1994). These community and organizational policies and practices must be evaluated, revised, and enforced in order to reduce teenage alcohol use.

Identifying Determinants

Research on adolescent alcohol and drug use that utilizes problem behavior and social influences theory suggests that factors within a teen's social environment, personality, and behavior are all important determinants of substance use. Alcohol and other drug use are viewed as the result of a complex interaction of influences at each of these levels (Jessor & Jessor, 1977). These environmental, intrapersonal, and behavioral factors, then, must be considered when identifying determinants associated with adolescent alcohol use.

Intrapersonal, interpersonal, and behavioral factors associated with adolescent alcohol use include parental influences, peer influences, self-efficacy, perceived access to alcohol, functional meanings, and previous alcohol or other drug use (Jessor & Jessor, 1977; Perry & Jessor, 1985). Parental influence is expressed through parent-child communication, parental supervision and monitoring of a child's activities, and rules at home. Research shows that associating with peers who drink is one of the strongest predictors of adolescent alcohol use (Jessor & Jessor, 1977). The world of older adolescents centers more and more around their peers and less around their families as they progress through high school (Perry, Kelder, & Komro, 1993). Functional meanings are the reasons for which teenagers use alcohol, such as stress, family problems, or socialization. Finally, previous alcohol or other drug use often predicts future behavior.

The determinants of community environmental conditions include the following: collective efficacy, collective knowledge, community norms, social support, opportunities, access, and enforcement. Important aspects of the process of community and citizen involvement are community ownership and empowerment (Rissel et al., 1996). Community empowerment is defined by participation in collective political action that results in a raised level of psychological empowerment and the achievement of some redistribution of resources or decision making sought by a community or subgroup (Bracht, 1999). Increasing individual and collective knowledge within the community, it is hypothesized, will lead to an increase in community efficacy (empowerment) and thus stimulate community action.

The determinants of organizational environmental conditions, such as characteristics of the high schools' organization, include students' self-efficacy, students' knowledge, social support or pressure, opportunities, resources, and school or community efficacy. Students must feel confident in their ability to be involved in changing the environmental conditions that contribute to underage alcohol use. Students are usually viewed as the targets for prevention programs rather than as active participants in the planning and implementation. Students' knowledge of the environmental conditions and ways to address them are critical to help them build their confidence and initiate changes.

Social support is especially necessary for students and school personnel involved in a new approach to an "old" problem. Social support is associated with self-efficacy and is critical for students' success. Students also need to be given the opportunity to be involved in reducing teenage alcohol use. As was mentioned, students are usually not asked to be actively engaged in setting school or community policies. Opportunities for alcohol-free activities are also important because these activities reduce access, provide alternatives, and potentially change norms. The availability of resources is critical to provide the opportunities and support needed for students to succeed. Without resources, students become easily discouraged and their involvement could easily falter as a result. Community efficacy is also important in creating change at the organizational level. Community and school change is closely linked, especially in locations where the school is the center of community activity. Community groups can contribute to environmental change as it relates to school activities.

Current Programs

The results of Project Northland–Phase I demonstrated the need to address the environmental conditions that contribute to adolescent alcohol use (Perry et al., 1996). Phase I of Project Northland was successful in reducing alcohol use, polydrug use, and psychosocial risks among adolescents in the intervention communities (Perry et al.). These changes were attributed to changes in intrapersonal and interpersonal determinants: peer influence, peer norms, parent-child communication, the functional meanings of alcohol use, and self-efficacy to refuse alcohol. However, during Phase I, no changes were detected in the larger community, such as in young people's ability to purchase beer without identification (Perry et al.).

School-based programs addressing individual characteristics and peer influence (e.g., demand reduction) are the most common approach to preventing onset of alcohol and other drug use (NIAAA, 1994). Early adolescence has been targeted for program focus because this developmental period is just prior to experimentation and there are not substantial pharmacological effects to counter. Also, early adolescents have not adopted some other behaviors that serve as cues for alcohol use. Few alcohol prevention programs have been developed for high school students, although such programs seem warranted given developmentally significant problems among older youth such as driving under the influence of alcohol (NIAAA). School-based demand reduction strategies increasingly are seen as necessary but not sufficient to reduce teenage alcohol use.

Needs Assessment Summary

The needs assessment indicated that Project Northland–Phase II should focus on significantly reducing the negative health consequences related to adolescent alcohol use by reducing alcohol use among older adolescents. The needs assessments conducted as part of Phase I and as baseline for Phase II showed underage youth could easily purchase alcohol in Project Northland's intervention communities (Forster et al., 1998) and that community norms and role models were the most potent predictors of alcohol use (Roski et al., 1997). Phase II, then, was designed to emphasize changes at the community level.

INTERVENTION MAPPING STEP 1: MATRICES OF PROXIMAL PROGRAM OBJECTIVES

Health-Related Behaviors and Environmental Conditions

As a result of Project Northland's Phase II interventions, high school students were expected to drink less alcohol. To accomplish this goal, it was critical to reduce teenage access to alcohol from both commercial sources (e.g., liquor stores and bars) and social sources (e.g., siblings and friends). Approaches such as increasing law enforcement and checks of age identification; establishing clear, consistent school and community policies that discourage adolescent alcohol use; reducing social access to alcohol; and increasing alcohol-free activities for youth can contribute to less alcohol use by teenagers in a community. Thus, the key environmental condition that needed to be addressed was reducing adolescents' access to alcohol. Policies related to underage alcohol use and enforcement of relevant laws are key factors in reducing access to alcohol. Each of these elements is linked to a community's acceptance of teenage alcohol use. Ease of access and lack of policy enforcement convey powerful messages to young people. Changes in school and community policies could help reduce adolescent alcohol use and were addressed in the Project Northland Phase I program. The goal, then, of the Project Northland community organizing and youth development programs was to reduce adolescents' access to alcohol and as a result reduce alcohol use by adolescents.

Performance Objectives

The following performance objectives were developed for the community level to reduce adolescent access to alcohol in the community.

- The community will develop capacity to address the issue of underage access to and use of alcohol.
- The community will reduce the number of commercial sources for alcohol that are available to adolescents.
- Policy makers and city government will strengthen the communities' alcohol policies and ordinances to prevent youth access to alcohol.
- The police and owners of retail stores will enforce policies, ordinances, and laws regarding underage drinking.

The first community-level performance objective was the basis of the direct action community-organizing model. One of the principles underpinning the model is a belief that fully informed individuals are better able to take active roles as citizens and to hold leaders accountable for decisions affecting public life (Hanna & Robinson, 1994). The model also assumes that increasing a community's capacity to address the issue of underage access and adolescent alcohol use will spur the community to take "action." A second principle underpinning the model is a belief that when people become aware of their values and find them in conflict with power structures, they can legitimately use that conflict to mobilize citizens to take action (Hanna & Robinson).

The remaining three objectives outline the specific actions that are sought to change the community environment in a way that reduces youth access to alcohol. The initiatives outlined in these three performance objectives address the following issues: Commercial sources are a primary source of alcohol for underage youth, as demonstrated by the needs assessment at Phase II baseline; new as well as existing policy implementation can reduce youth access to alcohol; and enforcement of new and existing policies is critical.

Based on what is known about adolescent alcohol use prevention, the following performance objectives were developed to change unclear and inconsistent enforcement of policies regarding students' alcohol use while involved in school activities such as sports, choir, band, and so on, or during school-sponsored events.

- Students will generate support in the school community (students, staff, and parents) for changes in school practices and policies.
- Students will work with school personnel (coaches, administrators, counselors, and teachers) to review and revise school policies and identify other solutions.
- Students will work with school personnel to establish an enforcement plan for school policies.
- Students or school personnel will inform the school community of policy changes and procedures.
- School personnel will enforce policies according to plan.
- Community groups, businesses, and parents will strengthen policies and norms to not allow alcohol use during prom, homecoming, and graduation.

Project Northland students entered Phase II of the program with knowledge regarding underage alcohol use and its consequences. They were well equipped with the resistance and decision-making skills needed to resist alcohol use because they had participated in Phase I of Project Northland (Perry et al., 1996). Given this exposure, students were prepared to be involved in creating policy change at the school and community levels.

Traditionally, school personnel and adult community leaders set school and community policies with little involvement from the students. The goal of Project Northland's youth development component was to change that dynamic to actively engage students in shaping school and community policies. The performance objectives reflected the need to challenge the status quo in order to have the students' voices heard. By having students involved in the process, the policies should have been viewed as more acceptable by their peers and would thus have increased the likelihood that they would be followed. This approach to peer leadership had been particularly effective during Phase I of the project, but the scope of peer involvement was expanded as seemed appropriate for 11th and 12th grade students (Komro et al., 1996; Komro, Perry, Veblen-Martenson, & Williams, 1994; Perry et al., 1996). The last two performance objectives acknowledge the need for school personnel and community involvement in implementing the changes initiated by the students. Without their support, the students' work could not succeed.

Determinants

Social cognitive theory was used to identify the determinants and develop the intervention components, which were designed to decrease alcohol use and related problems among adolescents through strategies to encourage adolescents not to drink and to reduce access to alcohol (Bandura, 1977, 1986; Baranowski, Perry, & Parcel, 1997; Jessor & Jessor, 1977; Perry & Jessor, 1985). Personal and external determinants were specified at both the organizational and community levels. The personal determinants were based on their ability to impact the chosen environmental conditions. Determinants were similar for the community level and organizational level.

At the community level, personal determinants included community members' knowledge about adolescent alcohol use in their community and about the process for changing community norms. Community members' knowledge about policies and ordinances was also identified as an important determinant. Important aspects of the process of community and citizen involvement are community ownership and empowerment (Rissel et al., 1996). Increasing these specific types of knowledge, it was hypothesized, would lead to an increase in community efficacy (empowerment) and would thus stimulate community action.

External determinants included social support from the community, opportunities to be involved in decision making, enforcement, and community norms (Perry & Jessor, 1985). The following actions were deemed important: mobilizing social support from the community, including media, merchants, law enforcement, parents, and schools; developing opportunities for adolescents to be involved in decision making and to be alcohol-free; enforcing existing or new laws that limit youth access to alcohol; and establishing community norms that set standards and behaviors that promote not giving or supplying alcohol to youth. Implementing alcohol-related policies and ordinances are a way to shift normative behavior within the community to promote a norm of no alcohol use by minors (Wagenaar & Perry, 1994).

At the organizational level, personal determinants of the students' ability to be involved with reviewing, revising, and enforcing school policies that would reduce students' alcohol use included not only self-efficacy to create change but also knowledge of school and community procedures. Again, because students were not traditionally part of policy formation or enforcement, a focus on self-efficacy and knowledge was particularly important. External determinants at the organizational level included social support from peers, school, family, and community; opportunities to be involved in decision making and to be alcohol-free; reinforcement of teen activities; and available resources. Students usually were not given the support, opportunities, or resources to be involved in addressing the issues that affect them. Focusing on these determinants could change the dynamic and improve the environmental conditions impacting alcohol use.

Key determinants of school personnel's management of school policies included self-efficacy to enforce policies, and knowledge about students' perspectives. External determinants of school personnel's management of school policies included social pressure and social support regarding enforcement of the policies created to reduce students' alcohol use while involved in school activities or during school-sponsored events. Community involvement in reducing adolescent alcohol use during prom, homecoming, and graduation was influenced by the knowledge of the environmental factors that contribute to adolescent alcohol use and of approaches to address those factors, by social support and social pressure to implement policies that would prevent teens from accessing alcohol, and by community efficacy.

Population Differentiation

The organizing process is a critical aspect of health action and is a kind of "glue" that maintains citizen interest, nourishes participation in the process and programs, and encourages support for long-term maintenance of successful intervention efforts (Bracht, 1999). The nature of an environmental intervention necessitates that the entire community be viewed as the target population, but various subgroups constitute critical aspects of the community that must be considered part of the population for the intervention itself.

The population differentiation for the Intervention Map was based on environmental levels. At the community level, we involved distinct sectors of the community, and at the organizational level, we addressed the school community, which included students, parents, and school personnel. Although there were different sectors (such as business and law enforcement) in each community, the determinants were consistent across groups. Therefore, one set of learning and change objectives was developed for the community organizing component and one for the youth development component. Differentiation was important in the development of the intervention to address the different subgroups of the community. These we addressed during the design and implementation of the program.

Matrices of Proximal Program Objectives

The proximal program objectives were the most immediate targets for change by the intervention and included learning and change objectives at both the community and organizational levels. The learning objectives were designed to address individual and community knowledge and efficacy important in supporting and initiating environmental change. The change objectives were designed to engage key community groups, students, and school personnel in the change process.

See Table 12.1 for a description of the proximal program objectives used to develop the community organizing intervention. See Table 12.2 for the youth

Table 12.1
Matrix of Proximal Program Objectives for the Community Level (Community Organizing) (Sample Cells)

	PERSONAL DETERMINANTS			EXTERNAL DETERMINANTS		
PERFORMANCE OBJECTIVES	Community efficacy	Knowledge	Social Support	Reinforcement	Enforcement	Community norms
Community members and organizers will increase the capacity of the community to address underage alcohol access and use	Express confidence to influence law enforcement, merchants, and policy makers in the community	Identify media advocacy and tactics	Build a base of support for implementing community alcohol prevention initiatives			There are norms or standards of behavior in the community (positive and negative) that are related to alcohol use and teens
	Express confidence to address underage access and teen alcohol use	Identify factors in the environment associated with alcohol use and teens	Identify "self-interest" of community members to increase involvement and participation in prevention initiatives			
Community members and organizers will establish resources to use in the organizing process	Express confidence to make changes to alcohol policies or ordinances	Identify sources of data about teens and alcohol use, and access to alcohol	Key community organizations and media are engaged in supporting alcohol access policies and ordinances			
		Identify models of alcohol access activities from other communities				
Community members and organizers will reduce number of commercial sources	Express confidence about reducing teen access to alcohol	Recognize the salience and importance of law enforcement measures (compliance checks) to reduce youth access to alcohol	Initiate law enforcement measures to elicit community support		Merchants are held accountable for violating alcohol-related laws	
Community members wil persuade merchants to comply with alcohol laws (check age, ID, recognize fake ID)						

(continued)

Table 12.1
Matrix of Proximal Program Objectives for the Community Level (Community Organizing) (Sample Cells) *(continued)*

PERFORMANCE OBJECTIVES	PERSONAL DETERMINANTS			EXTERNAL DETERMINANTS			
	Community efficacy	Knowledge	Social Support	Reinforcement	Enforcement	Community norms	
Policymakers and city government will increase and strengthen community policies to reduce youth access	Express confidence in being able to write and implement alcohol policies or ordinances	Identify steps in passing an ordinance	Policymakers support community initiatives	Community supports policymakers' efforts to pass policies to reduce access to alcohol		Establish alcohol-related policy or ordinance to the city council or policymakers	
Police and owners of retail stores will enforce policies and laws regarding underage drinking	Express confidence that the community can consistently enforce the laws Express confidence that access measures can reduce youth access to alcohol	Identify appropriate community enforcement measures	Enforcement measures are visible to the community	Results of laws, policies, and ordinances that reduce youth access to alcohol are shared with owners and police	Laws are enforced	Shift importance to enforcing policies as opposed to not enforcing policies	

Table 12.2
Matrix of Proximal Program Objectives for the Organizational Level (Youth Development) (Sample Cells)

PERFORMANCE OBJECTIVES	PERSONAL DETERMINANTS			EXTERNAL DETERMINANTS			
	Self-efficacy/ community efficacy	Knowledge	Social support/pressure	Reinforcement	Opportunities	Resources	
Students will increase school personnel's awareness of need to change policies	Students express confidence about educating others and shifting the focus of the debate to policy	Students identify environmental factors that contribute to adolescent alcohol use	An adult liaison will assist students with their tasks A core group of students will work together to support student efforts			An adult liaison is available to assist and advocate for students who are working on changing school policies	
Students review and revise school policies with school administrators	Students will feel confident to meet with school personnel and voice their opinions	Students identify options for revising school policies	An adult liaison will assist students with their tasks A core group of students will work together to support student efforts	School personnel acknowledge students' concerns about the school's alcohol policies	School administrators will invite students to participate in policy review and revisions and in enforcement plan development	An adult liaison is available to assist and advocate for students who are working on changing school policies	
Students will establish an enforcement plan with school administrators	Students express confidence about working with school personnel to create an enforcement plan	Students will identify enforcement options available for reducing adolescent alcohol use School personnel identify and acknowledge the negative consequences (perceptions, alcohol use) of not consistently enforcing the policies	School personnel listen to students and act on their suggestions	School personnel acknowledge students' concerns about the school's enforcement	School administrators invite students to participate in policy review and revisions and in enforcement plan development	An adult liaison is available to assist and advocate for students who are working on an enforcement plan	

(continued)

Table 12.2
Matrix of Proximal Program Objectives for the Organizational Level (Youth Development) *(continued)*

PERFORMANCE OBJECTIVES	PERSONAL DETERMINANTS			EXTERNAL DETERMINANTS			
	Self-efficacy/ community efficacy	Knowledge	Social support/pressure	Reinforcement	Opportunities	Resources	
Students will inform school and community of policy change	Students express confidence about presenting information to students, parents, and school staff Students feel confident that the policy changes will be acceptable to their peers	Students demonstrate how to prepare and present information to the school community	School personnel encourage students to plan and present information to others	Community and school recognition for student projects	School and community groups invite students to present information regarding policy changes and procedures in classrooms and at parent, staff, or community meetings	Resources will be available for an adult liaison to assist and advocate for students who are working on changing school policies	
School personnel enforce school policies	School personnel will feel confident that they can consistently enforce the rules		Parents, community members, and students support enforcement of the policies Parents, community members, and students advocate for school policies to be enforced				

Table 12.2
(continued)

PERFORMANCE OBJECTIVES	PERSONAL DETERMINANTS			EXTERNAL DETERMINANTS		
	Self-efficacy/ community efficacy	Knowledge	Social support/pressure	Reinforcement	Opportunities	Resources
Community groups revise policies and norms	Community groups, businesses, and parents believe that they can revise policies and norms that allow alcohol use during prom, homecoming, and graduation	Community members describe community policies and norms that restrict alcohol use during prom, homecoming, and graduation Community members explain policy options for reducing adolescent alcohol use during prom, homecoming, and graduation	Community members support changes in policies and norms that allow alcohol use during prom, homecoming, and graduation			

Intervention Mapping Step 1: Matrices of Proximal Program Objectives development objectives. These tables delineate the specific learning and change objectives for each of the major determinants.

INTERVENTION MAPPING STEP 2: THEORETICAL METHODS AND PRACTICAL STRATEGIES

Community Organizing Intervention

Four methods were utilized in the community organizing intervention during Phase II: (a) adoption of a direct action community organizing model; skills development of the community organizer and community action teams; (b) media advocacy; (c) policy and ordinance implementation; and (d) policy enforcement. These methods, delineated from previous research, have been found to be important in effecting change in the community environment (Wagenaar & Perry, 1994). Normative change within communities takes place when a shift occurs in the formal and informal rules that govern behavior. The shift applies not only to specific individuals but also to expectations governing behavior for the entire system or subsystem within which it occurs (Bracht, 1999). Community organizing, a way of eliciting large-scale social support, is a critical vehicle for shifting norms, in this case, to discourage availability of alcohol to underage youth. Building social support was critical, then, for engaging community members in the process and motivating them to continue to initiate change.

A direct action community organizing model supports the belief that a commitment to the democratic precept by large numbers of people can alter the typical balance of power held by the elite (Hanna & Robinson, 1994). The community organizing process itself, then, was key to the ability of the Project Northland action team to effect changes in communities' alcohol-related policies and ordinances as delineated by the performance objectives. Table 12.3 includes an overview of both the methods and the accompanying strategies that were developed to achieve the community organizing component's learning and change objectives.

Opportunities needed to be created to support the changes that were sought. For example, alcohol merchants within the community had to be able to provide training opportunities for their employees to increase compliance with the minimum age-of-sale laws. Limiting a teen's access to alcohol included creating barriers to young people's drinking by strengthening public policies and ordinances. Increased availability has been associated with increased alcohol consumption and related problems (Webb et al., 1997). The availability of alcohol directly affects the opportunities to drink and is also part of the environment that shapes normative expectations about appropriate alcohol consumption (Wagenaar & Perry, 1994).

To be effective, alcohol policies needed to be rigorously *enforced,* which was more likely to occur with a strong public consensus (Jeffery et al., 1990; Room, 1984). Education was also key to sustaining policy achievements. Citizens and

Table 12.3
Methods and Strategies for Community Organizing

METHOD	STRATEGIES
Community organizing and skill development	Form adult action teams in the community with a community organizer to support the group
	Train action team members in public participation, action strategies, advocacy, and policy implementation
	Use adult action teams to plan initiatives and activities to address issue of access
Media advocacy	Involve media to increase visibility of alcohol access issues and environmental strategy options in the community
	Provide media advocacy training for action team members
Policy or ordinance implementation	Use community organizing to shift power differential in community (groundwork for ordinance development)
	Provide training on alcohol policies and ordinances
	Provide responsible beverage service training and merchant training
Policy enforcement	Conduct educational compliance checks
	Conduct compliance checks with penalties
	Develop enforcement plan with law enforcement

government officials needed to be aware of new policies, and the law enforcement agencies needed to be responsible for their enforcement (Webb et al., 1997).

Youth Development Component

The methods used for the youth development component were based primarily on social cognitive theory. Six methods were selected from which to guide the development of program strategies: youth skills development, incentives, modeling, opportunities, peer participation, and creating norms for nonuse. These methods have the potential of engaging young people in prevention activities and creating the opportunities that young people need to socialize with peers and adults, develop skills that are relevant now and in the future, contribute to the community, belong to a valued group, and feel competent (Carnegie Council on Adolescent Development, 1992). Components that were important for effective prevention programs included a focus on changing norms, interaction among peers, and social skills training (Drug Strategies, 1996; Dusenbury & Falco, 1995). Table 12.4 includes an overview of both the methods and the accompanying strategies that were developed to achieve the youth development component's learning and change objectives.

Table 12.4
Methods and Strategies for Youth Development

METHOD	STRATEGIES
Youth development and skill development	Form youth action teams in the schools with an adult liaison to support the group
	Train students in public participation and action strategies
	Use youth action teams to plan projects and activities to address concerns
Incentives	Increase positive recognition of teens in the community
Modeling	Expose students to others their age who have taken action in their communities
Opportunities	Establish a grant-making system for students to receive funds for projects
Peer participation	Recruit students for youth action teams
	Create student-led teams
Norms for nonuse	Help students plan alcohol-free events and activities

INTERVENTION MAPPING STEP 3: PROGRAM DESIGN

Project Northland incorporated both intrapersonal (demand) factors and socioenvironmental (supply) factors into the interventions. However, there was a change in primary emphasis from intrapersonal factors during Phase I (1991–1994), when the cohort was in 6th to 8th grades, to socioenvironmental factors in Phase II (1996–1998), when the cohort was in 11th and 12th grades. The first phase of Project Northland was designed to address relevant intrapersonal and interpersonal factors that would lead a young person to have less of a desire (or "demand") to drink alcohol. Those factors included changing the meanings that young people place on alcohol, increasing teens' self-efficacy to refuse alcohol, and increasing communication around alcohol issues at home, school, and in the community (Perry, Williams, et al., 1993; Perry et al., 1996; Williams & Perry, 1998). Those factors were developmentally relevant and appropriate to address in interventions designed for young teens.

Although intrapersonal and interpersonal factors were still incorporated into the Project Northland interventions during Phase II, the emphasis of the interventions turned to strategies that were designed to reduce the supply of alcohol to teens. The focus was on changing community norms concerning the acceptability of underage drinking and on increasing community efficacy. This approach was thought to be more effective, because changing the environment relied less on changing the individual behavior of teens (many of whom had begun drinking) and more on changing the opportunities they had to obtain alcohol and to drink. In Phase II, then, changing practices of whole communities appeared to be most efficacious for this age group. Implementing policies and ordinances to reduce youth access to alcohol were the primary strategies to create those changes.

Community Program: Direct Action Community Organizing

Direct action community organizing was a systematic process for mobilizing community members to support, initiate, and establish policies to reduce youth access to alcohol. The key components that were vital to the organizing process were citizen participation, mobilizing and collective power, defining of self-interests, issue identification, relationships relevant to initiating and supporting policy change, and advocacy tactics with the media. The four primary stages to the community organizing were (a) gathering information; (b) recruiting and forming teams; (c) building team development and community awareness; and (d) establishing and enforcing policies.

Community organizers (local field directors) needed to have the experience and skill to work with diverse groups and coalitions and were the key facilitators of the organizing process. They had a basic understanding of community change processes and brought proven management experience to the local field effort. Good facilitation and listening skills were also important (Bracht, 1999). Training the organizers to facilitate the organizing process was the first step in implementing the direct action model. The community organizers received six core training sessions during Phase II. The primary topics covered were one-on-one interviews, community mobilizing, building a campaign around youth access initiatives, action team building, thinking strategically and politically, and policies and ordinances.

A significant part of the training was to help the organizers develop the skill to conduct one-on-one interviews. The model of direct action organizing utilizes this one-on-one approach during the first stage as a means of engaging the community in the process. The organizers interviewed from 40 to 100 citizens who represented a broad spectrum of the community (faith organizations, businesses, liquor merchants, medical organizations, educational organizations, etc.) and who had an interest in the prevention of adolescent alcohol use. These interviews were designed to build a broad base, encourage recognition of self-interest of the interviewees, and identify the community's social, economic, and political power structures.

The second stage of the organizing process involved the recruitment and formation of community action teams. The action teams played an important role in mobilizing the community to facilitate change in alcohol policies and ordinances. Team members were recruited based on interest in reducing underage access to alcohol, leadership ability, access to resources, and representation of a particular community sector. Eleven action teams, ranging from 5 to 12 members, were formed in Project Northland communities. Each team was facilitated and supported by the community organizer. Regional training sessions were held to support the work of the action teams and provide them with skills in public participation strategies, action strategies, advocacy, and policy implementation.

A community at large can be collectively mobilized to support initiatives. Thus, the community intervention component during Phase II relied heavily on the community organizing model to facilitate community-level change. The process of community organizing, that is, involving various key individuals and subgroups, was critical to the outcome of the project.

During the third stage, action teams were facilitated to develop a sense of ownership. A primary strategy during this stage was mobilizing the community through action team member presentations and encouraging team members to talk to members in the community utilizing the one-on-one method. Action teams needed to develop a sense of identity within the community and work to engage other community members in the process.

During the final stage of community organizing, teams were encouraged to develop action plans that indicated the methods and strategies they would use to decrease commercial availability in liquor stores, bars, and convenience stores. The community organizing provided the groundwork for shifting the power differential in the community and, thus, for ordinance and policy development and implementation. Teams received training on policy development and were provided with a menu of potential actions. The purpose of these training sessions was to foster community adoption of institutional or policy solutions to underage drinking rather than to focus on educational strategies directed at the adolescents.

During their first training, action teams were presented with a framework to apply to the strategies they adopted to ensure that they were pursuing initiatives that would effect the community environment. The framework consisted of three questions: How and where do high school students obtain alcohol? What barriers can communities create to keep high school students from obtaining alcohol? and How will my community know if changes take place at the community level? Action teams were continuously challenged to measure their initiatives against the following framework: "Changes target groups, not individuals; Changes are targeted to institutions, businesses, whole communities; Changes are long-term solutions and will benefit high school students now and in the future."

Training was also extended into community institutions. Each of the communities offered responsible beverage service training for bartenders, and several communities offered training for managers of bars and liquor stores including specific policy options they could implement within their stores to reduce youth access to alcohol. Engaging merchants in ownership of this issue promotes community efficacy and potential support for future initiatives around youth access.

There were a variety of strategies utilized during the final stage to encourage enforcement of existing policies and to encourage the adoption of new policies. Educational compliance checks (not for legal prosecution) of age-of-sale laws, coordinated with local law enforcement, were conducted in many of the intervention communities to inform the community and local alcohol merchants of the ease at which underage youth could purchase alcohol. Letters were sent to offending merchants notifying them of the compliance check and the failure of their staff to enforce the age-of-sale law. Merchants were warned that compliance checks would occur again, at random.

Successive compliance checks were conducted with penalties attached. The community action teams utilized both educational checks and those for prosecution as evidence for lack of enforcement of existing laws. This evidence was leveraged with city councils to initiate the adoption of community-wide compliance check ordinances and responsible beverage service training as well as administrative penalties for businesses that failed to comply with the age-of-sale law.

Community Program: Media Advocacy

The media have an important role in defining a health agenda within a community. Media are important in achieving the goals of public health, first, because they raise the public profile of issues in bringing them to the attention of the community. Second, they confer importance and legitimacy to the issues as relevant to community concerns. Third, they provide the frameworks of meaning within which to understand the issues (effective preventive actions, the need for behavioral norms, the need for public policy, etc.). Fourth, the media are capable of widespread public dissemination of, and exposure to, public health information (Bracht, 1999; Wallack, Dorfman, Jernigan, & Themba, 1993).

Involving media to increase the visibility of the issue of alcohol access and environmental strategy options in the community was key to supporting the community action teams' agendas. Community organizers and the action teams had media advocacy training available to them and were also provided with media support from the university in the form of written articles and a press package to give to their local media (newspapers). Radio and television were not utilized in the Phase II intervention because they might have led to contamination between intervention and control communities.

Youth Action Teams and Skill Development

The core strategy chosen to accomplish the youth development program's objectives was the formation of youth action teams in each of the Project Northland schools. These teams consisted of students who voluntarily participated in training sessions and project planning to reduce teenage alcohol use in their community. An adult coordinator was hired to work with each youth action team. The role of these coordinators was to recruit students and guide them through the process of learning about environmental conditions that contribute to alcohol use in their community and translating that knowledge into community action projects that would address those conditions.

Youth action team training sessions were conducted during both years of the Phase II intervention. Students from all Project Northland schools gathered at retreat centers for a day-long session. Students from all schools were brought together to share their experiences and ideas, to motivate each other to take action in their community, and to learn the skills needed to address environmental conditions. Educational topics included community-action (environmental change) approaches to alcohol-use prevention, use of the media, action plans and timelines, and motivations to reduce teenage alcohol use. The training sessions focused on increasing knowledge about the environmental factors, on options for revising school policies, on enforcement options, and on building students' confidence to work on this issue.

The adult coordinators met with youth action teams upon their return to the communities to identify the environmental conditions that contributed to alcohol use in each team's specific community. A practical manual was developed to help the youth action teams with this process. Each team then explored various strategies to address these conditions. Students were given the opportunity to choose projects that addressed a problem related to high school students' alcohol use and that changed something in the community or school environment. Although youth action teams implemented a variety of projects, only those that chose to focus on the school environment are covered so as to limit the breadth of this chapter.

After testing their project ideas for feasibility, youth action teams created action plans, which included steps that needed to be taken to change their school's policies. These steps included meeting with school personnel; sharing their opinions and ideas; drafting policy changes and enforcement procedures; finalizing changes; informing students, parents, and school community about the changes; and participating in enforcement of the policies.

The adult coordinator and university staff provided ongoing support for the youth action teams. A staff member visited each community at least once to help youth action teams identify feasible projects. Adult coordinators provided resource materials and ongoing communication to keep their action team on track and working on environmental approaches.

An important part of the Project Northland youth development component was to increase positive recognition of teens in the community. The media served as the main vehicle to accomplish this recognition. Youth action teams were encouraged to submit press releases, and university staff submitted several releases with pictures of the students at the youth action team training sessions. One press release included recommendations for their communities about how they could reduce teenage alcohol use. The students developed these recommendations at one of the training sessions. The training sessions also served as incentives for student participation because they were held during the school day and the coordinators provided food at most meetings. Students were also given the opportunity to plan alcohol-free social activities for their peers.

The training sessions exposed students to peers who had taken action in their communities. Youth speakers were invited to share stories about their involvement with tobacco use prevention, community development, and increasing opportunities for youth. The formation of youth action teams served as a vehicle for modeling as well. Students were allowed to join a team at any point during the two years of the intervention. Positive recognition of students and their activities helped recruit additional students to the action teams. Project Northland students also served as role models for students in lower grades by speaking in classrooms and at assemblies and by attending Project Northland training sessions and activities.

The formation of the youth action teams and the hiring of an adult coordinator provided the opportunity for students to be involved in reducing alcohol use in their community. The monetary support and resources that were provided by the research grant allowed students who were interested in this issue to take an active role. The adult liaisons also connected students with school personnel so they could express their concern about school policies. The school personnel benefited from these meetings as well because they recognized that they had student support for the new policies.

Youth action teams were given the opportunity to apply for minigrants to help implement their projects. This system was chosen to teach students about grant writing, timelines, and budgeting. On the grant application they were also asked to demonstrate collaborative efforts with community organizations. These efforts increased the students' ownership, exposure, and positive recognition as well.

The youth action teams were designed to be led by the students. The adult coordinator's role was to guide the students and support their activities. Students were given parameters in which to choose their projects, but without peer leadership, they would not have been as likely to participate. Many youth action teams elected spokespeople or leaders to conduct their meetings, to meet with school personnel and community members, and to present information to peers, school, and community groups.

Prom, homecoming, and graduation are key times of the year when students drink alcohol and community members often turn the other way. The youth development component wanted to address this critical issue because of the potential harm that can result in students' consuming large amounts of alcohol with implied consent from their parents and communities. The risks come from both the actual consumption and the message that is sent to the students.

Youth action teams were encouraged to identify important environmental conditions related to prom, homecoming, or graduation and to plan an event or a project that would address that condition. Minigrants were given for projects such as homecoming tailgate parties, postprom parties, preprom dinners, and graduation celebrations (Komro et al., 1996). The policies that were developed for these events explicitly stated the procedures for attending and what actions would be taken if a student was caught drinking. A major element to the success of these events was community support. Students proved that they were committed to working on the issue and educated community groups about the need for their involvement in addressing this problem. Community members, impressed with the students' initiative in planning these events on their own, donated items such as door prizes and food, gave volunteer support, and stimulated media coverage. Many of these events will now become annual celebrations because of the normative shift from one successful year.

INTERVENTION MAPPING STEP 4: ADOPTION AND IMPLEMENTATION

Linkage System

Project Northland received commitments from each of the school districts that were involved in the program prior to program implementation. This prior commitment, as well as each of the schools' past involvement with Project Northland during Phase I of the intervention, contributed to smooth program adoption and implementation. Positive experiences and the resulting outcomes of Phase I were strong influences for continued program adoption and implementation.

Past experience from Phase I demonstrated the need for several factors to successfully implement the community component. Building linkages between the school, community, parents, and students was critical for the success of this multifaceted project. The community organizers filled an important need by serving as the liaison between the university staff and the community. Given the distance between the university and the Project Northland communities (two to five hours), it was critical to have field staff who could form the community action teams and implement the policy strategies.

Policy Change Implementation Determinants and Strategies

A key factor that needed to be addressed was the communities' resistance to policy-level change. Policy change can be controversial and therefore risky, especially in smaller communities. As was mentioned, adolescent alcohol use is a widely accepted behavior, and most previous strategies focused on the individual behavior of the students. Shifting the focus to the community and adults had to be carefully considered. Several strategies were implemented to address this concern: keep the focus on adolescents and their safety and well-being; start with enforcement of existing policies; provide resources and support; and provide training to community members and merchants.

To ensure implementation of the youth development component, adult coordinators were hired to work with each youth action team. This step was important because the adults were needed to advocate for the students and to guide them through the process. The incentives—such as training held during classtime, food, and media coverage—addressed some of the other obstacles that arise when students are involved in a project. Given the voluntary nature of the program, it was critical to provide incentives to keep students interested and involved. Adult coordinators had to be flexible and supportive. Support from school personnel was also important in order to release students from class for training sessions and meetings, hold events on school grounds, and include students in shaping school policies.

Keeping the community informed of Project Northland activities was also an important part of both components. The media was the main tool used for this communication; monthly articles were submitted to each local newspaper.

Community action teams and youth were encouraged to submit news releases to announce their activities and accomplishments.

INTERVENTION MAPPING STEP 5: EVALUATION

Effect Evaluation

Evaluation of Phase II of Project Northland was notably complex, given the size of the project and its focus on both personal and environmental changes (Komro et al., in press). The first level of evaluation was to assess the effects of the intervention. Because the project was developed with the ultimate goal of reducing adolescent alcohol use, this assessment was done through a self-administered questionnaire with the Project Northland cohort members at the end of their 10th, 11th, and 12th grades. This questionnaire assessed students' use of alcohol—including quantity, frequency, and recency of use—as well as alcohol-related problems. Because of the design of the study, which included randomized education and reference communities, differences between groups on measures of these behaviors indicated the effect of the intervention.

The next level of evaluation focused on the determinants of change in high school students' alcohol use, as discussed in this chapter. This evaluation included measures of community and peer norms, community and personal efficacy, underage access to alcohol, opportunities to drink, and enforcement of community policies. These factors were measured by questions on the self-administered student survey and by telephone surveys of the cohort's parents, young adults (ages 18 to 24), high school principals, community leaders, police, and alcohol beverage merchants. These telephone surveys were conducted when the cohort was in the 10th grade and again after they graduated from high school in 1998. These surveys attempted to assess each group's perceptions of norms, efficacy, access, enforcement, and opportunities, so that the convergence of evidence would indicate how and with whom the intervention had been effective. A final assessment of underage access to alcohol was done by implementing alcohol purchase attempts (by young-looking 21-year-olds without age identification) in all the alcohol outlets in the Project Northland education and reference communities. Examination of the determinants will allow mediation analyses to assess how the intervention was or wasn't effective in reducing adolescent alcohol use.

Process Evaluation

Process evaluation was conducted on all the components of the Phase II intervention. For community organizing, this evaluation included organizers' assessment of their training sessions, computerized records of each community contact, action team minutes and attendance records, written assessments of community events and action team participation, city council meeting minutes, monthly status reports by organizers, and a survey of the organizers at the end of the intervention. For the youth development component, process evaluation consisted of students' assessments of their training sessions, the action team coordinators' assessments of their training sessions, project reports, monthly status reports, site visit reports, and a survey of the coordinators at the end of the intervention. Process data will provide information on exposure, compliance, and fidelity to the intervention components (Perry et al., 1997).

SUMMARY

Project Northland's Phase II project focused on change in the environmental context surrounding the drinking behavior of older adolescents. This chapter presents two items of particular note. One is that the chapter is a good example of an intervention that focuses on community and organizational-level change. The other is that this intervention empowered the at-risk group itself to make changes in circumstances important to the lives and health of its members. Furthermore, the intervention is a good example of mixing social cognitive theory concepts with community organization and group empowerment approaches.

REFERENCES

Adger, H., Jr. (1991). Problems of alcohol and other drug use and abuse in adolescents. *Journal of Adolescent Health, 12*(8), 606–613.

Bandura, A. (1977). *Social learning theory.* Englewood Cliffs, NJ: Prentice Hall.

Bandura, A. (1986). *Social foundations of thought and action: A social cognitive theory.* Englewood Cliffs, NJ: Prentice Hall.

Baranowski T., Perry, C. L., & Parcel, G. S. (1997). How individuals, environments, and health behavior interact: Social cognitive theory. In K. Glanz, F. M. Lewis, & B. K. Rimer (Eds.), *Health behavior and health education: Theory, research, and practice* (2nd ed., pp. 153–178). San Francisco: Jossey-Bass.

Bracht, N. (Ed.). (1999). *Health promotion at the community level 2: New advances.* Thousand Oaks, CA: Sage.

Brent, D. A., Perper, J. A., & Allman, C. J. (1987). Alcohol, firearms, and suicide among youth: Temporal trends in Allegheny County, Pennsylvania, 1960–1983. *Journal of the American Medical Association, 257*(24), 3369–3372.

Caces, M. F., Stinson, F. S., & Elliott, S. D. (1991). *U.S. alcohol epidemiologic data reference manual: Vol. 3. County alcohol problem indicators, 1979–1985* (3rd ed.) (DHHS Publication No. ADM 91-1740). Rockville, MD: National Institute on Alcohol Abuse and Alcoholism.

Carnegie Council on Adolescent Development. (1992). *A matter of time: Risk and opportunity in the nonschool hours.* New York: Carnegie Corporation.

Drug Strategies. (1996). *Making the grade: A guide to school drug prevention programs.* Washington, DC: Author.

Dryfoos, J. (1990). *Adolescents at risk: Prevalence and prevention.* New York: Oxford University Press.

Dusenbury, L., & Falco, M. (1995). Eleven components of effective drug abuse prevention curricula. *Journal of School Health, 65*(10), 420–425.

Forster, J. L., Murray, D. M., Wolfson, M., Blaine, T. M., Wagenaar, A. C., & Hennrikus, D. J. (1998). The effects of community policies to reduce youth access to tobacco. *American Journal of Public Health, 88*(8), 1193–1198.

Gardner, S. E., Green, P. F., & Marcus, C. (Eds). (1994). *Signs of effectiveness II. Prevention alcohol, tobacco, and other drug use: A risk factor/resiliency-based approach.* Rockville, MD: Center for Substance Abuse Prevention.

Grant, B. F., & Dawson, D. A. (1997). Age at onset of alcohol use and its association with DSM-IV alcohol abuse and dependence: Results from the National Longitudinal Alcohol Epidemiologic Survey. *Journal of Substance Abuse, 9,* 103–110.

Greenfield, T. (1996, July). *Consumption and risk patterns: Who buys and who pays?* Paper presented at the Winter School in the Sun, Brisbane, Australia.

Hanna, M. G., & Robinson, B. (1994). *Strategies for community empowerment.* Lewiston, NY: Edwin Mellen.

Jeffery, R. W., Forster, J. L., Schmid, T. L., McBride, C. M., Rooney, B. L., & Pirie, P. L. (1990). Community attitudes toward public policies to control alcohol, tobacco, and high-fat food consumption. *American Journal of Preventive Medicine, 6*(1), 12–19.

Jessor, R., & Jessor, S. (1977). *Problem behavior and psychosocial development.* New York: Academic Press.

Johnston, L. D., O'Malley, P. M., & Bachman, J. G. (1999). *National survey results on drug use from the Monitoring the Future study, 1975–1998.* Rockville, MD: U.S. Department of Health and Human Services, Public Health Service.

Kandel, D., & Yamaguchi, K. (1993). From beer to crack: Developmental patterns of drug involvement. *American Journal of Public Health, 83*(6), 851–855.

Komro, K. A., Perry, C. L., Murray, D., Veblen-Mortenson, S., Williams, C. L., & Anstine, P. (1996). Peer-planned social activities for preventing alcohol use among adolescents. *Journal of School Health, 66*(9), 328–334.

Komro, K. A., Perry, C. L., Veblen-Mortenson, S., & Williams, C. L. (1994). Peer participation in Project Northland: A community-wide alcohol use prevention project. *Journal of School Health, 64*(8), 318–322.

Komro, K. A., Perry, C. L., Williams, C. L., Veblen-Mortenson, S., Forster, J., Munson, K., Farbakhsh, K., Lachter, R. B., & Pratt, L. (in press). Research and evaluation design of a community-wide program to reduce adolescent alcohol use: Project Northland Phase II. In S. Casswell (Ed.), *1998 Kettil Bruun Society Thematic Meeting: Fourth Symposium on Community Action Research and the Prevention of Alcohol and Other Drug Problems.* Wellington, New Zealand: Alcoholic Advisory Council.

Kusserow, R. (1991). *Youth and alcohol: A national survey—Drinking habits, access, attitudes, and knowledge* (OEI Publication No. OEI-09-91-00652). Washington, DC: U.S. Department of Health and Human Services, Office of Inspector General.

National Highway Traffic Safety Administration. (1990). *Alcohol and highway safety 1989: A review of the state of knowledge.* Washington, DC: U.S. Department of Transportation.

National Institute on Alcohol Abuse and Alcoholism. (1994). *Eighth special report to the U.S. Congress on alcohol and health* (NIH Publication No. 94-3699). Washington, DC: U.S. Department of Health and Human Services.

Perry, C. L. (1999). *Creating health behavior change: How to develop community-wide programs for youth* (Developmental Clinical Psychology and Psychiatry No. 43). Thousand Oaks, CA: Sage.

Perry, C. L., & Jessor, R. (1985). The concept of health promotion and the prevention of adolescent drug abuse. *Health Education Quarterly, 12*(2), 169–184.

Perry, C. L., Kelder, S. H., & Komro, K. (1993). The social world of adolescents: Family, peers, schools, and community. In S. G. Millstein, A. C. Petersen, & E. O. Nightingale (Eds.), *Promoting the health of adolescents: New directions for the twenty-first century* (pp. 73–96). New York: Oxford University Press.

Perry, C. L., Sellers, D., Johnson, C., Pedersen, S., Bachman, K., Parcel, G., Stone, E., Luepker, R. V., Wu, M., Nader, P., & Cook, K. W. (1997). The Child and Adolescent Trial for Cardiovascular Health (CATCH): Intervention, implementation, and feasibility for elementary schools in the U.S. *Health Education and Behavior, 24*(6), 716–735.

Perry, C. L., Williams, C. L., Forster, J. L., Wolfson, M., Wagenaar, A. C., Finnegan, J. R., McGovern, P. G., Veblen-Mortenson, S., Komro, K. A., & Anstine, P. S. (1993). Background, conceptualization, and design of a community-wide research program on adolescent alcohol use: Project Northland. *Health Education Research: Theory and Practice, 8*(1), 125–136.

Perry, C. L., Williams, C. L., Veblen-Mortenson, S., Toomey, T., Komro, K., Anstine, P. S., McGovern, P., Finnegan, J. R., Forster, J. L., Wagenaar, A. C., & Wolfson, M. (1996). Outcomes of a community-wide alcohol use prevention program during early adolescence: Project Northland. *American Journal of Public Health, 86*(7), 956–965.

Rissel, C., Perry, C., Wagenaar, A., Wolfson, M., Finnegan, J., & Komro, K. (1996). Empowerment, alcohol, 8th grade students, and health promotion. *Journal of Alcohol and Drug Education, 41*(2), 105–119.

Room, R. (1984). Alcohol control and public health. *Annual Review of Public Health, 5,* 293–317.

Roski, J., Perry, C. L., McGovern, P. G., Williams, C. L., Farbakhsh, K., & Veblen-Mortenson, S. (1997). School and community influences on adolescent alcohol and drug use. *Health Education Research: Theory and Practice, 12*(2), 255–266.

Semlitz, L., & Gold, M. S. (1986). Adolescent drug abuse: Diagnosis, treatment, and prevention. *Psychiatric Clinics of North America, 9,* 455–473.

Trends in drug and alcohol use by youth in the USA. (1993, July–Sept.). *Statistical Bulletin, 74,* 19–27.

Wagenaar, A. C., & Perry, C. L. (1994). Community strategies for the reduction of youth drinking: Theory and application. *Journal of Research on Adolescence, 4*(2), 319–345.

Wallack, L., Dorfman, L., Jernigan, D., & Themba, M. (1993). *Media advocacy and public health: Power for prevention.* Thousand Oaks, CA: Sage.

Webb, R. J., Toomey, T. L., Short, B., Murray, D. M., Wagenaar, A., & Wolfson, M. (1997). Relationships among alcohol availability, drinking location, alcohol consumption, and drinking problems in adolescents. *Substance Use and Misuse, 32*(10), 1261–1285.

Williams, C. L., & Perry, C. L. (1998). Design and implementation of parent programs for a community-wide adolescent alcohol use prevention program. *Journal of Prevention and Intervention in the Community, 17*(2), 65–80.

CHAPTER 13

Theory and Context in Project PANDA: A Program to Help Postpartum Women Stay Off Cigarettes

Patricia Dolan Mullen, Carlo C. DiClemente, and L. Kay Bartholomew

READER OBJECTIVES

- Be better able to apply theory and evidence to define the intervention focus
- Develop and use design documents to communicate message intent
- Use target group context to improve intervention salience

Just as a life-threatening disease often sparks modification of health-related behaviors, pregnancy also motivates lifestyle changes by women and their partners (Johnson, McCarter, & Ferencz, 1987; Kruse, LeFevre, & Zweig, 1986). Although most changes are appropriate only for the duration of the pregnancy, some, such as smoking cessation, would confer health benefits to the woman and her child if they were maintained. Further, although pregnancy is often portrayed in the media through idealized images of happiness and family harmony, it is a highly salient experience for most women, and it has predictable stages and concerns. Fathers who are in a relationship with the woman are typically "on board" a little later, but also undergo an intense and broadly recognizable experience during the pregnancy and period immediately after the birth. An estimated one third of smokers quit sometime during pregnancy, usually in the first trimester (Floyd,

---

Project PANDA was funded by the National Cancer Institute (CA-27821 and 2R25CA57712-06).

Rimer, Giovino, Mullen, & Sullivan, 1993; Mullen, 1999; Quinn, Mullen, & Ershoff, 1991), and there have been numerous evaluations of programs to promote cessation during this time (Dolan-Mullen, Ramirez, & Groff, 1994; Mullen & Ramirez, in press). Interventions with parents who smoked had not been very effective. One study conducted in pediatrics offices about the same time as Project PANDA found a small increase in self-reported cessation by mothers who smoked, and a larger increase when the intervention was with a woman who had stopped smoking during pregnancy and whose intervention message was not to resume smoking (Wall, Severson, Andrews, Lichtenstein, & Zoref, 1995). However, at the time we developed the PANDA intervention, there had been no reports of programs to improve the rate of maintenance of cessation postpartum.

This chapter is a case study of Project PANDA (Parents and Newborns Developing and Adjusting), a program to decrease rates of return to smoking among pregnant women who have stopped smoking (DiClemente, Mullen, Pollak, Sockrider, & Stotts, 1998; Mullen, DiClemente, et al., 1999). The project is a good example of an explicit, rational approach to intervention design and is a particularly good model of the use of both theory and evidence very early in the design process to define the problem. The case also highlights the importance of understanding the context of the target groups and of designing messages to increase salience of the intervention by addressing the context in addition to the health risk. Finally, Project PANDA illustrates the successful use of detailed design documents to communicate message intent to the producers of program materials.

PERSPECTIVES IN THIS CASE

Using Theory to Define the Problem

This case provides an example of the role of reasoning with theory and evidence in the delineation of the actual problem to be solved. We discuss in detail the analysis by Mullen, later elaborated by the team, that went beyond the interpretation that the problem of women who returned to smoking after having quit during pregnancy was a problem of relapse (Marlatt & Gordon, 1985). Had these women really relapsed? Thinking of them as relapsers implies that they had intended to quit for good. But Mullen had worked with Ershoff and Quinn on a pregnancy smoking cessation trial in a health maintenance organization in Los Angeles, and when they followed up successful quitters 6 months postpartum, they heard statements from the women indicating no such resolve (Ershoff, Mullen, & Quinn, 1989; Mullen, Quinn, & Ershoff, 1990). Many of the women who returned to smoking right after the birth said they had not planned to quit for good. Virtually every woman who reported having returned to smoking added, "but I never smoke around the baby" (Mullen, Richardson, Quinn, & Ershoff, 1997). Thus, Mullen initiated the collaboration with DiClemente, co-developer of the transtheoretical model, reasoning that the model could accommodate women who might be in various stages with respect to postpartum smoking even though they had been abstinent for several months at least. The transtheoretical model encompassed relapse prevention, but it had a broader view of the process of change that allowed us to gain some evidence about the change process for these women.

Understanding the Importance of the Context

A second issue that is well explicated in this case study is the importance of the context of the pregnant women who are at risk for returning to smoking postpartum. What are the women's interests? Are they interested in changes in their bodies? changes in their relationships? babies? changes-to-come in daily schedules, jobs, and careers? creating an environment for a new baby? Is the possibility of return to cigarette smoking in this list of women's concerns? If it is, it may be only a vague concern. The PANDA development team reviewed lay and scientific literature to distill a list of the issues that may be of concern to women and their partners during the phases of pregnancy (Tables 13.1 and 13.2 give examples of these concerns). For example, at 28 weeks the couple may be participating in prepared childbirth classes together and they may begin to communicate more about the baby. Women report an upsurge in conflict with their partners (Saunders & Robins, 1987). "Nesting" also begins about this time (Joffe, 1989). Later, both the mother and father develop anxiety about the birth, with the man more focused on threats to the woman's well-being and the mother more focused on the baby (Arizmendi & Affonso, 1987).

Table 13.1
Concerns of Women and Their Partners During Pregnancy

28 WEEKS	34 WEEKS	36 WEEKS
Prepared childbirth classes: messages on labor and delivery, little on emotional or relationship transition (Imle, 1990)	Woman focuses on labor and delivery	Anxiety increases (Drake, Verhulst, & Fawcett, 1988)
	Beginning of worry about birth (about the well-being of baby; partner worries about woman's health and safety)	Physical discomfort may lessen when baby engages
"Nesting" begins for both parents (Joffe, 1989)		Focus may narrow to delivery (Joffe, 1989)
Beginning focus on woman's "bigness" (Arizmendi & Affonso, 1987)	Increase in communication between partners; increased conflict (Saunders & Robins, 1987)	Focus on time intensifies until delivery: "Haven't you had the baby yet?"
Woman feels better but anticipates having "old" body back	Poignancy about loss of couplehood	Planning for, and fantasies about, going to the hospital
Baby becomes more of a reality for partner	Partner participates in plans for birth of the baby; he is not anticipating decrease in opportunities for participation	Arranging for help with the newborn
	Motivated to learn infant caretaking skills (Bliss-Holtz, 1988)	Little information about recovery from delivery
	Physical discomforts heighten	

Table 13.2
Concerns of Women and Their Partners After the Birth

IMMEDIATELY POSTPARTUM	2 WEEKS POSTPARTUM	6 WEEKS POSTPARTUM
Woman is focused on physical recovery	Mother home alone with baby; mother thinking about whether to return to work	Feeling more competent as a mother
Sleep deprivation and possible depression	Baby is separate entity; mother and baby's health now separate	New schedule challenges: returning to work
Demand to learn many new skills	Partner may feel loss of woman	Negotiating child care
Overwhelmed and out of control	Focus of health care on baby; mother has lost supportive relationship with the obstetrician	Six-week checkup for mother
Lack of instrumental role for partner		May resume sexual intercourse
Extended family at home to "help"	First well-baby checkup	Most women who begin breastfeeding quit at this point
Attention on baby, not mother	Baby begins to have a schedule	Trauma of returning to work; emotional separation, longing, guilt (Lewis & Cooper, 1987)
Learning who infant is	Still sleep-deprived, but taking excursions out of the house	
Some movement back to old self		Return to old environment and smoking cues
Surprised at distance from old self		Second well-baby checkup
Partner may feel left out		Peak of baby's crying

Mullen and DiClemente then based the intervention on the issues of the mothers as a framework for including messages designed to promote continued abstinence. This case study is an excellent example of consideration of context, because the planning team was concerned from the very beginning of the project about how difficult it might be to get the women to attend to messages about the problem of return to smoking. However, the issue of context should actually be an important focus in all intervention development.

NEEDS ASSESSMENT

Epidemiologic Analysis

Approximately 20% of pregnant women smoke during pregnancy (U.S. Office on Smoking and Health, 1980). In 1994, more than 14 million U.S. women ages 15 to 45 years were smokers; 800,000 to one million of these women become pregnant each year. As with smoking generally, smoking during pregnancy is much more prevalent in women who are unmarried and have low income and education (Stockbauer & Land, 1991; U.S. Office on Smoking and Health).

In the industrialized world, cigarette smoking is the most powerful known determinant of fetal growth retardation, affecting 22% to 36% of all cases (Wen, Goldenberg, Cutter, Hoffman, & Cliver, 1989). The relationship between smoking and low birth weight is one of the most consistent findings in the epidemiology literature. Maternal smoking also is recognized as a significant risk factor for preterm birth (Wen et al.), sudden infant death syndrome (Malloy, Hoffman, & Peterson, 1992; Malloy, Kleinman, Land, & Schramm, 1988), spontaneous abortion (Windham, Swan, & Fenter, 1992), cleft palate/cleft lip, and mental retardation and impaired school performance (Cook, Peterson, & Moore, 1990; Lieberman, Gremy, Lang, & Cohen, 1994; U.S. Office on Smoking and Health, 1980).

It is well established that smoking increases risk for lung and heart disease, cancer, and stroke as the most serious and prevalent problems (U.S. Office on Smoking and Health, 1980, 1984a, 1984b, 1985). The prospect of hastening quitting in such a relatively young group is particularly important in light of these effects on the health of the woman herself.

Environmental tobacco smoke, or ETS, has been consistently reported to cause increased respiratory infections and risk for asthma and asthma exacerbation in children (Emerson et al., 1994; Murray & Morrison, 1989; Overpeck & Moss, 1991; Samet, Cain, & Leaderer, 1991). A study by Cuijpers, Swaen, Wesseling, Stumans, and Wouters (1995) found passive smoking (during a child's entire life) to be significantly correlated with impairments to all spirometry parameters tested, and others have argued that smoking in the child's environment is an irritant to airways and should be eliminated (Hovell et al., 1994). A study of urban children with asthma showed that exposure to environmental tobacco smoke is common; 59% of subjects' parents reported at least one smoker in the home. Additionally, at the study's baseline testing, 48% of children had a cotinine/creatinine ratio above 30 ng/mg, a level indicating significant exposure to ETS in the last 24 hours (Huss et al., 1994).

Quitting During Pregnancy and the Problem of Return to Smoking

Many smokers stop smoking early in pregnancy, either on their own or with assistance. As many as 40% of women who smoked prior to the pregnancy stop spontaneously by the time of their first visit for prenatal care (Quinn et al., 1991; Secker-Walker et al., 1995; Woodby, Windsor, Snyder, Kohler, & DiClemente, 1999). Brief counseling of 5 to 15 minutes plus pregnancy-oriented self-help materials almost doubles validated cessation over the 5% to 15% cessation rate that would have occurred with usual care after the first visit (Dolan-Mullen et al., 1994; Mullen & Ramirez, in press). Smoking cessation for pregnancy is important because of benefits to the baby. However, it is disappointing to know that 63% to 73% of mothers return to smoking within 6 months after the birth, putting the infant at risk for the effects of ETS and themselves back on the track to severe health consequences (Fingerhut, Kleinman, & Kendrick, 1990; Mullen et al., 1990; Pirie et al., 1992). Viewed as relapse, these rates are very similar to those measured for other addictive behaviors—including heroin—after the end of a treatment program (Hunt, Barnett, & Branch, 1971; see Figure 13.1).

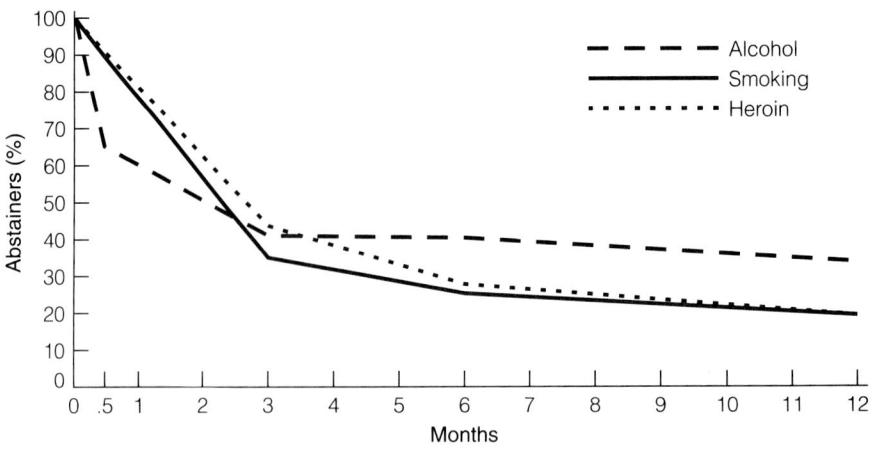

FIGURE 13.1 Relapse Curves (*Note.* From "Relapse Rates in Addiction Programs," by W. A. Hunt, L. W. Barnett, and L. G. Branch, 1971, *Journal of Clinical Psychology, 27*(4), 455–456.)

Factors Related to the Return to Smoking

The literature suggests several predictors of postpartum smoking, including not being completely abstinent ("taking puffs") during pregnancy; having a partner, friends, and family who smoke; having been more addicted before pregnancy; having lower self-efficacy in midpregnancy about maintaining cessation postpartum; and quitting but neglecting the use of coping strategies to resist the temptation to smoke. Study findings have been mixed with respect to level of smoking before the pregnancy as a predictor of postpartum smoking. Another issue, dissatisfaction with weight loss after the birth, has been shown to have a relationship to postpartum smoking, and postpartum exercise may be a protective factor (Mullen et al., 1997; Pirie et al., 1992; Severson, Andrews, Lichtenstein, Wall, & Zoref, 1995).

In addition to reviewing the literature, we used quantitative and qualitative data from the interviews mentioned earlier with women who had achieved biochemically validated cessation 6 months after the birth (Ershoff et al., 1989; Mullen et al., 1990, 1997). We also conducted focus groups with women and men in childbirth preparation classes and with pregnant women who had smoked prior to pregnancy and with their partners. Women and men were in separate groups with leaders of the same gender. We administered mail surveys once in mid to late pregnancy and again about six weeks after delivery to women who had been prepregnancy smokers and to their partners. The surveys addressed perceptions of pregnancy, perceived social support, sources of stress, concerns, and behavior change stimulated by the pregnancy (Pollak & Mullen, 1997; Richardson, Mullen, & DiClemente, 1993; Stotts, DiClemente, Carbonari, & Mullen, 1996; Taylor, Richardson, & Mullen, 1993). In the course of data collection, we learned that women were not sure about the seriousness of ETS or at what distance or under what conditions the baby is actually exposed. The women noted the benefits of smoking: It helps them control stress, concentrate, and take off the weight they still had by six weeks postpartum. Significantly, most women did not view quitting during pregnancy as a "success," and when we framed their stopping as a success, their attributions were to external, temporary causes (i.e., the baby, nausea). Further, new mothers expressed increased stress from such factors as sleep deprivation, dissatisfaction with slow postpartum weight loss, return to cues for smoking such as caffeine and alcohol consumption, and the perception that significant others no longer disapproved of smoking once the pregnancy was over.

Both from the literature and from our conversations with women who quit during pregnancy, we found that the role of the partner was important to relapse. A partner who smoked created not only an issue of social pressure but also a presence of stimuli for smoking and a ready access to cigarettes. Lastly, it was apparent that intervention should start in late pregnancy. Half of those women who would return to smoking by six months had already returned by the sixth postpartum week. The six-week postpartum checkup by the obstetrician gynecologist was too late, and for many mothers, so was the first pediatric visit.

How to Define the Problem—A Problem of Relapse or a Problem of Change?

We have recounted how Mullen came to understand the problem as more complex than relapse alone. This shift was an important one in describing desired behavior change and performance objectives; it would have profound effects on hypothetical determinants of performance. The relapse prevention model (Figure 13.2) seems to show that common reasons for relapse would relate to the presence of temptation or stimuli to smoke and the presence or absence of a coping

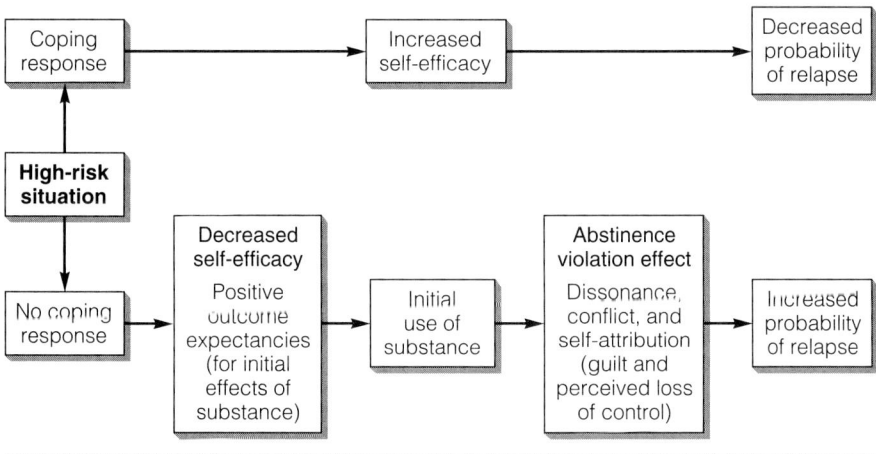

FIGURE 13.2 Relapse Prevention Model (*Note.* From *Relapse Prevention* by G. A. Marlatt and J. R. Gordon, 1985, New York: Guilford.)

response for dealing with the temptation (Marlatt & Gordon, 1985). It was clear that the women had reasons for return to smoking that spanned a much broader conceptual range than just temptation and coping.

In a new survey, Stotts, DiClemente, Carbonari, and Mullen (in press) asked women in late pregnancy their stage of change for continued abstinence after the birth. This survey produced a clearer idea of the women's perspective. Some women reported not intending to quit for good, believing that smoking is safe after birth if they keep smoke away from the baby. Others said that they "hoped" they wouldn't go back to smoking, although they had no specific plan to enable abstinence. Another group expressed resolve to make this quit "for good," although it was clear that even though they may have spent six months "in action," they had not been tested in the same way that smokers in the general population would have been.

Using stages of change from the transtheoretical model, Stotts et al. (in press) explored in more depth whether the women were conceptually in the action stage (having quit smoking) or were actually distributed over the earlier stages of precontemplation and contemplation with respect to postpregnancy smoking abstinence. The researchers based this analysis on what the women said about quitting during pregnancy and the processes they had used to quit as well as a staging algorithm. For example, women who had "really quit" probably would no longer be grappling with beliefs about the harm that cigarettes could cause themselves or their children, but some of these women were unconvinced about these issues. Real quitters would have high self-efficacy, determined at least partially by attributing successful quitting more to internal, stable causes—"I am the type of person who can give up cigarettes" (Marlatt & Gordon, 1985; Prochaska, Velicer, DiClemente, & Fava, 1988)—and not to unstable, external causes.

In other words, women who had really "quit" would have used many of the change processes described by Prochaska, DiClemente, and colleagues (DiClemente et al., 1991; Prochaska et al., 1988; Prochaska, Velicer, Guadagnoli, Rossi, & DiClemente, 1991). Processes of change in the transtheoretical model are described in the following way: Experiential processes peak in the contemplation stage, and behavioral processes peak in the preparation, or early action, stage (Prochaska et al., 1991). In contemplation, higher levels of experiential processing cause the pros of smoking to become less important than the cons of smoking. Yet, in an analysis of the survey data from this project compared with similar data for women who were not pregnant, pregnant quitters were seen as having lower process use (Stotts et al., 1996). Those women seemed to be in contemplation for abstinence postpartum because they used fewer experiential processes compared to women in the preparation stage.

These considerations led us to conclude that the transtheoretical model was an appropriate conceptual framework and that relapse prevention could be subsumed within it. Further, we were intrigued with the successful coping path of the relapse prevention model and saw that it had received less attention than unsuccessful coping had (Mullen, Pollak, & Kok, 1999). We also recognized the ambiguity of the role of attributions on the success path and of the general lack of

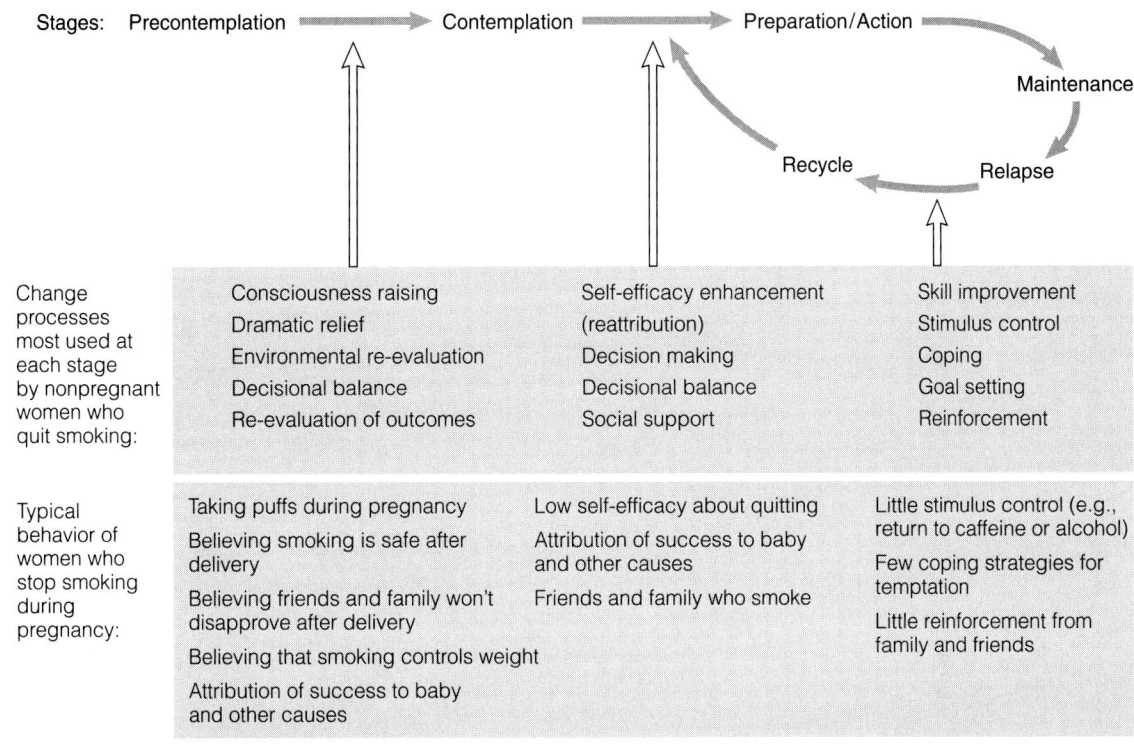

FIGURE 13.3 Stages, Processes of Change, and Evidence That Women Who Stop Smoking During Pregnancy Are Not "Quitting Smoking"

salience of success, particularly among women (Deaux & Farris, 1977; Reno, 1981; see Figure 13.3).

Under the conceptual framework of the transtheoretical model, the purpose of the program was to help women who had merely stopped smoking become real quitters. We hypothesized that among quitters at 28 weeks of pregnancy there would be precontemplators, contemplators, and women in action. (Preparation was included in action.) And even those women with six or more months of continuous abstinence were not classified as being in the maintenance stage, because of lower process use and less exposure to usual temptations.

Conclusions and Program Objectives

The focal factors from the needs assessment were the following:

- Moving women across the stages of change instead of assuming they were in the action phase
- Viewing men as important environmental influences who would need their own program

- Turning stopping for pregnancy into permanent cessation, focusing on the woman rather than ETS

Based on the needs assessment, program objectives for the women's program were as follows:

- Decrease return to smoking at 12 months postpartum by 10 percentage points
- Decrease infant ETS exposure by increasing nonsmoking by parents and other household members and by decreasing smoking in the home by parents who continued to smoke

Because of the important association of the prevalence of smoking in women's social networks (particularly their partners) with the likelihood of their return to smoking and with infant ETS exposure, we focused the program on men as well as women. The association of quitting and smoking by friends and family is ubiquitous in the smoking literature, yet interventions to increase social support through buddy contracts, tip sheets for quitters to give to significant others, and other such interventions had not produced the hoped-for results (Cohen et al., 1988). Thus, because the pregnancy presumably would be a time when some smoking fathers might be motivated to stop, Mullen and DiClemente decided that the intervention for fathers should be focused on quitting if the father was a smoker. This focus would have another benefit, because mothers are the number one source of ETS if they are smokers, but fathers who smoke are a significant source as well. Thus, one program objective for the men was as follows:

- Decrease the percentage of partners who smoke

INTERVENTION MAPPING STEP 1: MATRICES OF PROXIMAL PROGRAM OBJECTIVES

We had two major behavior change objectives for both women and their partners. The women were to remain abstinent and protect the infant from ETS. The men who smoked were to quit smoking; all the men were to protect the infant from ETS. Women and men were staged with respect to these objectives; they were in precontemplation, contemplation, or action. They were also differentiated by time-point in the pregnancy-to-parenthood transition. Table 13.3 shows the groups after the population was differentiated, and Figure 13.4 depicts the algorithm used to stage the women for staying off cigarettes postpartum.

Because of their primary role as environment for the women's smoking and because of their efforts at ETS control, men were considered a primary group for ETS and a secondary group for quitting. Further, we wanted men to provide instrumental, appraisal, and emotional social support to help the woman cope with postpartum stress and temptations to smoke (see Table 13.3).

Table 13.3
Population Differentiation

TARGET	PREGNANCY TRANSITION					
	29–30 weeks	32–34 weeks	34–36 weeks	Immediate postpartum	2 weeks postpartum	6 weeks postpartum
Women and smoking	Precontemplator or contemplator	Contemplator	Contemplator	Action	Action	Action
Women and ETS control	—	Contemplator	Action	Action	Action	Action
Men and smoking	Precontemplator or contemplator	Contemplator	Contemplator	Action	Action	Action
Men and ETS control and social support	Precontemplator or contemplator	Contemplator or action	Action	Action	Action	Action

Note. ETS = environmental tobacco smoke.

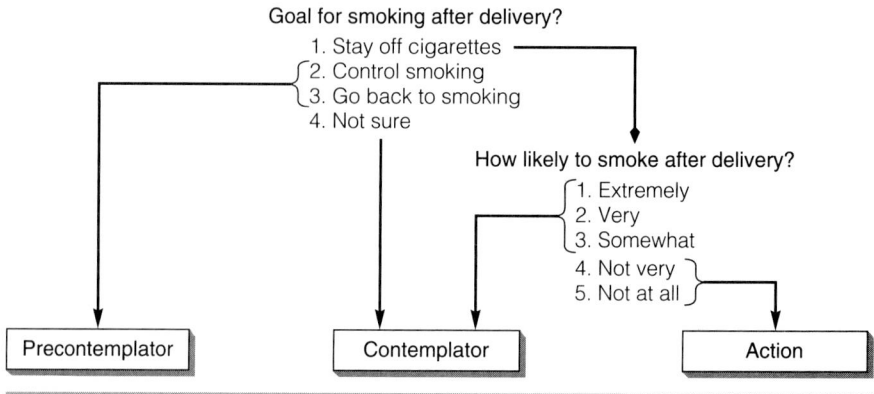

FIGURE 13.4 Stage of Change for Postpartum Smoking

Based on the transtheoretical model, there is actually one performance objective for each stage for the two behaviors (refraining from smoking and controlling ETS). For example, the performance objective for women in the contemplation stage for smoking is "Move to the action stage for remaining abstinent from cigarettes after the birth." For women in the action stage the performance object is "Continue to remain abstinent from cigarettes after the birth." Table 13.3 illustrates that, technically, every person times each pregnancy stage times behavior times stage of change is a separate matrix because the behaviors and determinants are different. This breakdown results in 27 matrices. However, each matrix has only one performance objective and few determinants or factors were hypothesized to influence the performance objective. Tables 13.4, 13.5, and 13.6 are sample matrices. Determinants were chosen with guidance from theory (from the change processes of the transtheoretical model in Figure 13.3 and from the literature). For example, Table 13.4 includes the decisional balance as an important determinant for moving from precontemplation to contemplation, whereas Table 13.5 includes attribution, decisional balance, skills, and social support as hypothesized determinants for moving from contemplation to action. Each matrix also includes notations about the salient pregnancy issues that will interact with the determinants.

INTERVENTION MAPPING STEP 2: METHODS AND STRATEGIES

Table 4.3 in Chapter 4 introduces processes of change that have been proposed as mechanisms that people use to get themselves from one stage of change to another. These processes of change are methods to influence stage shifts. For example, for people to move from precontemplation to contemplation, they need to become more aware through consciousness raising, dramatic relief, environmental re-evaluation, and increased perception of risks and benefits. They need

Table 13.4
Matrix for Smoking and ETS in Women Precontemplators at 29–30 Weeks (Sample Cells)

PERFORMANCE OBJECTIVES	DETERMINANTS	
	Attribution	Awareness and decisional balance
Smoking: Woman will move to the contemplation stage of remaining abstinent from cigarettes after the birth	Views stopping smoking as a success Views self as the kind of person who can successfully give up cigarettes	Believes that smoking is bad for self and baby Notices negative responses to smoking Develops long-term pros of not smoking for self Describes how smoking is bad for the baby after birth Describes possible improvements in health and self-image
ETS Control: Woman will move to the contemplation stage of protecting the infant from ETS	Sees self as the kind of person who would (and can) protect her child from environmental tobacco smoke	Increases awareness of effects of ETS on infants and children
Pregnancy issues: Beginning childbirth classes; many messages on labor and delivery; beginning to think about having old body back; baby becomes more of a reality for the partner; nesting begins for both parents.		

Note. ETS = environmental tobacco smoke.

to begin to tip the scales toward the pro side of making a change. To enable movement from contemplation to action, the experiential processes continue to tip the decisional balance with re-evaluation of self that focuses on important benefits and positive outcomes. Promoting movement between these stages must also include processes to enhance self-efficacy, such as skill building and trying out the new behavior. Social support becomes important at this point. As a person moves firmly into action, he or she continues to build skills, enhance self-efficacy, and exert control over the environment. Table 13.7 presents some of the theoretical methods and practical strategies used to correspond with the stage of change segments of the target groups for Project PANDA. For example, to raise their awareness of the benefits of not smoking and of protecting their baby from ETS, fathers first had to see themselves as important to the baby. Articles in the first newsletter delivered these messages. Figure 13.5 shows one of these articles.

This project was done for managed care settings, which now manage a large part of the prenatal care in the United States. In the HMOs in which the program would initially be implemented and evaluated, the average prenatal visit with a health care provider was scheduled for 7 minutes. Early in the project, developers recognized that counseling for maintaining abstinence probably could not fit within these time constraints. Therefore, we decided to use the mediated delivery

Table 13.5
Matrix for Smoking and ETS Control in Women Contemplators at 32–34 Weeks (Sample Cells)

PERFORMANCE OBJECTIVES	PERSONAL DETERMINANTS				EXTERNAL DETERMINANTS
	Attribution	Self-efficacy	Decisional balance	Skills	Social support
FOR SMOKING					
Woman will move to the action stage of remaining abstinent from cigarettes after birth	Views stopping smoking as a success Views self as the kind of person who can successfully give up cigarettes	Expresses confidence that she can remain off cigarettes postpartum Expresses confidence in being able to maintain relations where smoking has been a shared activity Expresses confidence in being able to return to normal postpartum without smoking	Notices negative responses to smoking Develops long-term pros of not smoking for self		Partner will not smoke around woman prepartum or postpartum
FOR ETS CONTROL					
Woman will move to the action stage of protecting the infant from ETS	Sees self as the kind of person who would (and can) protect her child from ETS	Expresses confidence in ability to ask family not to smoke	Increases awareness of effects of ETS on infants and children	Increases skills for negotiating with partner, friends, and family for not smoking around the baby	Partner negotiates about a smoke-free environment
Woman will deal with visitors and relatives who smoke		Expresses confidence in ability to ask partner not to smoke in the house			Partner begins to help develop smoke-free house rules
Woman will make house smoke free					
Woman will choose smoke-free environments outside of the home		Expresses confidence in ability to ask friends not to smoke around baby			

Pregnancy issues: Focusing more on labor and delivery; beginning to worry about the birth and the health of the baby; increased communication between couple; poignancy about loss of couplehood.

Note. ETS = environmental tobacco smoke.

Table 13.6
Matrix for Smoking and ETS and Social Support Action in Men Contemplators at 32–34 Weeks (Sample Cells)

PERFORMANCE OBJECTIVES FOR SMOKING	DETERMINANTS		
	Attribution	Self-efficacy	Decisional balance
Partner will move to the action stage for quitting smoking	Views self as the kind of person who can successfully give up cigarettes	Expresses confidence in ability to quit smoking	Notices negative responses to smoking. Increases awareness of effects of ETS on infants and children. Increases awareness of self as smoking role model for children and of self as an instrumental parent

PERFORMANCE OBJECTIVES FOR ETS AND SOCIAL SUPPORT ACTION	DETERMINANTS			
	Skills	Self-efficacy	Stimulus control	Coping
Partner will protect child from ETS	Discusses how to make home smoke free	Expresses confidence in ability to ask family not to smoke	Displays cues for smoke-free house	Has plan for how to cope with friends and family for not smoking around the baby or in the house
Partner will work with woman to make house smoke free	Practices routine for dealing with friends and relatives	Expresses confidence in ability to ask friends not to smoke around baby		
Partner will deal with friends and relatives regarding smoke-free house	Lists places outside of home that will be avoided with family	Expresses confidence in ability not to smoke in the house		
Partner will not smoke around the woman or child	Practices leaving the home environment to smoke			
Partner will choose smoke-free environments outside the house				

Pregnancy issues: Beginning to worry about birth and the woman's health and safety; participation in plans for the birth; not anticipating postpartum changes in participation; motivated to learn infant caretaking.

Note. ETS = environmental tobacco smoke.

Table 13.7
Brainstorming Methods and Strategies for Project PANDA

THEORETICAL METHODS	PRACTICAL STRATEGIES—WOMEN	PRACTICAL STRATEGIES—MEN
To move from precontemplation to contemplation:		
Persuasion of the benefits of not smoking	Newsletter article on risks and benefits	Articles pairing general parenting competence and expectation of being a participatory father with protecting the baby from ETS
Persuasion of the risks of smoking	Newsletter messages about attribution for quitting	
Persuasion of the costs of smoking and costs of a new baby		Videotape modeling moving to the role of fatherhood as one gets healthier and protects the infant
Persuasion of the risks of ETS to baby		
Modeling for reattribution training		Article stressing the benefits of taking care of own health and conveying the message that fathers should consider quitting
To move from contemplation to action:		
Modeling for reattribution training	Attribution article on becoming a good parent, including ETS protection	Newsletter articles teaching social support strategies and strategies to help fathers cope well enough to give support
Promotion of decisional balance shift		
Skill building	Article on skill building for dealing with stress without cigarettes	Attribution articles on becoming the type of father who will protect baby
Social support from partner and others	Persuasive articles about environmental control	
Cues for environmental control	Signs for environmental control	Skill building for environmental control
	Letter from the baby to reinforce environmental control	Article and videotape models that stress fathers as role models for their children
To support action and move toward maintenance:		
Skill building for coping with relapse temptations	Videotape with role models coping with temptation and recycling from relapse	Newsletter skill-building article for problem solving
Skill building for environmental control and social support		Newsletter skill-building article for stress management
Coping models	Newsletter role model story on preventing relapse	Skill building for infant protection
Social comparison	Newsletter skill-training article on coping with stress	
Skill training for coping with negative feelings	Newsletter articles to model a coping mom versus a mastery mom to enhance self-efficacy and lower stress	
Models for problem solving	Newsletter skill-training article for coping with negative feelings	
	Video modeling for enhancing social support	
	Newsletter article encouraging the building of social support	

THE SMOKE-FREE ZONE

Creating your own zone

You know the effects of passive smoke aren't good for you or your baby, but how about friends and family? Smoking is a habit people do without thinking. Often they will light up whenever they feel like it, whether or not you and your baby are present. To keep you and your baby smoke-free, you will need to take action.

First decide what "smoke-free" means. How big of a smoke-free zone do you need? Certainly, babies shouldn't be in a closed car or in the same room with someone smoking. But what about the next room? Or a house where someone has been smoking? Scientific studies tell us that the byproducts of cigarette smoke don't leave an area as quickly as we might think. Practical experience tells us the same thing. Airlines switched from no-smoking sections to a ban on smoking because cigarette smoke affected passengers throughout the plane.

Protecting your zone

Often a "no smoking" sign is enough to communicate the message that you don't want smoking in your house or car. Some smokers, however, may have to be told what your rules are. Say, for example, "I'd like you to smoke outside," or "I really feel tempted to smoke right now, and I want to remain a nonsmoker, so please don't smoke around me."

Friends and relatives

To her neighbor who was about to take a pack of cigarettes out of her purse, Amelia said: "If you want to smoke, please smoke on the balcony. There's a chair and an ashtray, and when you're finished, we'll have the iced tea I'm making."

Some situations are more complicated. Mothers we have talked to say that discouraging smoking by members of their husband's family, and in someone else's house, is especially touchy. They suggest a private talk before the visit or strategies like keeping the baby in another room. If the smokers are your partner's friends or family, maybe you can suggest that he talk to them.

Partner

We all know perfectly well that the most difficult situation in the no-smoke battle is having a husband or partner who smokes. His smoking may make it hard for you not to smoke. And, of course, smoking fathers are a big source of smoke exposure for their babies. Although to quit smoking entirely is best for him, he has to make that decision. While he is still smoking, you will need to be assertive, factual, and firm. Let him know how much you value his company. Don't be judgmental about his smoking habit or get into arguments. Focus on finding a solution together. Ask him how he would keep some part of the house smoke-free. Perhaps the establishment of a smoking area is one solution. The best place is outside. The garage or a room with the door closed is next-best.

After the birth of their twins, Amelia's husband decided he could not quit smoking. But, agreeing that protecting the babies was the priority, he smoked on the patio when he needed a cigarette. He worked on old cars in the garage, which they agreed to designate as a second smoking area.

Working together on solutions seems to be best for both partners. After establishing a smoke-free routine with family and friends, you will find that visits will be more enjoyable because both you and your visitors will be more relaxed.

Keeping you and your baby smoke-free takes effort. You will need to be assertive. Most mothers find they have hidden stores of strength when it comes to protecting their children.

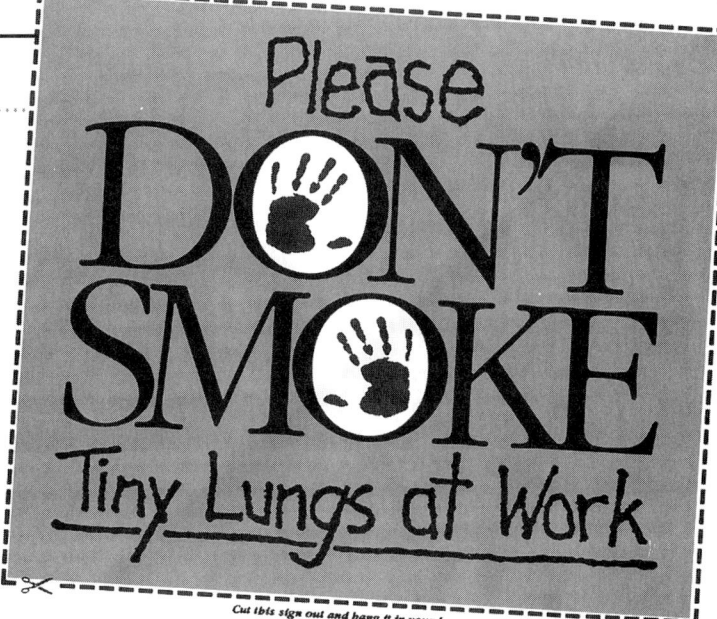

Cut this sign out and hang it in your home.

FIGURE 13.5 The Smoke-Free Zone

mechanisms of newsletters and videotapes mailed to the homes of program participants. In checking with various types of videotape rental businesses, we estimated that more than 90% of households in the United States have access to VCRs and that this rate could be expected to hold in this employed population. Further, the men who participated in focus groups expressed a preference to have their own materials (versus shared with the woman) mailed directly to them (versus delivered to him by the woman).

INTERVENTION MAPPING STEP 3: PROGRAM DESIGN

The challenge of the program development step is to translate the planning up to this point into a creative, deliverable program with a defined scope and sequence. Chapter 7 explains that program design documents are needed to communicate product characteristics within a design team and certainly when production people are vendors who may not have participated in the entire planning process. One of the defining characteristics of Project PANDA development was our careful use of design documents. Figure 13.6 shows a flow diagram for the preparation of the newsletters (the design document for which is shown in Chapter 7), and Figure 13.5 shows part of an article from a final newsletter.

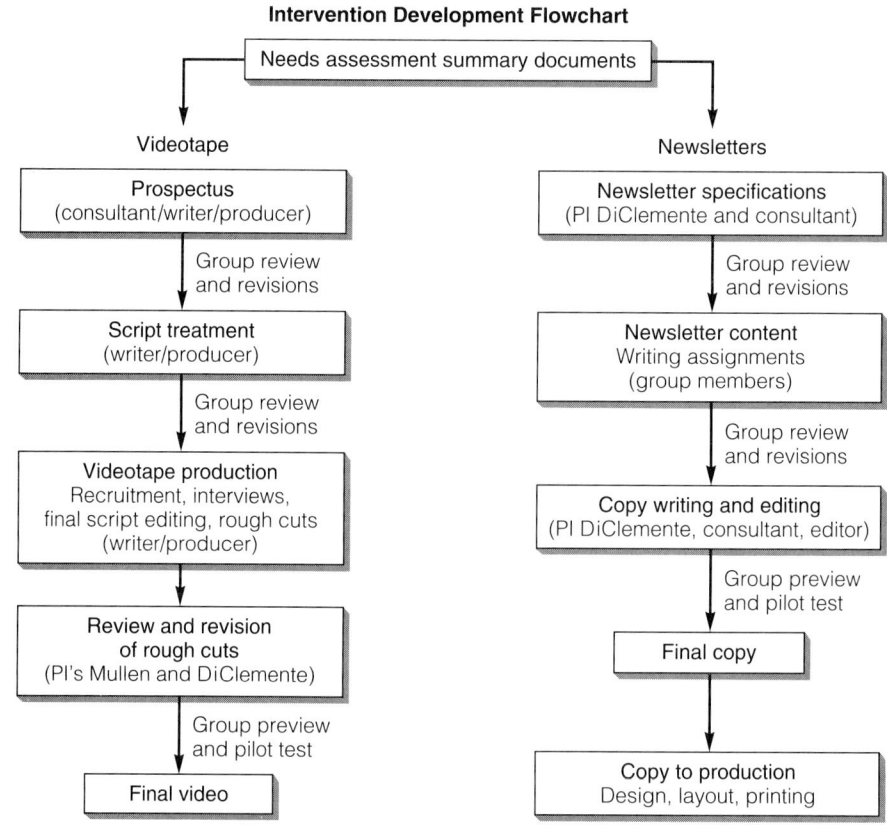

FIGURE 13.6 Intervention Development Flowchart

The video writer/producer, in addition to creating the design documents for the two videotapes that were part of the intervention, participated with the development team in conducting focus groups. In this way, she heard the concerns of women and their partners firsthand. We recommend involving outside vendors in as much of the planning and target group communication process as is possible and practical. Seeing and hearing the target group conveys much more than design documents alone (but even being in the entire process and communicating with the target group often does not take the place of a design document).

To pretest the Project PANDA materials, we engaged a panel of men and another of women from the target groups to review and respond to materials. The newsletters were presented in an almost-finished format with response boxes at the end of each article. Because each article, rather than each newsletter, was intended to have a specific impact, we wanted the panel members' responses to specific newsletter segments.

Videotapes were reviewed at the rough-cut stage. As was discussed in Chapter 7, the women's tape required significant changes because the role-model material abstracted from interviews by the video producer was overly positive and mastery focused. We needed to re-edit to find material that was closer to the psychological and physical state of a newly delivered woman who was trying to stay off cigarettes.

INTERVENTION MAPPING STEP 4: IMPLEMENTATION

Project PANDA entailed entirely mediated intervention components—newsletters and videotapes. However, the components were mailed to the homes of the women and their partners under the imprimatur of the women's health maintenance organizations. Therefore, an advisory committee from the HMOs worked with the project to review intervention development and to facilitate implementation.

INTERVENTION MAPPING STEP 5: EVALUATION

The evaluation model is presented in Figure 13.7. For this project, the evaluation of the validity of the hypothetical determinants was explored in a pilot project rather than in the randomized trial of smoking abstinence. Therefore, in the model, process extends to the determinants box and includes consideration of self-efficacy, the influence of attributions on self-efficacy, stress, social support, and use of the processes of change.

In the process evaluation, we looked at the implementation of the project via telephone interviews with the women. They were asked whether they and their partners received the videos and newsletters (women, 96%; partners, 90%) and

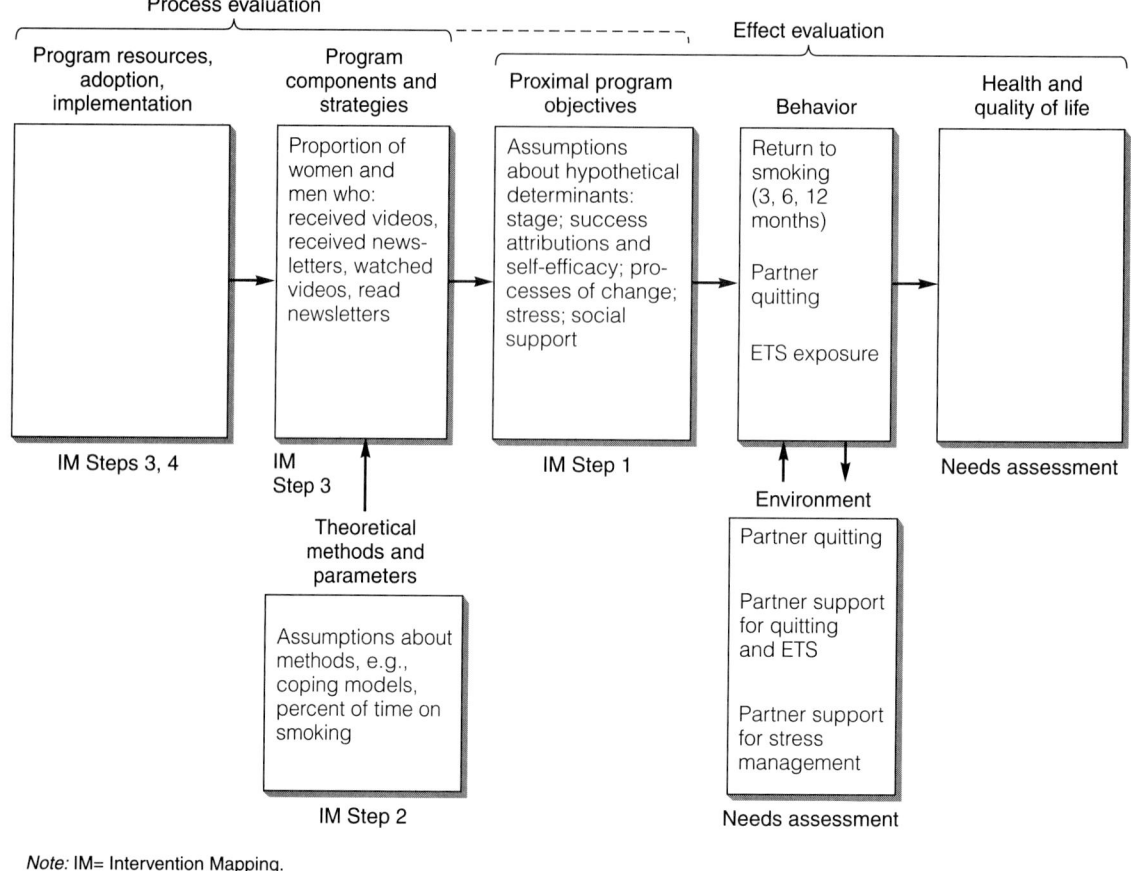

FIGURE 13.7 Evaluation Map

whether they read all the newsletters (women, 78%; partners, 59%) and watched the videos (women, 66%; men, 59%). We also explored aspects of the intervention components in terms of how well they met our assumptions about methods and strategies. We wanted to verify how much of our intent to respond to the pregnancy context of the women we had been able to operationalize. We wanted to confirm, for example, how much of the "airtime" in the videotapes and how much of the copy in the newsletters had been devoted to smoking and how much had been devoted to supportive topics for the new mothers and fathers. Figures 13.8 and 13.9 are graphs that show the percentage of time per minute devoted to smoking in the men's and women's videotape. The men's tape, which came to the men early in the program sequence when we expected them to be in early stages of change for smoking cessation and for protecting the baby from ETS, did not mention smoking at all until the 10th minute and focused on smoking in only 6 of 18 minutes of tape. The women's tape was delivered when most of the women were hypothesized to be in the action stage of continued abstinence and when the

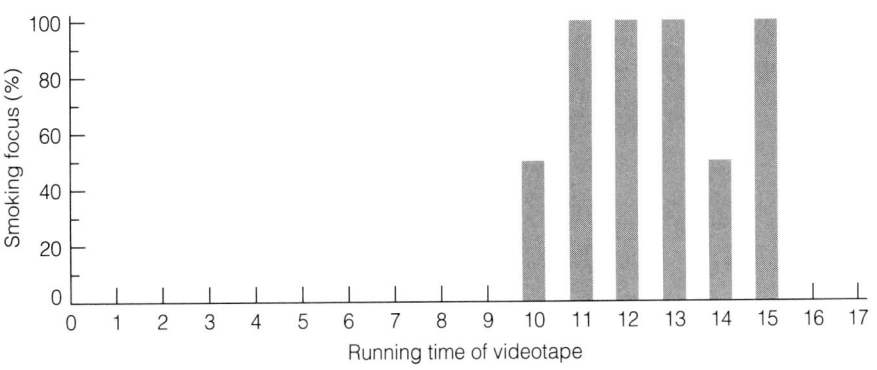

FIGURE 13.8 Percentage of Smoking Focus in Each Minute of Men's Video, Project PANDA

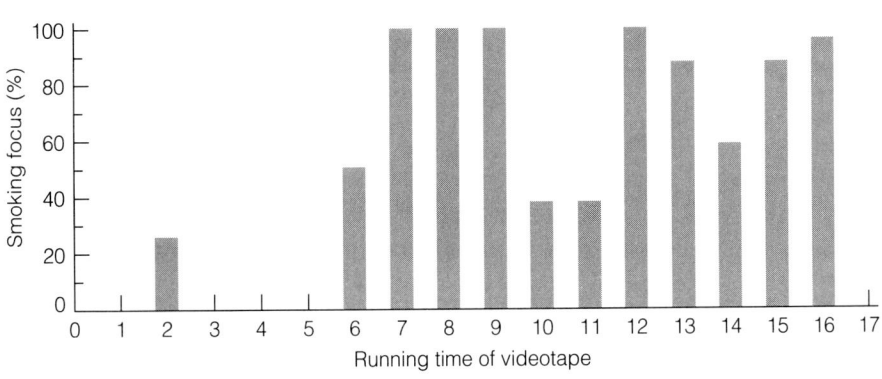

FIGURE 13.9 Percentage of Smoking Focus in Each Minute of Women's Video, Project PANDA

temptations to return to smoking immediately postpartum were particularly high. The women's tape focused almost entirely on smoking (12 of 19 minutes had a smoking focus), whereas the newsletters that preceded the tape were heavily devoted to pregnancy issues.

The effect evaluation of this project is being completed. As the evaluation model (Figure 13.7) indicates, the main outcome variable being measured is whether the woman is smoking at 6 weeks and at 3, 6, and 12 months. The measure in the woman is self-report with urine cotinine validation in a subsample. Women are also being asked to report on their partners' smoking without the validation measure. The other outcome measure is ETS protection, which is being measured by the placement of nicotine monitors in the room where the family reports spending the most time.

SUMMARY

Project PANDA is a good example of using theory to define the behavior of interest for a health education and promotion program and to tailor interventions to effect change in the behavior. Had program developers Mullen and DiClemente adopted the most obvious approach to addressing return to smoking among women who had quit postpartum (i.e., relapse prevention), they would have had a very different program. And in these differences the program would have lacked messages for a majority of the women (i.e., the precontemplators and contemplators for staying off cigarettes).

In addition, Project PANDA is a model for getting to know the target group for a program and using their input throughout program development. From the very beginning of thinking about the program, when the development team heard clues to an early stage of change and to lack of use of the processes of change, through the target group pretesting of the intervention materials, this project was guided by the women and men it sought to help.

REFERENCES

Arizmendi, T. G., & Affonso, D. D. (1987). Stressful events related to pregnancy and postpartum. *Journal of Psychosomatic Research, 31*(6), 743–756.

Bliss-Holtz, V. J. (1988). Primiparas' prenatal concern for learning infant care. *Nursing Research, 37*(1), 20–24.

Cohen, S., Lichtenstein, E., Kingsolver, K., Mermelstein, R., Baer, J. S., & Kamarck, T. W. (1988). Social support interventions for smoking cessation. In B. H. Gottlieb (Ed.), *Marshaling social support: Formats, processes, and effects* (pp. 211–240). Newbury Park, CA: Sage.

Cook, P. S., Peterson, R. C., & Moore, D. T. (1990). *Alcohol, tobacco, and other drugs may harm the unborn* (Report No. DHHS [ADM] 90-1711). Rockville, MD: U.S. Department of Health and Human Services.

Cuijpers, C., Swaen, G., Wesseling, G., Stumans, F., & Wouters, E. F. (1995). Adverse effects of the indoor environment on respiratory health in primary school children. *Environmental Research, 68*(1), 11–23.

Deaux, K., & Farris, E. (1977). Attributing causes for one's own performance: The effects of sex, norms, and outcome. *Journal of Research in Personality, 11*(1), 59–72.

DiClemente, C. C., Mullen, P. D., Pollak, K. I., Sockrider, M. M., & Stotts, A. L. (1998). *Intervention effects on pregnant quitters' partners' smoking.* Paper presented at the annual meeting of the Society of Behavioral Medicine, New Orleans, LA.

DiClemente, C. C., Prochaska, J. O., Fairhurst, S. K., Velicer, W. F., Velasquez, M. M., & Rossi, J. S. (1991). The process of smoking cessation: An analysis of precontemplation, contemplation, and preparation stages of change. *Journal of Consulting and Clinical Psychology, 59*(2), 295–304.

Dolan-Mullen, P., Ramirez, G., & Groff, J. Y. (1994). A meta-analysis of randomized trials of prenatal smoking cessation interventions. *American Journal of Obstetrics and Gynecology, 171*(5), 1328–1334.

Drake, M. L., Verhulst, D., & Fawcett, J. (1988). Physical and psychological symptoms experienced by Canadian women and their husbands during pregnancy and the postpartum. *Journal of Advanced Nursing, 13*(4), 436–440.

Emerson, J. A., Wahlgren, D. R., Hovell, M. F., Meltzer, S. B., Zakarian, J. M., & Hofstetter, C. R. (1994). Parent smoking and asthmatic children's exposure patterns: A behavioral epidemiology study. *Addictive Behaviors, 19*(6), 677–689.

Ershoff, D. H., Mullen, P. D., & Quinn, V. P. (1989). A randomized trial of a serialized self-help smoking cessation program for pregnant women in an HMO. *American Journal of Public Health, 79*(2), 182–187.

Fingerhut, L. A., Kleinman, J. C., & Kendrick, J. S. (1990). Smoking before, during, and after pregnancy. *American Journal of Public Health, 80*(5), 541–544.

Floyd, R. L., Rimer, B. K., Giovino, G. A., Mullen, P. D., & Sullivan, S. E. (1993). A review of smoking in pregnancy: Effects on pregnancy outcomes and cessation efforts. *Annual Review of Public Health, 14,* 379–411.

Hovell, M. F., Meltzer, S. B., Zakarian, J. M., Wahlgren, D. R., Emerson, J. A., Hofstetter, C. R., Leaderer, B. P., Meltzer, E. O., Zeiger, R. S., & O'Connor, R. D. (1994). Reduction of environmental tobacco smoke exposure among asthmatic children: A controlled trial. *Chest, 106*(2), 440–446.

Hunt, W. A., Barnett, L.W., & Branch, L. G. (1971). Relapse rates in addiction programs. *Journal of Clinical Psychology, 27*(4), 455–456.

Huss, K., Rand, C. S., Butz, A. M., Eggleston, P. A., Murigande, C., Thompson, L. C., Schneider, S., Weeks, K., & Malveaux, F. J. (1994). Home environmental risk factors in urban minority asthmatic children. *Annals of Allergy, 72*(2), 173–177.

Imle, M. A. (1990). Third trimester concerns of expectant parents in transition to parenthood. *Holistic Nurse Practitioner, 4*(3), 25–36.

Joffe, H. (1989). Emotional factors in pregnancy. *Australian Family Physician, 18*(5), 493–497.

Johnson, S., McCarter, R., & Ferencz, C. (1987). Changes in alcohol, cigarette, and recreational drug use during pregnancy: Implications for intervention. *American Journal of Epidemiology, 126*(4), 695–702.

Kruse, J., LeFevre, M., & Zweig, S. (1986). Changes in smoking and alcohol consumption during pregnancy: A population-based study in a rural area. *Obstetrics and Gynecology, 67*(5), 627–632.

Lewis, S. N., & Cooper, C. L. (1987). Stress in two-earner couples and stage in the lifecycle. *Journal of Occupational Psychology, 60*(4), 289–303.

Lieberman, E., Gremy, I., Lang, S. M., & Cohen, A. P. (1994). Low birthweight at term and the timing of fetal exposure to maternal smoking. *American Journal of Public Health, 84*(7), 1127–1131.

Malloy, M. H., Hoffman, H. J., & Peterson, D. R. (1992). Sudden Infant Death Syndrome and maternal smoking. *American Journal of Public Health, 82*(10), 1380–1382.

Malloy, M. H., Kleinman, J. C., Land, G. H., & Schramm, W. F. (1988). The association of maternal smoking with age and cause of infant deaths. *American Journal of Epidemiology, 128*(1), 46–55.

Marlatt, G. A., & Gordon, J. R. (1985). *Relapse prevention: Maintenance strategies in the treatment of addictive behaviors.* New York: Guilford.

Mullen, P. D. (1999). Smoking during pregnancy and intervention to promote cessation: A meta-analysis. In J. G. Spangler (Ed.), *Primary care: Clinics in office practice* (Vol. 6, pp. 577–589). Philadelphia: Saunders.

Mullen, P. D., DiClemente, C. C., Carbonari, J. P., Nicol, L., Richardson, M. A., Sockrider, M. M., & Taylor, W. C. (1999). *Project PANDA: Maintenance of prenatal smoking abstinence 12 months postpartum.* Manuscript submitted for publication.

Mullen, P. D., Pollak, K. I., & Kok, G. (1999). Success attributions for stopping smoking during pregnancy, self-efficacy, and postpartum maintenance. *Psychology of Addictive Behaviors, 13*(3), 198–206.

Mullen, P. D., Quinn, V. P., & Ershoff, D. H. (1990). Maintenance of nonsmoking postpartum by women who stopped during pregnancy. *American Journal of Public Health, 80*(8), 992–994.

Mullen, P. D., & Ramirez, G. (in press). Efforts to reduce tobacco use among women: Pregnant women and mothers. In U.S. Public Health Service: Office on Smoking and Health, *The health consequences of smoking for women: A report of the Surgeon General.* Rockville, MD: U.S. Department of Health and Human Services.

Mullen, P. D., Richardson, M. A., Quinn, V. P., & Ershoff, D. H. (1997). Postpartum return to smoking: Who is at risk and when. *American Journal of Health Promotion, 11*(5), 323–330.

Murray, A. B., & Morrison, B. J. (1989). Passive smoking by asthmatics: Its greater effect on boys than girls and older than younger children. *Pediatrics, 84*(3), 451–459.

Overpeck, M. D., & Moss, J. A. (1991). *Children's exposure to environmental cigarette smoke before and after birth: Advance data from Vital and Health Statistics #202.* (DHHS Publication No. 91-1250). Hyattsville, MD: National Center for Health Statistics.

Pirie, P. L., McBride, C. M., Hellerstedt, W., Jeffery, R. W., Hatsukami, D., Allen, S., & Lando, H. (1992). Smoking cessation in women concerned about weight. *American Journal of Public Health, 82*(9), 1238–1243.

Pollak, K. I., & Mullen, P. D. (1997). An exploration of the effects of partner smoking, type of social support, and stress on postpartum smoking in married women who stopped smoking during pregnancy. *Psychology of Addictive Behaviors, 11*(3), 182–189.

Prochaska, J. O., Velicer, W. F., DiClemente, C. C., & Fava, J. (1988). Measuring processes of change: Applications to the cessation of smoking. *Journal of Consulting and Clinical Psychology, 56*(4), 520–528.

Prochaska, J. O., Velicer, W. F., Guadagnoli, E., Rossi, J. S., & DiClemente, C. C. (1991). Patterns of change: Dynamic typology applied to smoking cessation. *Multivariate Behavioral Research, 26*(1), 83–107.

Quinn, V. P., Mullen, P. D., & Ershoff, D. H. (1991). Women who stop smoking spontaneously prior to prenatal care and predictors of relapse before delivery. *Addictive Behaviors, 16*(1–2), 29–40.

Reno, R. (1981). Sex differences in attribution for occupational success. *Journal of Research in Personality, 15*(1), 81–92.

Richardson, M. A., Mullen, P. D., & DiClemente, C. C. (1993, March). *Smoking during pregnancy: A man's perspective.* Poster presented at the Society of Behavioral Medicine annual meeting, San Francisco, CA.

Samet, J., Cain, W., & Leaderer, B. (1991). Environmental tobacco smoke. In J. Samet & Spengler (Eds.), *Indoor air pollution—A health perspective* (pp. 131–169). Baltimore: Johns Hopkins University Press.

Saunders, R. B., & Robins, E. (1987). Changes in the marital relationship during the first pregnancy. *Health Care for Women International, 8*(5/6), 361–377.

Secker-Walker, R. H., Solomon, L. J., Flynn, B. S., Skelly, J. M., Lepage, S. S., Goodwin, G. D., & Mead, P. B. (1995). Smoking relapse prevention counseling during prenatal and early postnatal care. *American Journal of Preventive Medicine, 11*(2), 86–93. (Published erratum in *American Journal of Preventive Medicine,* 1996, *12*(2), 71–72)

Severson, H. H., Andrews, J. A., Lichtenstein, E., Wall, M., & Zoref, L. (1995). Predictors of smoking during and after pregnancy: A survey of mothers of newborns. *Preventive Medicine, 24*(1), 23–28.

Stockbauer, J. W., & Land, G. H. (1991). Changes in characteristics of women who smoke during pregnancy: Missouri, 1978–1988. *Public Health Reports, 106,* 52–58.

Stotts, A. L., DiClemente, C. C., Carbonari, J. P., & Mullen, P. D. (1996). Pregnancy smoking cessation: A case of mistaken identity. *Addictive Behaviors, 21*(4), 459–471.

Stotts, A. L., DiClemente, C. C., Carbonari, J. P., & Mullen, P. D. (in press). Postpartum return to smoking: Staging a "suspended" behavior. *Health Psychology.*

Taylor, W. C., Richardson, M. A., & Mullen, P. D. (1993, March). *Intrinsic and extrinsic motivation: Implications for smoking cessation during pregnancy.* Poster presented at the Society of Behavioral Medicine annual meeting, San Francisco, CA.

U.S. Office on Smoking and Health. (1980). *The health consequences of smoking for women. A report of the Surgeon General.* Rockville, MD: Author.

U.S. Office on Smoking and Health. (1984a). *The health consequences of smoking: Cardiovascular disease. A report of the Surgeon General* (DHHS Publication No. PHS 84-50204). Rockville, MD: Author.

U.S. Office on Smoking and Health. (1984b). *The health consequences of smoking: Chronic obstructive lung disease. A report of the Surgeon General* (DHHS Publication No. PHS 84-50205). Rockville, MD: Author.

U.S. Office on Smoking and Health. (1985). *The health consequences of smoking: Cancer and chronic lung disease in the workplace. A report of the Surgeon General* (DHHS Publication No. 85-50207). Rockville, MD: Author.

Wall, M. A., Severson, H. H., Andrews, J. A., Lichtenstein, E., & Zoref, L. (1995). Pediatric office-based smoking intervention: Impact on maternal smoking and relapse. *Pediatrics, 96*(4, Pt. 1), 622–628.

Wen, S. W., Goldenberg, R. L., Cutter, G. R., Hoffman, H. J., & Cliver, S. P. (1989). Intrauterine growth retardation and preterm delivery: Risk factors in an indigent population. *American Journal of Obstetrics and Gynecology, 162*(1), 213–218.

Windham, G. C., Swan, S. H., & Fenter, L. (1992). Parental smoking and the risk of spontaneous abortion. *American Journal of Epidemiology, 35*(12), 1394–1403.

Woodby, L. L., Windsor, R. A., Snyder, S. W., Kohler, C. L., & DiClemente, C. C. (1999). Predictors of smoking cessation during pregnancy. *Addiction, 94*(2), 283–292.

CREDITS

CHAPTER 1 Fig. 1.1 Adapted from "Assessment of the Integration of the Ecological Approach in Health Programs," by J. Richard, L. Potvin, N. Kishchuk, H. Prlic, L. W. Green, 1996, *American Journal of Health Promotion*, 10(4), 318–328. Reprinted with permission from the publisher.

CHAPTER 2 Fig. 2.1 From A. Steckler, K. R. McLeroy, R. M. Goodman, S. T . Bird, L. M. McCormick, *Health Education Quarterly*, 1992, 19(1), 1–8. With permission from Plenum Publishing Corporation. Illustration 2.1 Copyright © 2000 Kay Bartholomew. Table 2.1 Copyright © 2000 Kay Bartholomew. Fig. 2.3 From L. W. Green and M. W. Kreuter, *Health Promotion Planning: An Educational and Ecological Approach, Third Edition*, Mayfield, 1999. Figs. 2.4, 2.6, 2.7, 2.8 Adapted from L. W. Green and M. W. Kreuter, *Health Promotion Planning: An Educational and Ecological Approach, Third Edition*, Mayfield, 1999.

CHAPTER 4 Table 4.8 From E. H. Schein, *Organizational Culture and Leadership, Second Edition*, Jossey-Bass, Inc., a subsidiary of John Wiley & Sons, Inc., 1992. Reprinted by permission of John Wiley & Sons, Inc. Fig. 4.1 From "Freirian Praxis in Health Education," *Health Education Research*, 1994, Vol. 9, No. 1, 105–118. Reprinted by permission of Oxford University Press. Fig. 4.2 From K. Glanz, F. M. Lewis, B. K. Rimer, eds., *Health Behavior and Health Education: Theory, Research, and Practice, Second Edition*, Jossey-Bass, 1997. Reprinted by permission of Jossey-Bass, Inc., a subsidiary of John Wiley & Sons, Inc. Fig. 4.3 From N. Milio, *Promoting Health Through Public Policy*, F. A. Davis, 1981. Reprinted with permission from the publisher.

CHAPTER 7 Fig. 7.2 From T. L. L. Temple Foundation Stroke Project, Lewis Morgenstern, M.D., Principal Investigator, Department of Neurology, University of Texas Medical School, 6431 Fannin, MSB 7.124, Houston, TX 77030. Reprinted with kind permission from Dr. Morgenstern. Fig. 7.3 With permission from The Regents of the University of California and Griffin Publishing Group. Figs. 7.4, 7.5 From the Cystic Fibrosis Family Education Program, funded by a grant from National Heart, Lung and Blood Institute, Dan K. Seilheimer, M.D., Principal Investigator. For further information contact Dr. Kay Bartholomew. Fig. 7.6 From Street Kids AIDS Training and Education Project, funded by a grant from the Centers for Disease Control. For more information contact Javier Amaya, HIV/STD Education Team, Seattle/ Kings County Department of Public Health, 400 Yesler Way, Third Floor, Seattle, WA 98104, (206) 296-4649. Fig. 7.7 From *Preventive Medicine*, Fig. 1, Vol. 25, 236–242, 1996. Copyright © 1996 by Academic Press. Reproduced by permission of the publisher. Fig. 7.8 From H. Z. Ramelson, R. H. Friedman, J. K. Ockene, "An Automated Telephone-Based Smoking Cessation Education and Counseling System," *Patient Education and Counseling*, 1999, Vol. 36(2), 131–144, Fig. 2. With permission from Elsevier Science. Fig. 7.11 With permission from Texas Department of Health. Fig. 7.12 Adapted from Gillian Kaye and Tom Wolff, *From the Ground Up: A Workbook on Coalition Building and Community Development*. With permission from AHEC/Community Partners, Amherst, MA. Fig. 7.13 From materials from Coalition Training Institute, The Center for Pediatric Research, Eastern Virginia Medical School. Reprinted by permission of Dr. Fran Butterfoss. Fig. 7.14 With permission from Project PANDA, Center for Health Promotion and Prevention Research, University of Texas–Houston School of Public Health. Table 7.2 Copyright © 2000 Kay Bartholomew. All rights reserved. Used with permission. Table 7.3 From

D. A. Lieberman, "Interactive Video Games for Health Promotion: Effects on Knowledge, Self-Efficacy, Social Support, and Health," Table 6.1, pp. 108–109, in R. Street, W. Gold, T. Manning, eds., *Health Promotion and Interactive Technology: Theoretical Applications and Future Directions*, Lawrence Erlbaum, 1997. With permission from the publisher.

CHAPTER 8 Fig. 8.2 From E. M. Rogers, *Diffusion of Innovations, Fourth Edition*, 1995, p. 262. Copyright © 1995 E. M. Rogers. Reprinted with permission from The Free Press, a division of Simon & Schuster. Fig. 8.3 From T. Paulussen, G. Kok, H. Schaalma, G. S. Parcel, "Diffusion of AIDS Curricula Among Dutch Secondary School Teachers," *Health Education Quarterly*, 22(2), 231. With permission from Plenum Publishing Company. Table 8.1 From L. K. Bartholomew, D. I. Czyzewski, P. R. Swank, L. McCormick, G. S. Parcel, "Maximizing the Impact of the Cystic Fibrosis Family Education Program: Variables Related to Diffusion," *Journal of Family and Community Health*, 22(4), 1–22, Table 1, 2000. Copyright © 2000 Aspen Publishers, Inc. With permission from the publisher. Table 8.2 From G. S. Parcel, W. C. Taylor, S. G. Brink, N. Gottlieb, K. Engquist, N. M. O'Hara, M. P. Eriksen, "Translating Theory into Practice: Intervention Strategies for the Diffusion of a Health Promotion Innovation," *Family and Community Health*, 1989, 12(3), 1–13. Copyright © 1989 Aspen Publishers, Inc. With permission from the publisher.

CHAPTER 9 Fig. 9.1 Adapted from Exhibit 3-G, p. 99 and Exhibit 3-H, p. 101 in P. H. Rossi, H. E. Freeman, M. W. Lipsey, *Evaluation: A Systematic Approach, Sixth Edition*, Sage, 1999. Copyright © 1999 Sage Publications, Inc. Reprinted by permission of the publisher.

CHAPTER 10 Fig. 10.1 From D. E. Montano, D. Kasprzyk, S. H. Taplin, "The Theory of Reasoned Action and the Theory of Planned Behavior," in K. Glanz, F. M. Lewis, B. K. Rimer, eds., *Health Behavior and Health Education: Theory, Research, and Practice, Second Edition*, p. 92, Jossey-Bass, 1997. Reprinted by permission of Jossey-Bass, a subsidiary of John Wiley & Sons, Inc.

CHAPTER 11 Fig. 11.1 From L. K. Bartholomew, R. Shegog, G. S. Parcel, M. Fernandez, R. S. Gold, D. I. Czyzewski, M. M. Sockrider, N. Berlin, "Watch, Discover, Think, and Act: A Model for Patient Education Program Development," *Patient Education and Counseling* 2000, 39(2–3), 253–268. With permission from Elsevier Science. Fig. 11.2 From Watch, Discover, Think, and Act of Partners in School Asthma Management Project funded by a grant from the National Heart, Lung and Blood Institute, NIH. Lead contractor Macro International, Calverton, MD. For further information contact Dr. Kay Bartholomew.

CHAPTER 12 Fig. 13.1 From W. A. Hunt, L. W. Barnett, L. G. Branch, "Relapse Rates in Addiction Programs," *Journal of Clinical Psychology*, 1971, Vol. 27, 355. Reprinted by permission of John Wiley & Sons, Inc. Fig. 13.2 From G. A. Marlatt, J. R. Gordon, *Relapse Prevention: Maintenance Strategies in the Treatment of Addictive Behaviors*, Guilford Press, 1985. Reprinted with permission of the publisher. Fig. 13.6 With permission from Project PANDA, Center for Health Promotion and Prevention Research, University of Texas–Houston School of Public Health. For further information contact Dr. Patricia Dolan Mullen.

NAME INDEX

Abbey, H., 392
Abe, K., 134
Abel, E., 135
Abraham, C., 94, 189, 190, 199, 368
Abrams, D., 368
Abramson, S. L., xviii, 96, 235, 249, 391, 392, 410
Adair, E. G., 22
Adger, H., Jr., 427
Affonso, D. D., 455, 455 table 13.1
Agars, J., 136
Aggleton, P. (ed.), 368
AIDS Community Demonstration Projects, 241
Ainsworth, B. E., 340
Ainsworth, T. H. (ed.), 100, 102, 102 table 4.7, 107, 108, 205, 206
Airhihenbuwa, C. O., 259
Ajzen, I., 60, 61, 65, 66, 83, 84, 94, 220, 309, 355, 357, 377
Alan Guttmacher Institute, 354
Alberts, M. J., 30
Alcoe, S. Y., 135
Alemi, F., 117
Alexander, M., 340
Allegrante, J., 188, 203
Allen, B. F., 156
Allen, D. B., 64
Allen, J., 107, 108, 109, 192
Allen, M. (ed.), 89
Allen, R., 107, 108
Allen, S., 457, 458
Allensworth, D., 201
Allman, C. J., 427
Altman, D., 203
Altman, D. G., 214, 215, 215 table 6.14, 216, 217 table 6.15, 242
Altpeter, M., 206
Altschuld, J. W., 18
American Psychological Association, Commission on Youth Violence, 49
American Society of Heating, Refrigerating, and Air-Conditioning Engineers, 391
Ammerman, A. S., 157, 182

Anda, R. F., 64
Anderson, E., 60
Anderson, J. R., 185
Anderson, S., 140
Andrews, J. A., 454, 458
Andriole, D. A., 104
Anstine, P. S., 432
Anstine, S., 425, 426, 430, 432, 442
Antolini, I., 391
Arfken, C., 20
Arfken, C. L., 104
Arizmendi, T. G., 455, 455 table 13.1
Armstrong, M. A., 340
Aronson, E. (ed.), 65, 81, 89, 90, 172, 180, 181, 189, 190, 194, 229, 281, 315, 367, 370
Arsham, G. M., 403
Ary, D., 52, 60
Atkin, C. K., 277, 278
Atkin, C. K. (ed.), 277, 278
Auslander, W., 20
Axner, M., 210
Axton, R. A., 135

Bachman, J. G., 425, 428
Bachman, K. J., 138, 235, 307, 450
Backbier, E., 84, 87, 87–88 table 4.3
Backial, M., 403
Baer, J. S., 103, 138, 462
Baglioni, A. J., Jr., 17
Bahir, A., 391
Bakeman, R., 24
Baker, D., 390
Baker, S., 49
Balabanis, M., 250
Balcazar, F. E., 214, 215, 215 table 6.14, 216, 217 table 6.15
Balderman, B., 261
Balding, J. (ed.), xviii
Bando, T., 134
Bandura, A., 33, 60, 68, 83, 84, 94, 96, 97, 98, 99, 100, 115, 147, 150, 180, 183, 190, 193, 194, 195, 196, 197, 281, 294, 309, 314, 315, 355, 357, 373, 401, 410, 433

481

Name Index

Bane, A. L., 84, 164, 196
Banspach, S., 339
Baranowski, T., xvii, 7, 12, 47, 96, 320, 321, 322, 332, 333, 340, 345, 433
Barbec, R. A., 390
Bargh, J. A. (ed.), 370–371
Barnett, L. W., 457, 458 fig. 13.1
Barron, K., 28, 34
Bartholomew, L. K., xviii, 25, 28, 34, 96, 139, 147, 156, 177, 182, 188, 234, 235, 237, 245, 249, 259, 291, 297, 299–300 table 8.1, 312, 321, 335, 391, 392, 395 fig. 11.1, 410, 417, 418
Basch, C. E., 22, 249, 354
Basen-Engquist, K. M., 7, 60, 305, 339, 373
Bassford, T. L., 25
Bast, R. C., Jr., 135
Baum, A. (ed.), 372
Bauman, K. E., 79, 85
Bauman, L. J., 22
Bebchuk, J., 139
Beck, B. M., 135
Becker, B. L., 16–17, 18
Becker, M. H., 64, 65, 93, 94, 367
Becker, M. H. (ed.), 47, 56, 297
Bee, D. E., 7
Belasquez, M. M., 460
Belk, R. (ed.), 278
Bell, D. E., 371
Bellingham, R., 107, 108, 109, 192
Bellis, J. M., 248, 249
Benne, K. D., 112
Bennett, P., 367–368
Bennis, W. G., 112
Bental, D. S., 247
Berg, B. L., 23
Bergman, A. B., 64
Berkley, J. Y., 110
Berkowitz, B., 210
Berkowitz, L. (ed.), 90, 91, 181, 367, 368, 370, 370–371, 372
Berlin, N., xviii, 96, 139, 147, 182, 235, 245, 259, 395 fig. 11.1, 410
Berry, C. C., 132, 134
Bertels, C., 30
Beyer, J. M., 105, 156, 182, 295
Bianchi, C., 22
Bibeau, D., xvii, 4, 79
Biddle, A. K., 64
Biesecker, G. E., 49
Biglan, A., 52, 60
Bijur, E., 387, 389, 392
Bird, S. T., 23, 24 fig. 2.1, 61, 62
Bishop-Townsend, V., 54, 60
Blaine, T. M., 430
Bliss-Holtz, V. J., 455 table 13.1
Bloom, J. R., 103
Bloom, S. R., 392
Bloom, S. S., 142

Boberg, E. W., 245
Boer, H., 94
Boles, S. M., 19, 332, 343
Bone, L. R., 292, 293 fig. 8.1, 301
Boner, A. L., 391
Bonnie, R. J. (ed.), 140
Boon, M. E., xviii
Booth, E. M., 142, 143
Borko, H., 378
Borne, D., 178, 179 table 6.2
Bosker, R. J., xviii, 328, 330, 335, 345, 346, 379
Bossert, T. J., 301
Bosworth, K., 245
Bouman, M., 203
Bowditch, J. L., 106, 107
Boyd, B., 101
Boyd, W. L., 109
Boyer, R., 84, 190
Bracht, N., 172, 301
Bracht, N. (ed.), 172, 290, 429, 434, 440, 443, 445
Brackbill, R., 64, 343
Bradac, J. J. (ed.), 368, 371
Bradet, R., 84
Bradford, L., 21
Brady, C. A., 315
Braeken, D., 355
Brager, G. A., 208, 209 table 6.12
Braithwaite, R. L., 22
Branch, L. G., 457, 458 fig. 13.1
Brandon, R., 140
Brannon, B. R., 370
Brasfield, T. L., 204
Brass, L. M., 30
Bratina, P., 30
Brennan, F. A., 245
Brennan, P., 245
Brent, D. A., 427
Brewer W. F. (ed.), 185
Bricker, E., 245
Briggs, L. J., 142
Bright, F., 303
Brink, S. G., xviii, 7, 293 fig. 8.1, 296, 305, 309, 310 table 8.2, 311
Britten, K. M., 392
Britton, B., 252, 274
Britton, M. G., 392
Brock, D. J. H., 135
Brooks, J. M., 30
Brown, J. E., 136
Brown, R., 203
Brown, R. W., 392
Brown, S. J., 245
Brownson, R. C., 139
Bruce, B. C. (ed.), 185
Brug, J., 83, 181–182, 182, 187, 248, 248 table 7.4, 249 fig. 7.7
Brugman, E., 353, 354, 360
Bruning, R. H., 185

Name Index

Bryant, F. B., 56, 59
Bulger, D. W., 92, 198, 412
Bull, F. C., 248 table 7.4
Bunker, J. F., xvii, 32, 76, 77
Bunton, R., 367–368
Buono, A. F., 106, 107
Burdine, J. N., 5, 203
Burge, H. (ed.), 389, 390
Burgoon, M., 368, 371
Burnett, J., 241 table 7.1, 252
Burns, K. L., 403
Burris, M. A., 19, 112, 213
Burrows, B., 390
Butterfoss, F. D., 109, 110, 182, 208
Butz, A. M., 392, 457
Byers, T., 340

Caces, M. F., 427
Cacioppo, J. T., 90, 91, 138, 181, 235, 244, 367, 368, 370–371
Cacioppo, J. T. (ed.), 64, 65, 94, 367, 370
Caffarella, R., 162 Table 5.6
Cain, W., 390, 457
Call, R. S., 390
Campbell, D. T., 22, 58, 259, 320, 345
Campbell, M. D., 16–17, 18
Campbell, M. K., 157, 182
Capra, A. M., 392
Carbonari, J., 59, 236, 454, 458, 460
Carey, K., 250
Carey, M., 339
Carnegie Council on Adolescent Development, 441
Carovano, K., 213
Carroll, J. S., 368
Carvajal, S., 341
Cassady, C. E., 292
Cassidy, A. (ed.), 208, 269, 272
Casswell, S. (ed.), 426
Catford, J., 118
Cats-Baril, W. L., 117
Cawsey, A., 247
CDC: AIDS Community Demonstration Projects Research Group, 241
CDC: Centers for Disease Control and Prevention, 24, 26, 52, 343, 387, 389
Center for Pediatric Research, 270
Centerwall, B. S., 49
Chaffe, S. H., 244
Chaiken, S., 90, 189, 190, 370, 370–371
Chalela, P., 238, 242, 315
Chamberlain, R. M., 137
Chang, C., 391
Chapman, M. D., 390
Charson, L., 403
Chavis, D., 110
Checkoway, B., 206
Chewning, B., 245
Chin, R., 112

Choi, W. S., 132, 134
Chorba, T. L., 64
Cialdini, R. B., 368
Clark, C. M., 378
Clark, N. M., xvii, 12, 47, 95, 95 table 4.5, 136, 147, 320, 321, 322, 332, 333, 340, 345, 392, 394, 395, 403
Clarke, W., 96
Cline, M. G., 390
Cliver, S., 456, 457
Coates, T. J., 207
Cobb, R. W., 117, 118, 119, 218, 219
Cochrane Collaboration, 59
Cohen, A., 457
Cohen, A. H., 391
Cohen, J. E., 79, 85
Cohen, R. (ed.), 259
Cohen, S., 103, 138, 462
Cohen, S. (ed.), 100, 102 table 4.7
Coie, J., 49
Coleman, J. S., 76
Collins, J., 361, 367
Combes, R., xviii, 96, 235, 410
Comings, J., 19, 112, 213, 214
COMMIT Research Group, 301
Comstock, G. (ed.), 367
Confino-Cohen, R., 391
Congdon, B., xviii, 156, 177, 188
Conner, M., 79, 83, 84
Conner, M. (ed.), 83, 84, 94
Contreras, J. M., 138
Cook, D. T., 22, 58, 320, 345
Cook, K., 138, 235, 307, 450
Cook, K. C., 139
Cook, S., 457
Cooper, C. L., 456 table 13.2
Cooper, H., 47, 55
Copps, T. J., 64
Corbett, J., 301
Corbett, K., 301
Corbin, J., 344
Corby, N. H., 241
Coss, S., 403
Costa, F. M., 54–55
Cotter, J., 391
Cotton, D., 87, 87–88 table 4.3, 189, 193
Cottrell, L., 25
Cowley, R. A., 64
Cox, D. J., 96
Cox, F. M. (ed.), 111, 112, 113, 202, 212
Coyle, K., 339
Crain, E. F., 387, 389, 390, 392
Craun, A. M., 136
Creholder, H., xviii, 342
Creer, T. L., 95 table 4.5, 394, 395, 403, 406
Cristinzio, S., 248, 248 table 7.4
Cropp, G., 403
Cuijpers, C., 390, 457
Cullen, K. W., xviii

483

Name Index

Cullinane, M., 250
Cummings, T. G., 192, 208
Cunningham, J., 389
Curry, S. J., 248 table 7.4
Cutrice, L., 117
Cutter, G., xvii, 12, 47, 320, 321, 322, 332, 333, 340, 345
Cutter, G. R., 456, 457
Cystic Fibrosis Foundation, 312
Czyzewski, D. I., xviii, 25, 34, 96, 139, 147, 156, 177, 182, 188, 235, 237, 245, 249, 259, 291, 297, 299–300 table 8.1, 312, 321, 335, 395 fig. 11.1, 410, 417, 418

Dahlquist, L., 28, 34
Daka-Mulwanda, V., 109, 208
Dana, G. S., 79, 85
Daniels, W. R., 21
Darby, A. L., 135
Davenport, M. G., 389
Davies, J. K. (ed.), 117
Davies, P. (ed.), 368
Davis, A., 392
Davis, C. A., 254
Davis, R. M., 139
Davis, S., 293 fig. 8.1
Dawson, D. A., 427
Dawson, D. V., 30
Dawson, K., 392
Dawson, L., 106
de la Sota, A., 403
de la Torre, J., 238, 242, 315
De Leeuw, E., 118
De Madres a Madres, 213
De Vries, H., xviii, 5, 23, 25, 47, 54, 61, 65, 83, 84, 87, 87–88 table 4.3, 89, 93, 173, 196, 248, 248 table 7.4, 249, 249 fig. 7.7
De Vries, N., 190
de Zapien, J. G., 104
Deaux, K., 461
Dede, C., 244
Deffenbacher, J. L., 136
Delamater, A. M., 396
Delbecq, A., 22
DeMuth, N. M., 138
Den Boer, D. J., 93, 157, 182, 196, 248, 248 table 7.4
Denzin, N. K. (ed.), 47
Derry, S. J. 185
Desvousges, W. H., 23
DeVellis, B. M., 92, 94, 157, 182, 198, 412
DeVellis, R. F., 157, 182, 340
Deven, F., 355
Diaz, Y. E., 204
DiClemente, C. C., xviii, 59, 86, 87, 87–88 table 4.3, 156, 183, 189, 190, 194, 197, 236, 248, 248 table 7.4, 249, 330, 454, 457, 458, 460
DiClemente, R. J., 24

Dijker, A. J., 176
Dijkstra, A., 248, 248 table 7.4, 294
Dijkstra, M., xviii, 23, 47, 84
Dillard, J., 66, 189
Dillworth, M. (ed.), 256
DiMatteo, M. R., 136
Dimeff, L. A., 199
Dimicco, A., 340
DiNicola, D. D., 136
Dishion, T., 49
Djukanovic, R., 392
Doak, C. C., 252–253, 273, 274
Doak, L. G., 252–253, 273, 274
Dockery, D. W., 389
Dodge, J. A., 136
Dodge, K., 49
Dolan-Mullen, D., 454, 457
Donnelly, J., 136
D'Onofrio, C. N. (ed.), 183
Donovan, J. E., 54–55
Dorfman, L., 119, 214, 216, 217–218, 445
Dow, L., 111, 213
Drake, M. L., 455 table 13.1
Drug Strategies, 441
Dryfoos, J., 425
DuBois, D. L., 138
Duggan, A. K., 49
Duhl, L., 25, 118, 119
Duncan, R., 156
Dungy, C. I., 391
Duroux, P., 392
Dusenbury, L., 441
Dusenbury, L. J., 303
Dutton, J., 250
Duzey, O., 403

Eagly, A. H., 189, 190, 370, 370–371
Earnshaw, J. S., 392
Earp, J. A., 5, 53, 138, 206
Eckhardt, L., 56
Edelman, B. (ed.), 60
Edling, C., 391
Eggleston, A., 390, 392, 457
Ehrhardt, A. A., 25
Eilat-Greenberg, S., 56
Eiser, C., 156
El-Askari, G., 115
El-Basel, N., 178, 179 table 6.2
Elder, C. D., 117, 118, 119, 218, 219
Elder, J., 142, 143, 241 table 7.1
Ell, K., 103
Elliott, S. D., 427
Ellis, J., 254
Ellison, R. C., xviii, 138
Emerson, J. A., 390, 457
Eng, E., 18, 19, 26, 104, 206
Engquist, K. E., xviii, 293 fig. 8.1, 309, 310 table 8.2, 311
Enguidanos, S. M., 241

Name Index

Ennett, S. T., 5, 53
Epstein, L. H., 138
Erickson, P., 117
Eriksen, M., xviii, 91, 132, 134, 139, 293 fig. 8.1, 296, 305, 309, 310 table 8.2, 311, 344
Erlich, J. L. (ed.), 18, 111, 112, 113, 202, 212
Eron, L. D., 49
Ershoff, D. H., 453–454, 454, 457, 458
Escobedo, L. G., 64
Evans, D., 392, 395, 403
Evans, R., III, 390
Evans, R. I., 84, 164, 196, 372, 374

Fairhurst, S. R., 460
Falco, M., 441
Fan, Y. C., 245
Farbakhsh, K., 426, 430
Farkas, A. J., 132, 134
Farrington, D., 49
Farris, E., 461
Fava, J., 460
Fava, J. L., 248, 249
Fawcett, J., 455 table 13.1
Fawcett, S., 26, 101, 139–140
Fawcett, S. B., 17, 110, 214, 215, 215 table 6.14, 216, 217 table 6.15
Fayad, B., 30
Fehir, J., 213
Feighery, E., 109, 132, 134
Feldman, C., 395
Feldman, C. H., 395, 403
Feldmann, E., 30
Fellin, P., 18
Fenter, L., 457
Ferencz, C., 453
Fernandez, M., xviii, 96, 139, 147, 182, 235, 245, 259, 291, 312, 392, 395 fig. 11.1, 410, 417, 418
Fernandez-Esquer, M. E., 238
Fetterman, D. M. (ed.), 324
Ffrench, M. L., 309
Field-Fass, M., 138
Fike, J. M., 64
Filbert, L., 109, 208
Finer, D., 140, 201
Fingerhut, L. A., 457
Fink, R., xviii, 25, 312
Fink, S. V., 245
Finkelstein, D., 392
Finkelstein, J. A., 392
Finnegan, J., 429, 433
Finnegan, J. R., 301, 425, 426, 430, 432, 442
Fiocoo, G., 390
Fireman, P., 403
Fischer, C. S., 212
Fishbein, M., 83, 241, 249, 330, 355, 357
Fisher, E. B., 104
Fisher, E. B., Jr., 20
Fisher, J. L., 110

Fisher, R., 144 table 5.1, 212
Fishman, S., 253
Fiske, S. T. (ed.), 79, 83, 91, 94, 182, 187, 190, 192, 197, 235
FitzGerald, S. J., 340
Flax, V., 206
Flay, B. R., 321, 367, 370
Fleisher, L., 248, 248 table 7.4
Flesch, R. F., 253
Flora, J. A., 132, 134, 157, 238, 244, 308
Florin, P., 110
Floyd, R. L., 453–454
Flynn, B. C., 117
Flynn, B. S., 79, 85, 457
Folkman, S., 95, 95 table 4.5
Fontana, L., 244
Forbing, S. E., 140
Forrest, J. D., 354
Forster, J., 426
Forster, J. L., 425, 426, 430, 432, 442
Forsyth, A. D., 339
Fortenberry, J. D., 54–55
Fortin, C., 84, 190
Fortmann, S., 308
Fowler, M. G., 389
Fox, C. L., 140
Francisco, V. T., 110
Frank, G. C., 134
Franklin, B. A. K., 157
Frankowski, R. F., 56
Freeman, H. E., 12, 40, 47, 297, 320, 321, 322, 323, 323 table 9.1, 324, 324 fig. 9.1, 325, 327, 337, 345
Freestone, J., 115
Freimouth, C., 277
Freimuth, V. S., 278
Freire, P., 22, 111, 212–213, 260
Frey, J. H., 23
Friday, G. A., 403
Friedman, R. H., 250, 251–252 fig. 7.8
Fry, E., 253
Fukao, A., 134
Fulk, J. B., 101
Fulton, J. E., 340
Fultz, P., 233
Funch, D., 103

Gadotti, M., 213
Gagne, R. M., 142
Galant, S., 391
Gallion, K. J., 204, 238, 242, 315
Gallup, J., 391
Ganster, D. C., 138
Gardner, S. E. (ed.), 426
Garg, R., 389
Gargreave, F. E., 392
Garza, I. R., 238, 242, 315
Gavin, M., 370
Gearon, S. A. N., 157

485

Name Index

Gedney, K., 233
Geller, E. S., 241 table 7.1
Gentry, E. M., 140
Gerards, F., 93, 196
Gergen, J., 387, 389, 390
German, D. F., 403
Germeny, B. A., 245
Gershwin, M. E., 391
Getz, J. G., 196, 372, 374
Ghatala, E., 186
Gilbert, D. T. (ed.), 79, 83, 91, 94, 182, 187, 190, 192, 197, 235
Gilbert, L., 178, 179 table 6.2
Gilchrist, L. D., 367, 373
Gilfillan, A., 135
Gilmore, G. D., 16–17, 18
Giloth, B. E. (ed.), 57, 57 fig. 3.2
Gilpin, E. A., 132, 134
Gingiss, L., 7
Ginsberg, M. B., 260
Ginsburg, M. J., 49
Giovino, G. A., 91, 132, 134, 453–454
Gira, C., 403
Gittelsohn, A. M., 395
Glanz, K., xvii, 4, 28, 61, 79, 181–182, 182, 187, 248, 248 table 7.4
Glanz, K. (ed.), xvii, 5, 7, 19, 61, 79, 83, 84, 93, 96, 101, 102, 103, 105, 106, 113, 138, 157, 172, 173, 182, 188, 191, 197, 204, 205, 206, 255, 290, 292, 293 fig. 8.1, 295, 296, 300, 302, 355, 376, 433
Glasgow, R., 92, 198, 412
Glasgow, R. E., 19, 136, 321, 332, 343
Gleason, J., 301
Gleason, L. R., 370
Glenday, M. C., 56
Global Initiative for Asthma, 391, 392
Glover, L. H., 185
Glowacz, K. M., 370
Glynn, S. M., 252, 274
Godard, P., 392
Godin, G., 79, 83, 84, 190
Goebel, J. B., 64
Goedhart, H., 353, 354, 360
Goeppinger, J., 17
Gold, M. S., 427
Gold, R. S., xviii, 96, 139, 147, 182, 235, 245, 259, 291, 312, 395 fig. 11.1, 410, 417, 418
Gold, W. (ed.), 244, 245, 247, 249
Goldberg, A., 391
Goldenberg, R. L., 456, 457
Goldmann, D. A., 392
Goldstein, A. O., 79, 85
Gollwitzer, M., 198
Gonder-Frederick, L., 96
Goodman, D. D., 213
Goodman, L. S., 157
Goodman, R. M., xvii, 7, 17, 23, 24 fig. 2.1, 26, 61, 62, 101, 105, 106, 109, 110, 139–140, 156, 173, 182, 188, 203, 204, 206, 208, 292, 293 fig. 8.1, 295, 296, 300, 301
Goodwin, G. D., 457
Gordon, J. R., 68, 87, 87–88 table 4.3, 93, 147, 454, 459 fig. 13.2, 460
Gordon, J. R. (ed.), 199
Gordon, N., 30
Gortamaker, S., 389, 390
Gottheil, E., 103
Gottlieb, B. H., 100
Gottlieb, B. H. (ed.), 138, 462
Gottlieb, N. H., xvii, xviii, 4, 7, 32, 64, 76, 79, 85, 100, 102, 102 table 4.7, 139, 205, 206, 208, 209 table 6.12, 292, 293, 293 fig. 8.1, 294, 296, 303, 305, 309, 310 table 8.2, 311
Goumans, M., 140
Gowland, G., 391
Graeff, J. A., 142, 143
Grant, B. F., 427
Green, F. (ed.), 426
Green, L. W., xvii, xviii, 2, 4, 5, 6 fig. 1.1, 7, 8, 12, 18, 19, 22, 27, 28, 29 fig. 2.3, 30, 33, 39, 47, 56, 75, 76, 84, 94, 101, 132,138, 148, 181, 182, 183, 206, 291, 293 fig. 8.1, 294, 296, 297, 305, 309, 311, 320, 322, 342, 344, 367, 388
Green, L. W. (ed.), 118
Greenbaum, T. L., 47
Greenberg, L., 30
Greene, J. C., 324
Greene, W. H., xvii, 4, 32, 76, 208, 209 table 6.12
Greenfield, T., 428
Greenhouse, J. B., 49
Greenspan, P., 392
Gregg, E. W., 340
Gremy, I., 457
Gritz, E., 341
Gritz, E. R., 137
Groff, J. Y., 234, 454, 457
Gronlund, E. E., 143
Grossman, W. (ed.), 208, 269, 272
Grothaus, L. C., 248 table 7.4
Grotta, J. C., 30
Guadagnoli, E., 460
Guba, E. G., 344
Guenther-Grey, C., 241
Guerin, J. C., 392
Guerra, N. G., 2, 6, 49
Gustafson, D. H., 22, 117, 245

Habana-Hafner, S., 110, 208
Haddix, A., 91, 132, 134
Haglund, B. J. A., 140, 201
Hale, J. L., 66, 189
Haley, N., 7, 19, 302, 376
Halfon, N., 390
Hall, A., 100, 102 table 4.7
Hall, G. E., 297
Halonen, M., 390

Name Index

Halpern, G., 391
Hamilton, M. A., 89
Hamilton, R., 186
Hampson, S. E., 136
Hancock, T., 22, 25, 117
Hanna, M. G., 431, 440
Hannafin, M. J., 244
Hansen, W. B., 84, 164, 196, 370
Hardcastle, D. M., 7, 290, 295, 296
Harkavy, J., 156
Harlan, C., 206
Harris, D. (ed.), xviii
Harris, E., 201
Harris, J. S. (ed.), 107, 108, 109, 192
Harris, K. J., 110
Harris, L. M. (ed.), 244
Harrison, D., 20
Harrison, J. A., 94
Harrist, R. B., 305
Hart, G. (ed.), 368
Haskell, W. L., 340
Hassan, H., 395
Hatch, J. W., 104
Hatry, H., 320
Hatry, H. (ed.), 292, 297, 321, 324, 325, 328
Hatsukami, D., 457, 458
Hauth, A. C., 204
Havelock, R. G., 302
Havis, J., 84, 164, 196
Hawkins, R., 245
Hawkins, R. (ed.), 244
Haynes, R. B. (ed.), 136
Hays, R. B., 207
Heaney, C. A., 101, 102, 103, 138, 205
Heather, N. (ed.), 156
Hedges, L. V., 47, 55
Hedlund, S., 303
Heitzmann, C. A., 212
Hellerstedt, W., 457, 458
Helman, C. G., 255
Henderson, A. M. (trans.), 202
Henderson, K. A., 340
Hendrick, R. E., 135
Hendricks, S. A., 64
Hendrickx, L., 367, 368
Hennessy, C. H., 343
Hennrikus, D. J., 430
Henry-Amar, M., 392
Henshaw, S. K., 354
Herman, C. (ed.), 90
Hermann, N. B., 137
Hersey, J. C., 104, 194
Hersh, M., 387, 389, 392
Hewstone, M. (ed.), 5, 54, 65, 84, 89, 173
Hiatt, R. A. (ed.), 183
Hickenbottom, S., 234
Higgins, C., 392
Higgins, C. A., 297
Higgins, D., 241

Hindi-Alexander, M. C., 403
Hirsch, B. J., 138
Hisamichi, S., 134
Hochbaum, G. M., 4, 5, 28
Hodgkins, S., 84
Hodgson, T., 389
Hoelscher, D. M., 340
Hoffman, H. J., 456, 457
Hofstetter, C. R., 390, 457
Holcomb, C., 254
Holgate, S. T., 392
Hollis, J., 321
Hollis, R., 104
Holloway, S., 208, 209 table 6.12
Holman, H., 47
Holtgrave, D. R., 87, 87–88 table 4.3, 188, 191
Homer, C. J., 392
Honsinger, R., 390
Hoover, S., 17
Horev, Z., 391
Hospers, H. J., 83, 93, 157, 182, 196, 197, 248, 248 table 7.4, 396
Hough, J. F., 343
House, J. S., 103, 138
Hovell, M. F., 241 table 7.1, 390, 457
Hovland, C. I., 371
Howard, M., 361, 367
Howarth, H., 392
Howe, C. Z., 340
Howe, H. E., Jr. (ed.), 380
Howell, J. M., 297
Hoyle, R. H., 292
Hoyt, K. B., 109
Hu, S., 238
Huberman, A. M., 23, 47, 105, 344
Huesman, L. R., 49
Hugentobler, M. K., 20
Hughes, G. W., 403
Humberto, A. H., 389, 392
Hunt, R. E., 156
Hunt, W. A., 457, 458 fig. 13.1
Hunter, J. E., 89
Hunter-Gamble, D., 24
Hurley, S. F., 135
Huss, K., 392, 457
Hutchinson, K., 19
Hyppolite, K., 250

Imai, Y., 134
Imle, M. A., 455 table 13.1
Ingram, J. M., 390
Irizarry, C., 115
Irwin, J. C., 391
Irwin, J. W., 254
Iscoe, I., 25
Isenberg, D. J., 372
Israel, A., 101, 102, 103, 138, 205
Israel, B. A., 20, 102 table 4.7, 103, 104, 138, 206

Name Index

Itoh, O., 134
Ivanoff, A., 178, 179 table 6.2
Iverson, D. C., 302

Jackson, C., 308
Jackson, K., 19
Jackson, R. E., 24
Jackson-Thompson, J., 20
Jacobs, A. M., 22, 395, 403
Jacobs, D. R., Jr., 340
Jacobs, I. J., 135
Jacobson, D. E., 138
James, C. (ed.), xviii
Janis, I. L., 147
Janz, N. K., 64, 65, 93, 94, 136, 367
Jeffery, R. W., 440, 457, 458
Jencks, C., 60
Jernigan, D., 119, 214, 216, 217–218, 445
Jessor, R., 49, 54–55, 428, 429, 433
Jette, A., 250
Joffe, H., 455, 455 table 13.1
Johnson, C., 138, 235, 307, 450
Johnson, C. A., 370
Johnson, C. C., 139
Johnson, J., 390
Johnson, K., 208, 269, 272
Johnson, S., 453
Johnson, S. B., 156
Johnson, W., 241
Johnston, J. J., 64
Johnston, L. D., 425, 428
Johnston, M., 190, 199
Johnston, P., 392
Jonas, J. R., 242, 269
Jones, E. F., 354
Jones, R., 247
Jorgensen, C., 203
Jorgensen, C. M., 140
Joswiak, M. L., 340
Julian, D. M., 96
Juniper, E. F., 392

Kaftarian, S. J. (ed.), 324
Kagan, S. L., 109
Kahneman, D., 368, 370
Kaldor, J. M., 135
Kalichman, S. C., 204
Kamarck, T., 103
Kamarck, T. W., 138, 462
Kandel, D., 427
Kang, B. C., 390
Kaplan, B. H., 64
Kaplan, D., 395, 403
Kaplan, M., 403
Kaplan, R. M., 212
Kaslow, R., 390
Kasprzyk, D., 83, 84, 355
Kattan, M., 390

Kay, L. S., 87, 87–88 table 4.3, 188, 191, 204, 241, 315
Kazdin, A. E., 33
Kazis, L. E., 250
Kegeles, S. M., 207
Kegler, M. C., 26, 101, 105, 106, 139–140, 173, 182, 188, 204, 206, 292, 293 fig. 8.1, 295, 300
Keintz, M. K., 248, 248 table 7.4
Kelder, S. H., 429
Kelley, M., 117
Kelley, M. (ed.), 117
Kelly, J. A., 204
Kelsey, E., 292, 303
Kendrick, J. S., 457
Keteyian, S., 136
Kiecolt-Glaser, J. K., 138
Kiely, M. C., 324
Kilburn, K. H., 132
Kingdon, J. W., 118, 119, 219
Kingsbury, L., 172
Kingsolver, K., 138, 462
Kirby, D., 339, 361, 367
Kirk, J., 344
Kirmil-Gray, K., 95 table 4.5, 394
Kirsch, I. S., 254
Kishchuk, N., 6 fig. 1.1, 18, 30, 75, 84
Klein, T., 109, 208
Kleinman, J. C., 457
Klibanoff, L. S., 104, 194
Kline, A., 392
Kling, J., 212
Kluckhohn, C., 255
Knoke, D. 118
Kobrin, S., 157, 182, 248, 248 table 7.4
Koch, G., 293 fig. 8.1
Koenning, G., 28, 34
Koffka, K., 184
Kohler, C. L., 457
Kok, G. J., xviii, 5, 7, 23, 25, 28, 47, 50, 54, 61, 65, 66, 79, 83, 84, 86, 89, 92, 93, 94, 156, 173, 176, 181–182, 182, 187, 189, 190, 196, 197, 198, 203, 248, 248 table 7.4, 290, 295, 296, 309, 311 fig. 8.3, 328, 330, 335, 345, 346, 355, 357, 360, 361, 367, 373, 374, 377, 378, 379, 380, 396, 412, 457, 460
Kolbe, L., 361, 367
Kolbe, L. J., 7, 182, 302
Komro, K., 429, 430, 432, 433, 442
Komro, K. A., 425, 426, 432, 442
Koob, J. J., 204
Koomen, W., 176
Kotses, H., 95 table 4.5, 394, 395, 406
Kozak, P. P., 391
Kraemer, H. C., 103
Kraft, C., 107, 108
Kraut, K. L., 115
Kresnow, M. J., 64

Name Index

Kretzmann, J., 17, 27, 212
Kreuger, R. A., 22, 47
Kreuter, Marshall W., xvii, 2, 4, 8, 19, 27, 28, 29 fig. 2.3, 33, 39, 40, 101, 132, 137, 148, 157, 182, 206, 248, 248 table 7.4, 249, 291, 322, 342, 388
Kreuter, Matthew W., 19, 27
Kromer, M. E., 389, 392
Kruse, J., 453
Kuo, A. R., 64
Kusserow, R., 428
Kuttner, M. J., 396

La Chance, A., 321
Labarthe, D. R., 134, 135
Labonte, R., 111
Lachter, R. B., 426
Ladner, J. (ed.), 60
Ladson-Billings, G., 212, 260
Lafond, A. K., 301
Lam, D. J., 104, 194
Land, G. H., 456, 457
Landers, C., 7, 19, 302, 376
Landis, K. R., 103, 138
Lando, H., 321, 457, 458
Lang, S. M., 457
Latham, G., 92, 198, 412
Laumann, E. O., 118
Lawson, E., 201
Lazarus, R. S., 95, 95 table 4.5, 96, 147
Lazarus, R. S. (ed.), 95, 95 table 4.5
Leaderer, B., 390, 457
Lechner, L., 83
Leenders, F. J., 378
Lefebvre, R. C., 157, 238
LeFevre, M., 453
Lefkowitz, M. M., 49
Leickly, F., 390
Leippe, M. R., 371
Lenderink, T., 182, 187
Lepage, S. S., 457
Lepper, M., 134
Lepper, M. R., 410
Lerman, C., 188
Leung, P., 403
Leventhal, H., 367, 370
Leventhal, J. M., 392
Levin, B., 392, 395
Levin, S., 340
Levine, D. M., 138
Levine, S. R., 30
Levinson, R. A., 55, 60
Levison, M. J., 392, 395, 403
Leviton, L., 157
Lewin, K., 76, 208
Lewinsohn, M., 136
Lewis, C. E., 403
Lewis, F. M., xvii, 12, 22, 28, 47, 61, 320, 322

Lewis, F. M. (ed.), xvii, 5, 7, 19, 61, 79, 83, 84, 93, 96, 101, 102, 103, 105, 106, 113, 138, 157, 172, 173, 182, 188, 191, 197, 204, 205, 206, 255, 290, 292, 293 fig. 8.1, 294, 295, 296, 300, 302, 355, 376, 433
Lewis, M. (ed.), 49
Lewis, M. A., 403
Lewis, M. J., 7
Lewis, P., 95 table 4.5, 395
Lewis, R. K., 110
Lewis, S. N., 456 table 13.2
Lezin, N. A., 19, 27
Li, G., 49
Liberman, A., 370–371
Lichtenstein, E. 103, 138, 301, 454, 458, 462
Lichtman, R. R., 103
Lieberman, D. A., 245, 247
Lieberman, E., 457
Lieu, T. A., 392
Lincoln, Y. S., 344
Lincoln, Y. S. (ed.), 47
Lindsay, M. (ed.), 89, 90, 172, 180, 181, 189, 190, 194, 229, 281, 315, 367, 370
Lindsteadt, J. F., 157
Lindzey, G. (ed.), 65, 79, 81, 83, 91, 94, 182, 187, 190, 192, 197, 235, 255
Ling, J. C., 157
Linn, M., 245
Lipsey, M. W., 12, 40, 47, 297, 320, 321, 322, 323, 323 table 9.1, 324 fig. 9.1, 325, 327, 337, 345
Littlefield, D., 308
Liu, S., 134
Livingston, C., 378
Livingstone, J., 135
Locke, D. C., 256, 257
Locke, E. A., 92, 198, 412
Loeber, R., 49
Loomes, G., 371
Lorig, K., 4, 5, 28, 47
Loucks, S. F., 297
Loughrey, K., 157
Louie, D., 248 table 7.4
Lovato, C. Y., xviii, 7, 293 fig. 8.1, 296, 305, 309, 311, 344
Luepker, R. V., xviii, 134, 138, 139, 235, 307, 450
Lugg, C. A., 109
Lumb, J. R., 24
Lurie, D., 157
Lux, K. M., 60
Lynch, B. S. (ed.), 140
Lynn, H., 390
Lynn, L. E. (ed.), 60

Maas, L., 203
Madden, T. J., 61
Mager, R. F., 143
Mahoney, C. A., 340

Name Index

Maibach, E. (ed.), 66, 81, 83, 182, 189, 190
Maibach, E. W. (ed.), xvii, 76, 87, 87–88 table 4.3, 172, 189, 193, 197, 339
Mains, D. A., 56, 181, 182, 183
Majumdar, B., 261
Mak, H., 392
Malloy, M. H., 457
Malveaux, F. J., 390, 392, 457
Mandelberg, A., 391
Mangelsdorf, S. C., 138
Mann, L., 147
Manning, D., 274
Manning, T. (ed.), 244, 245, 247, 249
Manson, A., 395
Manstead, T., 84
Marcus, C. (ed.), 426
Marion, R. J., 403
Mariotto, M., xviii, 25, 312
Mark, M. M., 324
Markham, C., 391, 392
Marks, D., 368
Marlatt, G. A., 68, 87, 87–88 table 4.3, 93, 147, 199, 454, 459 fig. 13.2, 460
Marlatt, G. A. (ed.), 86, 87, 87–88 table 4.3, 183, 189, 190, 194, 197, 199
Martin, J., 134
Martin, K. E., 392
Martinez, F. D., 390
Martinez-Ramirez, M., 25
Mashiyama, S. T., 115
Mâsse, L. C., 339, 340
Maurer, T. J., 339
Mayer, J. A., 56, 241 table 7.1
Mayer, R. E., 185
Mayer, S. E., 60
Mayne, L., 206
Mayo, K., 340
McAlister, A. L., 64, 204, 238, 241, 242, 315
McAllister, J., 211
McBride, C., 248 table 7.4
McBride, C. M., 440, 457, 458
McCalister, L., 212
McCallum, M., 156
McCarter, R., 453
McConnaughy, K., 394
McCormick, L. K., xviii, 7, 23, 24 fig. 2.1, 25, 61, 62, 106, 237, 297, 299–300 table 8.1, 305, 321, 335, 341
McCray, E., 24
McCuan, R. A., 64
McDaniel, J. E., 256
McFarlane, J., 213
McGeary, M. (ed.), 60
McGovern, P. G., 425, 426, 430, 432, 442
McGrath, J., 76, 189
McGuire, L. W., 65, 81
McGuire, W. J., 89, 90, 172, 180, 181, 189, 190, 194, 229, 281, 315, 367, 370, 372
McKinlay, S. M., xviii

McKnight, J. L., 17, 27, 212
McLeroy, K., 26, 101, 139–140
McLeroy, K. R., xvii, 4, 5, 7, 23, 24 fig. 2.1, 61, 62, 79, 100, 102, 102 table 4.7, 106, 205, 206, 292, 293 fig. 8.1
McMurray, A., 136
McNabb, W. L., 22, 395, 403
McNiff-Mortimer, K., 390
McPherson, R. S., 340
McRae, S. G., 321
McTavish, F., 245
Mead, B., 457
Meertens, R. M., xviii, 92, 198, 342, 412
Meibach, E. (ed.), 87, 87–88 table 4.3, 188, 191
Meister, J. S., 104
Mekori, Y. A., 391
Mellins, R. B., 392, 395, 403
Melton, R. J., 308
Meltzer, E. O., 390, 457
Meltzer, S. B., 390, 457
Mendoza, G. R., 392
Mennie, M., 135
Mermelstein, R., 103, 138, 462
Merriam, S. B., 47
Merrit, R. K., 91, 132, 134
Mesters, I., xviii, 342
Mettlin, C., 103
Metzler, C. W., 52, 60
Meyerowitz, B. E., 370
Michaels, L., 403
Michaud, F., 84
Miczek, K., 2
Miklich, D. R., 403
Miles, M. B., 23, 47, 105, 344
Milio, N., 116, 116 fig. 4.3, 117, 119
Miller, B., 361, 367
Miller, M. L., 344
Miller, S. M. (ed.), 49
Miller, W. (ed.), 156
Miller, W. R., 250
Millstein, S. G. (ed.), 429
Minami, N., 134
Minkler, M., 7, 17, 22, 80, 104, 111, 113, 113 fig. 4.1, 114, 114 fig. 4.2, 139–140, 201, 211, 213
Minkler, M. (ed.), 17, 22, 103, 104, 111, 113, 114, 114 fig. 4.2, 139–140, 201, 211, 212, 213
Mishan, E. J., 322
Mitchell, H., 390
Mittelmark, M. B., 84, 164, 196
Mogilner, A., 254
Monahan, J., 190, 292, 296
Monakir, D., 391
Monat, A. (ed.), 95, 95 table 4.5
Monsees, B. S., 104
Montaño, D. E., 83, 84, 355
Montano, G., 25
Montgomery, K., 278

Name Index

Moore, D. T., 457
Moore, S., 245
Morag, H., 391
Morgan, D. L., 22, 47
Morgan, M. A., 115
Morgan, M. G., 204
Morgenstern, L., 234
Moriarty, D. G., 343
Moriarty, S., 241 table 7.1, 252
Morisky, D., 28
Morisky, D. E., 138
Morrill, C., 403
Morris, E., 390
Morrison, B. J., 390, 457
Morrison, K., 255
Mosenthal, B., 254
Moss, J. A., 390, 457
Mrazek, P., 157
Mudde, A. N., 93, 196
Mullen, D., xviii, 7, 47, 56, 57 fig. 3.2, 59, 64, 94, 181, 182, 183, 236, 249, 293, 453–454, 454, 457, 458, 460
Mullen, D. (ed.), 47, 56
Mullen, L. R., 7, 293
Mulvihill, C. K., 60
Munger, M. C., 79, 85
Munro, J., 20
Munson, K., 426
Murigande, C., 392, 457
Murphy, D. A., 339
Murphy, S., 367–368
Murray, A. B., 390, 391, 457
Murray, D., 432
Murray, D. M., 340, 430, 440, 441
Musick, J. S., 60
Mussman, M., 395

Nader, R., xviii, 138, 235, 307, 403, 450
Nagai, K., 134
Nan Kammen, W., 49
Naroll, R. (ed.), 259
National Cancer Institute, 90, 253, 340
National Health Strategy, 201
National Heart, Lung, and Blood Institute, 389, 390, 391, 392, 397
National Highway Traffic Safety Administration, 427
National Institute of Neurological Disorders and Stroke, 30
National Institute on Alcohol Abuse and Alcoholism, 427, 430
Natowicz, M. R., 135
Nazareno, F., 30
NCAB [Nationale Commissie AIDS Bestrijding], 353
Needleman, H. L., 49
Nercsmar, C., 390
Nettekoven, L., 301
Neuberger, J. S., 391

Newacheck, W., 389, 390
Newcomer, K. E., 320
Newcomer, K. E. (ed.), 292, 297, 321, 324, 325, 328
Newkirk, D. D., 391
Nichols, D. C., 315
Nicholson, L., 201
Nicol, L., 59, 236, 454
Nightingale, E. O. (ed.), 429
Nodora, J., 52, 339
Noell, J., 52, 60
Norback, D., 391
Norcross, J. C., 86, 87, 87–88 table 4.3, 183, 189, 190, 194, 197
Normal, A. L., 391
Norman, P., 79
Norman, P. (ed.), 83, 84, 94
Northouse, L. L., 103
Noviski, N., 391
Nutbeam, D., 201

Oberman, A., 340
O'Brien, K., 23
O'Byrne, M., 392
Ockene, J. K., 250, 251–252 fig. 7.8
O'Connor, R. D., 390, 457
Oden, S., 136
O'Donnell, M. (ed.), 100, 102, 102 table 4.7, 107, 108, 109, 192, 205, 206
O'Hara, N. M., xviii, 7, 293 fig. 8.1, 309, 310 table 8.2, 311
O'Hara-Tompkins, N. M., 7, 305
Ohkubo, T., 134
Oldenburg, B. F., 7, 290, 295, 296, 309
Olkin, I., 47
Olsen, J. M. (ed.), 90
O'Malley, M., 425, 428
O'Neill, M., 49
Oram, D. H., 135
Orbell, S., 84
O'Reilly, K., 204, 241, 315
Orlandi, M. A., 7, 19, 302, 317, 376
Orleans, C. T., 248, 248 table 7.4
Orum, A. M., 202
Ory, M. G., 138
Osterlind, S. J., 340
Ostrander, L., 136
Otten, W., 64, 187
Ottoson, J. M., 297
Overpeck, M. D., 390, 457
Ovrebo, B., 19
Owen, N., 309
Owens, B., 245
Owens, N. J., 20
Ownby, D., 390

Page, M. M. (ed.), 380
Paine-Andrews, A., 110
Pakula, L. C., 49

Name Index

Palmer, J. B., 392
Palmer, R. C., 56
Palmo, A. J. (ed.), 256
Papineau, D., 324
Parcel, G. S., xvii, xviii, 5, 7, 25, 28, 32, 34, 54, 60, 65, 76, 77, 79, 84, 86, 89, 96, 137, 138, 139, 147, 156, 173, 177, 182, 188, 235, 237, 245, 259, 290, 291, 293 fig. 8.1, 294, 296, 297, 299–300 table 8.1, 305, 307, 309, 310 table 8.2, 311, 311 fig. 8.3, 312, 321, 328, 330, 335, 339, 341, 345, 346, 355, 373, 377, 378, 379, 392, 395 fig. 11.1, 403, 410, 417, 418, 433, 450
Parker, D., 84
Parker, E. 18, 26, 101, 104, 139–140, 206
Parker, E. A., 104
Parker, L. E., 410
Parker, R. C., 252, 273
Parrott, R. L., xvii, 172, 189, 197
Parrott, R. L. (ed.), 66, 76, 81, 83, 87, 87–88 table 4.3, 182, 188, 189, 190, 191, 193
Parsons, T. (trans.), 202
Pasick, R. J., 255
Pasick, R. J. (ed.), 183
Pasmore, W. A. (ed.), 173
Pasta, D. J., 245
Pasteur, W., 30
Patrick, D. L., 117
Patterson, D., 156
Patterson, G. R., 49
Patterson, R. (ed.), 389, 390
Patton B., 144 table 5.1
Patton, M. Q., 23, 47, 320, 325, 331
Paul, O., 134
Paulussen, T., xviii, 5, 7, 54, 65, 84, 86, 89, 173, 296, 309, 311 fig. 8.3, 335, 355, 377, 378
Pedersen, S., 138, 235, 307, 450
Pereira, M. A., 340
Peroni, D. G., 391
Perper, J. A., 427
Perrin, J. M., 392
Perry, C. L., xviii, 49, 96, 138, 139, 235, 290, 307, 425, 426, 428, 429, 430, 432, 433, 440, 442, 450
Perry, D. G., 49
Persinger, G. S., 181, 182, 183
Peters, L., xviii, 328, 330, 335, 345, 346, 357, 360, 361, 373, 379, 380
Petersen, A. C. (ed.), 429
Peters-Golden, H., 103
Peterson, D. R., 457
Peterson, L., 378
Peterson, R. C., 457
Petosa, R., 60
Pettersson, B., 140, 201
Petty, R. E., 90, 91, 181, 190, 192, 235, 244, 367, 368, 370–371
Petty, R. E. (ed.), 64, 65, 94, 367, 370

Pierce, H. R., 339
Pierce, J., 132, 134, 250
Pierrel, E., xviii, 96, 235, 410
Pieterse, M., 66
Pilisuk, M., 211
Pingree, S., 245
Pingree, S. (ed.), 244
Piontek, M. E., 322, 324
Pirie, F. L., 440
Pirie, L., 457, 458
Platts-Mills, T. A., 390
Poelman, J., xviii, 328, 330, 335, 345, 346, 374, 379
Poland, B. (ed.), 118
Pollack, R. H., 371
Pollak, K. I., 454, 457, 458, 460
Pollak, R. T., 156
Pollart Squillace, S., 390
Pollart, S. M., 390
Pollay, R. W., 91, 132, 134
Pope, A. (ed.), 389, 390
Porras, J. I., 173
Portes, A., 101
Posner, B. A., 250
Potvin, L., 6 fig. 1.1, 7, 18, 30, 75, 84
Pratt, L., 426
Preiss, R. W. (ed.), 89
Prence, E. M., 135
Preskill, H. S., 322, 324
Prihoda, T. J., 389, 392
Prlic, H., 6 fig. 1.1, 18, 30, 75, 84
Prochaska, J. O., 86, 87, 87–88 table 4.3, 156, 183, 189, 190, 194, 197, 248, 248 table 7.4, 249, 330, 460
Prokhorov, A. V., 340
Pryor, B. J. (ed.), 64, 187
Public Health Service, 387
Pulley, L. V., 204, 238, 241, 315
Pumariega, A. J., xviii, 25, 28
Putnam, R. D., 27, 101
Pyke, S. D., 135

Quesenberry, C., Jr., 392
Quine, L. (ed.), 335, 346, 367, 374
Quinn, V., 453–454, 454, 457, 458
Quintana, J. M., 392

Rachelefsky, G., 403
Rafaeli, S., 244
Raines, B. S., 196, 372, 374
Rakowski, W., 136
Ramachandran, R., 135
Ramelson, H. Z., 250, 251–252 fig. 7.8
Ramirez, A. G., 204, 238, 242, 315, 454, 457
Ramirez, G., 47, 56, 454, 457
Ramirez, V., 238, 242, 315
Ramsdale, E. H., 392
Rand, C. S., 392, 457

Name Index

Rauch, H. J., 156
Raynor, W. J., Jr., 134
Redline, S., 390
Reed, H. B., 110, 208
Reeder, G. D. (ed.), 64, 187
Reinders, J., xviii, 156, 328, 330, 335, 345, 346, 374, 379
Reineke, R. A., 323
Reis, J., 249
Reiss, A., 2
Reiss, J. A., 49
Remington, L., 64
Reno, R., 461
Renon, D., 392
Resch, N., 248, 248 table 7.4
Reynolds, K. D., 368
Rezmovic, E. L., 7
Rhodes, F., 249
Rhodes, J. E., 138
Rice, R. E. (ed.), 277
Rich, R., 110
Richard, L., 6 fig. 1.1, 7, 18, 30, 75, 84
Richard R., 64, 187, 190
Richardson, M. A., 59, 236, 454, 458
Richter, K., 110
Rigler, S., 391
Rimal, R. N., 244
Rimer, B. K. (ed.), xvii, 5, 7, 19, 28, 61, 79, 83, 84, 93, 96, 101, 102, 103, 105, 106, 113, 138, 157, 172, 173, 182, 188, 191, 197, 204, 205, 206, 248, 248 table 7.4, 255, 290, 292, 293 fig. 8.1, 295, 296, 300, 302, 355, 376, 433, 453–454
Rios, R. A., 256
Ripich, S., 245
Rips, J., 395, 403
Rissel, C., 301, 429, 433
Rivas, R. F., 21
Roberts, J., 261
Roberts-Gray, C., 292, 303
Robertson, A., 7
Robertson, J., 173
Robins, E., 455, 455 table 13.1
Robinson, B., 431, 440
Roche, W. R., 392
Rochlin, L., 157
Rodewald, L., 392
Rodin, J., 83, 94, 182, 187, 190, 197
Rogers, E. M., 203, 292, 293, 293 fig. 8.1, 294, 294 fig. 8.2, 295, 296, 297, 301, 306
Rogers, R., 64, 65, 94, 367, 370
Rogers, R. W., 94
Rogers, T., 109
Roijackers, J. G., 248, 248 table 7.4
Roizen, M. F., 188
Rokeach, M., 380
Rollnick, S., 250
Ronning, R. R., 185

Room, R., 440
Rooney, B. L., 440
Root, J. H., 252–253, 273, 274
Rootman, I. (ed.), 118
Rosbrook, B., 250
Rose, G., 390
Rosen, R. H., 201
Rosen, Y., 391
Rosenbloom, A. L., 156
Rosenstock, I. M., 28, 65, 93, 94, 182, 191, 197, 395
Rosenstreich, D. L., 390
Roser, C., 244
Roski, J., 430
Rossi, J. S., 248, 248 table 7.4, 249, 460
Rossi, H., 12, 40, 47, 297, 320, 321, 322, 323, 323 table 9.1, 324, 324 fig. 9.1, 325, 327, 337, 345
Roth, J., 2
Rothman, A. J., 83, 94, 182, 187, 190, 197
Rothman, J., 111, 112, 113, 202, 211, 212
Rothman, J. (ed.), 18, 111, 112, 113, 202, 212
Rounds, K. A., 103
Rowling, L., 201
Rozelle, R. M., 84, 164, 196
Rudd, R. E., 19, 112, 213, 214
Rugg, D., 361, 367
Ruhl, R., 391
Ruiter, R., 94, 189
Rumelhart, D. E., 185
Russell, J., 64
Russell, M. L., 64
Rutledge, J. H., 135
Rutter, D. R. (ed.), 335, 346, 367, 374
Ryan, M., 19
Ryan, W. J., 340

Sabini, J., 79
Sackett, D. L., 136
Sackett, D. L. (ed.), 136
Sadler, G., 250
Saidi, A. A., 64
Saint-Germain, M. A., 25
St. Lawrence, J. S., 204
Sakuma, M., 134
Sallis, J. F., 56, 309
Salmeron, S., 392
Salovey, P., 83, 94, 182, 187, 190, 197
Samet, J., 390, 457
Samet, J. (ed.), 390, 457
Sanchez-Merki, V., 111, 112, 213
Sandelowski, M., 344
Sanderson, L., 64
Sandler, R. S., 157, 182
Santiago, J. V., 396
Sarsfield, J. K., 391
Satoh, H., 134
Saunders, R. B., 455, 455 table 13.1

Name Index

Savage, J., 340
Savard, J., 84, 190
Sawaya, K., 30
Scamagas, P., 403
Scanlon, K. S., 340
Schaalma, H., xviii, 5, 7, 54, 65, 84, 86, 89, 156, 173, 296, 309, 311 fig. 8.3, 328, 330, 335, 345, 346, 355, 357, 360, 361, 373, 374, 378, 379, 380
Schaffer, L. C., 244
Scharff, D., 248 table 7.4
Schein, E. H., 107, 108 table 4.8
Scheirer, M. A., 7, 156, 292, 296, 297, 321, 325
Scherr, A., 343
Schidlow, V., xviii, 25, 312
Schilling, R. F., 178, 179 table 6.2
Schinke, S., 367, 373
Schmid, J. L., 440
Schmid, T. L., 303
Schneider, L. C., 392
Schooler, C., 132, 134
Schopman, M., 355
Schramm, W. F., 457
Schultz, J. A., 110
Schulz, A. J., 104
Schulz, A., 206
Schunk, D. H., 96
Schunk, D. H. (ed.), 96
Schurman, S. J., 20
Schwartz, R., 17, 303
Schwartzman, D. F., 368
Schwarzer, R. (ed.), 93, 196
Secker-Walker, R. H., 457
Seekins, T. M., 214, 215, 215 table 6.14, 216, 217 table 6.15
Seijts, G. H., 92, 198, 412
Seilheimer, D. K., xviii, 25, 28, 147, 156, 177, 188, 312
Sellers, D. E., 138, 139, 235, 307, 450
Semlitz, L., 427
Serdula, M. K., 340
Severson, H. H., 454, 458
Seydel, E. R., 94
Shaffer, R., 213
Sharpe, A., 136
Sharpe, C., 392
Shavelson, R. J., 378
Shediac, M. C., 292
Shediac-Rizkallah, M. C., 292, 293 fig. 8.1, 301
Sheeran, P., 84, 190, 199
Shegog, R., xviii, 96, 139, 147, 182, 235, 245, 249, 259, 291, 312, 395 fig. 11.1, 410, 417, 418
Shekelle, R. B., 134
Shephard, R. J., 135
Sherif, M., 371
Sherman, C. B., 390
Sherman, S. J., 368
Shiffman, S., 199

Short, B., 440, 441
Short, L., 361, 367
Shotland, R. L., 324
Shryock, A. M., 134
Siddarth, S., 91, 132, 134
Sidney, S., 340
Siegel, M., 91, 132, 134
Siero, F., xviii
Siero, S., xviii
Silverman, J., 354
Silverstein, J. H., 156
Simonds, S. (ed.), 47, 56
Simons-Morton, B. G., xvii, 4, 7, 32, 76, 77, 182, 208, 209 table 6.12
Simons-Morton, D. G., 5, 56
Singer, D. G., 244
Singer, J. (ed.), 372
Singer, J. L., 244
Singh, G. K., 2
Skelly, J. M., 457
Skinner, B. F., 33
Skinner, C. S., 104, 157, 182, 248, 248 table 7.4, 249
Slaby, R. G., 49
Slattery, M. L., 340
Slavin, R. G., 390
Smalley, R., 245
Smart, C. R., 135
Smelser, N. J., 203
Smelser, N. J. (ed.), 202, 203
Smigelski, C., 250
Smith, C., 303
Smith, C. K., 372
Smith, D. W., 7, 106
Smith, J., 104, 206
Smith, M. B., 250
Smith, R. A., 135
Smith, S. R., 26, 101, 139–140
Smith, T. F., 390
Smolkowski, K., 52, 60
Snider, J., 308
Snow, J. C., 136
Snyder, S. W., 457
Sobol, A., 389, 390
Sobol, D. F., 370
Sockrider, M. M., xviii, 25, 59, 96, 139, 147, 156, 182, 235, 236, 245, 249, 259, 291, 312, 391, 392, 395 fig. 11.1, 410, 417, 418, 454
Soet, J. E., 249
Solomon, L. J., 79, 85, 457
Solomon, T., 292, 303
Sonenstein, F., 361, 367
Sorel, M. E., 392
Sorenson, J. R., 4, 5
Soriano, F. I., 18
Spangler, J. G. (ed.), 453–454
Sparks, P., 83, 84
Spears, R., 368
Speers, M. A., 26, 101, 139–140, 303

Name Index

Speizer, F. E., 389, 390
Spengler, J. (ed.), 390, 457
Spiegel, D., 103
Spiegel, D. C., 370
Spillar, R., 156
Spinelli, S. H., xviii, 25, 28, 147, 156, 177, 188
Spiro, R. J. (ed.), 185
Sporik, R., 390
Springett, J., 140
Stake, R. E., 47
Stamler, J., 134
Stamm, K., 238, 242, 315
Stanley, J. C., 320, 345
Starfield, B., 395
Starr-Schneidkraut, N. J., 394
Staub, L., 234
Steckler, A. B., xvii, 4, 7, 17, 23, 24 fig. 2.1, 61, 62, 79, 105, 106, 156, 173, 182, 188, 203, 204, 206, 292, 293 fig. 8.1, 295, 296, 300, 301
Steenhuis, I., 248, 248 table 7.4, 249 fig. 7.7
Steiger, J. H., 248, 249
Stein, R. E., 387, 389, 392
Sterling, T. D., 26, 101, 139–140
Stern, P., 378
Sternfeld, B., 340
Steuart, G. W., 75
Stevenson, L. Y., 204
Stewart, J., 245
Stinson, F. S., 427
Stockbauer, J. W., 456
Stokking, K. M., 378
Stokols, D., 5
Stollerman, J. E., 250
Stone, E. J., xviii, 138, 139, 235, 307, 450
Stoto, M., 157
Stotts, A. L., 454, 458, 460
Stout, C., 394
Stouthamer-Loeber, M., 49
Stowell, L., 256
Strauss, A., 344
Strauss, A. L., 23
Strecher, V. J., 65, 92, 93, 94, 157, 182, 191, 198, 247, 248, 248 table 7.4, 396, 412
Street, R. (ed.), 244, 245, 247, 249
Street, R. L., Jr., 244
Stroebe, W. (ed.), 5, 54, 65, 84, 89, 173
Strong, L. V., 252
Strunk, R. C., 20
Stumans, F., 390, 457
Suarez, L., 204, 315
Sugden, R., 371
Sulayman, R. F., 64
Sullivan, S. E., 453–454
Suls, J., 315, 367, 371
Suminski, R. R., 340
Susser, E., 181
Sussman, L. K., 20
Sussman, S., 367, 370

Sutton, S. M., xvii
Swaen, G., 390, 457
Swan, S. H., 457
Swank, R., xviii, 25, 96, 139, 147, 182, 237, 245, 291, 297, 299–300 table 8.1, 312, 321, 335, 417, 418
Swanson, M., 390
Sykes, R. K., 20, 104
Sylvia, S., 20
Syme, L. (ed.), 100, 102 table 4.7
Syme, S. L., 114
Szilagyi, P., 392
Szklo, M., 395

Tabak, E. R., 56
Tager, I. B., 390
Talamo, R. C., 392
Tanner, W. M., 371
Tao, Z. W., 213
Taplin, S., 403
Taplin, S. H., 83, 84, 355
Taylor, D. W. (ed.), 136
Taylor, J., 245
Taylor, R. L., 104, 194
Taylor, S. E., 22, 103
Taylor, S. E. (ed.), 372
Taylor, W. C., xviii, 59, 236, 290, 293 fig. 8.1, 309, 310 table 8.2, 311, 454, 458
Taylor, W. R., 389
Taytard, A., 392
Telepchak, J., 248, 248 table 7.4
Texas Department of Health Coalition Task Force, 208, 210 table 6.13
Themba, M., 119, 214, 216, 217–218, 445
Thombs, D. L., 340
Thompson, B., 301
Thompson, E. J., 64
Thompson, F. E., 340
Thompson, L. C., 392, 457
Thompson, P., 390
Thompson, S. G., 135
Thoresen, C. E., 95 table 4.5, 394
Thornburg, K. R., 109, 208
Thorpe, A., 391
Tiernan, K., 403
Tillgren, P., 140, 201
Tinsley, B. J., 87, 87–88 table 4.3, 188, 191
Tobin, M. J., 49
Tolan, H., 2, 6
Toobert, D. J., 136
Toomey, T. L., 430, 432, 440, 441, 442
Torgen, M., 391
Torgerson, J., 250
Torrence, D. R., 274
Torrence, J. A., 274
Torres, A., 354
Torres, I., 238
Torres, J., 181
Torres, R. T., 322, 324

Tortolero, S. R., 340, 391, 392
Toseland, R. W., 21
Tosteson, T. D., 390
Toy, R., 391
Trapini, F., 253
Trevino, F., 238
Triandis, H. C., 255, 257, 259
Trice, H. M., 105, 156, 182, 295
Tripp, J. H., 156
Tripp, M., 341
Tripp, M. K., 137
Tropman, J. E. (ed.), 18, 111, 112, 113, 202, 212
Tryon, W. W., 340
Tsuji, I., 134
Tufte, E. R., 254
Turkeltaub, C., 390
Turner, J. C., 367
Tversky, A., 368, 370
Tyrrell, S., 391

Uchino, B. N., 138
Uleman, J. S. (ed.), 370–371
Ulene, A. L., 370
Ullman, S., 403
Umberson, D., 103, 138
University of Texas Health Science Center–Houston, 390
Ury, W., 144 table 5.1
U.S. Department of Health and Human Services, 134, 135, 164, 254, 331, 376
U.S. Department of Justice, 2
U.S. Environmental Protection Agency, Indoor Air Division, 391
U.S. Office on Smoking and Health [U.S. DHHS], 134, 454, 456, 457
U.S. Preventive Services Task Force, 135
Utter, A. C., 340

Vaden, A., 134
Valencia, E., 181
Vallone, G., 391
Van Asperen, P., 392
Van Assema, P., 181–182, 182, 187, 248, 248 table 7.4, 249 fig. 7.7
Van Breukelen, G. J., 84, 181–182, 248, 248 table 7.4
Van de Ven, A. H., 22
Van den Bos, G. R. (ed.), 86, 87, 87–88 table 4.3, 183, 189, 190, 194, 197
Van der Pligt, J., 64, 187, 190, 367
Van der Velde, F., 64, 187
van der Vliet, R., 353, 354, 360
Van Horn, L., 340
van Nunen, M., 342
Van Zessen, G., 353, 354, 360
Vanzieleghem, M. A., 392
Veblen-Mortenson, S., 301, 425, 426, 430, 432, 442

Veen, P., 5, 50, 53, 59
Velez, R., 181, 182, 183
Velicer, W. F., 248, 248 table 7.4, 249, 460
Verbeek, J., 66
Veres-Throner, C., 390
Verhulst, D., 455 table 13.1
Viadro, C. I., 206
Victor, B., 138
Vierthaler, W. A., 403
Villarreal, R., 204, 238
Vincus, A. A., 206
Vogels, T., 353, 354, 360
Vogt, T. M., 19, 332, 343

Wagenaar, A. C., 425, 426, 428, 429, 430, 432, 433, 440, 441, 442
Wagener, D. K., 387
Wagner, E. H., 248 table 7.4
Wagner, W. W., 142
Wahlgren, D. R., 390, 457
Walater, C. H., 211
Walder, L. O., 49
Wall, M. A., 454, 458
Wallace, D. G., 135
Wallace, R. B. (ed.), 132, 134
Wallack, L., 119, 214, 216, 217–218, 445
Wallack, L. (ed.), 278
Wallerstein, N. B., 7, 17, 26, 101, 111, 112, 113, 114, 114 fig. 4.2, 139–140, 201, 211, 213
Walls, A. F., 392
Walmsley, S. A., 253
Walter, R. S., 64
Walton, S., 115
Wandersman, A., 109, 110, 182, 208
Wandersman, A. (ed.), 324
Wang, C., 19, 112, 213
Wang, C. C., 213
Ward, W. B. (ed.), 47, 56, 294, 297
Warner, J. O., 391
Warner, K. E., 139
Warren, R. L. (ed.), 25
Wasilewski, Y., 392, 395, 403
Watanabe, N., 134
Webb, R. J., 440, 441
Webber, G. C., 244
Webber, L. S., xviii, 138
Weber, M., 202
Webster, D. W., 49
Wedner, H. J., 390
Weeks, K., 392, 457
Wegener, D. T., 91, 190, 192, 235
Weijts, W., 23, 25, 47, 61
Weikel, W. J. (ed.), 256
Wein, T. H., 234
Weinberg, L., 157
Weiner, B., 92, 196, 396, 410
Weinstein, N. D., 64, 93, 367, 368
Weinstein, R., 344

Name Index

Weisbrod, R., 301
Weiss, K. B., 387, 389, 390, 392
Weiss, S. T., 390, 392
Weitzman, M., 389, 390
Wellman, B., 100, 102 table 4.7
Wells, W., 241 table 7.1, 252
Wen, S. W., 456, 457
Werner, O., 259
Wesseling, G., 390, 457
Westbrook, L., 387, 389, 392
Westen, D., 81
Weston, R., 7, 19, 302, 376
Wheeler, F., 303
Wheeler, J. R., 136
Whitbeck, J., 340
White, J. V., 252, 273
Whitehead, L., 391
Whitley, N., 24
Whitney-Saltiel, D. A., 370
Wholey, J. S., 320, 324, 328
Wholey, J. S. (ed.), 292, 297, 321, 324, 325, 328
Wiemann, J. M. (ed.), 244
Wigal, J. K., 95 table 4.5, 406
Williams, C. L., 425, 426, 430, 432, 442
Williams, E. L., 110
Williams, R., 252, 273
Williams, R. M., Jr., 256–257
Wills, T. A., 315, 367, 371
Wilson, D. M., 245
Wilson, J. W., 392
Wilson, M. E., 49
Wilson, S. J., 392
Wilson-Pessano, S. R., 22, 395, 403
Winder, J. A., 394
Windham, G. C., 457
Windsor, R. A., xvii, 12, 47, 320, 321, 322, 332, 333, 340, 345, 457
Wing, R. R. 138
Wingood, G. M., 24
Wise, M., 245
Wiseman, R. L. (ed.), 255
Wissow, S., 395
Witkin, R. B., 18
Witte, K., 81, 83, 182, 255
Wittrock, M. C. (ed.), 378
Wlodkowski, R. J., 260
Wohlfeiler, D., 103
Wolberg, W., 245
Wolcott, H. F., 23

Wolfson, M., 425, 426, 429, 430, 432, 433, 440, 441, 442
Wood, A. H., 104
Wood, C., 391
Wood, D. A., 135
Wood, J. V., 103
Wood, R., 389, 392
Woodby, L. L., 457
Woodman, R. W. (ed.), 173
World Health Organization, 7, 19, 117
Worley, C. G., 192, 208
Wortman, M., 56, 59
Wortman, M. (ed.), 56, 59
Wouters, E. F., 390, 457
Wu, M., 138, 235, 307, 450
Wyche, J., 201

Yamaguchi, K., 427
Yates, B. T., 322
Yazdgerdi, S., 392
Yeaton, W. H. (ed.), 56, 59
Yi, W. K., 213
Yin, R. K., 47, 301, 344
Yingling, S., 25
Yoshikawa, H., 49
Young, J. Q., 214, 215, 215 table 6.14, 216, 217 table 6.15
Young, R., 19
Yu, S. M., 2

Zabin, L. S., 361, 367
Zack, M. M., 343
Zajonc, R. B., 82, 371
Zakarian, J. M., 390, 457
Zaltman, G., 156
Zanna, M. (ed.), 90
Zastawney, A. L., 250
Zawadzki, R., 25
Zeiger, R. S., 390, 457
Zhang, Q., 238
Zhu, S. H., 250
Zimbardo, G., 371
Zimmerman, B. J., 95, 95 table 4.5, 136, 147
Zimmerman, B. J. (ed.), 96
Zimmerman, M. A., 114, 206
Zmuda, J. M., 340
Zoref, L., 454, 458
Zweig, S., 453

SUBJECT INDEX

Acres Homes Community, 17
Active learning, 100, 197, 299
Activities of daily living (ADL), 337
Adherence, 136
Adolescent Social Action Program, 112, 213
Adoption, program, 293 fig. 8.1, 306
   determinants of, 86, 309–314, 416
   and evaluation, 323 table 9.1, 335
   matrices for, 12, 313–314
   organizational change and, 105–106, 208
   performance objectives for, 306–308, 313–314
   planning for, 7, 9, 290–291
   process of, 204, 292–295, 306
   theories and, 79, 309
   See also Intervention Mapping Step 4
Advocacy, 214
   guidelines for effective, 217 table 6.15
   life cycle of issues in, 219
   as method, 120, 198, 201 fig. 6.2, 207 table 6.11
   of policies, 218–220
   setting the agenda in, 216, 218
   strategy and tactics of, 214–216, 270–271, 275 fig. 7.13
   as vehicle for change, 242
   See also Advocacy, media; Policy windows
Advocacy, media, 68, 207 table 6.11, 216–218
Affirmation of beliefs and values, 101–102
Agenda-building theory, 118–119
   use of theory, 75 table 4.1, 80 table 4.2
   See also Advocacy
Agenda setting
   in advocacy, 216, 218
   and innovations, 295
Agents, change, 32, 106
Agents, environmental
   decision-making, 77, 86, 106
   determinants' influence on, 77
   examples of, 19, 32–33, 68, 77, 145
   as intervention group, 19, 33, 106, 109, 145
   organizational, 77, 105, 106, 109

   and theory of planned behavior, 86
Agents, linking, 101–102
   See also Program champions
AIDS/HIV
   determinants of safe sex, 355–360
   epidemiology, 353–355
   indicators for evaluation, 342
   screening for, 135
   among women, 24–25
   See also Intervention, prevention
Air quality and health, 132
Alcohol abuse, epidemiology of, 425, 427
   See also Intervention, adolescent alcohol use (Project Northland)
Alcoholics Anonymous, 104
Alinsky method organizing, 212
Alma-Ata Declaration, 19
Alzheimer disease, 245
American Heart Association, 292, 303
America Responds to AIDS, 140
Analysis, behavioral, 29–30
Analysis, environmental, 30
Analysis of determinants. *See* Determinants
Anticipatory regret, 84, 190
Appraisal, 101, 188
Asbestos, 213
Assessment, needs. *See* Needs assessment
Asthma
   action plans, 397, 401 table 11.3, 404, 406, 407, 412, 415, 417
   agents of change for, 397
   epidemiology of childhood, 387, 389–390
   health-promoting behaviors for, 95–96
   management, 388, 391–393, 397
   PRECEDE model of, 34–35, 35 fig. 2.5
   risk factors, 390–391
   See also Intervention, asthma
A Su Salud program, 238, 242
At-risk group. *See* Population, at-risk
Attention, 66, 89, 98
Attitudes, 190
   as determinant, 65, 66, 83, 106, 120, 299

Subject Index

Attitudes *(continued)*
  measures of, 83
  methods to change, 91, 190–193, 191 table 6.6, 246, 367
  motivation, 84, 85, 98
  and persuasion communication model, 89, 90–91
  and self-regulatory theories, 96
  surveys to determine, 357, 358 table 10.2
  and theory of planned behavior, 83, 86
Attribution theory, 92–93
  and determinants, 395–396, 398–400, 465–467
  dimensions (stable, controllable), 93, 196, 197
  examples of method, 406 table 11.7, 461 fig. 13.3
  reattribution training, 197
  and relapse prevention, 199
  use of theory, 80 table 4.2
Awareness
  methods to change, 187–188, 187 table 6.5
  and theory of planned behavior, 83

Barriers, 94, 183, 200
  and attributional theory, 93
  as determinants, 404 table 11.5
  to environmental change, 413
  and health belief model, 94, 95
  methods to reduce, 191
  to program implementation, 309, 335
  and self-efficacy, 197
  and social cognitive theory, 100
  and theory of planned behavior, 86
  and transtheoretical model, 87
Behavior, 66, 83, 134, 340,
  and attributional theory, 93
  and evaluation, 321, 326, 327, 335, 336
  and goal-setting theory, 92
  indicators of, 34 table 2.2
  and learning theories, 82
  methods for changing, 100
  and organizational change, 109
  perceived, 194, 309
  and performance objectives, 142
  and persuasion communication model, 89–91
  and PRECEDE, 39
  precursors to, 195
  and self-regulatory theories, 96
  and social cognitive theory, 96, 99–100
  and theory of planned behavior, 86
  and transtheoretical model, 87
  See also types of behavior; Change, behavior
Behavior, health and health-related, 79, 94, 133, 134
  as outcomes, 201 fig. 6.2
  See also Adherence

Behavior, health-promoting, 34, 134, 135
  determinants of, 74
  examples of, 35–36, 142
  and health belief model, 95
  as outcomes, 137
  perceived, 97, 98, 100, 340
  and self-regulatory theories, 95
  and transtheoretical model, 86
  understanding using theory, 74
  See also Adherence
Behavior, risk, 132, 134–135
  changing, 135, 330
  and environmental factors, 137
  examples of, 17, 134
  methods to change, 74
  and perception of risk, 25
  and PRECEDE, 36
  restating as health-promoting behavior, 134–135
  theory to define, 75 table 4.1
  See also Factors, behavioral
Behavioral analysis, 29–30
Behavioral capability, 98, 100, 401
  as determinant in asthma, 398–401, 404–405
  as determinant of behavior, 106, 120
  methods to change, 100, 195–198
  and program implementation, 298, 300, 309
  and social cognitive theory, 97, 98, 100
Behavioral control, perceived. *See* Self-efficacy
Behavioral factors. *See* Factors, behavioral
Behavioral intentions, 84, 85, 197, 198–199
Behavioral journalism, 203
  See also Mass media
Behavioral Risk Factor Surveillance System, 33, 34 table 2.2, 343
Behavior change. *See* Change, behavior
Beliefs, 79, 83–86, 182
  changing, 182
  and theory of planned behavior, 86
Benefits, perceived, 94, 95
  See also Outcome expectations
Boycotts, 212
Brainstorming, 53–54, 230, 232, 233, 309, 314
BRFSS. *See* Behavioral Risk Factor Surveillance System
Buddy systems, 104, 201 fig. 6.2

Cancer, 135
  See also Intervention, skin cancer
Cardiovascular disease, 135
  See also Intervention, cardiovascular disease
CATCH. *See* Intervention, cardiovascular disease
Centers for Disease Control and Prevention, 33, 34 table 2.2, 343
  See also name index
Champion, program. *See* Program champion
Change, behavior, 79–80, 87, 89, 92

Subject Index

and health belief model, 94
methods for, 100
and social cognitive theory, 96, 99–100
specifying, 130
See also Stages of change; Transtheoretical model
Change, environmental, 132, 201 fig. 6.2, 213, 268
specifying, 130
as strategy, 204
Change agents. *See* Agents, change
Change objectives. *See* Objectives
Change teams, internal, as strategy, 201 fig. 6.2
Channels and vehicles, 237–242, 249–250, 266, 277–278
Child and Adolescent Trial for Cardiovascular Health. *See* Intervention, cardiovascular disease
China, interventions in, 213
Chunking, 184–185
Classical conditioning, 81–82
Coaching, as strategy, 204
Coalitions, 76, 109–111, 208
as channels, 242–243
design documents for, 266, 269, 270, 272 fig. 7.12, 275 fig. 7.13
development, stages of, 110, 208, 210 table 6.13
and empowerment, 110–111
guidelines for, 242–243
and interorganizational relationships theory, 109–111
recruiting members, 270 fig. 7.11
stages of change in, 182
as strategies, 201 fig. 6.2, 212
visualization exercise for, 269
See also Organizations
Cochrane Collaboration, 59
Cognitive support. *See* Social support.
Collective efficacy. *See* Efficacy, collective
Commitment, public, 198
Communication
within a culture, 258–259
McGuire communication matrix, 229
as method, 120
methods to improve, 246
of risks, 188
skills training, 178
See also Channels and vehicles; Elaboration likelihood model; Negotiation; Persuasion communication model
Communities, 18, 25, 111
assessment of, 20
change in, 115, 173–174
as intervention groups, 112
as networks, 100
as program planners, participation, 183
social capital of, 101

Community Action Programs, 212
Community building. *See* Community organization
Community capacity, 26–28
assessment of, 16, 17, 25
building, 207, 301
and collaborative planning, 19
and community change, 115
and social networks, 101
See also Needs assessment; Intervention Mapping Task 4
Community competence, 19, 25–26
Community organization
community building, 211–212
community development, 208–212, 309, 330
as method, 201 fig. 6.2
methods, 195
models and theories, 38, 111–116, 173
and social action, 212, 213
social planning model and policy, 118
use of, 80 table 4.2
See also Coalitions
Community resources. *See* Community capacity
Complexity, 5–8, 132, 133, 143
of causation, 5, 18, 330
and goal-setting, 198
of planning, 8, 229
Compliance. *See* Adherence
Comprehension, 66, 89
Comprehensive Health Enhancement Support System (CHESS), 245
Computer-assisted interventions, 241 table 7.1, 244–249, 251–252
See also Intervention, asthma
Conditions, behavioral. *See* Factors, behavioral
Conditions, environmental. *See* Factors, environmental
Condoms
availability as environmental risk factor, 355
focus group on, 357 table 10.1
performance objectives for use, 144 table 5.1
surveys regarding use, 357
use as health-promoting behavior, 134, 143
use as program objective, 328, 329, 336, 346, 348
Congruity theory, 369 table 10.5
Conscientization, 111–112
as method, 207 table 6.11, 212–214
use of theory, 75 table 4.1, 80 table 4.2
Consciousness raising
as method, 187 table 6.5, 408 table 11.9, 413
methods for, 189
as process of change, 461 fig. 13.3
Consistency. *See* Measures
Construct-related approach to literature, 177
Construct validity, 50, 58–59, 337–340, 344

501

Subject Index

Subject Index

Constructs, theoretical
  and empirical evidence, 66
  and indicators and measures, 336–337, 339
  and levels of intervention, 174
Context of behavior, 199
Context of innovations, 297
Context of program participants, 17–18, 181, 229, 232, 304, 455, 459, 464–467
Contingency management, 68, 197, 198
Contra Costa County Health Services Department, 115
Control, perceived behavioral. *See* Self-efficacy
Coping behavior
  and attributional theory, 93
  and relapse, 199, 459 fig. 13.2, 461 fig. 13.3
  and self-regulatory theories, 96
  See also Intervention, cystic fibrosis
Coping model. *See* Role model
Copyright, 253
Core processes, 9, 47–50, 51 fig. 3.1, 131
  and causal model, 328
  for choosing methods and strategies, 314
  for determinants, 52–53, 62
  example of, 62–68, 355–356, 367
  formulate working answers, 62
  research with intervention population, 176, 177 fig. 6.1
Core processes: brainstorming, 53–54, 230, 232, 233, 309, 314
Core processes: determining need for new data, 61–62
Core processes: posing questions, 50–53
Core processes: searching the empirical literature, 50, 53, 54–59, 174–176, 177 fig. 6.1
  evaluating literature, 55, 58, 78
  examples of review, 403, 406, 455
  on program implementation, 309, 314
  in program planning, 4, 47, 147
  synthesis of, 47
Core processes: searching the theoretical literature, 48–50, 54, 59–61, 174–176, 177 fig. 6.1
Cost-benefit analysis, 94, 321–322
  See also Efficiency, program; Theory of economic decision making
Cost effectiveness, 321–322
Counterconditioning, 197–198
Critical incident technique, 34 table 2.2
Cues
  to action, 91, 94, 95, 178, 198, 412
  control of, 461 fig. 13.3, 467 table 13.6
  examples of cues, 182, 339
  to memory, 186
  as method, 299, 406–409 tables 11.7–11.9
  self-monitoring of responses, 199
  stimulus control, 197, 198, 268
Cultural competence, 182–183, 212, 230–231
  definition of, 107, 255

  developing, 255–258, 260–261
  evaluating materials for, 251–253
  inclusivity, checking for, 272 fig. 7.12
  and personal ethnocentrism, 254, 255–258
  and teaching and learning, 260–261
  See also Culture and ethnicity; Translation
Culture and ethnicity, 5, 213, 255
  and communication, 258–259
  as cues, 182
  embedding mechanisms, 108 table 4.8
  and health, 81, 254, 255
  and information processing, 186
  organizing across, 212
  tailoring on, 178, 183, 409–410
  See also Cultural competence; Populations, Intervention, differentiation of; Organizational culture; Translation
Cystic fibrosis, 135
  See also Intervention, cystic fibrosis

Data
  as basis of intervention, 4–5, 9, 20, 41, 66
  sources of, 33–34, 34 table 2.2
  See also Methods, qualitative and quantitative
Decentering, 259. *See also* Translation
Decisional balance, 461 fig. 13.3, 464, 465–467 tables 13.4–13.6
Delivery, program, 8, 325
Demonstrations (political), 201 fig. 6.2, 212
Desensitization, 198
Design documents, 261–277
  for abstract vehicles, 266, 269–271
  examples, 267–269, 272 fig. 7.12, 275 fig. 7.13
  for print pieces, 271–273
  for program parameters, 262–263
  for videotapes, 274–277
  writing, 263, 266
Determinants, 1, 17, 65, 66, 77, 96, 178
  analysis of, 33, 59, 61–62
  and attribution theory, 92, 93
  changing, 74, 81, 131, 330
  of environmental conditions, 1, 9, 77, 133
  and evaluation, 321, 326, 327, 335, 336, 339
  external, 5, 199–220, 398–400 table 11.2, 401, 403
  and goal-setting theory, 92
  and health belief model, 94, 95
  indicators of, 34 table 2.2
  and learning theory, 82
  and matrices, 9
  of organizational change, 106
  personal, 133, 152–157
  and persuasion communication model, 91
  of program diffusion, 299–300
  of program implementation, 298, 308–313
  of program institutionalization, 313
  ranking of, 81, 311–312

Subject Index

of self-efficacy, 92–93
and self-regulatory theories, 96
of sexual risk-taking, 24–25
and social cognitive theory, 92, 97, 100
and theory of planned behavior, 83, 84
and transtheoretical model, 87, 89
using theory with, 8, 75 table 4.1
See also specific interventions; Intervention Mapping Step 1
Differentiation. *See* Populations, intervention
Diffusion, program, 7, 25, 26 fig. 2.2, 86, 106, 292
  example of plan, 299–300, 310 table 8.2
  planning for, 302–306
  and social cognitive theory, 294–295
  stages of, 105–106, 299–300
  See also Adoption; Diffusion of innovations theory; Implementation
Diffusion of innovations theory, 292, 294
  in organizations, 295–297
  use of, 75 table 4.1, 80 table 4.2
  See also Diffusion, program
Disease management, 33–34, 246
Dissonance reduction, 299
Domains. *See* Measures
Dramatic relief, 187 table 6.5, 189, 461 fig. 13.3
Dutch Foundation for Traffic and Safety, 62
  See also Intervention, child restraint devices; Intervention, traffic

Ecological approach, 4–6, 6 fig. 1.1, 138
  framework for planning interventions, 132
  levels, 130–133, 138–139
  theories for each level, 80 table 4.2, 81
  See also Ecological levels
Ecological levels
  of causation, multiple, 7
  change in, 76
  community, 18, 30
  and determinants, 5
  of health, 7
  individual, 18
  interaction of, 5, 6, 30
  interpersonal, 18
  intervention, 18, 75
  measures of quality of life, 342, 343
  organizational, 10, 18
  and PRECEDE, 30
  schematic of, 6 fig. 1.1
  societal, 18
  supranation, 18
  as target of intervention, 75–76, 80–81
  theories for, 79, 80 table 4.2
  theory of planned behavior and, 86
  See also Ecological approach
Economics. *See* Cost-benefit analysis
Effect evaluation. *See* Evaluation, effect
Effectiveness, program, 321, 331
Efficacy, collective, 99, 112, 198

Efficacy, intervention, 7, 321
Efficacy, self. *See* Self-efficacy
Efficiency, program, 321–322
Elaboration, as aid to memory, 186
Elaboration likelihood model, 90, 181, 192, 369 table 10.5
  See also Communication
Emotional appeals, 190
Emotional support. *See* Social support
Empirical evidence. *See* Evidence, types of
Employee assistance programs, 105
Empowerment, 19, 68, 110–114, 198, 324, 330
Environment, 5, 7, 33–34, 36, 91, 92, 201
  community, 139–140
  health care, 34
  interpersonal, 138–139, 461
  organizational, 109, 139
  physical, 34, 99, 100
  social, 5, 99, 100, 138
  societal, 140
Environmental levels. *See* Ecological approach
Environmental re-engineering, 198
Environmental re-evaluation, 191
Environmental report cards, 413, 414 fig. 11.3, 415, 417
  See also Intervention, asthma
Environmental tobacco smoke (ETS) 191–192, 457, 459, 462
  controlling, as outcome measure, 473
  controlling, as performance objective, 465–467 tables 13.4–13.6
  See also Intervention, smoking cessation (Project PANDA)
Epidemiology. *See* Needs assessment
Ethnographic interviews, 34 table 2.2
Ethnomedical systems, 255
Evaluation, effect, 12–13, 320, 321, 335
  for asthma, 417
  for HIV, 328, 330, 336, 348
  questions for, 336, 345
  See also Evaluation, program
Evaluation, formative, 277, 322, 332
Evaluation, process, 12–13, 320–321, 331–332
  for AIDS prevention, 328–330, 347
  for asthma intervention, 417
  for diabetes intervention, 332–334
  and program failure, 331
  and program fidelity, 332, 334–335
  and program implementation, 322, 330
  and program reach, 332, 335
  questions for, 332
  for smoking cessation, 471–476
  See also Evaluation, program; Implementation, program; Performance standards
Evaluation, program, 321, 324, 325, 327, 328
  "black box", 331
  experimental design, 345–346
  generation of plan, as step, 9, 10 fig. 1.2, 320

Evaluation, program *(continued)*
    for HIV intervention, 328–330, 347–348
    model of, 325
    and needs assessment, 321
    plan for, 19, 346
    purpose and use of, 322, 331, 349
    qualitative and quantitative methods in, 23–25, 26 fig. 2.2
    texts for, 345
    time frame of, 328, 330, 331, 343
    See also Evaluation map; Intervention Mapping Step 5
Evaluation, summative, 322, 332
Evaluation map, 325–327, 331
    for asthma intervention, 417 fig. 11.4
    for HIV intervention, 329
    model, 327 fig. 9.3
    for smoking intervention, 472 fig. 13.7
Evidence, types of, 5, 9, 17, 41
Expert systems, 247, 248–249, 250

Facilitation, 183, 409 table 11.9
Factors, behavioral, 1–2, 7, 31–33, 87
    in PRECEDE, 29 fig. 2.3, 39, 39 fig. 2.8
    questions to ask in defining, 52
    See also Behavior, risk
Factors, enabling
    cultural elements, 139
    definition of, 33
    identifying, through needs assessment, 132
    in PRECEDE, 29 fig. 2.3
    in stroke, 31–32 table 2.1
Factors, environmental, 75 table 4.1, 98, 133, 137–138
    analysis of, 32, 138
    as basis of matrices, 9
    behavior, interaction with, 138
    change, methods to, 74
    change agents of, 32, 33
    change outcome and, 140
    as context of health, 132–133
    determinants of, 33, 74
    and effect evaluation, 321, 326, 327, 335, 336
    and evaluation of health, 342
    and evaluation of quality of life, 342
    interpersonal environment, 138
    and levels of environment, 30 fig. 2.4
    MATCH model, 32
    and matrices, 9
    needs assessment and, 137
    performance objectives and, 133, 144
    in PRECEDE, 29 fig. 2.3, 39, 39 fig. 2.8
    ranking of, 137
    and self-regulatory theories, 96
    and social cognitive theory, 97
    stating, 140
    in stroke, 31–32 table 2.1
    sun exposure and, 139
    and transtheoretical model, 87
    use of theory with respect to, 74, 75 table 4.1
Factors, predisposing, 29 fig. 2.3, 31–33, 132
Factors, reinforcing, 29 fig. 2.3, 31–33, 132
Factors, risk, 35–36, 134
Fatalismo, 255, 256
Fear arousal, 187 table 6.5, 188–190, 369 table 10.5, 370
Feedback, 183
    in changing organizational culture, 109
    from computers, 244, 249
    and consciousness raising, 189
    as method, 98, 183, 195–196, 197, 198, 201 fig. 6.2
    in social support, 101
Fidelity and reach, program. *See* Evaluation, process; Implementation, program
Fluoridation, adoption of, 192–193
Focus groups, 23, 24, 233, 259, 311
    in pretesting, 278, 279
Framing (the issue), 214, 217
Framing (loss or gain), 187, 188, 190
Freire, Paulo, 212
    Freirian question posing, 34, 112, 212–213
    See also name index; Conscientization
Functional status, 336–337
Funding agencies, 323 table 9.1

Gatekeepers, 76–77, 200, 281, 291
Goal-setting, 94, 197–199
    theory, 91–92
    use of theory, 80 table 4.2, 327, 406–409 tables 11.7–11.9, 461 fig. 13.3
"Good Friends Make Good Medicine," 103–104
Graphics in program materials, 253, 254
Grassroots organizing, as strategy, 201 fig. 6.2, 211–212
Grounded theory. *See* Methods, qualitative and quantitative research
Group discussion, as strategy, 201 fig. 6.2
Group polarization, 369 table 10.5, 372
Guatemala, hand-washing intervention in, 142–143

Health belief model, 64, 65, 93–95
    use of, 75 table 4.1, 80 table 4.2
Health Care Forum, 208
Health care providers and facilities
    as channels, 239, 242
    as determinant of program implementation, 300
    as environmental agents, 19
    as intervention group, 19, 201 fig. 6.2, 234, 243 table 7.2
    and program planning, 20
    as stakeholders, 242
    See also Environment, health care
Health education. *See* Health promotion
Health outcomes. *See* Outcomes, health

Subject Index

Health problems
  defining, 50–52
  indicators of, 34
  in PRECEDE, 29 fig. 2.3, 36, 37–38
  program objectives related to, 40–41
Health promotion (term), 1, 11
Health-related quality of life (HRQOL) indices, 343
Healthy Cities, 117, 140
Healthy Neighborhoods Project, 115
Healthy People 2010, 254
Heart Partners program, 292
HIV. See AIDS
Hotlines, 249
HRQOL indices. See Health-related quality of life

Imagery, 185–186, 191
Impact, program, 7
Impact evaluation. See Evaluation, effect
Impact pathways. See Program pathways
Implementation, program, 7, 8, 11, 19, 290–292, 297–298
  of diabetes intervention, 332–335
  of HIV intervention, 335
  evaluation of, 321, 344
  factors affecting, 7, 86, 308–314
  guidelines, 335
  index, 332–334, 333 table 9.3 (diabetes), 334
  matrices for, 12, 313–314
  performance objectives for, 306–308, 313–314
  planning for, 19, 290–291
  pretesting and, 281
  reinvention in, 297
  terms for, 293 fig. 8.1
  use of theories in, 79, 86, 309
  See also Intervention Mapping Step 4
Incentives, 98, 100
Individualization, 182
  See also Tailoring
Information processing (human), 90–91, 180–181, 192, 244
  theory, 184–186
  when using computer, 245–246
  See also Elaboration likelihood model
Innovations. See Diffusion of innovations theory
Institutionalization, 105, 300–302, 308
  See also Sustainability, program
Intentions. See Behavioral intentions
Interactive multimedia. See Computer-assisted interventions
Internet as source of materials, 253
Interorganizational relationship theory. See Organizations
Intervention, adolescent alcohol and substance abuse (other)
  Adolescent Social Action Program, 112

Intervention, adolescent alcohol use (Project Northland)
  behavioral conditions, 428
  community change, 426, 427, 435–436, 443
  community norms, 430, 435, 439, 440, 442–443
  community organizing, 431, 440–441, 443, 444
  determinants, 428–429, 433–434, 435–439
  differentiation of population, 434
  evaluation, effect and process 449–450
  factors, demand and supply, 426–427, 435 table 12.1
  individual change, 427
  intervention population, involvement of, 432, 442 table 12.4
  laws, enforcement of, 435–436, 441, 444–445
  linkage system, 448
  matrices, 432, 434, 435–439
  media, use of, 441, 445, 446, 448–449
  methods and strategies, 280–281, 430, 441, 442, 446–447
  needs assessment, 427–428
  performance objectives, 431–432, 435–439
  policies regarding, 428, 431, 432, 437–439, 440–448
  review of existing programs, 427, 430
  risk factors, 427
  social cognitive theory, 433, 441
  youth development, 426, 432, 441–442, 445–447
Intervention, advanced AIDS, 245
Intervention, asthma (expert system), 249
Intervention, asthma (Health Hero), 245–246
Intervention, asthma (Watch, Discover, Think, and Act)
  action plan, asthma, 412–413, 415, 417
  adoption and implementation factors, 416
  advisory and other committees, 304, 408, 413, 415, 416
  agents of change, 397
  characteristics, desired program, 406, 409
  computer game, 245, 409–412, 414, 415, 417–418
  conceptual framework, 394, 395
  determinants, 395, 398–401, 403–405
  differentiation of population, 396–397
  environmental factors, 388, 389–391, 397, 402, 413, 415
  environmental report card, 413, 414 fig. 11.3, 415, 417
  evaluation, 417–418
  health and quality of life, 389–390, 393, 417
  implementation of, 291
  intervention population, 139, 393
  levels of intervention, 388, 393, 397
  linkage system, 304
  linkage to physicians, 412, 415
  linkage to schools, 413, 415, 416, 417

Intervention, asthma (Watch, Discover, Think, and Act) *(continued)*
  literature review, 403, 406
  measures, 336–337, 338–339
  matrices, 397, 417
  methods and strategies, 403, 406–409, 410–412, 418
  motif, 410
  needs assessment, 388–393, 417
  performance objectives, 394, 396, 398–402
  policy, district-level, 413, 415 table 11.10
  PRECEDE model for, 34–35, 388–389
  pretesting of program, 304
  program components, 388, 409, 414, 415
  program materials, review of, 414
  program objectives, 393, 394, 417
  review of existing programs, 403, 406
  risk factors, 390–393
  self-management training, 415, 417
  self-regulation skills in, 96, 394
  strategies. *See* methods and strategies
  surveys, 415, 417
  tailoring, 182, 246, 409, 410, 418
  telephone calls, 415
  theme, 410
  translation into Spanish, 259
  videos, 412, 417
  See also Asthma
Intervention, breast cancer
  lay health advisors in, 206
  social networks in, 103
Intervention, cancer detection
  specific for populations, 183
Intervention, cardiovascular disease (CATCH)
  determinants in, 36
  environmental intervention, 138, 139
  evaluation, health outcomes, 342
  implementation, 298, 307–308
  intervention population, 138
  motif, 235, 236
  performance objectives, 144, 308
  risk factors, 17, 35–36
Intervention, cardiovascular disease (Heart Partners)
  linkage system, 303
  program champions, 292
Intervention, child restraint devices
  causal model for use, hypothetical, 67, 325
  child's behavior and, 66, 68
  core processes, as example, 62–68
  determinants of use, 63, 66–68
  survey of parents, 66
Intervention, culture change, 107–109
Intervention, cystic fibrosis (CF Family Education Program)
  adoption of, 312–313
  coping behaviors in, 96, 97

diffusion intervention plan, 299–300, 312–313
disease-management model, 33–34
evaluation of, 312, 327
fidelity, program, 335
focus groups, use of, 278
goal-setting in, 92, 327
implementation of, 177, 297, 298, 312–313, 335
institutionalization of, 313
motifs in, 235, 238 fig. 7.5
performance objectives, 96, 97 table 4.6, 147–148
qualitative and quantitative methods in, 25, 26 fig. 2.2
reinvention of, 297
self-regulatory theories and, 96
strategies, 177
themes in, 235, 237 fig. 7.4
Intervention, diabetes
  Health Hero program, 245–246
  implementation index, 334
  performance standards, 334
  process evaluation, 332–334
Intervention, dietary
  environmental change, 140
  goals, 135
  measures, 340
  telephone use in, 250
Intervention, dietary (school cafeteria)
  adoption and implementation, 12
  effect evaluation, 340
  matrices, 11, 340
  methods and strategies, 11, 12
  performance objectives, 144
  program components, 12
Intervention, hand-washing, 142–143
Intervention, health crisis (CHESS), 245
Intervention, HIV prevention
  America Responds to AIDS, 140
  cultural groups, 261
  evaluation, 328, 329, 336, 342
  natural helpers in, 204
  pretest data, 282
  process evaluation, 335
  role-model story, 241, 242
  STOP AIDS Project, 103–104
  social support, 103
  wrong message in, 231
Intervention, HIV prevention (Dutch school program)
  adoption and implementation, 309, 311, 376–379
  behavioral and environmental risk factors, 32, 354–360, 362
  definition of health problem, 52
  determinants of safe sex, 355–360, 362–364, 371

determinants of program adoption and implementation, 309, 311, 378
differentiation of population, 359, 360–361
diffusion, 382
effect evaluation, 380
evaluation plan, 329, 339, 347–348, 379–382
fear-arousing messages, 370
focus group interview, 356, 357
group discussions, 372
group norms, 371
impact of behavioral experience, 357, 358–360, 361, 363
implementation, fidelity in, 335
knowledge, 363, 364, 365–366, 367, 368
and learning theories, 82
linkage system, 303, 376–377
literature review, 355–356, 367
matrices, 365–366
methods, 367, 369, 370–373
needs assessment, 353–360, 363
outcome expectations, 367
perceived social influence, 357, 359–360, 362–367, 369, 371
performance objectives, 144, 362, 365–366
planning and implementation issues, 373–374
pretesting of materials, 375–376
process evaluation, 381–382
program plan 373–375, 375
program production, 376
risk perceptions, 364, 365–366, 368, 369
self-efficacy, 363, 364, 365–366, 367, 369
skill training, 371, 373, 374
social pressure, resisting, 372
strategies, 367–368, 369, 370–372, 375
support materials, 374, 378
surveys, 357, 377–378, 380, 381
theory of planned behavior, 309, 311, 355
Intervention, HIV prevention (homeless men)
methods, 181
Sex, Games, and Videotapes, 181
Intervention, HIV prevention (Mpowerment Project),
outreach team, 207
social networks, use of, 207
Intervention, HIV prevention (women in jail)
determinants, 178, 179
methods and strategies, 178–180
negotiation skills, 178–179
personal triggers, 178, 179
program components, 178
Intervention, measles, 301
Intervention, parenting (never implemented), 331
Intervention, physical activity
measures, 340
telephone use in, 250

Walk Texas! program, 242, 269, 270 fig. 7.11
Intervention, skin cancer (Project SPF)
behavioral and environmental conditions, 139, 140, 141, 146
environmental agents and, 137, 146 table 5.2
environmental changes, 140–141, 340
health-promoting behaviors, 137
intervention populations, 137, 141
matrices, 137, 339
measures, 339, 341
performance objectives, 140, 145, 146, 341
slogan, 185
Intervention, smallpox eradication (WHO), 301
Intervention, smoking and tobacco
diffusion, 105–106
evaluation, 345
Health Hero program, 245–246
implementation process, 344
measures, 340
methods, 199, 213
organizational change, 182
social support in, 103
strategies, 198
telephone use in, 250, 251–252
Intervention, smoking cessation (Mexican Americans, *A Su Salud*)
use of media, 238
use of volunteers, 238, 242
Intervention, smoking cessation (pregnant women, Project PANDA)
attributions, 460, 465–467
context, pregnancy as, 454–456, 464, 465–467
coping, 459, 460
cues for smoking, 459
decisional balance, 465–467
definition of problem, 454–455, 457, 459–461
design documents, 267–268, 454, 470
determinants, 464, 465–467
differentiation of population, 462, 463
environmental re-evaluation, 191
focus groups, surveys, and interviews, 454, 458–460, 469–471, 474
framing success, 459, 460–461
literature review, 58–59
materials, development of, 470–471
matrices, 464–467
methods and strategies, 468
needs assessment, 453–454, 456–457, 458
newsletters, 465, 468, 469 fig. 13.5, 470 fig. 13.6
partner's role, 459, 461, 467
performance objectives, 464, 465–467
physical environment, 99
pretesting of materials, 278, 280, 470, 471

507

Subject Index

Intervention, smoking cessation (pregnant women, Project PANDA) *(continued)*
  processes of change, 460, 461 fig. 13.3
  program components, 471
  program evaluation, 471–473
  program objectives, 461–462
  qualitative and quantitative research methods, 458
  risk factors for relapse, 458
  social environment, 99, 458, 459, 462
  theme, 236
  transtheoretical model, 434 fig. 13.4, 454–455, 459, 460, 461, 463
  using theory and evidence, 454
  videotapes, 277, 465, 468–470
  See also Interventions, smoking and tobacco
Intervention, smoking prevention, adolescent (Smart Choices)
  adoption and implementation, 309
  diffusion intervention plan, 310–311
  linkage system, 305–306
  performance objectives for adoption, 306–307, 310 table 8.2
Intervention, stroke (T.L.L. Temple Foundation), 234–235, 242, 298
  behavioral factors, 29–30
  change agents, 32
  environmental factors, 30
  epidemiological analysis, 29
  mass media, use of, 234, 235
  matrices, 234
  message development guide, 243
  PRECEDE model, 31–32
  program vehicles, 243–244
  scope and sequence, 234
  skill training in, 234
  theme, 235
Intervention, sunscreen. *See* Intervention, skin cancer
Intervention, traffic, 50–52, 115
Intervention levels. *See* Ecological levels
Intervention Mapping, 1, 5, 8–13, 120, 426
  core processes of. *See* Core processes
  as iterative process, 13
  overview, 9–13
  preparation for. *See* Needs assessment; PRECEDE
  See also individual steps
Intervention Mapping Step 1: matrices
  defining environmental conditions, 133
  defining health behaviors, 133
  task 1, define what needs to change, 133–142
  task 2, write performance objectives, 142–148
  task 3, select determinants, 148–150
  task 4, create matrices, 150–151, 156–159, 162–164
  writing performance objectives, 133

See also Objectives, proximal program
Intervention Mapping Step 2: methods and strategies
  causal chain, 172–173
  definitions, 171–172
  and determinants, 172, 173
  examples of, at interpersonal level, 407 table 11.8
  examples of, at organizational level, 408–409 table 11.9
  examples of, at personal level, 406 table 11.7
  and levels of intervention, 172, 173
  task 1, brainstorm methods, 174–176
  task 2, translate methods into practical strategies, 176–178
  task 3, organize by learning objectives, 243 table 7.2
  See also Methods, intervention; Strategies
Intervention Mapping Step 3: Program and materials
  task 1, create program plan, 232–261
  task 2, develop design documents, 261–277
  task 3, pretest, 277–282
Intervention Mapping Step 4: adoption and implementation plans
  conceptual framework for, 292
  find end product of, 10 fig. 1.2, 12
  task 1, develop linkage system, 302–306
  task 2, create matrices for adoption and implementation, 306–314
  task 3, select methods and strategies, 314–315
  task 4, write a plan, 315
  See also Adoption; Implementation; Linkage systems
Intervention Mapping Step 5: evaluation plans
  definition and examples, 321, 329, 417–418, 472
  evaluation map, 325–327, 331
  task 1, form model and develop map, 324
  task 2, state process and effect questions, 331
  task 3, choose indicators and measures, 336
  task 4, design study and write plan, 343
  See also Evaluation, program

Knowledge
  and behavior change, 184
  methods to increase, 184–185, 185 table 6.4

Lay health advisors, 201, 205–206
Learned helplessness and self-efficacy, 66
Learning objectives. *See* Objectives, learning
Learning theories, 81–82, 369, 371
  examples of, 33, 68, 81
Linkage systems, 19–20, 302–306, 309, 412
Literacy, 178, 212–213, 250–251, 274
  evaluating reading levels, 253–254, 279

Subject Index

writing for comprehension, 273–274
Literature, health education and promotion. *See* Core processes

Maintenance, program. *See* Sustainability, program
Mass media
   advocacy, methods of, 216–218
   advocacy, theories of, 68
   as agent, 77
   as communication vehicle, 239–241, 277–278, 314–315
   gatekeepers of, 189, 291
   market segmentation techniques for, 238
   and persuasion communication model, 89–90
   as strategy, 195, 201, 203, 234, 238
Mastery learning, 98
Mastery model. *See* Role model
MATCH model, 32–33, 76
Materials, program
   community involvement in planning, 19
   evaluating existing, 250–254
   See also Production of program materials
Matrices, 1, 9–11, 131, 132, 306
   See also Intervention Mapping Step 1; Intervention Mapping Step 4
Measures, 337, 338–339
   baseline, 345
   of behavior, 340–342
   choosing, 338–339, 340–341
   definition, 337
   of determinants, 338–340
   domains in, 338–339, 341
   of environmental factors, 340–342
   followup, 345
   of health, 342–343, 346
   of quality of life, 342–343, 346
   reliability of, 337, 338, 344
   of skills, 346
   texts on, 340
   validity of, 337, 338
Media advocacy. *See* Mass media
Medicaid, 412
Memory, 184–186
Mentor programs, 104, 201 fig. 6.2
Methods, intervention, 11, 171–173, 176, 178–180, 243 table 7.2, 367, 406–409
   attitudes, 190–193
   attributional theory, 93
   awareness, 187 table 6.5
   behavioral capability, 195–198
   coalitions, 111
   community change, 116
   evaluation of, 321, 326
   external determinants, 199–220
   fear arousal, 189–190
   general, 178, 181
   goal-setting theory, 92
   health belief model, 95
   higher ecological levels, 201 fig. 6.2
   identification of, 75
   knowledge, 184–186
   learning theory, 82
   objectives, 176
   organizational change, 109, 111
   parameters of, 180, 229, 369 table 10.5
   personal determinants, 184–199
   persuasion communication model, 91
   program adoption and implementation, 314–315
   risk perception, 187–188
   self-efficacy, 195–198
   self-regulatory theories, 96
   skills, 195–198
   smoking cessation, 199, 465, 468
   social capital, 204–207
   social influence, 193–195
   social networks, 104
   social norms, 203–204
   stage theory of organizational change, 106
   strategies, 172, 243 table 7.2, 335
   texts on methods and strategies, 172
   themes, 235
   theory-based, 9, 75 table 4.1
   theory of planned behavior, 86
   translation into programs, 9
   transtheoretical model, 87, 89
   See also Intervention Mapping Step 2; Strategies
Methods, qualitative and quantitative research
   characteristics of, 23
   in Cystic Fibrosis Family Education Program, 25, 26 fig. 2.2
   with determinants, 84, 310–311
   examples of, 22, 344
   reliability and validity of data, 344
   texts on, 22–23, 47
   and theories, 61–62
   uses, 22–25, 84, 310–311, 343–344
Mister Roger's Neighborhood, 244
Model, causal, 325
Model, evaluation, 324. *See also* Intervention Mapping Step 5, task 1
Modeling, 98–100, 103, 197
   communication channels for, 239–241, 280–281
   coping versus mastery, 277
   criteria for effective, 195
   examples of use, 243, 406–412, 418
   in mass media, 203
   as method for program diffusion, 299
   as social influence, 65
   social support and, 138
   use of, 11, 68, 81
   See also Role model

Subject Index

Motifs, program, 235, 236 fig. 7.3, 238 fig. 7.5, 410
Motivation. *See* Attitudes
Mpowerment Project, 207

National Asthma Education and Prevention Program (NAEPP), 397, 412
National Center for Health Statistics, 33
National Cooperative Inner-City Asthma Study, 390
National Health Interview Survey, 33
National Health Interview Survey on Child Health, 389
Natural helpers, 104, 201, 204, 205–206
Need recognition. *See* Awareness
Needs assessment, 8, 16–41
    causal model from, 132
    community involvement in, 19
    data, 20, 22–25, 34 table 2.2
    environmental conditions and, 137, 342
    and evaluation, 236, 321
    and health outcomes, 342
    and PRECEDE model, 28
    product of, 131, 132, 133
    use of findings, 130, 131
    use of qualitative and quantitative methods in, 23–25
Negotiation, 178, 179
Networking, as strategy, 201 fig. 6.2
Networks, social. *See* Social networks
Nominal group technique, 34 table 2.2
Normative beliefs, 79, 84, 85
Normative influences, 85
Norms, personal moral, 84
Norms, social, 200
    causation, influence on, 6
    creation and transmission, 79, 203
    as determinant, 203, 243 table 7.2
    examples of, 339
    levels of, 6
    methods to change, 203–204, 207
Norms, subjective, 65, 83, 309
    See also Social expectations, perceived
North Carolina Breast Cancer Screening Program, 206
Northern Virginia HIV Consortium, 271
Northland, Project. *See* Intervention, adolescent alcohol use
Novelty, 192, 244, 250

Objectives, learning and change. *See* Objectives, proximal program
Objectives, performance, 96, 133, 142–145, 147–148
    for asthma, 402, 404, 405
    behavioral outcomes and, 133, 142, 322
    for environmental change, 402 table 11.4
    and evaluation, 321, 327, 340
    examples of, 146, 152–154, 160–161, 340
    for program diffusion and use, 299–300, 306–308, 327
Objectives, program, 10, 39–41, 336
    behavior, 41
    environmental, 41
    and evaluation, 322
    formulation, examples of, 81
    health and quality of life, 40–41, 133
Objectives, proximal program, 9–10, 40, 130, 143
    and behaviors, 133–137
    change, 131–133, 243, 321–322
    and determinants, 243 table 7.2
    and environmental conditions, 133, 137–141
    and evaluation, 321, 326, 327, 335
    learning, 131–133, 158–159, 162 table 5.6, 321–322
    matrices of, 9, 150–151, 159, 162–164
    and methods, 180, 243
    ranking of, 130–131
Operant conditioning, 33, 68, 81, 82
Organizational change
    behaviors in, 106
    from innovation, 7, 104–111
    as method, 207, 234–235
    and program adoption and implementation, 295–296, 309
    stages and tasks, 188, 208, 209 table 6.12
    strategies for, 195
    tailoring in, 182
    theory and models, 104–111
    use of theory, 75 table 4.1, 80 table 4.2
    See also Program champions
Organizational culture, 107–109
    as determinant, 200
    methods and strategies to change, 201 fig. 6.2
    of school districts, 416
    See also Organizational change
Organizational development, 106, 192, 201 fig. 6.2
    theory, 106–109
    use of theory, 75 table 4.1, 80 table 4.2
Organizations, 18, 19
    Interorganizational relationship theory (IRT), 109–111
    IRT, use of theory, 80 table 4.2
    mobilizing, as method, 203 table 6.9
    as target of intervention, 201 fig. 6.2
    See also Coalitions; Organizational development
Ottawa Charter, 117
Outcome evaluation. *See* Evaluation, effect
Outcome expectancies, 83
    definition of, 97
    as determinants, 309
    and social cognitive theory, 97
Outcome expectations, 82–84
    definition of, 97
    as determinant, 243, 398–400, 401, 404, 405

as determinant of program adoption and
use, 299, 300, 309
and fear arousal, 189–190
and health belief model, 95
methods to change, 194–195
and self-efficacy, 98, 197
and social cognitive theory, 97, 100, 194–195
Outcomes, 131, 132, 140
behavioral, 132, 134, 137, 142, 322, 342
environmental, 132, 134, 322
health, 132, 133, 321, 327, 330–331, 336, 342
quality of life, 31–32 table 2.1, 343–343

PANDA, Project. *See* Intervention, smoking cessation
Parameters of methods. *See* Methods
Pathways to Early Cancer Detection project, 183
Patient education, 136
See also Health promotion
Perceived behavioral control. *See* Self-efficacy
Performance objectives. *See* Objectives, performance
Performance standards, 332, 334
Persistence, 198
Persuasion, 100, 120, 192–193, 197
communication channels for, 239–241
as method for program diffusion, 299
See also Communication
Persuasion communication model, 65, 81, 89–91, 180–181
examples of use, 369 table 10.5, 382
matrix, 89, 90 table 4.4
use of model, 75 table 4.1, 80 table 4.2
Persuasive communication
examples of method, 406–409 tables 11.7–11.9, 412
Photonovels, 213–214
Pilot testing. *See* Pretesting
Policy windows, 219–220
theory, 119, 120
use of theory, 80 table 4.2
Population, at-risk
definition, 17–19
and evaluation, 324
intervention effect on, 19, 76, 321
as intervention population, 137
pretesting with, 231–232
See also Populations, intervention
Populations, intervention
agents as, 109
and attributional theory, 93
children as, 137
coalitions as, 111
communities as, 115
definition and examples, 19
differentiation of, 91, 183, 367, 396–397, 462, 463 table 13.3
differentiation of, for mass media, 238

end users (participants) as, 20
and evaluation, 321, 326
as evaluation stakeholders, 323 table 9.1
as experts on subjective meaning, 8
and goal-setting theory, 92
and health belief model, 95
identifying health-related behaviors of, 134
intermediate users (implementers) as, 20
and learning theories, 82
marginalized populations as, 112
networks as, 104
organizations as, 109, 111
and persuasion communication model, 91
policy-makers as, 120
resource system (developers) as, 20
and self-regulatory theories, 96
for social support interventions, 104
and theory of planned behavior, 86
and transtheoretical model, 87
use of theory in defining, 74, 75 table 4.1
and utilization plan, 325
See also Population, at-risk
Power, 80, 172, 202, 212
power relationships, 293
power with and power over, 113, 202, 207 table 6.11, 212
Practice, guided, 81, 100, 178, 299–300
Praxis, 213
Precaution adoption theory, 64, 87
PRECEDE/PROCEED model, 8, 28–29
assumption of, underlying, 132
for asthma, 34–35
and disease management models, 33–34
as risk model, 33
self-management programs, use in planning, 34
use of, in asthma intervention, 388
where to enter, 36–39
Pretesting, 278–282
methods, 279, 281
necessity of, 231
and persuasion communication model, 90
of program as a whole, 304
of program materials, 230, 253, 278, 280
steps in, 90
using data from, 281–282
Prevention, 19, 29–30, 135, 139
Process evaluation. *See* Evaluation, process
Process pathways. *See* Program pathways
Production of program materials
abstract vehicles, 266–267
hiring creative resources, 261–262
print pieces, 264, 271–274
specifying project parameters, 262–263, 266
videotapes, 265, 274–277
See also Materials, program
Program aims. *See* Objectives, program; Objectives, proximal program

Program champions, 106, 292, 296–297, 299–300, 321
Program delivery, 8, 325
Program materials. *See* Production of program materials
Program pathways, 324 fig. 9.1, 325, 328
Project Northland. *See* Intervention, adolescent alcohol use
Project PANDA. *See* Intervention, smoking cessation
Project SPF. *See* Intervention, skin cancer
Protection-motivation theory, 64, 65, 94
Proximal program objectives. *See* Objectives, proximal program
Psychological expectancy-value models, 93, 192
Public service announcements (PSAs), 234, 241 table 7.1
Punishment. *See* Reinforcement

Qualitative data. *See* Data
Qualitative methods. *See* Methods, qualitative and quantitative
Quality of life
  in asthma, 34
  and behavioral and environmental conditions, 132
  determinants, external, of, 5
  and evaluation, 321, 327, 336
  and health, 7
  in HIV, 245
  indicators of, 34 table 2.2, 40–41
  measures of, 342–343
  objectives, 40–41
  as outcome, 245
  in PRECEDE, 29 fig. 2.3, 36–37, 37 fig. 2.6
  See also Outcomes, quality of life
Quantitative data. *See* Data
Quantitative methods. *See* Methods, qualitative and quantitative
Quasi-experimental designs, 345
Questions. *See* Core processes
Questionnaires. *See* Surveys

Randomization, 345
Reading levels. *See* Literacy
Reattribution. *See* Attribution theory
Reciprocal determinism, 97
Redundancy and novelty, 244
Refusal skills. *See* Skills
Reinforcement, 100, 183, 198
  of behavior, 82
  communication channels for, 239–241
  as determinant, 200, 243 table 7.2, 398–400 table 11.2, 405 table 11.6
  as method, 100, 204, 300 table 8.1, 406–407, 411–412, 461 fig. 13.3
  as method for program diffusion and use, 299, 300

and modeling, 100
and motivation, 98
negative, 401–402
positive, 183
and program use, 298, 300, 309
punishment, 183
self-reinforcement, 183
and social cognitive theory, 100, 197
social support and, 138
vicarious, 100, 183
Reinvention, 297
Relapse prevention, 267
  and attributional theory, 93
  examples of use, 178
  methods for, 198, 199
  model, 459 fig. 13.2
  theory, 68, 199
Relaxation, as strategy, 198
Reliability. *See* Measures
Resources, access to
  methods and strategies to change, 207 table 6.11
Risk, perception of, 25, 63–64
  and health belief model, 94
  and intervention methods, 367
  methods to change, 187–188, 187 table 6.5
  models of, 65
  theories relating to, 64, 80, 87
  unrealistic optimism, 64, 187, 367, 368
  use of theory, example of, 369 table 10.5
Risk factors
  behavioral. *See* Behavior, risk
  environmental, 17
  physiological, 17, 134
  See also Determinants
Role model, 299–300, 314–315
  communication channels for, 239–241, 314–315
  coping model, 98
  leader as, 204
  mastery model, 98
  selecting, 98
  stories, 241–242
  See also Modeling
Role plays, 180, 299

Schemas, 185
Scope and sequence of program, 232–233
Self-determination, principle of, 19
Self-efficacy expectations, 65, 82, 85, 94, 98, 401
  and attribution theory, 92–93, 196–197
  as barrier, 189
  and barriers, 100
  behavioral capability, distinction from, 98
  as determinant, 65, 66, 83, 92, 94
  as determinant of asthma management, 398–400 table 11.2, 401

Subject Index

as determinant of environmental change, 405 table 11.6
as determinant of implementation, 298
as determinant of physician behavior, 404 table 11.5
as determinant of program adoption and implementation, 299, 300, 309, 314
as determinant of safe sex, 357
determinants of, 92–93
and experience, 196
and fear arousal, 189–190
and feedback, 66
and goal-setting theory, 92
and health belief model, 95
and learned helplessness, 66
and learning objectives, 339
measures of, 84
methods to change, 100, 195–199, 245–246, 330, 461 fig. 13.3
and outcome expectations, 98, 197
and persuasion communication model, 89
and problem-solving skills, 188
and relapse prevention, 199
and social cognitive theory, 97, 98, 194, 314
and theory of planned behavior, 86
Self-liberation, 197–198
Self-management, 95, 96, 136, 188
in cystic fibrosis. *See* Intervention, cystic fibrosis
skills, teaching with computers, 245
use of PRECEDE in planning programs for, 34 table 2.2
See also Self-regulatory theories
Self-monitoring, 199, 406–407
Self-regulation, 190, 235
Self-regulatory theories, 95–96
constructs in, 95 table 4.5
examples of use, 388, 394
steps in process, 95–96
use of theory, 75 table 4.1, 80 table 4.2
See also Self-management
Sesame Street, 244
Severity, perceived, 94
and health belief model, 94, 95
Sex, Games, and Videotapes, 181
Skills and skill training
communication channels for, 239–241
as determinants, 298, 299, 466–467
examples of method, 234, 406–409, 461
as method for program diffusion, 299
methods for skills training, 197–198
refusal skills, 179
and self-regulatory theories, 96
social skills, 196
and social support interventions, 103, 104
as strategy, 299
types, 195–196
See also Communication; Negotiation

Slogans, 185, 214, 268
Smoking, 132–135, 139, 453, 456–459
See also Environmental tobacco smoke; Intervention, cardiovascular; Intervention, smoking cessation
Social action. *See* Community organization
Social capital, 27, 101, 104
methods to change, 204–207
See also Community capacity; Social networks
Social cognitive theory, 33, 64, 68, 79, 81–82, 87, 96–100, 194
and diffusion of innovations, 294–295, 309
examples of use, 178, 367, 369 table 10.5, 401
methods from, 195–196
and self-efficacy, 314
use of theory, 75 table 4.1, 80 table 4.2
Social comparison, 102
theory, 369 table 10.5, 371
Social ecological approach. *See* Ecological approach
Social environment. *See* Environment
Social exchange theory, 76
Social expectations, 83–84
perceived, 81, 86, 98
and theory of planned behavior, 86
Social influences
methods to change, 193–195
methods to deal with, 367
norms as determinant of, 203
and persuasion communication model, 89
theory, example of, 367
as type of determinant, 65, 94, 200, 357
Social inoculation theory, 369 table 10.5, 372
Social judgment theory, 369 table 10.5, 371
Social learning theory. *See* Social cognitive theory
Social liberation, 197, 198
Social networks, 101–104, 201–207
as method, 201 fig. 6.2, 203 table 6.9, 204
methods to change, 204–205
stategies for, 204–205
theories, 100–104
use of theories, 80 table 4.2
See also Social support
Social norms. *See* Norms, social
Social support, 101–104, 138
benefit, 204
collective action, 201 fig. 6.2
determinant, 66, 200, 464, 466 table 13.5
dimension of community competence, 26
methods, 194, 204–205, 246, 299, 300
and smoking, 458, 461 fig. 13.3, 462
strategy, 204–205, 299–300
theories, 100–104
use of theories, 75 table 4.1, 80 table 4.2
use with computers, 245
See also Natural helpers; Social networks

Subject Index

Societal and government theories, 116–120
Specifications, communicating program, 9, 12
  See also Design documents
SPF, Project. *See* Intervention, skin cancer
Stages of change, 86–88
  methods for moving through, 190–191
  organizational, 106, 182
  processes of change, 86–88, 464, 465, 471 table 13.7
  and relapse prevention theory, 199
  in smoking cessation, 267, 454–455, 461
  See also Transtheoretical model
Stanford Five-City Project, 308
Stimulus. *See* Classical conditioning
Stimulus control. *See* Cues
STOP AIDS Project, 103–104
Strategies, 11, 171–172, 176, 220
  for adoption, 7
  choosing, 9, 367
  for dramatic relief, 189
  ecological levels, 198, 201 fig. 6.2, 406–409
  evaluation, 321, 327
  examples of, 11, 171–172, 176, 178, 367–369
  operationalizing, 177–178, 325
  for smoking cessation, 198
  texts on strategies and methods, 172
  translation of methods into, 75 table 4.1
  See also Intervention Mapping Step 2; Methods, intervention
Stroke. *See* Intervention, stroke
Sunscreen intervention. *See* Intervention, skin cancer
Support. *See* Social support
Surveys, 357
  in asthma intervention, 415, 417
  attitudes, to determine, 357, 358 table 10.2
  in CRD intervention, 66
  in HIV intervention, 357, 377–378, 380, 381
  national, 33, 389
  norms, to determine, 204
  in smoking cessation intervention, 454, 458–460, 469–471, 474
  in smoking prevention intervention, 84–85
  as strategy, 201 fig. 6.2
Susceptibility, perceived, 94
  as determinant, 398–400
  and fear arousal, 189–190
  and health belief model, 94, 95, 187
Sustainability, program, 7, 301–302, 306–308

Tailoring, 247–249
  on beliefs, 181, 182
  conditions for effectiveness, 182
  on culture and ethnicity, 178, 409–410
  on disease characteristics, 246
  examples of, 173, 182, 409–410
  and health belief model, 95
  as method to increase knowledge, 185 table 6.4
  and organizational change, 182
  on personal characteristics, 181–182
  and societal and governmental interventions, 120
  on stage of change, 181, 249
  and transtheoretical model, 87
  See also Individualization
Target, 6, 19. *See also* Populations, program
Tay-Sachs, 135
Telephone Linked Communication system, 250
Telephones as program vehicle, 249–252
Tenderloin Senior Organizing Project, 104
Testimonies, public, 198, 243 table 7.2
T-groups, 107
Themes, 232, 235, 236
  examples of, 235 fig. 7.2, 237 fig. 7.4, 410
Theories, specific, 80 table 4.2
  coalition formation, 68
  communication, 79
  community development, 68
  coping, 68
  empowerment, 68
  learning, 68
  media advocacy, 68
  organizational change, 75 table 4.1
  organizational development, 75 table 4.1
  policy-making, 81
  theory of economic decision making, 188, 369 table 10.5, 371
  theory of planned behavior, 75, 79–81, 83–86, 98, 193–194, 309, 355
  theory of reasoned action, 83
  transtheoretical model, 75, 80, 86–89, 188–189, 249, 454–455
  See also Stages of change
Theories, types
  action, theories of, 75, 81, 106, 325
  behavior-oriented, 79
  change-oriented, 80
  environment-oriented, 79
  general, 61, 65
  health education–oriented, 80
  health-oriented, 80
  problem, theories of, 75, 81, 91–92, 173
  program, theories of the, 325, 328
  social psychological, 80
  training, 68
Theories, use, 4–5, 8, 9, 75 table 4.1, 120
  approaches to, 59–61
  comfortable, 78
  determinants of, 80
  development of, 48
  at ecological levels, 79, 80 table 4.2
  with factors, 33
  finding, 47–50, 59–61
  by level, 80 table 4.2

and performance objectives, 147
in program planning, 4, 5, 9, 47–49
textbooks on, 79
topic approach, 59–60
See also individual theories; Core processes; Intervention Mapping Step 2
Translation and back translation, 259, 415

Unrealistic optimism, 64, 187, 367, 368
Utilization plan, 325

Validity
of constructs, 339, 344
external, 58
internal, 58, 59, 344
of measures, 337–338
of performance objectives, 147–148
of qualitative data, 344
types of, in the literature, 58, 59
types of, in measures, 337
Vehicles. *See* Channels and vehicles
Vicarious learning, 98
See also Modeling

Vicarious reinforcement, 195, 243 table 7.2
See also Modeling
Videotape
access to VCRs, 469
criteria for use, 241 table 7.1
examples of use, 171, 173, 176–177, 179, 300, 412
in Project Northland, 280–281
as vehicle for modeling, 180
Vision, creating a, 201 fig. 6.2, 204, 211, 269
Volunteers, 3, 234, 238, 239

Walk Texas! program, 242, 269, 270 fig. 7.11
Watch, Discover, Think, and Act. *See* Intervention, asthma
WHO (World Health Organization), 142, 301
Alma-Ata Declaration, 19
definition of health, 7
definition of healthy community, 25
Ottawa Charter, 117
Work sites, 201 fig. 6.2, 204

DAYNA M. MANICCIA